FRONT LINES OF THORACIC SURGERY

Edited by **Stefano Nazari**

Front Lines of Thoracic Surgery
Edited by Stefano Nazari

Published by InTech
Janeza Trdine 9, 51000 Rijeka, Croatia

Publishing Process Manager Vedran Greblo

Technical Editor Teodora Smiljanic

Cover Designer InTech Design Team

Additional hard copies can be obtained from orders@intechopen.com

Front Lines of Thoracic Surgery, Edited by Stefano Nazari
p. cm.
ISBN 978-953-307-915-8

For EU product safety concerns:
IN TECH d.o.o., Prolaz Marije Krucifikse Kozulić 3, 51000 Rijeka, Croatia,
info@intechopen.com or visit our website at intechopen.com.

Meet the editor

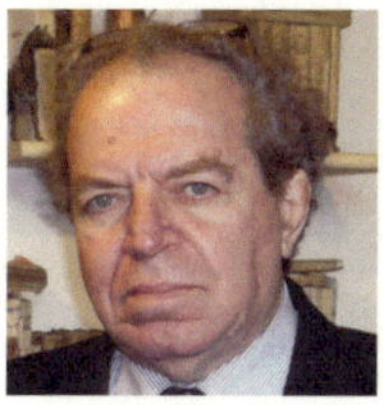

Stefano Nazari was born in Venice on Jan 2, 1949. His Classic Education was in Como (Liceo A. Volta 1968) and his Medical Education at Pavia University (MD 1974, residency in Surgery 1980) and at Turin University (residency in General Thoracic Surgery 1983). His clinical activity was nearly entirely dedicated to Thoracic Surgery at the Department of Surgery of IRCCS San Matteo Pavia Hospital until 2005 and in private structures thereafter. He was also deeply involved in experimental surgery research at the research unit lab of the Deptartment of Surgery at Pavia University, focused in particular on: nutritional status evaluation, one lung anesthesia (new endobronchial tube), lung transplant (funded by Italian Ministry of Health: bronchial art. revascularization, extracorporeal lung preservation, vascular stapler for pulmonary artery anastomosis), lung cancer surgery (SVCava and Pancoast t. resections, bronchoplastic procedures), and aortic surgery (endovascular "net" prosthesis, expandable anastomotic devices). He had stages at the Division of Organ Transplantation Univ. of Cincinnati (1973), Cardiothoracic Division of Hannover University (1987), Thoracic Surgery Div. Toronto GH (1988) and Cardiovascular Surgery at H. Broussais, Paris (1996/7). In 1997 he founded the Fondazione Alexis Carrel (not for profit, act 1532/906, Pavia) for thoracic and cardiovascular research.

Contents

Preface

Res ipsa loquitur
(The thing speaks for itself)
(*Cicero, Pro Milone, 53*)

It has indeed been a great privilege to be the Editor of the new book *Front Lines of Thoracic Surgery*, with the efficient assistance of the InTech technical team.

In this original and promising editorial format, the book collects the up-to-date contributions on some of the most debated topics in today's clinical practice of cardiac, aortic and general thoracic surgery and anesthesia, as viewed by authors personally involved in their evolution.

The strong and genuine enthusiasm of the authors was clearly perceptible in all their contributions, and I'm sure that will further stimulate the reader to understand their messages. Moreover, the strict adhesion of the authors' original observations and findings to the evidence base proved that facts are the best guarantee of their scientific value.

Unfortunately however, no matter how strong their rational theoretical basis and evidence may be, new ideas and hypothesis are not usually accepted as easily and as quickly as any author would expect. That is the case in science in general and in surgery in particular.

This is probably most related to "tradition", which is obviously widely recognized as the most important founding value of any culture. However, tradition is apparently resistant to innovations in different science fields in inverse proportion to the complexity of their own theoretical content.

This places surgery in an unfavorable position since, even though extensive theoretical and technological research precedes and justifies any surgical treatment, performance of any surgical act relies on very few, elementary, "mechanical" principles.

In considering the evolution of the vascular anastomosis technique, it is interesting to note that the famous Carrel "triangulation" original sketch still reported straight, not an atraumatic needle, similar to that in use then for gastrointestinal suture. That was in fact the necessary scenario for "triangulation" to stand for a very significant technical advancement at that point in time. Nonetheless, in spite of its persisting fame, "triangulation" was made obsolete by the advent of curved and proportionally dimensioned needles as well as of many other technical refinements.

After a century-long path, apparently pulverizing the retaining force of "tradition", the extreme evolution of surgical technique has today reached man-driven robotic surgery, suggesting that the theoretically insurmountable limits other science fields have (like absolute zero for lowest temperature, or light speed for highest velocity) do not seem to have been yet identified in surgery!

However the new "thing" brought to the final surgical act by the complex, highly technologic and expensive robot apparatus is, essentially, at this point in time, the significantly increased precision of the surgical act resulting from the amplification of the surgeon's hand movement in relation to that transferred to the activated instrument in the operative field. Mini-access and magnified operative field view in fact were options already brought to clinical practice by video assisted, mini-invasive surgery.

All together these new technical modifications of the final surgical act are advantageous enough to justify the sacrifice, at least for selected surgical conditions, of the still unparalleled versatility of the direct hand movements in the operative field.

Sometimes in my work on vascular anastomosis devices, I thought that proposing innovations in this basic surgical ambit could be quite similar to trying to popularize the use of the fork and knife in China. The thorough analysis and explanation of the many details that provide that a fork and knife are a better and easier method of controlling food than chopsticks for anyone, independently from his own local tradition, is as ingenuous and almost stupid as it is ineffective.

In surgery however, it is just the full and clear understanding of the little technical "things", that can reveal the expected and very relevant final effects to the patient and thus can eventually urge someone to accept the difficult, monopolizing and often bitter, but always exciting, challenge of bringing it into clinical practice.

I'm grateful to Dr Giuseppe Rescigno, Division of Cardiac Surgery, Lancisi Hospital, Ancona for the review of Dr H. Hiroshi's Chapter on Off Pump CABG.

Dr. Stefano Nazari
Fondazione Alexis Carrel
Milan, Italy

Part 1

Adult Cardiac Surgery

1

Mitral Valve Subvalvular Apparatus Repair with Artificial Neochords Application

Sergey Y. Boldyrev, Kirill O. Barbukhatty,
Olga A. Rossokha and Vladimir A. Porhanov
Department of Adult Cardiac Surgery, Regional Clinic Hospital #1, Krasnodar,
Kuban State Medical University, Krasnodar,
Russian Federation

1. Introduction

Degenerative mitral valve (MV) disease is a common disorder affecting around 2% of the population (Enriquez-Sarano M et al., 2009). The most common ending in patients with degenerative valve disease is leaflet rolapsed due to elongation or rupture of the chordal apparatus, resulting in varying degrees of MV regurgitation due to leaflet malcoaptation during ventricular contraction. The emphasis of clinical decision-making in patients with degenerative disease centres around the severity of regurgitation and its impact on symptom status, ventricular function and dimension, the sequelae of systolic flow reversal such as atrial dilatation/fibrillation and secondary pulmonary hypertension (PH), and the risk of sudden death (1-4). Current standard of care for MV rolapsed with severe mitral regurgitation (MR) is surgical MV repair (Adams et al., 2010). Implantation of neo-chordae with the use of expanded polytetrafluoroethylene (ePTFE) sutures (Gore Associates, Flagstaff, AZ, USA) has since its introduction into clinical practice by Frater et al. proven to be a valuable technique for contemporary MV repair. Chordal replacement enables preservation of native valve anatomy, physiological leaflet motion and creation of large mitral orifice area. Furthermore, it has contributed to the reparability independent of valve complexity (Seeburger et al., 2007).

2. Functional anatomy of the mitral valve

Historically, the mitral valve is described as composed of the leaflets, chordae, and papillary muscles. However, the mitral valve structurally and functionally is part of the left ventricle and intimately associated with the atrium and fibrous skeleton of the heart. Thus, alterations to the fibrous skeleton and ventricular and atrial muscle contribute to and affect valvular function.

2.1 Leaflets

The leaflets are the valve component that creates the division between the atrium and ventricle. There are two distinct leaflets: the anterior or aortic and posterior or mural. The anterior leaflet is usually comprised of a single trapezoidal-shaped unit. The posterior leaflet is punctuated with multiple slits and clefts that define usually three, but up to six, distinct scallops (Fig. 1). The anterior and posterior leaflets are separated at the commissures but there is usually some continuity of the valve tissue close to the annulus. Further, if one looks at the chordal distribution, at the commissures, chordae are distributed to both leaflets from a common structural source—so the leaflets form a single functional unit. Nevertheless, it is useful for the purposes of valve repair to differentiate anterior from posterior. However, one must remember that multiple separately suspended distinct units come together to make the valve competent. To describe components of mitral valve repair it is useful to label the scallops by position (Fig. 1); posteriorly from left to right P1, P2, P3, with corresponding regions of the anterior leaflet A1, A2, and A3.

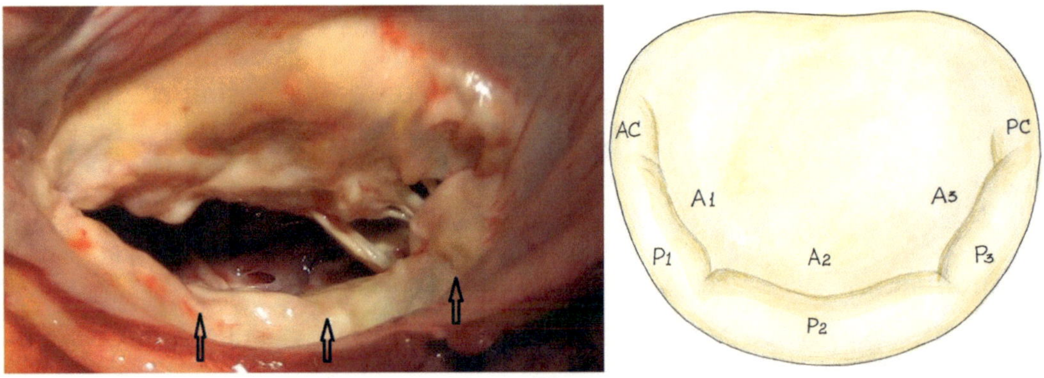

Fig. 1. Photograph of the mitral valve. Note multiple clefts in the posterior leaflet (arrows). The posterior leaflet is divided into 3 scallops or segments (lateral, middle, and medial scallops) identified as P1, P2, and P3. The corresponding segments of the anterior leaflet are labeled A1, A2, and A3.

When in the closed position, the orifice is obscured by the anterior and posterior leaflets. The anterior comprises about one half to two thirds of this area, the posterior comprises about one third to one half of this area. The point of attachment of the anterior leaflet comprises one third of the circumference of the annulus (the fibrous area) and the posterior leaflets comprises two thirds of the circumference of the annulus (the muscular area). The fibrous support of the anterior leaflet is fixed, the muscular support of the posterior leaflet can enlarge and does so when annular dilatation is associated with mitral regurgitation. The leaflets themselves are comprised of clear and rough zones. The clear zone is between the line of closure and the annulus and can be quite thin, almost transparent. The rough zone extends from the line of closure to the free edge, characterized by thicker, nodular ridges which promote sealing of the orifice on valve closure.

2.2 Annulus

Of the four heart valves, the mitral valve is the only valve that has a distinguishable annulus. However, the presence of a fibrous annular structure is variable and discontinuous. The firmest site of support for the mitral valve is the region of fibrous continuity between the aortic and mitral valves, the extent of which is delineated by the right and left fibrous trigones (Fig. 2). Nevertheless, for surgical purposes, the annulus is considered the area of attachment of the valve leaflets to the atrial muscle. The annulus is a functional component of the mitral valve. The annulus is quite flexible and changes shape throughout the cardiac cycle. With normal systolic function, the annulus will reduce in size by 20% to 40%. Functionally the mitral annulus is not two-dimensional but in fact three-dimensional assuming a saddle shape. The curvature imposed by the saddle shape reduces mechanical stress on the leaflets. The curvature of the saddle shape or height of the "saddle horn" is reduced in a model of ischemic mitral regurgitation. This may have implications in choosing techniques for annular reduction and stabilization.

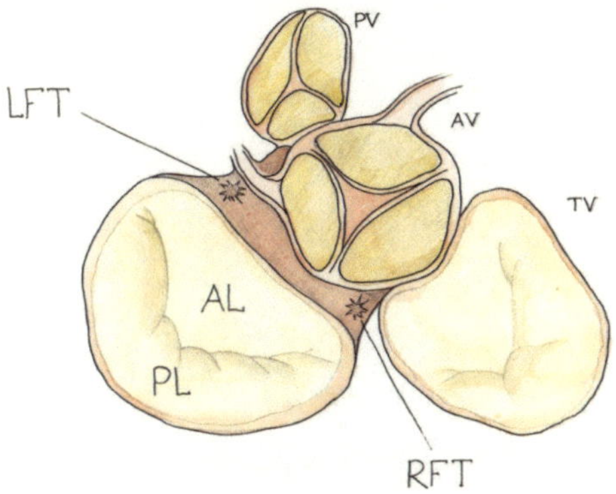

Fig. 2. Relational anatomy of the mitral valve: left and right fibrous trigones (LFT and RFT); anterior and posterior mitral leaflets (AL and PL); pulmonic, aortic, and tricuspid valves (PV, AV, and TV).

2.3 Tendinous chords

The tendinous chords, as functional extensions of the papillary muscles, perform the dual function of maintaining valvular competence by preventing leaflet prolapse and maintaining ventricular geometry by providing cross-ventricular support. The chords originate from the apical portions of the papillary muscles or directly from the posterior ventricular wall. They insert either into the free edge of the leaflets or on their ventricular surface. Chords have been characterized a number of ways. The most useful for repair purposes is to describe the first-degree chords as those inserting into the valve edge and the second-degree chords as those inserting into the underside of the leaflet. Both first-degree and second-degree chords originate from the papillary muscles and third-degree chords originate from the ventricular wall and insert into the base of the posterior leaflet.

2.4 Papillary muscles

There are two papillary muscles associated with the mitral valve (Fig. 3) When looking from the atrial side, the anterolateral is to the left and the posteromedial is to the right. The muscles are located under their respective commissures. They originate from the lower third of the left ventricular free wall. The papillary muscles are extensions of the ventricular muscle from which they originate. The chords originate from the fibrous tips of these muscles, extending to insert on the mitral leaflets. The blood supply of the anterolateral papillary muscle derives from the left circumflex and/or diagonal systems. The blood supply of the posteromedial papillary muscle derives from the posterolateral coronary branches whether it originates from the left or right coronary system. The papillary muscles adjust tension and stabilize the valve during the cardiac cycle, rather than pulling the chords and leaflets into position. The function of the papillary muscles and their position is greatly dependent on the status of the ventricular myocardium underlying it. Displacement of the papillary muscle by distorted ventricular geometry is one mechanism for the creation of mitral regurgitation.

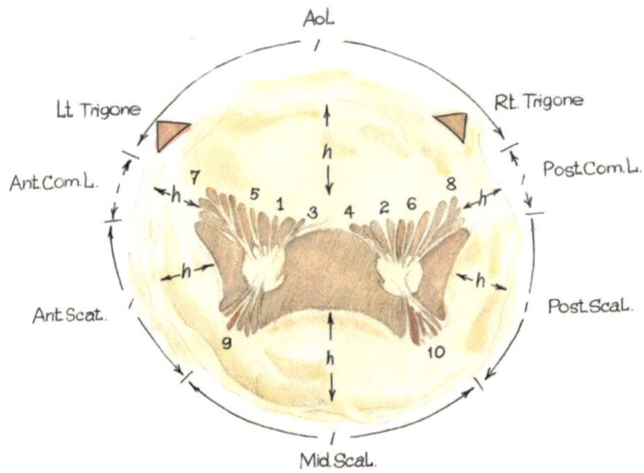

Fig. 3. Mitral apparatus. ALPM, Anterolateral papillary muscle; PMPM, posteromedial papillary muscle; AoL, aortic leaflet; Ant.Com.L., anterior commissural leaflet; Post.Com.L., posterior commissural leaflet; Ant.Scal. , anterior scallop; Mid.Scal ., middle scallop; h, height of a leaflet; l, length of the attachment of a leaflet; Post.Scal. , posterior scallop; Rt. Trigone, right fibrous trigone; Lt. Trigone, left fibrous trigone; 1, anterior main chorda; 2, posterior main chorda; 3, anterior paramedial chorda; 4, posterior paramedial chorda; 5, anterior paracommissural chorda; 6, posterior paracommissural chorda; 7, anterior commissural chorda; 8, posterior commissural chorda; 9, anterior cleft chorda; 10, posterior cleft chorda.

3. Pathophysiology

Today, multiple terminologies used to describe mitral pathology. Terms such as prolapse, flail, partial flail, redundant, overshooting, stretching, elongation, floppy, billowing, ballooning, Barlow, dysplasia, myxoid, and myxomatous, for example, have different meanings for different specialists. The confusion comes first from the fact that several of these terms are synonyms. For example, flail leaflet, overshooting leaflet and leaflet prolapse are synonyms. Other synonyms are Barlow, billowing, ballooning, myxomatous valve, and mitral valve prolapse. Another source of confusion comes from the fact that for some specialists a given term such as « prolapse» means a disfunction (leaflet prolapsed) while for others it refers to a disease (mitral valve prolapse). The same chaotic situation applies to the term « floppy valve», which is used to define either a valve morphology, or dysfunction, or a disease. Similar confusion exists in tricuspid and aortic valve diseases, in which many of previously listed terms are used without clear distinction. Clarification can be obtained by using a pathophysiological triad with a sound distinction between the terms describing valve etiology (i.e., the cause of the disease), valve lesions resulting from the disease, and valve dysfunction resulting from the lesions.

Etiology - The cause of the disease

↓

Lesions - Result from the disease

↓

Dysfunction - Result from the lesions

The pathophysiological triad facilitates communication between cardiologists, echocardiographers and surgeons and greatly clarifies clinical investigation.

4. Etiology

Cardiac valves can be affected by numerous disease (Tab # 1). Primary valve disease involve the valvular tissue. Secondary valve disease affect the supporting of the valves – that is, the ventricles for the mitral and tricuspid valves and the aorta and pulmonary artery for the aortic and pulmonary valves, respectively. The determination of the etiology of valvular disease is important because it helps to establish the medical treatment, which should precede or follow valve reconstruction.

Primary valve Disease	Secondary to Myocardial Disease
• Congenital malformation • Inflammatory disease Rheumatic Lupus erythematoses Valve sclerosis • Degenerative disease Barlow, s disease Marfan,s disease Fibroelastic deficiency • Infective endocarditis • Valvular or annular calcification • Trauma • Valvular tumors	• Ischemic cardiomyopathy • Dilated cardiomyopathy • Hypertrophic obstructive cardiomyopathy • Myocardial sarcoidosis • Endomyocardial fibrosis • Myocardial tumors

Table 1. Etiology of valvular disease.

5. Lesions

Any of the previously listed disease can cause lesions affecting one or several components of the heart valves: the annulus, the leaflets, and the supporting structures (Table #2).

Mitral\ Tricuspid Valves	Aortic\Pulmonary Valves
Annular dilatation	Annular dilatation
Leaflet perforation	Leaflet perforation
Leaflet tear	Leaflet distension
Leaflet thickening	Vegetations
Vegetations	Commissure detachment
Commissure fusion	Commissure fusion
Calcification	Calcification
Chordae rupture	Sino-tubular dilatation
Chordae elongation	
Chordae thickening	
Chordae fusion	
Papillary muscle rupture	
Papillary muscle elongation	
Ventricular aneurysm	
Ventricular fibrous plaque	
Ventricular dilatation	

Table 2. Valvular Lesions.

6. Valve dysfunction: The «Functional classification»

The pioneering cardiac surgeon Alain Carpentier, MD, PhD, developed a functional classification to reflect the underlying pathological changes that contributed to MR (*Carpentier A. 1983)* (Figure 4). As described in this classification, type I MR is characterized as normal leaflet motion but with annular dilatation or leaflet perforation; type II lesions are related to leaflet prolapse and may be caused by myxomatous disease, such as chord rupture or elongation, or by papillary muscle rupture or elongation; and type III lesions are caused by restricted leaflet motion. Type IIIA is typically caused by rheumatic valve disease with normal ventricular motion and subvalvular fibrosis and calcification; type IIIB is typically caused by ischemic or idiopathic cardiomyopathy with impaired ventricular function and dilation but a "normal" morphology to the leaflets, chords, and papillary muscles, frequently with restriction at the P3 segment. Type I MR may occur with billowing myxomatous leaflets but without elongated chordae and prolapse (type II), if extensive annular dilatation leads to inadequate leaflet coaptation (*Fornes P et al., 1999).*

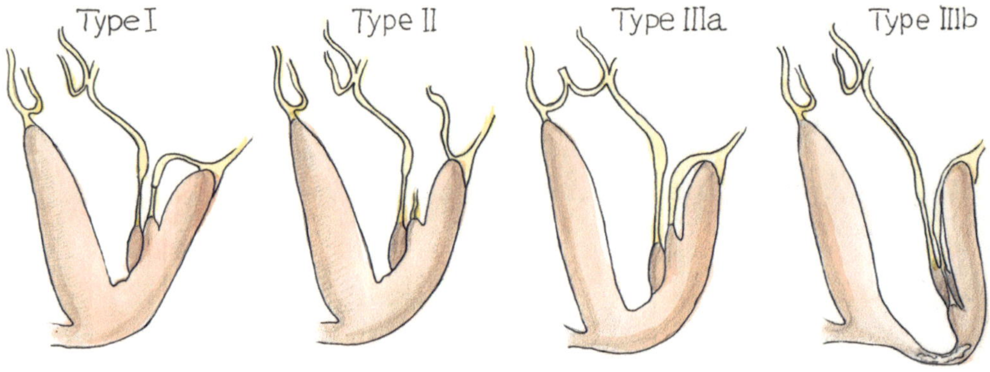

Fig. 4. Functional classification.

7. Degenerative valvular disease

The tree main types of degenerative valvular disease are Barlow,s disease, fibroelastoc deficiency, and Marfan,s disease.

7.1 Myxomatous mitral valve disease (Barlow's disease)

Barlow's disease is the most frequent degenerative valvular disease with a prevalence of 4% to 5 % in the general population, generally appears early in life. Patients present with a prolonged history of a murmur, thickened leaflets, substantial excess tissue, and a dilated annulus, which may be calcified (1). Chordae may be elongated and thinned. Often isolated ruptures are present, contributing to the focal prolapse. Classically, the most common abnormality is focal enlargement of the posterior central scallop (P2) with an associated ruptured chorda. Mills et al. comparing unileaflet versus bileaflet prolapse, found that patients with unileaflet prolapse were younger and had a higher incidence of flail leaflets (3). Patients with bileaflet prolapse were less likely to be hypertensive and had mechanically stronger chordae though leaflet strength was similar to patients with unileaflet prolapse.

7.2 Marfan's disease

Marfan's syndrome of the mitral valve is characterized by excess tissue, thickened leaflets, and a dilated annulus. Patients with Marfan syndrome have a shortened life expectancy because of cardiovascular complication, 80% of them developing mitral valve regurgitation.

7.3 Fibroelastic deficiency

Fibroelastic deficiency occurs mostly in the elderly with a short history of valvular dysfunction. The leaflets are transparent, and except for the prolapsing segment there is no excess tissue. The chordae are thin, fragile, and elongated. The annulus is dilated and often infiltrated with calcium (Table #3).

Key Differences Between Barlow's Disease and Fibroelastic Deficiency at Time of Surgical Presentation

	Barlow's Disease	Fibroelastic Deficiency
Pathology	Myxoid infiltration	Impaired production of connective tissue
Typical age	Young (<60 years)	Older (60+ years)
Duration of known mitral disease	Several years to decades	Months
Long history of murmur	Usually	No
Familial history	Sometimes	No
Marfanoid features	Sometimes	No
Auscultation	Midsystolic click and late systolic murmur	Holosystolic murmur
Echocardiography	Bulky, billowing leaflets, multi-segmental prolapse	Thin leaflets, prolapse of single segment, ruptured chord(s)
Surgical lesions	Excess tissue, thickened and tall leaflets, chordal thickening or thinning, chordal elongation or rupture, atrialization of leaflets, fusion, fibrosis or calcification of chords, papillary muscle calcification, annular calcification	Thin leaflets, thickening and excess tissue (if present) limited to prolapsing segment, ruptured chordae
Mitral valve repair	More complex	Less complex

Table 3. Key differences between Barlow,s disease and fibroelastic deficiency

7.4 Pathologic anatomy of degenerative mitral valve disease

According to A. Marc Gillinov and coworkers, pathologic anatomy of degenerative mitral valve disease is presented in group of 1072 patients as follows (Table #4).

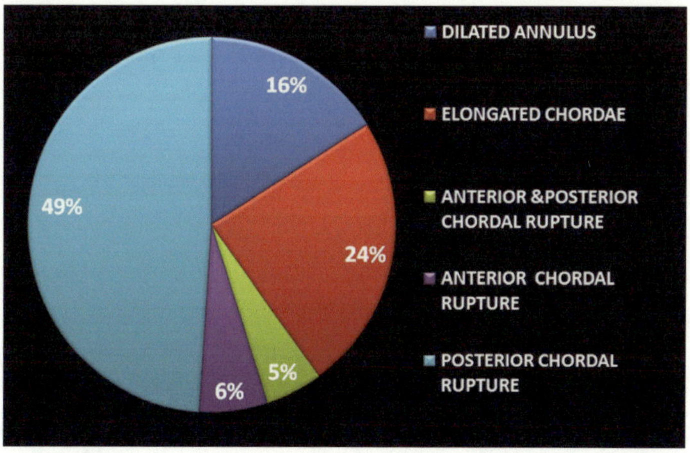

Table 4. Pathologic anatomy of degenerative mitral valve disease (n = 1072).

8. Surgical treatment

8.1 Principles of valve reconstruction

Guided by functional valve analysis, the surgeon should indentify all the lesions. The ultimate aim of valve reconstruction is to restore durable normal valve function. Three basic conditions are required to achieve this goal: preserving or restoring normal leaflet motion of all valve segments, creating a large surface of leaflet coaptation, remodeling the mitral valve orifice. Ideally correct application of repair techniques will produce appropriate coaptation. The rough zones of the leaflet should be in contact. The ratio of leaflet surface area to valve orifice area should be corrected to its natural 2:1 ratio. Because annular dilatation is a component of chronic mitral regurgitation, some type of annular support is necessary. Annuloplasty often completes the repair but cannot compensate for an inadequate repair. Echocardiography with color flow and spectral Doppler evaluation is an important noninvasive method for assessing the significance of cardiac murmurs. Information regarding valve morphology and function, chamber size, wall thickness, ventricular function, pulmonary and hepatic vein flow, and estimates of pulmonary artery pressures can be readily integrated. Zoghbi et al., 2003 presented qualitative and quantitative parameters useful in grading mitral regurgitation severity (Table#5).

Qualitative and quantitative parameters useful in grading mitral regurgitation severity

	Mild	Moderate	Severe
Structural parameters			
LA size	Normal*	Normal or dilated	Usually dilated**
LV size	Normal*	Normal or dilated	Usually dilated**
Mitral leaflets or support apparatus	Normal or abnormal	Normal or abnormal	Abnormal/ Flail leaflet/ Ruptured papillary muscle
Doppler parameters			
Color flow jet area^ξ	Small, central jet (usually < 4 cm^2 or < 20% of LA area)	Variable	Large central jet (usually > 10 cm^2 or > 40% of LA area) or variable size wall-impinging jet swirling in LA
Mitral inflow -PW	A wave dominant^♣	Variable	E wave dominant^♣ (E usually 1.2 m/s)
Jet density -CW	Incomplete or faint	Dense	Dense
Jet contour -CW	Parabolic	Usually parabolic	Early peaking-triangular
Pulmonary vein flow	Systolic dominance^§	Systolic blunting^§	Systolic flow reversal†
Quantitative parameters^♦			
VC width (cm)	< 0.3	0.3-0.69	≥ 0.7
R Vol (ml/beat)	< 30	30-44 45-59	≥ 60
RF (%)	< 30	30-39 40-49	≥ 50
EROA (cm^2)	< 0.20	0.20-0.29 0.30-0.39	≥ 0.40

CW, Continuous wave; *LA*, left atrium; *EROA*, effective regurgitant orifice area; *LV*, left ventricle; *PW*, pulsed wave; *RF*, regurgitant fraction; *R Vol*, regurgitant volume; *VC*, vena contracta.

* Unless there are other reasons for LA or LV dilation. Normal 2D measurements: LV minor axis ≤ 2.8 cm/m^2, LV end-diastolic volume ≤ 82 ml/m^2, maximal LA antero-posterior diameter ≤ 2 cm/m^2, maximal LA volume ≤ 36 ml/m^2 (2,33,35).

** Exception: acute mitral regurgitation.

ξ At a Nyquist limit of 50-60 cm/s.

† Pulmonary venous systolic flow reversal is specific but not sensitive for severe MR.

♣ Usually above 50 years of age or in conditions of impaired relaxation, in the absence of mitral stenosis or other causes of elevated LA pressure.

§ Unless other reasons for systolic blunting (eg. atrial fibrillation, elevated left atrial pressure).

♦ Quantitative parameters can help sub-classify the moderate regurgitation group into mild-to-moderate and moderate-to-severe.

Table 5. Qualitative and quantitative parameters useful in grading mitral regurgitation severity.

Three different MV operations are currently used for correction of MR: 1) MV repair; 2) MV replacement with preservation of part or all of the mitral apparatus; and 3) MV replacement with removal of the mitral apparatus. Each procedure has its advantages and disadvantages, and therefore, the indications for each procedure are somewhat different (Bonow et al., 2008).

In most cases, MV repair is the operation of choice when the valve is suitable for repair and appropriate surgical skill and expertise are available. This procedure preserves the patient's native valve without a prosthesis and therefore avoids the risk of chronic anticoagulation (except in patients in atrial fibrillation) or prosthetic valve failure late after surgery. Additionally, preservation of the mitral apparatus leads to better postoperative LV function and survival than in cases in which the apparatus is disrupted. Improved postoperative function occurs with repair because the mitral apparatus is an integral part of the left ventricle that is essential for maintenance of normal shape, volume, and function of the left ventricle. However, MV repair is technically more demanding than MV replacement, may require longer extracorporeal circulation time, and may occasionally fail. In USA (Savage et al., 2003) and Europe (Lung et al., 2003) the valve with MV regurgitation is repaired in only 50% of cases. Valve morphology and surgical expertise are of critical importance for the success of valve repair. The reoperation rate after MV repair is similar to the reoperation rate after MV replacement. There is a 7% to 10% reoperation rate at 10 years in patients undergoing MV repair, usually for severe recurrent MR. Approximately 70% of the recurrent MR is thought to be due to the initial procedure and 30% to progressive valve disease. The reoperation rate is lower in those patients who had the initial operation for posterior leaflet abnormalities than in those who had bileaflet or anterior leaflet abnormalities. In many cases, the type of operation, MV repair versus replacement, is important in timing surgery. In fact, although the type of surgery to be performed is never actually established until the operation, many situations lend themselves to preoperative prediction of the operation that can be performed. This prediction is based on the skill and experience of the surgeon in performing repair and on the location and type of MV disease that caused the MR. Nonrheumatic posterior leaflet prolapse due to degenerative MV disease or a ruptured chordae tendineae can usually be repaired using a resection of the portion of the valve and an annuloplasty. Involvement of the anterior leaflet or both anterior and posterior leaflets diminishes the likelihood of repair because the operation requires other interventions, such as chordal shortening, chordal transfer, and innovative anatomic repairs. Consequently, the skill and experience of the surgeon are probably the most important determinants of the eventual operation that will be performed.

8.2 Surgical approach

According to M. Scorsin (Scorsin et al., 2010), in 90% cases of posterior mitral valve prolapse is repaired with standart techniques: 1 - quadrangular \ triangular resection + placation of annulus, sliding, folding; 2- artificial chordate sutures. Current techniques for anterior leaflet prolapsed include valvular and subvalvular approach. In turn, valvular approach include papillary muscle placation, chordal shortening, leaflet resection, transposition of chordate. Subvalvular approach include artificial chordate. Among several repair techniques chordal replacement using ePTFE sutures has been introduced into clinical practise by Frater. There are several advantages to use of ePTFE suture for chordal replacement - preservation of native valve anatomy, physiological leaflet motion and creation of large mitral orifice area. Properly inserted, ePTFE sutures restore stress on the valve leaflet to a normal range. Long-term studies in experimental animals and in humans show that ePTFE chordae do not shrink or stiffen; indeed, these artificial chordae become covered by a fibrosis and intima simulating true chordae.

8.3 Evolution of modern valve repair techniques with artificial chordae

Medical literature describes numerous techniques to create and to determine ideal length for artificial chordae. Bizzarri et al has analysed evolution of modern valve repair techniques with artificial chordae (Bizzarri et al., 2010). **Morita et al., 1996** were the first to use 4-0 PTFE figure of 8 to repair both leaflets prolapse passing from the papillary body to the leaflet and back adding a Kay annuloplasty at the end of the procedure. **Zussa, 1997**, one of the pioneers of this technique, repaired an anterior leaflet with PTFE strings passing through the head of the papillary muscle and tying over a reinforcing autologous pericardial pledget. The strings were then anchored to the free margin of the anterior mitral leaflet at the unsupported areas and reinforced with a small autologous pericardial pledget. The two strands were tied after filling the ventricular cavity with saline solution for adjusting the chordal length. **Murakami et al., 1998** approached the anterior leaflet prolapse using mattress e-PTFE suture with Teflon or autologous pledget passed through the free margin of the leaflet from the ventricular side to the atrial side. The two arms of the suture, reinforced with pledgets, were brought down to the papillary muscle and passed through it. The length of the e-PTFE chordae was then adjusted by approximating the coapting area of the opposite leaflet and the ends of the sutures were then tied together (Figure 5).

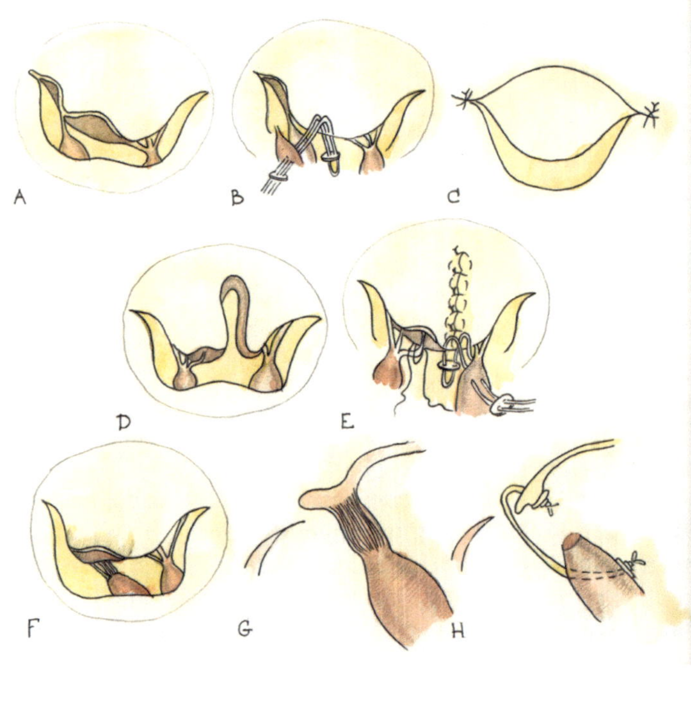

Fig. 5.

Chordae tendinae reconstruction, in patients with prolapsed of anterior leaflet was done by **Matsumoto et al., 1999** in children using the following technique: double-armed mattress e-PTFE sutures were passed through the free prolapsed edge from the ventricular side to the atrial side and then the two ends were passed through the papillary muscle at 3 to 4 mm from its top, drawing the free edge down to the entry point on the papillary muscle of the two ends of the suture. The sutures were passed through a pledget, which would be on the side where the sutures emerged from the papillary muscle. The knot was tied at the level of the opposing normal leaflet. The new chorda was pulled back through the papillary muscle until the pledget came up against the muscle. Another e-PTFE suture was placed in the same fashion. A Kay-Reed annuloplasty was added (Figure 6).

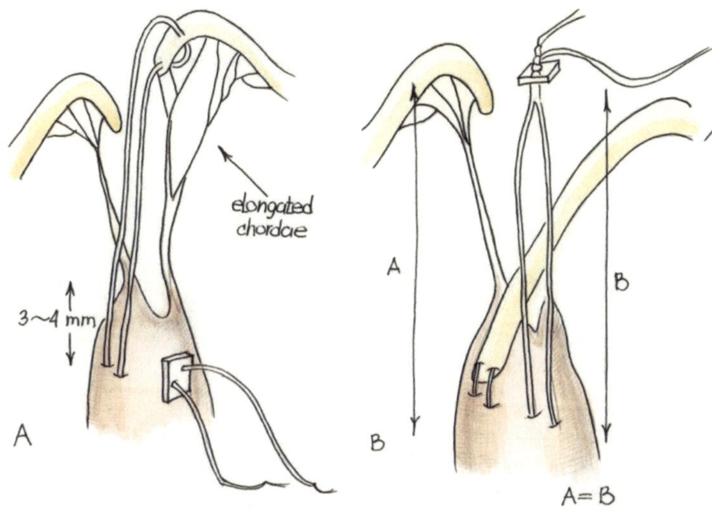

Fig. 6.

Kawahira et al., 1999 used 4-0 e-PTFE sutures through the prolapsed leaflet from its ventricular to atrial aspect, placing pledgets for reinforcement on the ventricular surface of the leaflet. The sutures were anchored to the papillary muscles in a mattress fashion. This maneuver could be carried out in reverse order: attaching e- PTFE suture initially to the papillary muscle, subsequently passing it through the leaflet from it's ventricular to atrial aspect. In this circumstance, the knot would be placed on the atrial aspect of the mitral valve. **Adams et al., 2001** placed one or more 4-0 Gore- Tex sutures into the head of the papillary muscle. Papillary muscle exposure was enhanced after quadrangular posterior leaflet resection. Before annuloplasty poor leaflet apposition is present in all leaflet segments with saline testing and segmental anterior leaflet prolapse is best identified by height comparison with a normal reference point. After ring annuloplasty symmetric leaflet apposition limits leaflet incompetence to the prolapsing anterior leaflet segment. Both arms of the previously placed Gore-Tex suture are passed through the margin of the prolapsing leaflet segment. Passing the suture through the free edge of the cusp twice as well as starting with a surgeon's knot are techniques to prevent overaggressive sliding of the knots when tying the Gore-Tex suture (Figure 7).

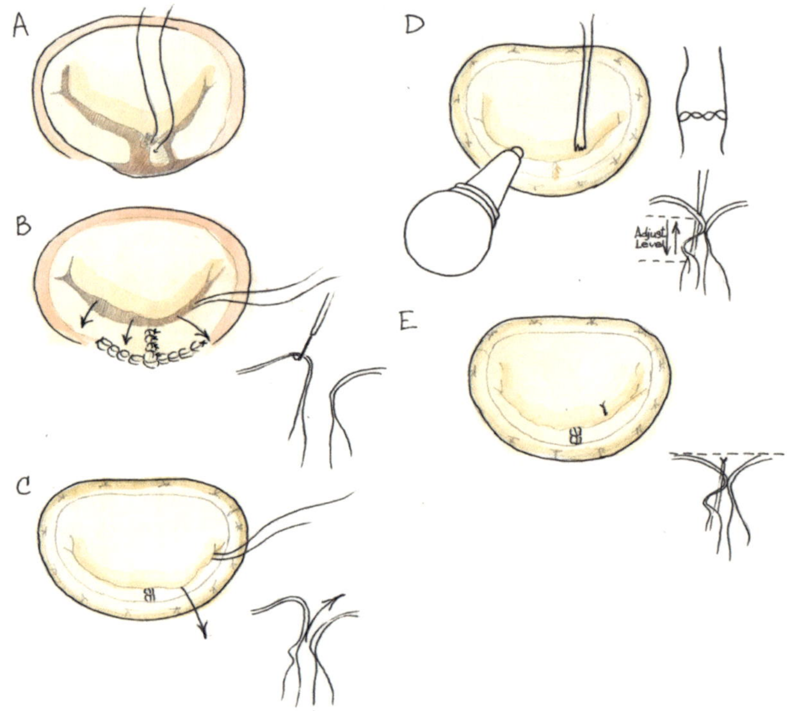

Fig. 7.

Tomita, 2002 applied the method of David to use the reconstruction of the valve with CV-4 e-PTFE sutures. The double armed suture is passed twice through the fibrous portion of the papillary muscle head that anchors the elongated or ruptured chordae and is tied down (seven or eight knots are needed for this type of suture material). The two arms of the suture are then brought up to the free margin of the leaflet and passed through the point where the original chorda was attached (thickened portion of the leaflet). The needle is brought from the ventricular side of the leaflet to its atrial side and then passed once through the leaflet. The length of the PTFE chordae is adjusted by approving the coating area of the opposite leaflet. Then both ends of the suture are passed through the leaflet again and tied together on the ventricular side. Another PTFE suture is placed when the prolapsed portion is wide. Kay's annuloplasty is added at the end.

With time, it appeared mandatory to find the correct technique to determine the length of the artificial chordae. **Sarsam et al., 2002** passed one or more 5-0 e-PTFE sutures, supported by a felt pledget through the fibrous portion of the papillary muscle. The suture was left untied. The two arms of the suture were then passed once through the rough free edge of the prolapsing leaflet from the ventricular to the atrial side. If the native chorda to the corresponding part of the opposing leaflet are normal, the edges of the anterior and posterior leaflet are temporarily approximated by a simple or figure 8 suture and then the suture is tied against the temporary suture. Three knots are used. The suture in passed again through the edge of the leaflet from the ventricular to the atrial side and tied permanently. The temporary suture is then removed (Figure 8).

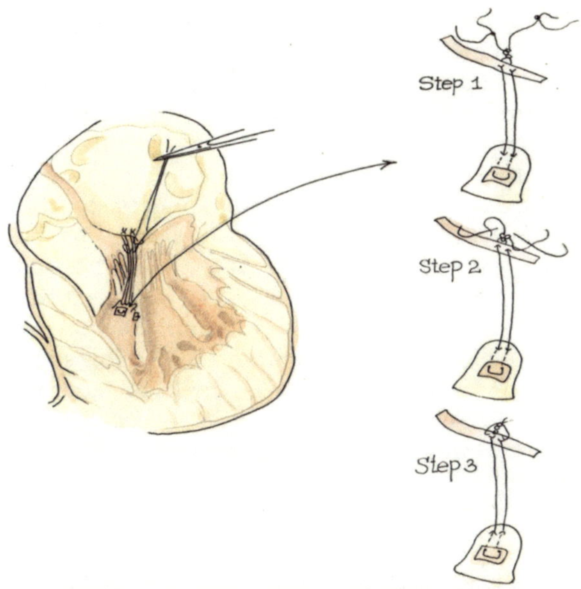

Fig. 8.

Soga, 2003 made a resection of both the anterior and posterior mitral leaflets and subvalvular apparatus and placed two 3-0 e-PTFE mattress sutures: one placed and tied at the tip of the anterior papillary muscle, and one at the tip of the posterior papillary muscle. The suture of the anterior PM is placed at the 9-10 o'clock position on the mitral annulus (as defined by mid-anterior annulus to be 0 o'clock), and the suture for the posterior PM at the 5-6 o'clock. According to the authors, the length of the artificial CT can be determined during intraoperative cardiac arrest, and may be suitable if the sutures are tied just less than taut before insertion of the prosthetic. After the valve replacement, the motion of the prosthetic leaflets is examined to ensure that the leaf let are not entrapped by the 3-0 e-PTFE sutures (Figure 9).

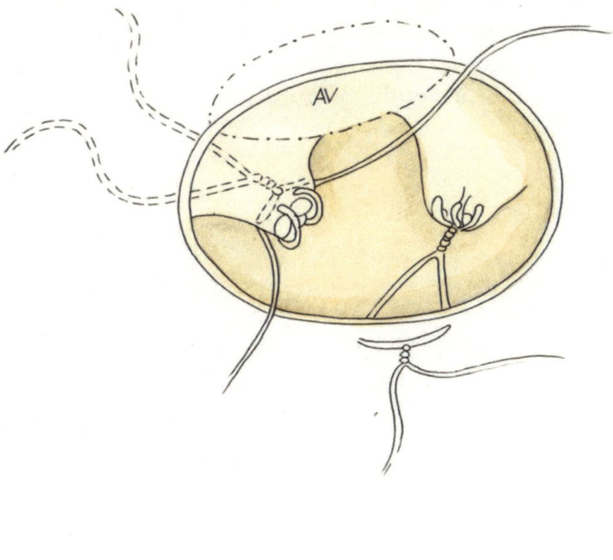

Fig. 9.

Tomita, 2005 repaired chordae tendinae with CV-4 e-PTFE sutures. Double armed sutures are passed twice through the fibrous portion of the PM head that anchors the elongated or ruptured chordae and are tied down (7 or 8 knots are needed for this suture material). The two arms of the suture are brought up to the free margin of the leaflet and passed through the point where the original chorda was attached (thickened portion of the leaflet). The needle is brought from the ventricular side of the leaflet to its atrial side and passed once more through the leaflet. The length of PTFE chordae is adjusted by referring the contact area of the opposite leaflet and then both ends of the suture are passed through the leaflet again and tied together on the ventricular side. When the prolapsed portion became wide, another PTFE suture was placed in the same fashion. At the end Kay's suture annuloplasty (n = 24) or ring annuloplasty was performed. **Minami, 2005** used double armed mattress sutures of 4-0, 5- 0 or 6-0 e-PTFE placed to reinforce with felt pledgets between the PM and free margin of the anterior leaflet. The length of the PTFE sutures was adjusted with the adjacent normal anterior leaflet or facing posterior leaflet. When the prolapsed portion became wide, another suture was placed in the same fashion. The number of sutures ranged from 1 to 3. In addition, Kay annuloplasty was perfomed.

Matsui, 2005 employed a new device (Matsuda Ika-Kogyo, Tokyo, Japan) consisting of two metallic tubes with a circular, hook shaped distal tip made entirely of stainless steel. The distal tip, which is perpendicularly attached to the inner tube, was designed to hold the Gore-Tex thread at the reference point on the PM immovable. The outer tube could slide on the surface of the inner tube to measure the length from the tip of inner tube to the hook of outer tube. A 4-0 or 5-0 Gore-Tex mattress suture, reinforced with a felt pledget, was placed into the head of the PM. Both arms of the suture where left untied. Length was determined by measuring the distance between the leaflet edge and the site of implantation of the artificial chordae on the PM, using a normal valve segment adjacent to the prolapsing segment as a reference. The distal tip of the inner tube of the device was placed at the sutured site of the artificial chordae on the PM. The proximal hook of the outer tube was slid to the edge of the adjacent non prolapsing leaflet and then fixed at that point after reading the distance between the distal tip and proximal hook to the device. Devices were then moved to the prolapsed segments so as to hold an edge of the prolapsed leaflet with a proximal hook. As the determined distance and edge of the leaflet were fixed with the device, the Gore-Tex suture could be tied in the usual manner without knot slipping. The action of knot-tying itself works to immobilize the device by its strength. After removing the device, followed by saline testing, a Carpenter- Edwards annuloplasty ring was attached according to the size of the mitral annulus (Figure 10).

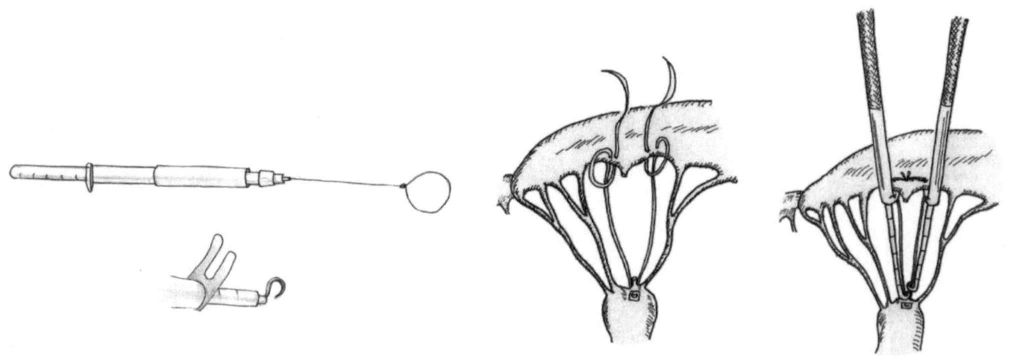

Fig. 10.

Prêtre et al., 2006 applied the artificial chordae to the mitral valve using an approach through the aortic valve for an anterior and posterior leaflet prolaps. In the anterior repair an atriotomy was performed first, the artificial chordae was placed in the usual manner, and then a flexible annular ring was tied on the mitral annulus. An aortotomy was performed to expose the native chordae and to calibrate the length of the artificial chordae that were locked but not tied down. The mitral valve was inspected through the atriotomy while saline water was injected through the aortotomy in the left ventricle. The chordae were tied from the aortotomy and the incisions closed in the usual fashion. In the posterior leaflet prolapse, repair was done and a ring was inserted using a classical atrial incision. The ascending aorta was opened and the artificial chordae were set on the papillary muscles and the anterior leaflet was calibrated. The valve was re-inspected through the atriotomy with instillation of saline in the left ventricle for adjusting the chordae until they were definitively secured Figure 11.

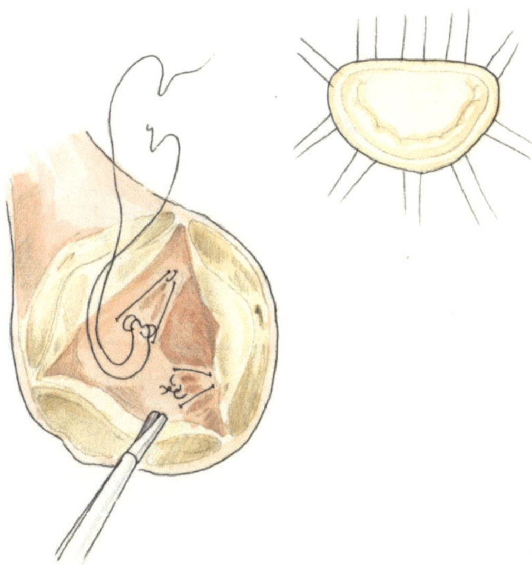

Fig. 11.

Lawrie et al., 2006 published their experience on 152 consecutive patients. 5-0 PTFE sutures were placed into the bases of the papillary muscles in a figure-8 fashion, and were brought through the free edge of the prolapsing segment. Dots were made to mark the desired final line of leaflet apposition. The left ventricle was inflated with saline solution and the chordal length was adjusted to align the edges of the leaflets. Leaflet alignment was checked and the PTFE was tied down. The knot was locked with a 6-0 polypropylene stitch which was tied over the end of the PTFE to prevent sliding of the PTFE knots. An annuloplasty ring was then implanted.

Calafiore, 2006 in the anterior leaflet prolapse passed 4-0 PTFE sutures through the fibrous tip of the papillary muscle and fixed the sutures. The new chorda was passed in the border of the anterior leaflet in the proper place and its final length was measured with a ruler. A mark was applied to indicate this distance and the suture was tied with the aid of a nerve hook (Figure 12).

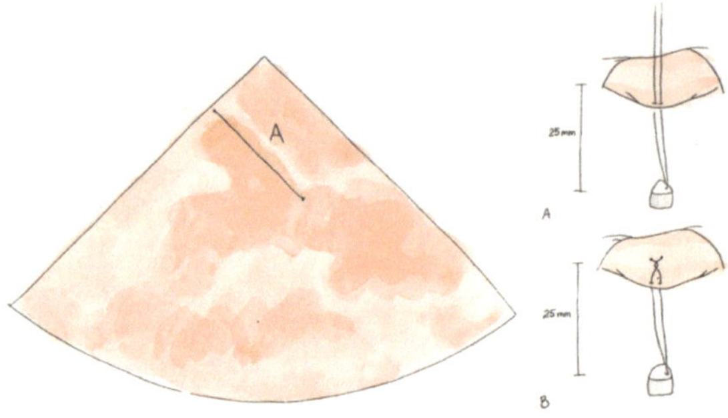

Fig. 12.

Rankin, 2006 in the anterior and/or posterior leaflet prolapsed placed 4-0 prolene pledgetted horizontal mattress sutures longitudinally into each papillary muscle, passing one arm through the fibrous tip, and tying firmly; through this anchor suture, a double-armed Gortex suture was passed but not tied. A Carpentier annuloplasty ring was sutured. With the ring in position, the chordae were retrieved from the ventricle, and both needles were woven into the prolapsing segment, straddling the point of maximal prolapse. Two or three bites were taken through the coaptation surface to the line of coaptation. The two arms of the suture were tied on the atrial surface with a slip-knot to bring the leaflet to the annular plane, and a clip was placed across the knot. Pericardial pledgets could be used if the leaflet tissue seems fragile. Cold saline solution was infused to check the length of the suture; once the valve was competent, eight more knot were tied tightly against the clip, the suture was cut, and the clip was removed (Figure 13).

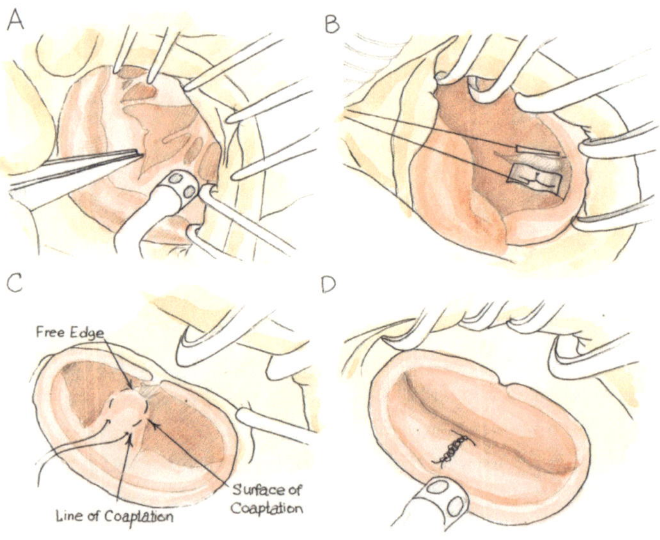

Fig. 13.

Tam, 2006 used the following technique for any prolapsing segment. A calliper was used to measure the length of the reference chordae. A 4-0 ePTFE suture was used to create loops around the calliper. Non-sliding knots were placed at the end of each loop while still on the calliper. After making a desired number of loops, the needles were passed through the loops and tied. Two needles at the end of the sutures were passed through an ePTFE pledget, which was now ready to be secured to the papillary muscle. The ePTFE chordae were secured at the tip of the papillary muscle with two pledgets and attached to the edge of the prolapsing mitral leaflet using eight 5-0 ePTFE sutures (Figure 14).

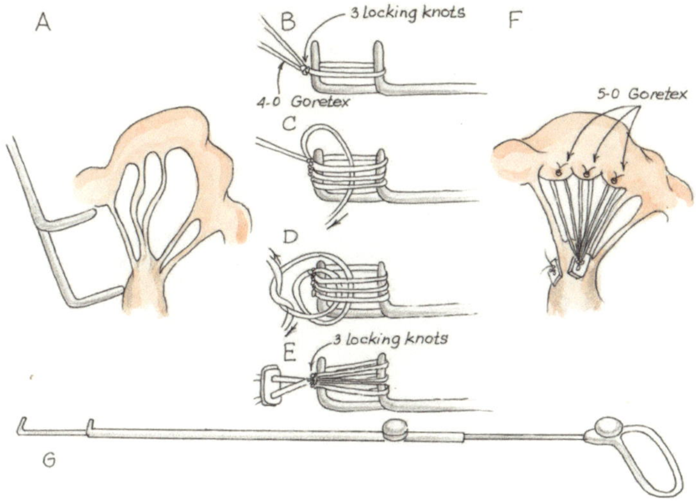

Fig. 14.

Mandegar, 2007 for any leaflet prolapse used following technique. During preoperative transesophageal echocardiography, a line was drawn between the base of the anterior and posterior mitral leaflet to measure the distance between the head of the posterior papillary muscle and the plane at the co-optation of the leaflets; this measured the artificial chordal length. During surgery, 4-0 Gore- Tex was passed through the fibrous tip of the papillary muscle with a pledget and was fixed with a loose knot. Two tight reverse knots were made for every millimeter of 4-0 Gore-Tex that was required. The needles were passed through the edge of the anterior leaflet at the prolapsing portion, and the Gore-Tex was knotted onto a strip of pericardium so that the final knot could be placed at the atrial side of the leaflet (Figure 15).

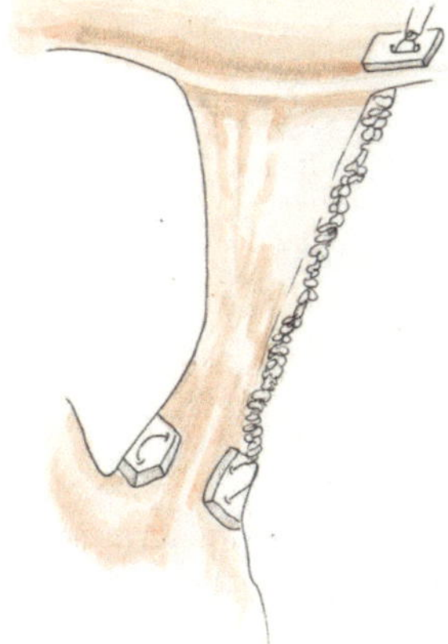

Fig. 15.

Gillinov, 2007 describe a technique for reparing anterior leaflet prolapse. Chordal length was determined with a calliper, and ePTFE chordae were constructed making loops around it. A pledget was used to prepare the number of 5-0 ePTFE loops that were needed. When all chordal loops were constructed, each needle was passed through the head of the papillary muscle, and was affixed to the free edge of the anterior leaflet with a figure 8 suture of CV-5 ePTFE (Figure 16).

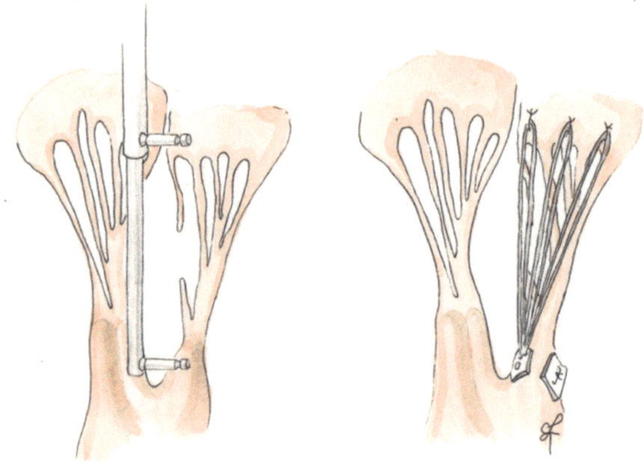

Fig. 16.

Scorsin et al., 2007: any leaflet prolapse. Artificial chordae system device was composed of 2 sets of 4 artificial chordae, attached to a 3-mm strip of knitted polyester 18 mm wide, leaving 4 mm between each chorda. The device was applied by suturing the strip to the free edge of the prolapsed leaflet by continuous suture. Each array was anchored to the tip of the correspondent papillary muscle by only one stitch. After this procedure, a prosthetic annuloplasty ring was inserted (Figure 17).

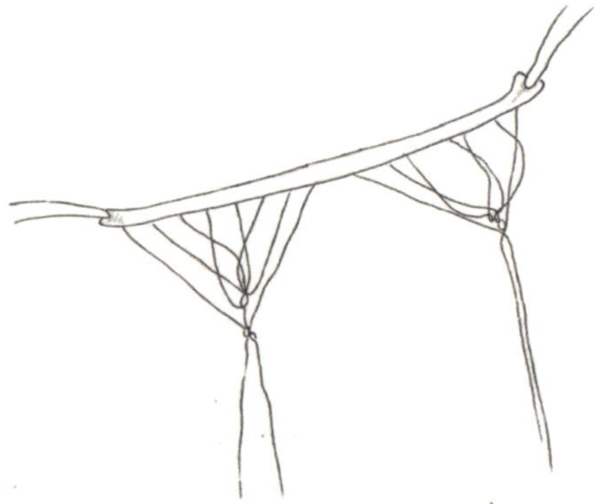

Fig. 17.

Maselli and De Paulis, 2007 used a novel system to repair the valve consisting of two components: leaflet component and the papillary component. The first one was achieved with a CV-5 PTFE suture. A circular loop was obtained at the middle of the suture by tying it around a Hegar dilator with a diameter of 13 mm. Flattened loop's length should equals half the circumference. Given a circumference of approximately 4 cm for a circle with a diameter of 13 mm the length of the loop would be approximately 2 cm. Papillary component was obtained by cutting a CV-4 PTFE suture in 2 halves; 5 double knots were placed at a distance of 2 mm at the needleless tip of each CV-4 semisuture. The needleless tip of the suture was anchored on a drape; knots were placed with the help of forceps and a needle holder and slid into definitive position by inserting the tip of the needle or a nerve hook in the knot itself. To realize papillary component for each neochorda 2 CV-4 half sutures with knots were needed. After the assessment of the mitral valve lesions, the papillary component was set in place by first fixing 2 semisutures to a papillary head and tying the sutures so that the papillary head was "sandwiched" between 2 e-PTFE pledgets to reduce trauma. Two CV-5 loops were fixed on the desired leaflet 2 to 3 mm apart from the leaflet's edge, passing the needle from the atrial to the ventricular side and leaving knots on the ventricular aspect of the leaflet. A single PTFE pledget was interposed on the atrial side. To obtain reversible coupling of the leaflet component with the papillary, a loop which could be tightened and loosened as many times as required, was placed in the leaflet component with the help of forceps and a curved instrument. The papillary component passed inside the loop and the loop was tightened. The loop had to fall in the gap between two knots. Chordal length was fixed by closing the loop under the selected reference knot of the papillary component. Same steps were repeated for the other chordae. To shorten or elongate the neochorda without touching its papillary or leaflet anchoring, the loop was released and slid under a reference knot respectively closer or farther from the papillary muscle tip, and tightened again (Figure 18).

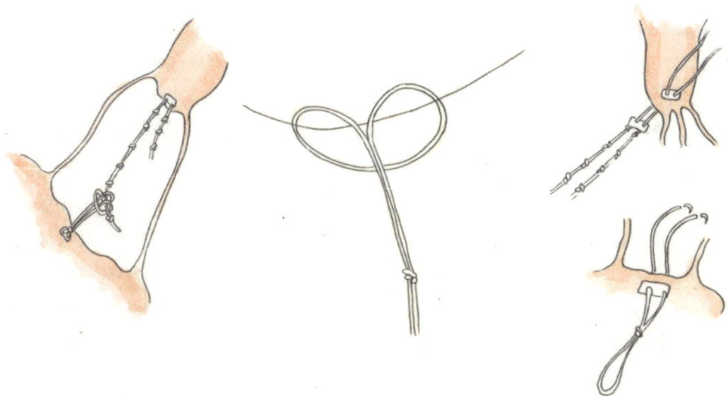

Fig. 18.

Boon et al., 2007 used CV-5 e-PTFE sutures for older children, while CV-7 was typically used in neonates and small infants. The suture was first tied to the fibrous tip of the PM and the two ends were fixed to the free edge of the valve leaflet in a V-shape. For the anterior leaflet, a new chord length was measured by bringing the free edge of the valve to the level of the anterior annulus. The length could also be compared to healthy non-elongated native chords in the adjacent area. Then both ends of the sutures would be passed again through the free edge and tied on the ventricular side of the leaflet, to prevent the knot from interfering with the co-optation zone. Because the sutures are placed in a V-shape, one suture accounts for 2 new artificial chords. In addition, ring annuloplasty or Wooler-Kay bilateral commissural plication annuloplasty was performed. **Chan, 2008**: for anterior leaflet prolapse a 4-0 Gore-Tex suture with pledgets was used. The suture was first passed through the papillary muscle and secured with 6 to 8 knots. Both braids were then passed through the prolapsed leaflet edge no more than 4 mm apart. The suture was then tensed up. The non-prolapsing posterior leaflet was used to check the reference length. A single-arm rubber- protected artery forceps was clipped on the mark, and knots were tied on it.

Salvador, 2008: for anterior leaflet prolapse repair a e-PTFE double-armed suture (GORE-TEX CV-5) were passed through the PM with a mattress technique and reinforced with autologous pericardial pledgets (rarely, GORE-TEX pledgets), on both sides of the muscle. Each end of the suture were fixed to the free margin of the prolapsed leaflet and reinforced with a small autologous pericardial pledget or a small GORE-TEX pledget. The length of the artificial chordae was adjusted to maintain the corresponding free margin of the leaflet at the desired level in the ventricular cavity. To determine the correct length of the artificial chordae, the neochordae were tied at the end of all the other repair procedures after the ventricular cavity is filled with saline solution. **Smith and Stein, 2008** made the first endoscopic placement of multiple pre-measured artificial chordae with Robotic assistance and nitinol clip fixation. Robotic bileaflet mitral valve repair used a more lateral approach and 5 right thoracoscopic ports, ranging in size from 8 to 20 mm. Left atriotomy was perform to expose mitral valve using a robotically controlled EndoWrist atrial retractor (Intuitive Surgical Inc.). The prolapsing segment was identified with valve hooks. The "ski-tip" style ends of the robotic retractor blades are longed into the anterior leaflet, then the atrial septum is lifted to visualize PM. The length of the artificial chordae loops were determined with the measure of the distance between the correct plane of apposition on an adjacent normal non-prolapsing segment of the mitral leaflet and the respective PM (done with a More Suture Ruler device). Artificial chordae, with 4 loops each, were constructed of 4-0 PTFE GORE-TEX per the technique by von Oppel and Mohr. A single felt pledget constructed the platform with multiple neochords of definite length extending from its base. Both free suture needles from the pledget platform were passed through the respective PM with 2 robotic large needle drivers. After the correct placement in the muscle head, the needles were retrieved and the neochordae platform was secured with extracorporeal knots tied by the assistant using a closed knot pusher. Each neochordae loop was attached to the edge of the prolapsing leaflet by applying a single-armed V60 U-clip per loop. The singlearmed U-clip was placed in the leaflet edge with a robotic large needle holder and the neochordae loop was captured in the open clip circle. The U-clip was deployed by pulling the needle off the clip portion, securing the neochordae loop to the leaflet. Additional reduction of the leaflet height could be achieved by folding the leaflet edge toward the ventricle before deploying the U-clip. The remaining loops were distributed at equal distance along the edge of the prolapsed segment by applying the same technique. After the pledget platform was secured, the 2 free suture needles were placed through the anterior prolapse. The correct apposition was confirmed with saline test. The assistan, at the patient side, tied the knots. Annuloplasty was performed at the surgeon's discretion. For concomitant left atrial ablation a SurgiFlex XL probe was applied endocardially. Lastly the heart was de-aired and the left atrium was closed with a running suture line (Figure 19).

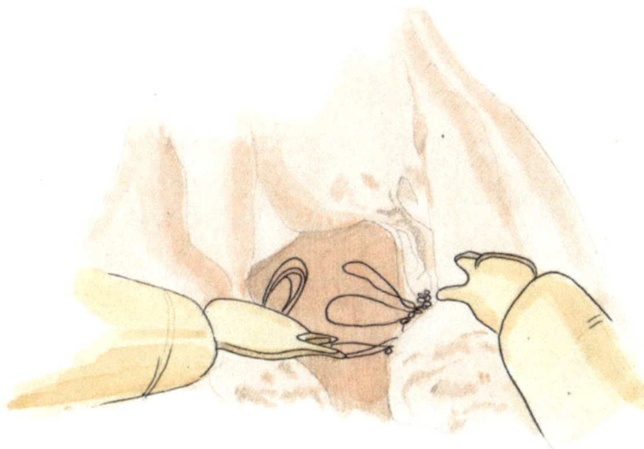

Fig. 19.

Doi, 2009 measured the length of the chordae of the posterior leaflet, opposing the prolapsing portion of the anterior leaflet by TEE. The length of chordae was a measurement of the distance between the head of the PM and the free edge of the posterior leaflet. Length of the opposing chordae of the posterior leaflet was measured directly by using a calliper. Double-armed mattress sutures with CV-5 GORE-TEX were placed at the fibrous tip of the PM using PTFE on both sides and tied down firmly. In all cases Doi performed Duran ring annuloplasty. Thereafter, the ePTFE suture is placed through the anterior leaflet. The needles were passed through the rough zone of the prolapsing portion from the atrial to the ventricular side, and again through the free margin of the leaflet from the ventricular to the atrial side. The caliper that was fixed at the length of the opposing chordae was inserted inside the loop created by the ePTFE suture. The suture was easily tied at the exact length of the opposing chordae and the anterior leaflet was fixed at the height of the posterior leaflet (Figure 20).

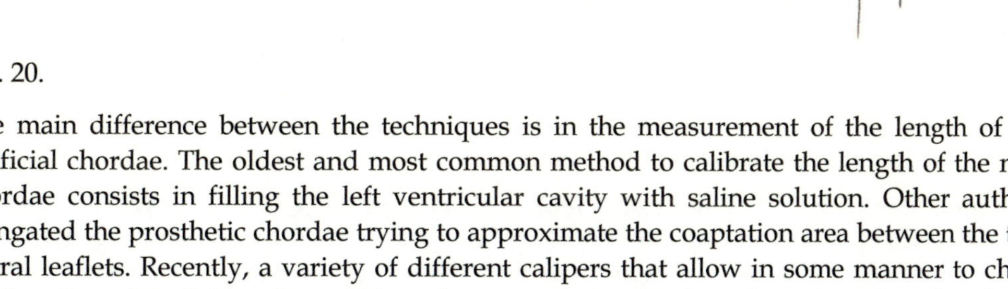

Fig. 20.

The main difference between the techniques is in the measurement of the length of the artificial chordae. The oldest and most common method to calibrate the length of the neo-chordae consists in filling the left ventricular cavity with saline solution. Other authors elongated the prosthetic chordae trying to approximate the coaptation area between the two mitral leaflets. Recently, a variety of different calipers that allow in some manner to check the length and to tighten the number of necessary chordae have been introduced to better define the adequacy of the PTFE chordae implantation.

8.4 New device

In our Cardiothoracic Surgery Center we worked out our own device to measure proper length of chords and multiple loops formation (Figure 21).

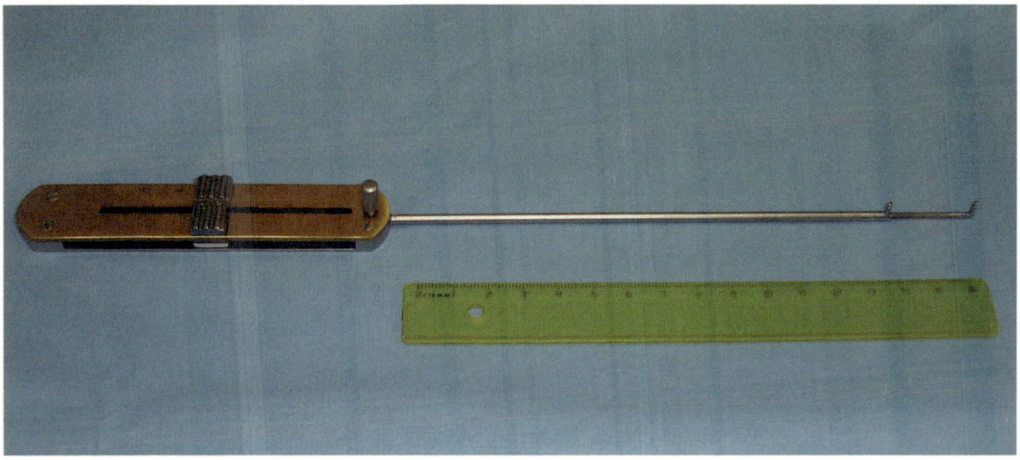

Fig. 21. Boldyrev - Barbukhatty- Porhanov device.

The gist of the given model is that on the end of the working body we placed props located perpendicularly to the plane of the graduated scale and fitted with circular cuttings for loop fixation, and on a scale there is a core clamp.By means of our appliance one is able to perform at the same time intraoperative measurement of the chordal apparatus and to generate necessary quantity of loops for chord prosthetic repair. This device is in process of patenting in the Russian Federation (request № 2011101697\14(002183), January 18, 2011)

8.5 South Russian experience

Material and Methods: From 2008 to 2011 we have treated 30 patients with moderately severe (3+) or severe (4+) mitral regurgitation. Echocardiographic findings are showed in the Table 6.

MV regurgitation grade by color Doppler	3 ± 0,44
Regurgitation volume, ml	109 ± 19,4
MV EF,%	57 ± 5,4
Left atrium size, mm	51,4 ± 6,8
Left ventricular end diastolic dimension, mm	60,9 ± 5,2
Left ventricular end diastolic volume, ml	199,5 ± 38,4
LV EF, %	49,2 ± 8,5
Pulmonary hypertension, mm Hg	49,2 ± 8,5

Table 6. Preoperative echocardiographic data.

They all underwent MV chord system repair. There were 17 male and 13 female patients. Age range was from 16 to 70 years (mean age 55,3 ± 13). Mean ejection fraction was 49%, and minimal - 35% (3 cases). Etiology 20 (66%) patient had fibroelastoc deficiency, 2 (7%) - ischemic heart disease, 3 (10%) had Barlow,s disease, 2 (7%) had Marfan,s disease, and 3 (10%) had mitral valve malformation. 7 (23%) patients were found to have posterior leaflet prolapse, 5 (17%) patients - bileaflet prolapse, and 18 (60%) - anterior leaflet prolapse. We performed 7 posterior mitral valve leaflet chord reconstructions, in 4 cases with multiple loops. Anterior mitral leaflet chord repair was carried out in 18 (60%) patients (including multiple loops in 10 cases). 5 (17%) patient had total AML chord repair (Figure 22, 23).

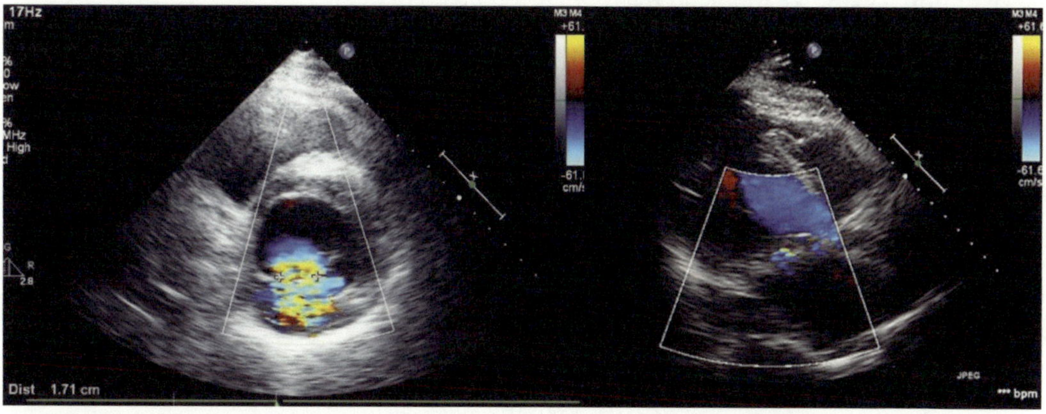

Fig. 22. Patient Ch. Preoperative echocardiography (left, two-chambered position at the mitral valve level) and postoperative view (right, four-chambered position).

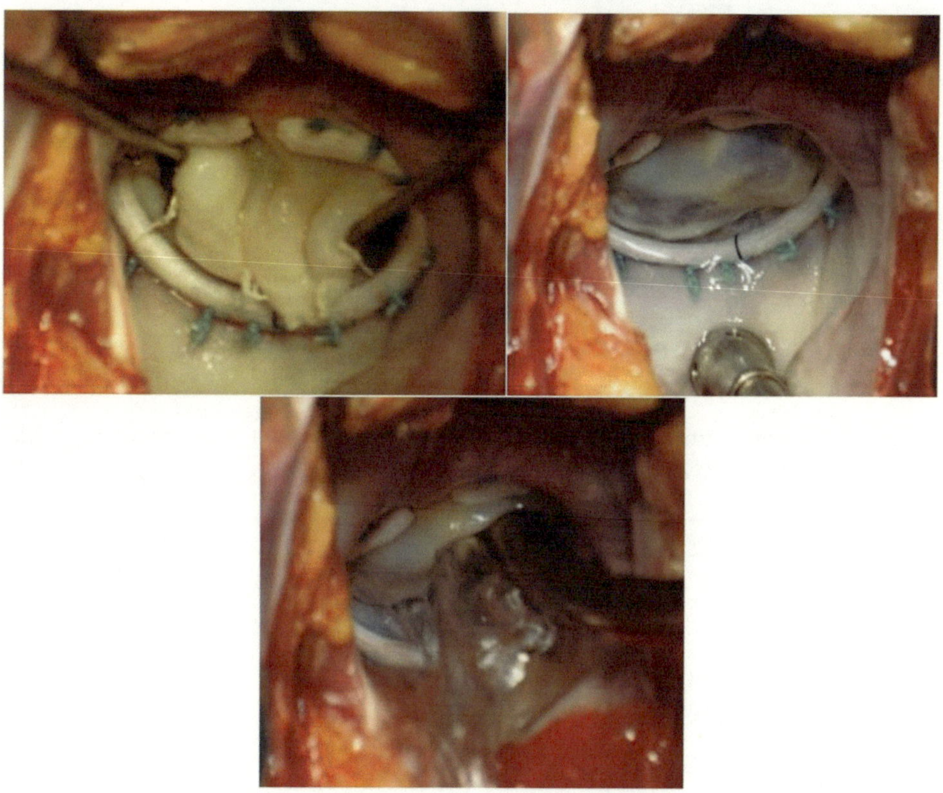

Fig. 23. Patient Ch. Intraoperative photo total anterior mitral leaflet chord repair.

1(3%) patient underwent total chordae replacement (anterior and posterior leaflets). We applied quadrangular resection with leaflet height adjustment of posterior leaflet for bileaflet prolapses with AMV chord repair. When we carried out repair with multiple loops we used a device (proper modification) to measure length and formation of neochords. To make multiple loops we followed the sequence showed in Figure 24.

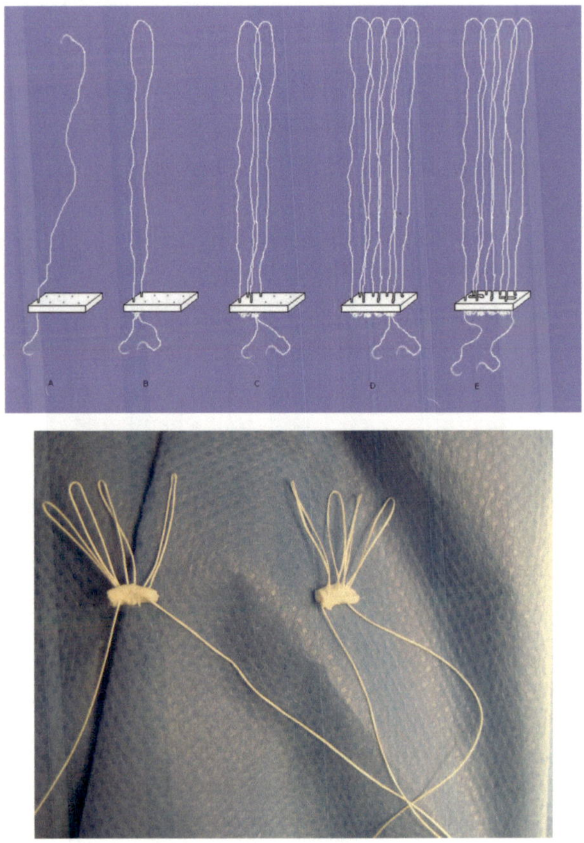

Fig. 24. Scheme of multiple loops performance (from A to E).

All patients underwent suturing annuloplasty or were implanted supporting rings MedIng. Results: All patients survived. Operative results were assessed by echocardiography (Table 7).

MV regurgitation grade by color Doppler	1,14 ± 0,8
Regurgitation volume, ml	20 ± 11,8
MV EF,%	20 ± 11,8
Left atrium size, mm	42,6 ± 4,2
Left ventricular end diastolic dimension, mm	51,8 ± 7,4
Left ventricular end diastolic volume, ml	51,8 ± 7,4
LV EF, %	54,6 ± 9,6
Pulmonary hypertension, mm Hg	34,8 ± 7,1

Table 7. Postoperative echocardiographic data.

We believe the quantitative assessment of regurgitation described by Zoghbi and co-authors (Zoghbi W et al, 2003) is the most unbiased. In immediate postoperative period in 1 patient we noticed systolic anterior motion syndrome with further release. In the follow-up period ranging from 1 to 30 months, 1 patient required reoperation in 4 months for 3 + mitral regurgitation; the mechanism of recurrent mitral regurgitation showed AL chords tearing off with high arterial hypertension (Table № 8).

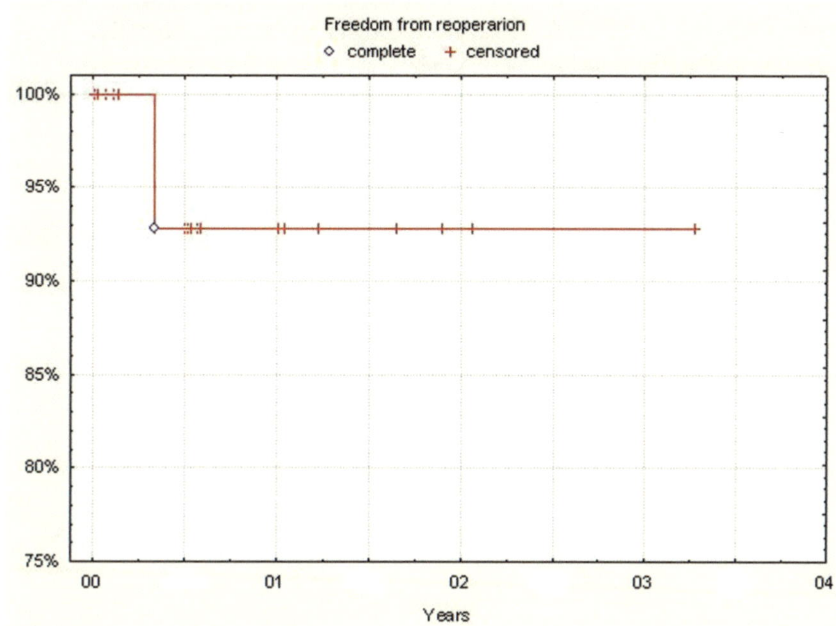

Table 8. Freedom from reoperation.

9. Conclusions

On the basis of our results we state that artificial chords are rather attractive method for MV repair in patients with abnormal chord apparatus. Despite some difficulty while selecting proper neochords, this technique is applicable and reliable in most cases. Mitral valve repair is a challenging technique deserving continuous attention over time. In the future we are waiting for more novel procedures to ensure better results in mid and long term morbidity.

10. References

Barbukhatty K., Boldyrev S, Rossoha O, Strigina O, Sapunov V. Mitral valve subvalvular apparatus reconstruction with ePTFE sutures. Cardiovascular diseases. Baculev's SCCVS ballot of RAMS. Volume 11, #6, November - December, 2010, oral report. The 10th Congress of Cardiovascular surgeons.

Bizzarri F, Tudisco A, Ricci M, Rose D, Frati G (2010). Journal of Cardiothoracic Surgery 2010, 5:22

Bonow RO, Carabello BA, Chatterjee K, de Leon AC Jr, Faxon DP, Freed MD,Gaasch WH, Lytle BW, Nishimura RA, O'Gara PT, O'Rourke RA, Otto CM, Shah PM, Shanewise

JS. 2008 focused update incorporated into the ACC/AHA 2006 guidelines for the management of patients with valvular heart disease: a report of the American College of Cardiology/American Heart Association Task Force on Practice Guidelines (Writing Committee to revise the 1998 guidelines for the management of patients with valvular heart disease). Endorsed by the Society of Cardiovascular Anesthesiologists, Society for Cardiovascular Angiography and Interventions, and Society of Thoracic Surgeons. J AmColl Cardiol 2008;52:e1–e142.

Carpentier A.; Adams D; Filsoufi F. (2010). Carpentier's Reconstructive Valve Surgery, Elsevier, ISBN: 978-0-7216-9168-8 USA

Savage E; Bolling S, (2006). Atlas of Mitral Valve Repair, Lippincott Williams & Wilkins, ISBN - 13:978-0-7817-4692-2 USA

2

Post Myocardial Infarction Ventricular Septal Defect

Michael S. Firstenberg and Jason Rousseau
Division of Cardiac Surgery, The Ohio State University Medical Center, Columbus, USA

1. Introduction

With advances in the management of acute myocardial infarction (AMI) the incidence of mechanical complications continues to decline. Nevertheless, when they occur, unfortunately, despite similar advances and growing experiences in the surgical management of these problems, morbidity and mortality remain high. Post-myocardial infarction ventricular septal defects (PI-VSD) have fascinated and challenged clinicians for years. The timing of presentation can be quite variable, as they tend to occur in patients several days after their initial cardiovascular insult (acute PI-VSD) - and unfortunately, they can occur in patients who appear to have been making significance progress on the road to recovery. In addition, although more rare, some patients might not present until weeks, if not longer, after their infarction with symptoms that prompt the discovery of a chronic PI-VSD. Early PI-VSDs tend to be catastrophic and typically result in early death. The pathophysiology is also variable and complex, but common themes include: 1) worsening cardiac output, often with manifestations of shock and end-organ damage, from acute left ventricular (LV) dysfunction and from increased left-right shunting, 2) acute right ventricular (RV) dysfunction from a sudden increase in pressure, volume, and flow from left to right shunts, and 3) pulmonary hypertension also from the increase in RV flow. Definitive management remains surgical, however controversies continue to exist regarding the timing of surgery and the role of concomitant coronary revascularization. Unfortunately, despite early repair and standardization of techniques, both short and long-term outcomes remain less than ideal.

2. History

As with many cardiovascular conditions, post-myocardial infarction ventricular septal defects (PI-VSD) were described first at autopsy (Latham, 1845) and then pre-mortum in 1923, many years before the pathophysiology was understood (Brunn, 1923). It was not until 1934 that the association with coronary artery disease was described (Sager, 1934). The first report of a surgical repair came in 1956 when Denton Cooley described the surgical management in a patient 9 weeks after the initial diagnosis (Cooley, 1956). With advances in cardiovascular surgery and peri-operative management of the cardiac surgery patient there were increasing reports of survival in what was previously felt to be a lethal problem. Most of the successful cases occurred in patients who presented in congestive heart failure many weeks after their initial acute event. It was these experiences that set the foundation for the belief that operative management should be delayed as long as possible to allow for scarring of the necrotic myocardium to provide for a more stable repair. As experiences grew – in terms of the initial diagnosis and surgical management – early repair was advocated, particularly in patients who were stable before hemodynamic deterioration and subsequent end-organ failure.

3. Clinical presentation

The incidence of PI-VSD has decreased considerably over the years with advances in myocardial reperfusion strategies. Historically, up to 5% of all myocardial infractions were associated with mechanical complications such free-wall rupture, papillary muscle rupture, and PI-VSD (Agnihotri, 2008). With current treatment algorithms that advocate early and aggressive attempts at revascularization of the acute ischemic myocardial – such as thrombolytic therapy, early percutanous interventions with coronary stenting (PCI), and, less frequently, emergent coronary artery bypass surgery (CABG) – the overall incidence has dropped significantly. Large multi-centers studies evaluating the pathophysiologies of acute myocardial infarctions have shown a current incidence of approximately 0.2% of all AMI. With delays in therapies, or late clinical presentation, and the resulting increase in myocardial damage, this incidence increases up to 2%. Despite the relatively low risk of developing a PI-VSD, it account for a disproportionally high risk of mortality. Over 5% of all early deaths after AMI are attributed directly to the pathophysiologic complications of PI-VSD (Poulsen, 2008).

The timing of the development of a PI-VSD can be quite variable with the average time to clinical presentation is between 2 and 4 days, however presentation can be as few as a few hours after AMI or as long as several weeks.

Patient risk factors include gender, with men at a greater risk than women (3:2 ratio), increasing age, and current smoking history. The mean age of presentation in GUSTO was 62.5 years and ranged from 44 to 81 years (Crenshaw, 2000).

4. Diagnosis

The diagnosis of a PI-VSD must be considered in the differential in any patient presenting with hemodynamic impairment, particularly in the context of a sudden deterioration in a patient who otherwise had been doing well, either during or after an AMI. As a PI-VSD presents in a similar manner as other mechanical complications of AMI, such a papillary muscle rupture (with acute mitral regurgitation), free wall rupture (with contained tamponade), or severe LV failure and pulmonary edema the initial diagnosis is often suspected during initial investigations and confirmed with additional imaging.

The typical presentation occurs in a patient who is otherwise recovering after initial management of an uncomplicated AMI. Patients often complain of recurrent chest pain from what is most likely new onset or recurrence of myocardial necrosis and will develop a new systolic murmur that can be harsh, pansystolic, and often-best ascultated at the left lower sternal border. Patients can often have a bundle branch block from disruption of the septal conduction system and will quickly deteriorate hemodynamically with findings suggestive of acute cardiogenic shock.

With the acute clinical deterioration, a rapid assessment of the etiology is critical. Unlike other mechanical complications, such as papillary muscle rupture, PI-VSDs will have imagining confirming a left to right shunt - such as contrast injected into the left ventricle during catheterization crossing the defect into the RV and entering into the pulmonary arteries (Figure 1). Likewise, oxymetric assessment with right heart catheterization will demonstrate a "step-off" from the mixing of de-oxygenated RV blood with the oxygenation LV blood. Quantitative assessment of Qp:Qs will correlate with the size of defect.

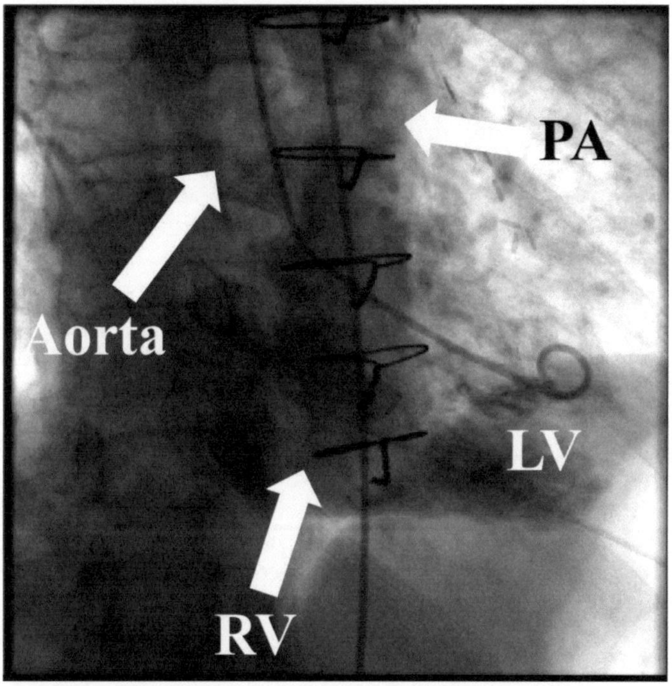

Fig. 1. Representative cardiac catheterization in which contrast is injected into the left ventricular cavity and then crosses the defect into the right ventricle. Contrast flowing into the pulmonary artery is then diagnostic for a ventricular septal defect.

4.1 Echocardiography

Transthoracic echocardiography (TTE) remains the cornerstone of the non-invasive assessment of PI-VSD (Kishon, 1993). TTE is indicated in any patient who presents with evidence of acutely impaired ventricular function or in unexplained hemodynamic deterioration suggests a mechanical complication following an acute myocardial infarction (Buda, 1991). Echocardiography has the benefit of being able to assess both left and right ventricular function, the presence of potentially co-existing and confounding valvular diseases - typically mitral regurgitation, and with color flow imaging it can be 100% specific and sensitive in diagnosing a PI-VSD. Despite the utility of TEE in the acute assessment of a deterioritating patient, a high index of suspicion is needed when looking for a PI-VSD as traditional echo windows might miss a small or apical defect. Large pericardial effusions might suggest an associated free wall rupture.

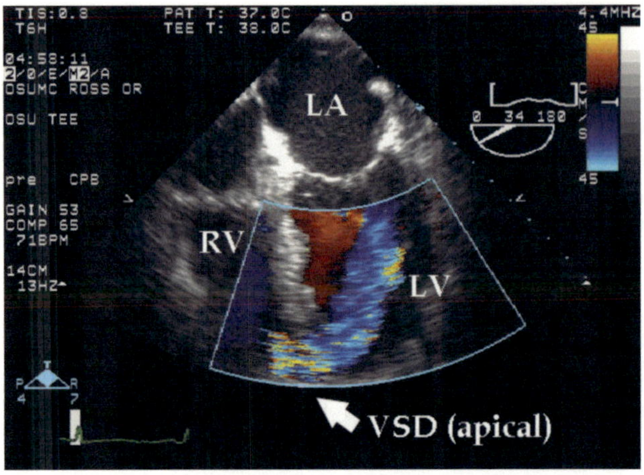

Fig. 2. Transesophageal echo, 4-chamber view, demonstration an apical VSD with from from the left ventricle (LV) to the right ventricle (RV). The left atrium (LA) is also shown to illustrate the typical relationship of the defect to the mitral valve.

4.2 Cardiac catheterization

Since patients who present with ECG and laboratory evidence of myocardial ischemia often undergo early cardiac catheterization with coronary angiography, this test often represents the initial study to suggest or confirm a diagnosis. Because the pathophysiology typically is associated with extensive and acute ischemia of a large territory of myocardium, it is not surprising that the findings at catheterization are often different than what would be expected for patients with a history of chronic coronary artery disease in which compensatory development of septal collaterals has had time to developed. During the acute presentation, the findings often suggest a complete occlusion of a large coronary artery in the setting of relatively minimal disease. Single vessel disease is found in 64% of patients and since the left anterior descending (LAD) artery is often the culprit vessel this explains why antero-apical septal VSDs are found in 60% of cases. Conversely, acute occlusions of a dominant right coronary or circumflex artery accounts for the remaining cases that occur in the posterior septum. Seven percent have concomitant double vessel disease, and 29% have triple vessel disease.

More importantly is that the cardiac catheterization might be the initial confirming diagnostic test. As mentioned above, quantitative assessment of oxygen step-offs, when performed, will demonstrate an increase in the partial pressure of oxygen (PaO_2) between the right atrium and ventricle - diagnostic of the left to right shunt. Left ventricular contrast injections, although less likely to be performed in a deteriorating patient secondary to the concern that additional contrast might further injure an already compromised renal function, is critical in patients with a suspected PI-VSD. Contrast injected into the LV will cross the defect (left-right shunt) and enter into the pulmonary arterial tree. This "pulmonary arteriogram" is characteristic for a VSD (Figure 1, see above).

Despite what may be perceived as the obvious value of early catheterization, the value is debatable. Opponents of mandatory catheterization advocate that in a clinically deteriorating patient in whom the diagnosis is clear it delays surgical management, the dye load may worsen already impaired renal function, and some reports suggest that considering the patterns of coronary disease typically encountered that coronary revascularization is actually a risk factor for a poor outcome (Muehrcke DD , 1992). Despite these theoretically arguments, from a practical standpoint it is hard to argue the clear benefits of defining the coronary anatomy prior to a surgical intervention aimed at treating a complication of coronary – particularly given the long-established importance of optimal or complete revascularization. Again, since these patients have already undergone catheterization as part of the initial management of their initial ischemic event the question whether to proceed with catheterization is rarely encountered. However, as many of the patients develop septal rupture several days (or weeks) after their initial acute coronary insult, it is hard to argue the need for repeat cardiac catheterization if the diagnosis is clear, particularly if the nuances of the coronary anatomy have recently been determined. Conversely, in less clear clinical situations, repeat catheterization might suggest an alternative, and potentially more likely, diagnosis such as acute stent thrombosis or disruption of an already unstable plaque.

4.3 Magnetic Resonance Imaging

Although the diagnosis is often made at the time of initial cardiac catheterization or echocardiography, occasionally a PI-VSD may be encountered during other diagnostic imaging. While patients might be too hemodynamically unstable or the presence of an intra-aortic balloon pump (or other ferrous containing or non-MRI safe device) might preclude MRI, with the growing indications and utilization of MRI for operative planning, PI-VSD might be encountered. Patients with low ejection fractions, cardiomyopathies, or suspicion for unusual cardiac anatomy, might have MRI performed to assess for myocardial viability, fibrosis, or valvular pathology. In these patients a PI-VSD may be an unsuspected finding (Figure 3). Although there is little literature describing the utility of MRI in PI-VSDs, using concepts derived from the literature on congenital shunts and pathology, MRI might be of value in assisting in defining the extent of the defect, the shunt fraction, right ventricular function, and other associated pathophysiology (Didier, 1986). MRI might be of additive value in cases of questionable catheterization or echocardiographic studies or in assessing the post-operative patient in which a residual shunt is suspected. Nevertheless, MRI is, in general, not considered a first-line imagining diagnostic tool.

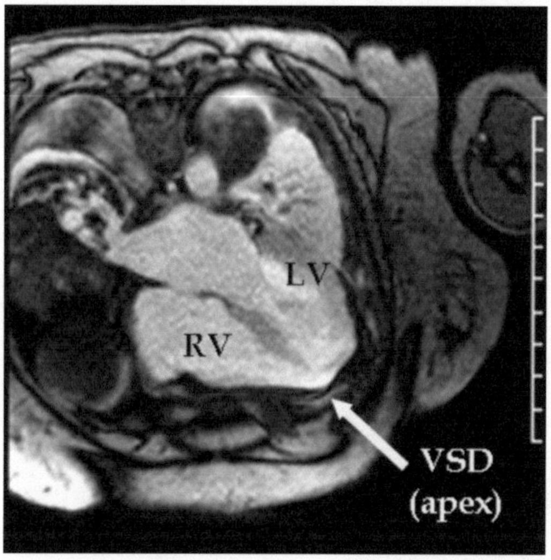

Fig. 3. Cardiac MRI demonstrating an apical defect. Gated cine images indicated a left to right shunt in which quantitative assessment can be used to determine the shunt fractions and size of the defect.

5. Pathogensis

The pathogensis reflects two different types of rupture. The first, a simple rupture, is a direct through-and-through defect that is typically located anteriorly (when associated with a LAD territory infarct). Conversely, complex ruptures are believed to result from tracking of blood as it dissects thru the septum with left ventricular entry sites remote from right ventricular exit sites - these tracks then enlarge over time due to the pressure gradient between the left and right ventricle. Multiple defects are found in 5-11% of cases and emphasized the need for a complex pre-operative and intra-operative assessment of all pathways to insure a complete repair (Edwards, 1984). Incomplete closure of residual or secondary defects can account for post-operative recurrences. Transmural infarcts can be quite extensive with defects developing to several centimeters in diameter and can often involve extensive areas of the left ventricular free wall. For complex defects, as blood dissects through the necrotic myocardium there can be further expansion and damage with loss of cellular integrity. With local cellular destruction there is fragmentation with degeneration of myocytes with enzymatic digestion and destruction. In patients who survive the acute presentation, up to 66% develop chronic ventricular aneurysms and a third will have significant functional mitral regurgitation from the secondary effects on the ventricular free wall.

The pathologic consequences and outcomes of surgery of anterior and posterior defects appear to be different in ways beyond what can be explained by the degree of shunting. Earlier autopsy studies have shown that anterior PI-VSDs were associated with 33% of the LV and only 10% of the RV being infarcted, while posterior defects were associated with only 20% of the LV and 33% of the RV being infarcted (Cummings, 1977). Particularly considering the acute pressure/volume overload and associated RV failure, it becomes understandable why posterior based defects have a worse prognosis.

6. Natural history

The natural history of untreated PI-VSD is also poorly understood. As advances in the acute and chronic management of coronary artery disease continues to evolve, so does complications of CAD. In general, 25% of patients with PI-VSDs die within the first 24 hours (Berger, 1992). Death is most likely a function of pre-existing comoribidites and potentially irreversible and catastrophic heart failure that comes from not only the acute pump failure from the precipitating infarct but also the massive acute left to right heart shunting that compromises systemic perfusion further. The sudden increase in pulmonary overcirculation also contributes to the development of significant right heart failure. For those patients who survive the acute event, 1, 2, and 4-week survival is 50%, 35%, and 20% respectively (Lemery, 1992). It is easy to appreciate that those patients who survive the first month may have inherently favorable factors that might further self-select for a good post-operative outcome. Prolonged untreated survival has been reported with up to 7% of patient surviving to 1 year - obviously the physiologic insult and over-circulation is minimal.

7. Timing/indications for surgery

The mere presence of a PI-VSD is considered an indication for surgery with the majority of patients undergoing urgent or emergent operative intervention. The primary goal of VSD closure is to reduce the end-organ damage from the combined insults of acute right ventricular overload/failure and systemic cardiogenic shock.

As soon as the diagnosis is made an intra-aortic balloon pump should be placed. Coronary augmentation will assist the ischemic and compromised myocardium, but more importantly it will unload the left ventricle and improve cardiac output, end-organ perfusion, and reduce pulmonary shunting and over-circulation. However, the physiologic improvements with IABP and other inotropic or vasoactive medications should only be viewed as transient and allow for finishing the pre-operative assessment.

Although some advocate a strategy of delayed repair, this approach is rarely successful. The theory is to give the friable necrotic myocardium time (3-6 weeks) to fibrosis thereby allowing for an easier and more secure repair. The scarred tissue will better hold suture and less likely to tear apart and result in an early post-operative failure. This approach appears reasonable, but it is rare that patients remain stable or can be support during this time period. While guidelines for delayed surgical management are lacking, this might be an option in those who are hemodynamically/physiologically stable with a delayed presentation, have no or minimal signs of pulmonary hypertension or over-circulation, and have a stable fluid balance with good renal function. Unfortunately, such patients are rare and less than 5-10% of all PI-VSD patients will survive to allow for delayed repair. Such an approach may represent a "survival of the fittest" perspective in those with minimal shunting and with strict attention to medical comorbidities and nutrition a period of close watchful waiting may work. This approach may also be used to justify waiting in patients who have other severe comordities preclude intervention and would in theory require optimization prior to surgery. Nevertheless, it is hard to argue that any other problem would improve to the point of making surgery safer in the setting of worsening right ventricular heart failure - a problem that by itself is very difficult to treat both pre and post-operatively. Although, one can argue that in these patients, unless early surgical repair is clearly contraindicated, that their physiologic reserve combined to a minimal pathophysiologic insult predisposes to a good outcome regardless of whether an early or late repair is performed.

8. Operative management

The initial attempts at repairing PI-VSD followed a surgical approach similar to that for congenital VSDs - through a ventriculotomy in the right ventricular outflow track (RVOT) (Cooley, 1957). It was quickly appreciated the significant limitations of this approach. Firstly, in an already compromised right ventricle, the outflow tract incision only further reduced residual RV function. In addition, while suited for many common types congenital VSD's near the aortic valve, the RVOT incision offered poor exposure of defects that tended to be much further down the septum towards the apex. Most importantly, because the patch and suture line was on the RV side, the defect was still exposed to LV pressures and consequently was at increased risk for patch dehiscence, early recurrence, and extension of the defect. Pioneering work by animal studies by Heimbecker in 1968 advocated an approach to the VSD thru the left ventricle in the region of the culprit vessel through infarcted myocardium - i.e., anterior defects approached through the anterior wall while posterior defects through the inferior wall. These techniques addressed the deficiencies of a RVOT approach (Heimbecker, 1968). The benefits of these animal studies were subsequently validated clinically within several years (Javid, 1972)(Buckley, 1971)

8.1 General considerations

After the patient arrives in the operating room, the patient is routinely anesthetized and pharmacologically paralyzed. If not already in place, all patients should have arterial monitoring lines and a pulmonary artery (Swan-Ganz) catheter inserted. Pressures and oxygen saturations should be obtained to determine shunt fractions and to assist in determining the completeness of repair at the end of the procedure. Given that this subset of patients possesses a left-to-right shunt, it is of upmost importance to avoid pharmacologic agents that cause pulmonary vasodilation, thus worsening the shunt, increasing pulmonary over-circulation, and potentially worsening right heart dysfunction. Preoperative antibiotics including a first generation cephalosporin, such as cefazolin, and vancomycin are administered. In cases of antibiotic allergies, appropriate alternatives should be chosen.

Median sternotomy is performed and the patient is prepared for cardiopulmonary bypass. Minimally invasive techniques are typically not advocated for this type of extensive and complex procedure in which complete exposure of heart is helpful. However, in situations of re-operative surgery, depending on surgeon preferences, consideration should be given to peripheral cannulation (i.e. femoral or axillary) prior to sternotomy as a re-entry injury to an already compromised and dilated RV can be catastrophic. The patient is heparized prior to standard aortic - right atrial cannulation. Some advocate routine bicaval venous drainage, but typically, as procedures on the tricuspid or mitral valves are not performed, this is not necessary. Cold-blood antegrade and retrograde cardioplegia is delivered via conventional root and coronary sinus catheters. Topical cooling to further reduce the metabolic demands of the already compromised heart is also liberally used. This author also routinely uses ice-slush wrapped in gauze to further cool the right ventricle to assist in reducing the temperature and thereby assisting in myocardial protection. Active or passive systemic cooling is performed with an ideal temperature of 25°-28°C to further assist end-organ protection.

In general, once the defect is identified, a piece of either glutaraldehyde-fixed bovine pericardium or Dacron is cut to not only cover the defect but a generous rim of surrounding, and potentially non-viable, myocardium. Continuous suture or interrupted pledgeted sutures are used to suture the patch to the residual septum. Tension on the repair must be avoided to minimize the risk of the sutures tearing through once the ventricle is pressurized and begins to contract. For posterior defects the patch might require anchoring to the annulus of the mitral valve. For cases in which the annulus of the mitral valve and/or peri-valvular tissues is involved, mitral valve replacement may be required.

The intra-operative approach and management of the defect is based upon the location of the VSD and, the need for concomitant procedures. The pre-operative assessment of the location of the defect is critical in determining the optimal approach to closing it.

8.2 Apical defects

Apical septal ruptures involve the cardiac apex, which includes the apical portion of the right ventricle, septum, and the left ventricle. Daggett and colleagues described the technique of apical amputation and repair of the PI-VSD in 1970. The initial incision is created through the infracted tissue of the cardiac apex. The necrotic myocardium is then

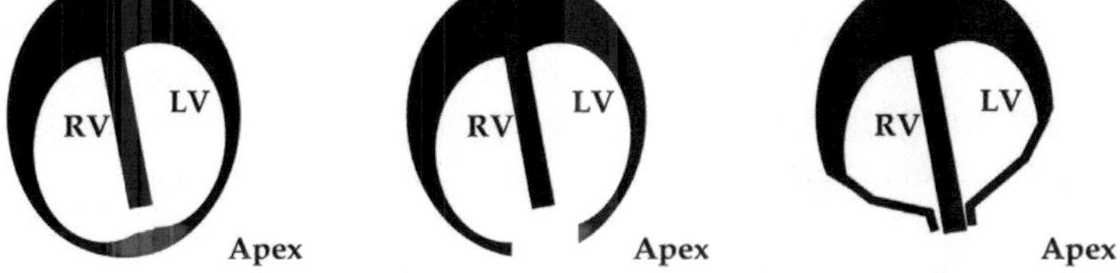

Fig. 4. Repair of apical repair involves excising the apical defect and bringing together the residual edges of the left and right ventricular walls using a primary repair reinforced with pledgets.

excised until healthy muscle is exposed and deemed adequate for repair. The healthy tissues of the right and left ventricle are then approximated to the septum using interrupted, felt pledgeted, heavy Tycron suture in a mattress fashion (Figure 4). Felt strips are placed along the right and left septal walls during this process to create a 'felt sandwich'. The apical repair can be reinforced with a second layer of suture. Meticulous hemostasis is critical.

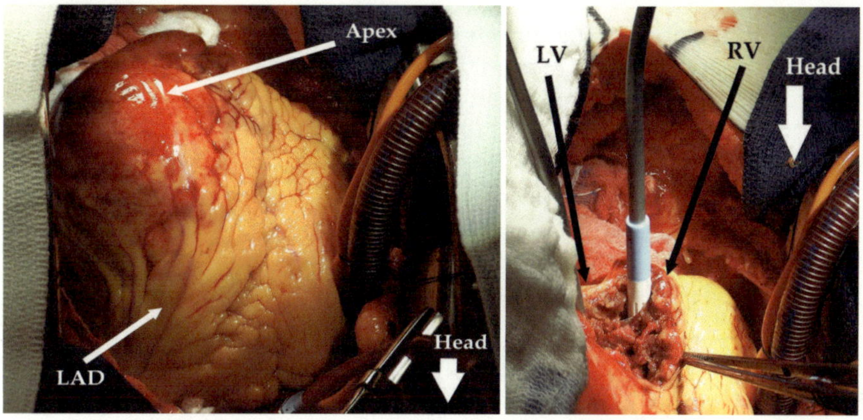

Fig. 5. Left: Intra-operative view of the extensive apical infarction that has resulted in the the echocardiographic findings demonstrated in Figure 2. The left anterior descending artery (LAD) is shown. Right: The same patient after opening and debridement of the infracted apex. The necrotic septum is visualized with a probe in the left ventricle (LV) and the bypass "pump sucker" is in the right ventricle (RV).

8.3 Anterior defects

The anterior septal rupture involves the anterior septum as well as the anterior left ventricular free wall. This, as discussed earlier, is a typically a result of acute infarct of the LAD territory. The initial approach is via an incision in the infarcted left ventricular myocardium. The infarcted area is then excised and debrided back to healthy, viable myocardium. The septum is then inspected and necrotic tissue is excised in the same fashion. This is can be straightforward in a single, obvious defect. However, great care must be taken if the defect is noted to be tracking through the myocardium - a finding that might not be obvious and hence a larger patch may be used than what would be employed to cover the defect.

Small defects can be plicated to the right ventricular free wall using interrupted, pledgeted suture as first suggested by Shumacker (Shumaker, 1972). For anything other than very small (<1.0 cm) defects, most anterior septal infarcts will require repair with a patch. This is created in a fashion that will allow for a tension-free repair. Excess tension in the repair can lead to devastating consequences and a return trip to the operating room.

The more complex approaches use a prosthetic patch that is anchored to the posterior wall of the septum using interrupted, pledgeted Tycron or Proline suture. The suture is passed from a right to left direction so that the patch-septum interface lies in the left ventricle, as opposed to the right. The anterior sutures are placed through the right ventricular free wall and tagged with hemostats (Figure 6). All sutures are placed prior to placing them through the patch. They can now be placed through the designated anterior region of the prosthetic patch and then through a second pledget if desired prior to tying the suture knots. The left ventricular free wall is then re-approximated using interrupted, mattress suture. A second layer of running suture is placed for reinforcement.

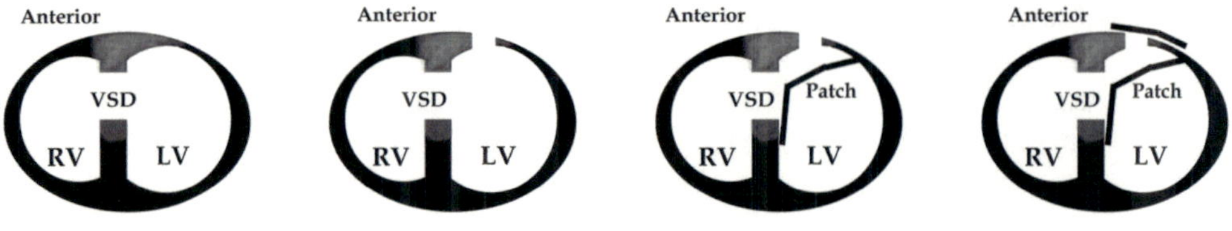

Fig. 6. Picture representation of the various steps used to repair an anterior defect with the patch excluding the necrotic septum from the higher pressure left ventricular cavity. The incision is through the infracted muscle on the anterior wall, parallel to the left anterior descending artery.

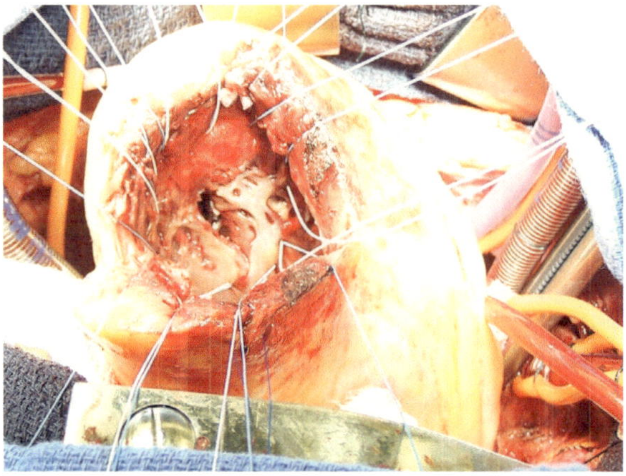

Fig. 7. Intra-operative picture with the apex of the heart elevated (head and aortic cannula to the right). The incision is through the infarcted anterior wall. The septal defect is shown in the middle of the cavity with circumferential sutures around a wide margin. The sutures will then be placed through a pericardial patch to exclude the infracted septal muscle and defect from the left ventricular cavity. Note: This is from a different patient than from the images above

8.4 Posterior defects

The posterior or inferior septal rupture involves a transmural infarction of the myocardium in the posterior descending arterial distribution. The inferior wall is often thin and after infarction, is quite friable. For this reason, primary repair is not a durable option and is rarely successful. Attempt at primary repair, in which the myocardium is placed under tension, can have disastrous and immediate, and potentially fatal, consequences. Hence, posterior/inferior septal ruptures are the most technically demanding of the PI-VSDs.

After the heart is arrested, the inferior wall is lifted out of the pericardial well and exposed. The transmural infarct may involve both ventricles, or the septum and left ventricle alone. The transinfarct incision is created in a longitudinal fashion in the left ventricle. The nonviable myocardium is excised, which will create adequate exposure of the septal defect. The papillary muscles are inspected. If the base is involved in the infarct resulting in ruptured papillary muscle, then mitral valve replacement is warranted. If a small posterior VSD (<1.0 cm) is identified, primary repair to the ventricular free wall using pledgetted suture as described earlier is satisfactory – but this situation is very rare and placement of a small patch may result in a more durable outcome than risking a primary repair involving ischemic myocardial tissue.

Large defects will require a tension free repair by utilizing a patch closure. This technique often necessitates the use of two separate patches, one dedicated to the septal repair and the other to the wall of the ventricle. Principles as described previously apply. The pledgetted mattress sutures are placed from the right ventricle to the left along the circumference of the VSD. The sutures are passed through the contoured patch and tied down. Great care should be taken to avoid lacerating the myocardium. Some authors suggest placing a second pledget on the patch side of the repair to minimize this risk. The posterior ventricular wall is repaired with the second patch using mattress sutures. Occasionally, depending on the size and quality of free wall myocardium, the free-edges can be approximated and closed primarily (and re-enforced with a pericardial or felt strip) rather than using a second patch.

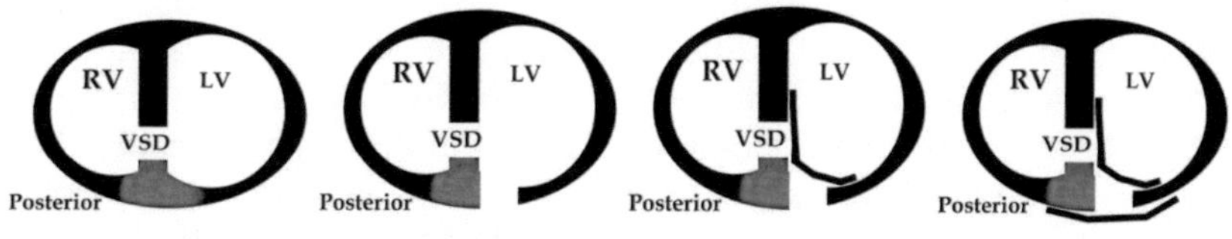

Fig. 8. Similar to anterior repairs, the high pressure left ventricular cavity is isolated from the necrotic septum with a patch repair. The incision is along the distal right coronary along and parallel to the posterior descending artery through the infracted basal muscle.

8.5 General principles

Closure of the ventriculotomy is performed by folding the free edge of the patch to the edge of the ventricle to exclude it from the circulation. The ventriculotomy repair is then closed with a primary closure re-enforced with strips of either Teflon felt or pericardium. Exclusion of the necrotic myocardium from the left ventricular is also important in minimizing the risk of small debris breaking off at any point and causing a systemic embolism.

Regardless of the location of the ventriculotomy, it cannot be emphasized enough the importance of a tension free closure. Any unnecessary tension through injuried or friable myocardium may predispose to catastrophic and potentially fatal post-operative bleeding once the ventricle becomes pressurized. In extreme cases involving extensive myocardial (free wall and septal) damage, temporary mechanical support with either extra-corporeal membrane oxygenation (ECMO) or a left ventricular assist device may help unload the ventricle to assist in recovery. The hypothesis behind this approach is by reducing the LV pressure, it will encourage recovery, reduce the pressure on the repair, and allow for further decision making in patients in whom there is extensive ventricular destruction and residual ventricular function may not be adequate to support physiologic needs (Firstenberg, 2009).

Although the benefits of concomintant revascularization on long-term outcomes are debatable, complete coronary revascularization, if possible, is typically advocated (Heitmiller, 1986). As with other risk models for outcomes after surgery (e.g. EuroScore and STS models), it is the need for revascularization and the extent of underlying CAD that defines the long-term outcome rather than the actual performing of the procedure. Overall, the paradigm of complete and/or optimal revascularization should apply in cases of PI-VSD management. It is hard to argue the conceptual benefits of revascularization in the setting of an already acutely and chronically compromised myocardium.

9. Post-operation management

The post-operative management of patients following successful repair should be similar to that of other high-risk surgical patients. However, there are several key points that need to be considered. As these patients often present and are taken to the operating room in acute decompensated heart failure, strict attention to optimizing biventricular function is critical. Post-operative left ventricular dysfunction is not uncommon and, unless already in place, there should be a low threshold for placement of an intra-aortic balloon pump (IABP). While, as discussed later, the use of an IABP is often associated with worse outcomes, the relationship is the need for it and the potential delaying in initiating it's use rather than the therapy itself that influences the outcomes. Right heart failure is common and often these patients require considerable therapies directed specifically at assisting in right heart recovery. Conventional intravenous agents such as epinephrine, milrinone, and dobutamine are often required - and sometimes at high doses. Inhaled agents that selectively reduce pulmonary vascular resistance and assist in reducing RV afterload such as inhaled nitric oxide (20-80 ppm) or Epoprostenol (2,500 - 20,000 ng/min) may be required (Rich, 1993). Ventricular arrhythmias are also common from the residual ischemic/necrotic myocardium (as well as secondary to the ventriculotomy) and anti-arrhythmic medications, such as Amiodarone, should be used liberally. In addition, as the repaired septal defect and free wall are often quite friable, strict attention to avoid hypertension is critical as even transient elevations in blood pressure can result in disruptions in the patch repair that might precipitate uncontrolled and fatal LV bleeding. Any acute increase in chest tube drainage should raise the concern for ventricular suture line dehiscensce and there should be a low threshold for returning the patient to the operating room for re-exploration - however, excess manipulation of the heart in the search for bleeding should be avoiding at the risk of catastrophic suture-line tearing in a beating and pressurized ventricle. Although recovery in these patients is unpredictable and may be prolonged and a slow wean of inotropes may be required, there should be a low threshold for repeat and/or frequent echocardiographic assessment in a patient who is not improving as predicted. Repeat echocardiophy might show a residual shunt or valvular dysfunction, more importantly would be identification easy to correct problems, such as tamponade.

10. Outcomes: predictors of survival

The increasing rarity of PI-VSD implies that few centers are able to report an extensive series. While several large single center experiences and outcomes have been reported, most summarize years of experience and may not consider the ongoing evolution in the peri-operative management and improvement in surgical skills and judgment of these critically ill patients.

Deja and colleagues reported their experience with 117 patients from the Glenfield General Hospital in England. The mean age was 65 ± 8 years and there were 43 females. Of the 117, 76 were anterior defects while 34 were posterior. One third of patients presented in cardiogenic shock. The average time from AMI to the development (or diagnosis) of a PI-VSD was 6 days and there was an additional 9-day average interval before surgical intervention. There overall mortality was 37% - not including a 6.4% intra-operative mortality. 40% have evidence of a residual left-right shunt with 13 patients undergoing early re-operation with 30% mortality in the re-op group. Table 1 summarizes their overall results. Their overall predictors of post-operative mortality include: shock at time of surgery, clinical deterioration while awaiting surgery, need for concomitant CABG, and pre-operative renal failure (as a marker for shock and organ failure). Criticisms of these results include that earlier surgical intervention after initial diagnosis might have resulted in less end-organ damage and an already compromised patient (Deja MA, 2002).

Overall surgical mortality (%)	37%
Intra-operative mortality (%)	6.4 %
ICU Stay (days)	4.8 days
Major inotropic support	90 %
Used of Intra-aortic balloon pump	75 %
Need for extra-corporeal membrane oxygenation (ECMO)	2 %
Ventilator Time (hours)	40 hours
Tracheostomy	5%
Continuous renal replacement	16 %
Re-exploration/bleeding	5 %
Stroke	5 %
Residual shunt	40%

Table 1. Post-Operative Complications Following Surgical Repair (From Deja MA, 2002)

National registry data has proven useful to define the real-world experiences with the presentation and management of PI-VSD. In the report of 189 patients from Sweden, several factors were able to predictable favorable vs unfavorable short (<30 days) and long-term (>30) outcomes (Tables 2 and 3) (Jeppsson, 2005).

Favorable Predictors	Unfavorable Predictors	No effect on outcome
Short time from MI to Dx	IABP	Age
Short time from Dx to OR	Stroke/Coma	Gender
Short time from MI to OR	Renal failure	Pre-OP IABP
Pre-operative catheterization	Re-op for bleeding	Pre-OP Lytic therapy
Anterior rupture		Concomitant CABG
		Residual shunt

Table 2. Predictors of short-term (<30-day) survival based on National Swedish Experience (Adapted from Jeppsson et al. Euro J Cardiothor Surg 2005;27:216-221). CABG: Coronary artery bypass surgery, Dx: Diagnosis, IABP: Intra-aortic balloon pump, MI: Myocardial infarction.

Favorable Predictors	Unfavorable Predictors	No effect on outcome
Younger age	Pre-Op IABP	Anterior rupture
	Pre-Op Cath	Time from MI to OR
	Need for CABG	Post-Op stroke
	Renal Failure requiring dialysis	Pre-OP Lytic therapy
	Residual shunt	Post-Op IABP
		Re-op for bleeding

Table 3. Predictors of Long-Term (>30 day). See above for legend.

In a similar national registry experience, Cerin and colleagues reported the outcomes in 58 patients treated with PI-VSD from 1992 to 2000 in Italy (Cerin, 2003). The mean age was 73 years/old. Thirty-six percent presented in acute renal failure, 33% were in atrial fibrillation, and 22% were insulin dependent diabetics. 57% were in NYHA Class IV heart failure with 41% in cardiogenic shock. Intra-aortic balloon pumps were used in only 20% of patients and 60% presented with significant mitral regurgitation. The timing of surgery was 14 ± 12 days from the acute event with 76% undergoing surgery within the first 3 weeks and 31% within the first 24 hours. A key point is again emphasizing the importance of early diagnosis and surgery before the onset of shock and organ failure (Table 4).

	Survivors (n=28)	**Death (n=30)**
Time to OR (d)	21 ± 13	11 ± 8
OR < 24hrs	18 %	43 %
Pre-Shock	28 %	57 %
Pre-sPAP (mmHg)	42 ± 11	56 ± 14
CPB time (time)	95 ± 28	126 ± 35
Post-IABP	39 %	90 %
Post-LVEF (%)	45 ± 2	29 ± 2
Post-Op Renal Failure	25 %	66 %

Table 4. Italian Registry Data. Legend: CPB: Cardiopulmonary bypass, IABP: Intra-aortic balloon pump, LVEF: Left ventricular ejection fraction, sPAP: Systolic pulmonary artery pressures. Table adapted from Cerin et al. Inter Soc Cardiovasc Surg 2003;11:149-154

More recently, Mantovani et al reported their 19-year, single center, experience in 50 patients. Between 1983 and 2002, 50 consecutive patients with a mean age of 66 ± 9 years (range: 45-81) who presented with either anterior (n=30, 60%) or posterior (n=20, 40%) PI-VSDs. Patients developed their defects on average 4 days post-AMI with most within the first week (76%) and only 2 patients presenting after 2 days. Cardiac catheterization was performed in 98% of patients (51% single vessel disease, 35% double, and 14% triple). 56% of patients required a pre-operative IABP and 74% underwent emergent surgery on average 2 days after diagnosis of a PI-VSD. Operative mortality (within 30 days) was 36% with 6 dying in the operating room. Posterior defects were associated with 50% mortality versus 25% for anterior. Other univariate risk factors for early death included: emergent surgery (p=0.02); cross-clamp time >100 minutes (p=0.035); and delayed surgical intervention (>3 days post diagnosis, p=0.0055). Interestingly, in their experience factors not associated with operative mortality included: gender, extent of CAD (single vs triple vessel disease), need for CABG, age (>65 years), or the year of operation (before/after 1992). In a logistic regression analysis, only emergent surgery (odds ration: 10.23) and a delayed treatment (OR: 4.03) were the only predictors of early mortality. Long-term survival was 76.5 ± 7.8 and 56.1 ± 11.5% at 5 and 10 years. No obvious predictors of long-term survival were found in their analysis although patients with residual myocardium at risk from unrevascularized regions tended to have a worse long-term prognosis (Mantovani, 2006).

In the GUSTO trial in which 41,021 patients were randomized to different strategies of reperfusion during AMI, 84 developed a PI-VSD. 34 of these were managed surgically, with 31 (90%) undergoing early treated and 3 (10%) undergoing delayed surgery. Survival in the surgical group was 53% at 30 days and 47% at 1 year. Conversely, for those treated medically, as an indicator of the lethality of this problem, survival at 30 days and 1 year was 6% and 3%, respectively (Crenshaw, 2000). All patients who presented in Class III or IV heart failure died.

11. Controversial topics

11.1 Percutaneous closure devices

Successful application of closure devices in children with congenital VSDs combined with the morbidity and mortality associated with surgical management has prompted enthusiasm for the use of percutaneous closure devices. The role of such devices has been proposed for both the primary closure of acute defects and to assist in the closure of recurrent or residual shunts (Shah, 2005).

While conceptually promising, initial experiences were discouraging and improvements in outcomes were not observed (Pienvichit, 2001). Difficulties in covering not only the actual defect, but also the residual necrotic myocardium predisposed to early recurrence. Early devices tended not to be large enough and were very difficult to position (or re-position if necessary).

In addition, the lack of a overall survival benefit further illustrates that clinical outcomes are not only dictated by closure of the VSD, but sometimes more importantly, a function of the extend of the myocardial infarction - which might be inherently so extensive as to preclude survival.

11.2 Mechanical support

As discussed, despite advances in surgical and post-operative management, operative mortality is still 10-60%. Even with early intervention biventricular failure is often a significant factor in early post-operative deaths. Short and long-term mechanical support, beyond intra-aortic balloon counterpulsation, is a reasonable option in patients with post-operative ventricular (left, right, or bi) failure and who are felt to be salvagable. Short-term support may be required as a bridge to recovery, while long-term device may be indicated for those with irreversible ventricular failure.

In cases in which there is extensive ventricular infarction/failure, associated free-wall rupture, or when there is excessive bleeding or tension from the ventriculotomy temporary left ventricular support should be considered. With LVAD inflow drainage from the left atrium, the LV is unloaded (i.e. 'atrialized') and may allow time for recovery/healing prior to exposing the injured LV to system pressures and contractile function (Firstenberg 2009).

Right ventricular support is also difficult following the acute volume/pressure overload of a PI-VSD with recovery unpredictable and potentially prolonged. Unfortunately, there is little data to support this use in this application other than clinical judgment and center experience.

Residual shunts after repair pose a unique challenge for patient's requiring mechanical support. Careful attention to left and right ventricular flows and pressures are critical to compensate for the residual shunt - and prevent worsening of over-circulation (Sai-Sudhakar, 2006). If residual shunts are significant then biventricular support may allow for a period of recovery and stabilization prior to an attempted repair in an otherwise very high-risk surgical patient.

The need for mechanical support, while attractive in unstable post-operative patients, is also associated with difficult problems. Often there is need for aggressive anti-coagulation, the need for multiple surgical procedures (i.e. device change-outs, explants, etc), and overall patient recovery is more difficult when tethered to external VAD controllers.

A total artificial heart precludes native cardiac recovery and obligates transplantation, nevertheless, it may be an option with appropriate resources and experience in highly selected patient with few other comorbidities.

11.3 Residual/recurrent defects

Residual shunts are found in up to 25% of patients after definitive repair (Skillington, 1990). The etiology of residual shunts is either a missed defect at the time of initial repair, dehiscence of a patch (sewn to necrotic or friable tissue), or further extension of the initial defect. Fortunately, most residual shunts tend to be physiologically tolerated and spontaneous closure has been reported. Operative re-intervention is associated with a >60% mortality (Jeppsson, 2005) and surgery is reserved for patients in heart failure failing medical management or those with large shunts (Qp:Qs>2.0) (Murashita, 2010). Because of the high operative mortality with repairing residual or recurrent shunts there has been interest, but limited success, with percutanous closure devices (Shah, 2005). Nevertheless, the role of percutaneous closure and the ideal devices are undefined (Pienvichit, 2001) and probably best reserved for use in those centers with extensive experience in the closure of congenital VSDs.

12. Conclusions

Post-myocardial infarction ventricular septal defects complicate up to 0.02% of acute myocardial infarctions. Despite advances in the surgical care of these moribund patients, operative mortality still approaches 50% with major risks including cardiogenic shock, renal failure, right and/or left ventricular failure, size of VSD, posterior/inferior locations, and residual VSD. While some patient may present late or benefit from a delayed repair, typically surgical intervention is indicated prior to irreversible end-organ damage. Repair techniques emphasize closure of the defect and protecting the injured septum from left ventricular pressures. Post-operative management is typically challenging considering the inherent pre-operative biventricular dysfunction and associated end-organ damage. Those who survive there initial event and operation tend to have favorable 5 and 10-year survivals.

13. Conflicts of interest

The authors have no conflicts of interest or disclosures related to any of the topics or technologies discussed in this manuscript.

14. References

Agnihotri AK, Madsen JC, Daggett WM. Surgical Treatment of Complications of Acute Myocardial Infarction: Postinfarction Ventricular Septal Defect and Free Wall Rupture. Cohn L, ed. Cardiac Surgery in the Adult. New York: McGraw-Hill, 2008:753-784.

Berger TJ, Blackstone EH, Kirklin JW. Postinfarction ventricular septal defect, in Kirklin JW, Barratt-Boyes BG (eds): Cardiac Surgery. New York, Churchill Livingstone, 1993; p 403.

Brunn F. Diagnostik der erworbenen ruptur der kammerscheidewand des herzens. *Wien Arch Inn Med* 1923; 6:533.

Buckley MJ, Mundth ED, Daggett WM, DeSanctis RW, Sanders CA, Austen WG. Surgical therapy for early complications of myocardial infarction. *Surgery*. 1971;70(6):814-20

Buda AJ. The role of echocardiography in the evaluation of mechanical complications of acute myocardial infarction. *Circulation*. 1991;84(3 Suppl):I109-21.

Cerin G, Di Donato M, Dimulescu D, Montericcio V, Menicanti L, Frigiola A, De Ambroggi L. Surgical treatment of ventricular septal defect complicating acute myocardial infarction. Experience of a north Italian referral hospital. Cardiovasc Surg. 2003 Apr;11(2):149-54.

Cooley DA, Belmonte BA, Zeis LB, Schnur S. Surgical repair of ruptured interventricular septum following acute myocardial infarction. *Surgery*. 1957;41(6):930-7.

Crenshaw BS, Granger CB, Birnbaum Y. et al. Risk factors, angiographic patterns and outcomes in patients with ventricular septal defect complicating acute myocardial infaction. GUSTO-1 (Global Utilization of Streptokinase and TPA for Occluded Coronary Arteries). Trial Investigators. *Circulation*. 2000; 101(1):27-32.

Cummings RG, Califf R, Jones RN, Reimer KA, King YH, Lowe JE. Correlates of survival in patients with postinfarction ventricular septal defect. *Ann Thorac Surg* 1989;47:824-30 (update: 1997;63:1508-9).

Cummings RG, Reimer KA, Califf R, Hackel D, Boswick J, Lowe JE. Quantitative analysis of right and left ventricular infarction in the presence of postinfarction ventricular septal defect. *Circulation*. 1988;77(1):33-42.

Deja MA, Szostek J, Widenka K, et al. Post infarction ventricular septal defect—can we do better? *Eur J Cardiothorac Surg*. 2000; 18:194

Didier D, Higgins CB. Identification and localization of ventricular septal defect by gated magnetic resonance imaging. *Am J Cardiol*. 1986;57(15):1363-8.

Edwards BS, Edwards WD, Edwards JE. Ventricular septal rupture complicating acute myocardial infarction: identification of simple and complex types in 53 autopsied hearts. *Am J Cardiol*. 1984; 54:1201.

Firstenberg MS, Blais D, Crestanello J, Sai-Sudhakar C, Sirak J, Louis LB, Vesco P, Sun B. Long-term mechanical support for complex left ventricular postinfarct pseudoaneurysms. *Heart Surg Forum*. 2009;12(5):E291-3.

Heimbecker RO, Lemire G, Chen C. Surgery for massive myocardial infarction. An experimental study of emergency infarctectomy with a preliminary report on the clinical application. *Circulation*. 1968;37(4 Suppl):II3-11.

Heitmiller R, Jacobs ML, Daggett WM. Surgical Management of Postinfarction Ventricular Septal Rupture. *Ann Thorac Surg*. 1986; 41(6):683-691.

Javid H, Hunter JA, Naiafi H, Dye WS, Julian OC. Left ventricular approach for the repair of ventricular septal perforation and infarctectomy. *J Thorac Cardiovasc Surg*. 1972 Jan;63(1):14-24.

Jeppsson A, Liden H, Johnsson P, Hartford M, Radegran K. Surgical repair of post infarction ventricular septal defects: a national experience. *Euro J Cardiothor Surg*. 2005;27: 216-221.

Kishon Y, Iqbal A, Oh JK, Gersh BJ, Freeman WK, Seward JB, Tajik AJ. Evolution of echocardiographic modalities in detection of postmyocardial infarction ventricular septal defect and papillary muscle rupture: study of 62 patients. *Am Heart J.* 1993;126(3 Pt 1):667-75.

Labrousse L, Choukroun E, Chevalier JM, et al. Surgery for post- infarction ventricular septal defect (VSD): risk factors for hospital death and long term results. *Euro J Cardiothor Surg.* 2002;21:725-732.

Latham PM. Lectures on Subjects Connected with Clinical Medicine Comprising Diseases of the Heart. London, Longman Rees, 1845.

Lemery R, Smith HC, Giuliani ER, Gersh BJ. Prognosis in rupture of the ventricular septum after acute myocardial infarction and role of early surgical intervention. *Am J Cardiol.* 1992; 70:147

Mantovani V, Mariscalco G, Leva C, Blanzola C, Sala A. Surgical repair of post-infarction ventricular septal defect: 19 years of experience. *International Journal of Cardiology.* 2006;108: 202-206.

Muehrcke DD, Daggett WM, Buckley MJ, et al: Postinfarct ventricular septal defect repair: effect of coronary artery bypass grafting. *Ann Thorac Surg.* 1992; 54:876.

Murashita T, Komiya T, Tamura N, Sakaguchi G, Kobayashi T, Sunagawa G. The clinical challenge to reduce the postoperative residual shunt in surgical repair of postinfarction ventricular septal perforation. *Interact Cardiovasc Thorac Surg.* 2010;11(1):38-41.

Pienvichit P, Piemonte TC. Percutaneous closure of postmyocardial infarction ventricular septal defect with the CardioSEAL septal occluder implant. *Catheterization and Cardiovascular Interventions.* 2001;54:490-494.

Poulsen SH, Praestholm M, Munk, Wierup P, Egeblad H, Nielsen-Knudsk JE. Ventricular septal rupture complicating acute myocardial infarction: Clinical characteristics and contemporary outcome. *Ann Thorac Surg.* 2008;85:1591–1596.

Rich GF, Murphy GD Jr, Roos CM, Johns RA. Inhaled nitric oxide. Selective pulmonary vasodilation in cardiac surgical patients. *Anesthesiology.* 1993;78(6):1028-35.

Sai-Sudhakar CB, Firstenberg MS, Sun B. Biventricular mechanical assist for complex, acute post-infarction ventricular septal defect. *J Thorac Cardiovasc Surg.* 2006;132(5):1238-9

Sager R. Coronary thrombosis: perforation of the infarcted interventricular septum. *Arch Intern Med.* 1934; 53:140

Shah NR, Goldstein JA, Balzer DT, Lasala JM, Moazami N. Transcatheter repair of recurrent postinfarct ventricular septal defects. *Ann Thorac Surg.* 2005;80(5):1907-9.

Shumacker H. Suggestions concerning operative management of postinfarction ventricular septal defects. *J Thorac Cardiovasc Surg.* 1972; 64:452

Skillington PD, Davies RH, Luff AJ, et al. Surgical treatment for infarct-related ventricular septal defects. Improved early results combined with analysis of late functional status. *J Thorac Cardiovasc Surg.* 1990;99(5):798-808.

3

Current Trend of Off-Pump Coronary Artery Bypass Grafting

Hitoshi Hirose
Division of Cardiothoracic Surgery, Department of Surgery
Thomas Jefferson University, Philaelphia PA,
USA

1. Introduction

Coronary artery bypass grafting (CABG) using cardiopulmonary bypass (CPB) and cardioplegic arrest has been performed safely over several decades. Cardiac surgery under cardiac arrest provides a bloodless stable operative field, that can facilitate anastomosis. In last decade, CABG without CPB, off-pump CABG (OPCAB) has become more common with advances in surgical instruments and technique. This chapter summarizes the surgical technique, risks and benefits of OPCAB.

2. Technical aspects

2.1 Anesthesia

After standard sternotomy and appropriate graft harvesting, a pericardial well is created. A standard dose of heparin is administered by the anaesthesiologist. The anaesthesia team should be prepared to perform appropriate hemodynamic monitoring. We use transesophageal echocardiography and Swan-Gantz catheters to monitor cardiac function in all patients. Activated clotting time above 350 is sufficient to perform OPCAB; however, a full dose of heparin may be given in cases undergoing emergent conversion to CABG using CPB. The anaesthesiologist should inform the surgical team any abrupt decrease in blood pressure, ST changes on EKG and arrhythmia, because these are signs for possible emergent conversion to CPB.

2.2 Retropericardial suture

The patient is placed in the Trendelenburg position and the sternal retractor is open widely. Right side stitches holding the pericardial well are released to minimize compression of the right heart. While the apex of the heart is gently elevated using one hand, retropericardial sutures are placed to support the heart (Figure 1). To minimize hemodynamic instability, we place the first retropericardial stitch into the mid-portion of the diaphragm. The stitch is pulled out to the right side of the lower edge of the skin incision and tightly secured so that the heart is somewhat elevated. The second deep pericardial stitch is applied to the midportion between the inferior vena cava and the left lower pulmonary vein, and the stitch is passed though a rubber catheter so that the heart will not be injured by the retropericardial sutures.

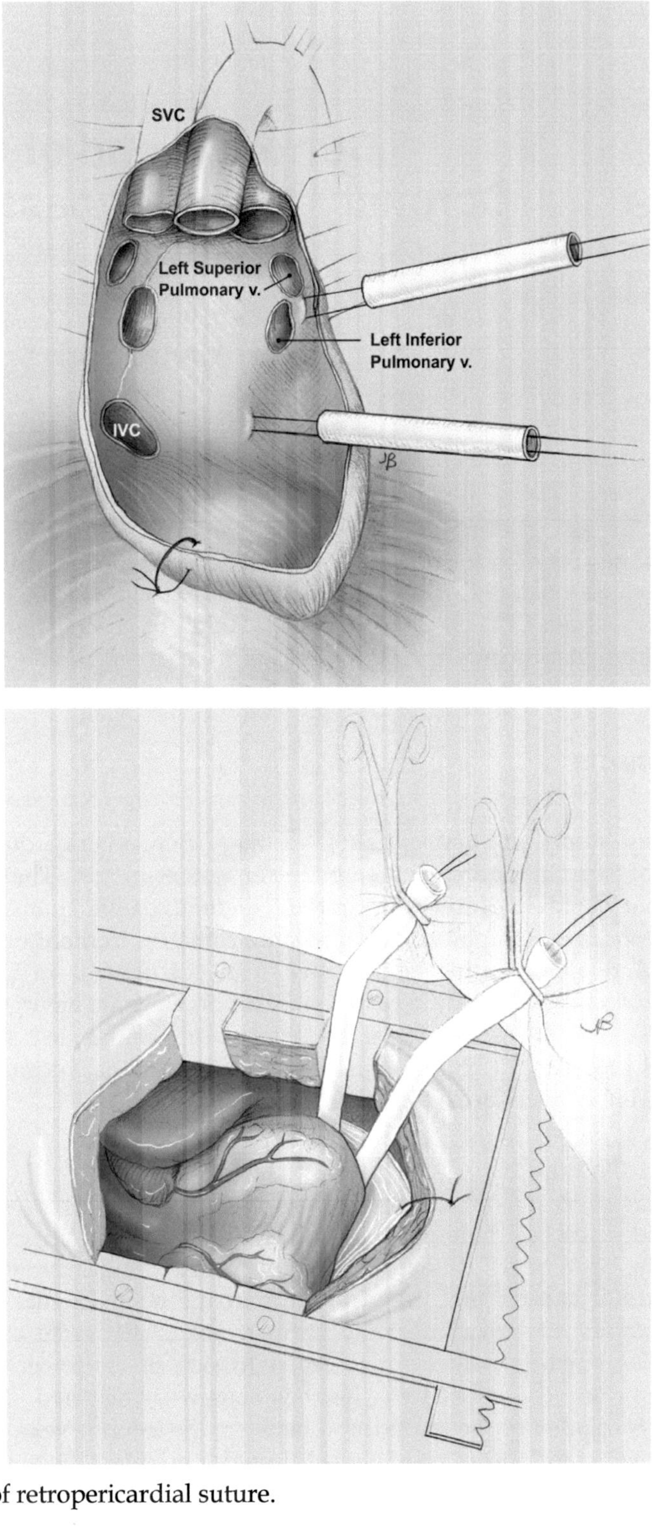

Fig. 1. A model of retropericardial suture.

The third stitch is applied inferior to the left upper pulmonary vein and is also passed through a rubber catheter. Usually three retropericardial sutures are sufficient to support the heart; however, an additional retropericardial suture can be added between the last two retropericardial sutures. An abrupt drop in blood pressure may occur during retropericardial suture placement. This hemodynamics instability is usually transient and injection of a small dose of vasoconstrictor or volume management will be enough to regain blood pressure. ST segment changes on EKG during the heart displacement is often observed in patients with severe left main disease. Preoperative intra-aortic balloon pump (IABP) placement would be helpful to maintain hemodynamic stability. If there is a persistent drop in blood pressure, ST-segment changes, and/or ventricular arrhythmia occurs during the manipulation of the heart, it is an indication to abort the OPCAB and convert to on-pump CABG. If the patient is not tolerating the short period of heart displacement during retropericardial suture placement, the patient most likely would not tolerate a longer period of heart displacement while performing anastomoses. Some surgeons may use suction-cup device to place the heart in an appropriate position. The use of a suction cup device and the use of retropericardial sutures have been proven to have similar effects (Gunnert et al., 2008).

2.3 Anterior wall revascularization

Anastomosis to the left anterior descending artery (LAD) using the internal mammary artery (IMA) graft is key to the success of OPCAB so that the LAD can be perfused after anastomosis. Without the Trendelenburg position, minimal elevation of the left heart with one or two sponges is usually sufficient to approach to the LAD. If the right ventricle is compressed and venous return is decreased, a significant decrease in blood pressure can occur. To avoid stress on the right system, the right pleura may be opened. This allows the heart to herniate into the right pleural space during heart displacement and minimizes the hemodynamic compromise.. After exposure of the target vessel, a suction type coronary stabilizer is placed on the target vessel. Before making coronary arteriotomy, a proximal snare is placed to the coronary artery slightly proximal to the anastomosis area using a silicone suture (Figure 2 top). EKG and blood pressure are carefully monitored by anesthesiologists. An arteriotomy is made on the target. Then a intracoronary shunt is quickly inserted into the coronary artery (Figure 2 middle) and the proximal snare is released (Figure 3 bottom) (Emmiler et al., 2008).

The sizing of the shunt is important. If a larger shunt is selected relative to the coronary artery size, the surgeon may encounter difficulty in placing the shunt into the coronary artery; moreover, vigorous forceful insertion of the shunt may cause injury or local dissection of the coronary artery. On the contrary, if a smaller shunt relative to the coronary artery is selected, the surgeon may experience excessive amount of bleeding from the anastomosis site, and smaller shunt may not able to supply enough blood distally. A CO2 mister-blower helps to provide a bloodless operative field. Anastomosis is performed in the standard manner; however additional care is always taken not to place a suture into the shunt. Right before completion of the anastomosis the proximal snare is tightened, the shunt is removed, and then the sutures are tied. Removal of the proximal snare allows abrupt restoration of distal coronary flow. In some cases of a small target coronary artery, the anastomosis can be performed without a shunt using a proximal snare only. If the target vessel is totally occluded vessel, the proximal snare is not necessary because of lack of forward blood flow. The IMA flow should be checked with ultrasound doppler before posterior or inferior wall revascularization.

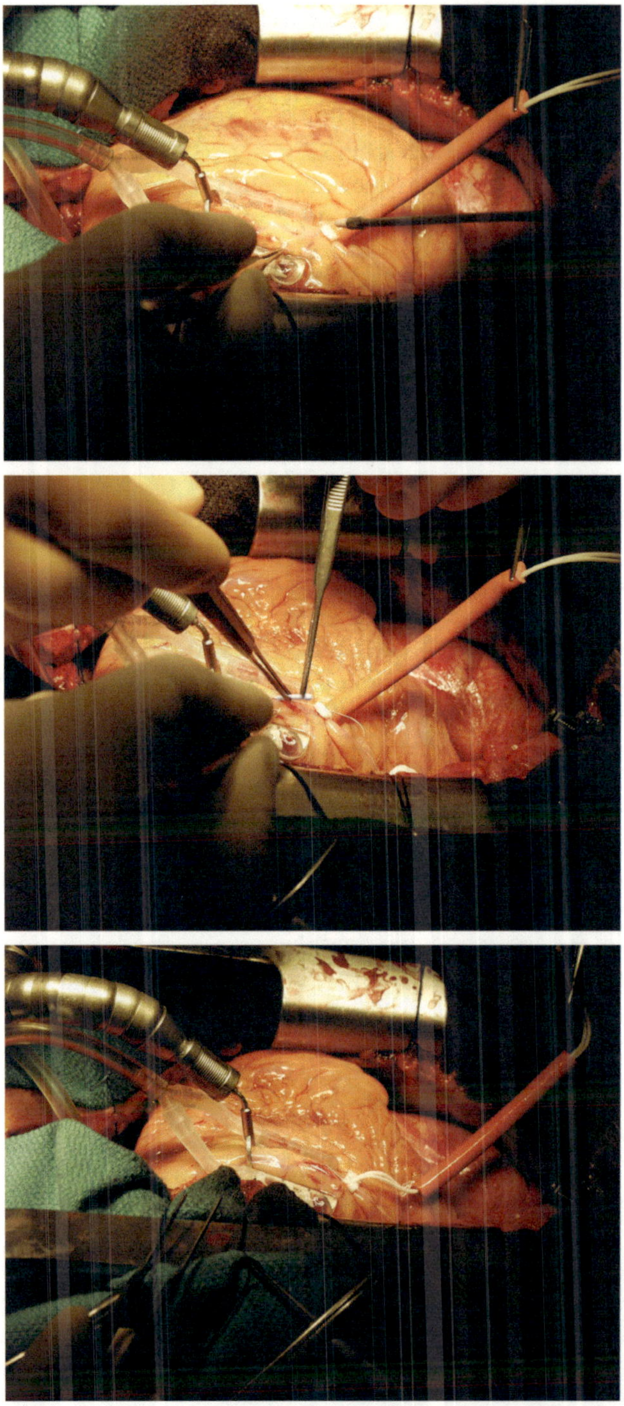

Fig. 2. Suction stabilizer and proximal snare is placed on to the target vessel (top). A shunt tube is placed thought the arteriotomy (middle). Proximal snare is open after shunt tube placement and the coronary vessel is ready to anastomose (bottom)

2.4 Posterior and inferior wall revascularization

After IMA-LAD anastomosis, anastomoses to the obtuse marginal branch (OM) or posterior descending artery can be performed. Prior to the OM anastomosis, the patient is placed in a steep Trendelenburg and left side up position on the operating table. The heart is gently elevated using a hand and then the heart can be rested on the retropericardial sutures. If the blood pressure drops, the heart is placed back into the natural position and wait for recovery. The previous IMA-LAD graft should stay open and this IMA-LAD flow will help the hemodynamics during the OM anastomosis is completed. Phenylephrine is a first drug of choice for hypotension during the anastomosis, because phenylephrine increase blood pressure without causing tachycardia. If persistent hypotension occurs, conversion to on-pump should be considered. However, we found most of patient with normal left ventricular function will tolerate displacement of the heart during the anastomoses. After adequate exposure of the target vessel, a stabilizer is placed onto the target. Confirmation of stable hemodynamics is necessary prior to making an arteriotomy. In a sequential manner, proximal snare placement, arteriotomy, shunt placement, release of the proximal snare, and then anastomosis are performed. Arterial blood drawn by the anesthetist should be avoided during the anastomosis of the posterior wall. After the OM anastomosis, the position of the operating table is returned to zero and maintain the Trendelenburg position. Anastomosis to the inferior wall is performed in a similar manner.

2.5 Proximal anastomosis

Proximal anastomoses are performed after all distal anastomoses. The patient is placed in a slight reverse Trendelenburg position, systolic blood pressure is controlled by anesthesia with a target of 110 mm Hg, so that the proximal clamp is not dislodged during the proximal anastomosis. Displacement of the proximal clamp during the proximal anastomosis is dangerous and may cause massive exsanguination, and may also cause aortic dissection. After achieving an adequate blood pressure, a side-biting clamp is gently applied to the ascending aorta. An aortotomy is made and proximal anastomosis is completed in the standard manner. The side-biting clamp is removed and the grafts are de-aired. Proximal anastomosis of the graft may be performed before the distal anastomosis, especially if a proximal automatic anastomosis device is used. The automatic proximal anastomosis device is useful for the patient with severe calcification of the aorta.

2.6 Doppler assessment to the grafts

After completion of all anastomoses, the blood flow of the grafts should be accessed using an ultrasound flow probe. A poor graft flow mandates additional attention to the anastomosis and consider revision of the graft anastomosis (Kim et al., 2005). Protamine is administered after confirmation of the graft flow and then the chest is closed in the standard manner.

2.7 Postoperative management

Without using CPB, the fibrinolytic activity of the patient who undergo OPCAB is lower than those who undergo conventional CABG using CPB. After OPCAB surgery, patient may develop a hypercoagulable state. To avoid platelet aggregation at the anastomosis site, clopidogrel is started as early as postoperative day 0 (Quigley et al, 2003). Other postoperative managements are similar to those after on-pump CABG.

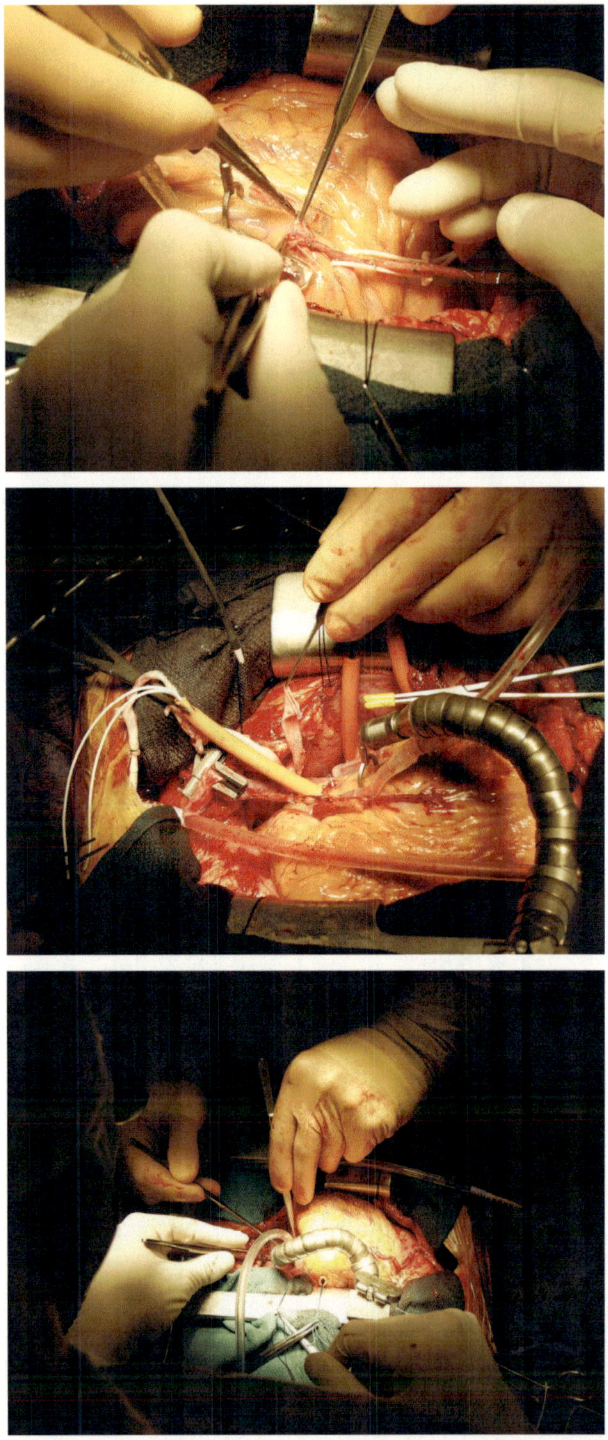

Fig. 3. Examples of anterior (top), posterolateral (middle), and inferior (bottom) revascularization.

3. Advantages of OPCAB

In general, those who are considered to be contraindicated for on-pump CABG, such as patients with calcified aorta, advanced age, and significant comorbidities, can be a candidate for OPCAB. OPCAB does not require CPB and theoretically eliminates all CBP-related complications. OPCAB can reduce blood loss and the need of transfusion. OPCAB has known to provide less myocardial enzyme release, fewer incidence of neurocognitive dysfunction and postoperative renal injury than conventional CABG. Studies found OPCAB can make patient recovery time shorter as well. Table 1 summarizes the best candidates for OPCAB.

Calcified aorta
Advanced age
Significant comorbidities
Recent stroke
Severe carotid disease
Renal dysfunction
Severer chronic lung disease
Jehovah's Witness

Table 1. The patients that benefit most from CABG

3.1 Mortalities

Studies have shown that postoperative mortality is favorable to OPCAB (Puskas et al., 2003, Cleveland et al., 2001, Puskas et al., 2008). Mortality benefit from OPCAB is more obvious in high risk patients. (Hirose et al., 2010). The reasons are multifactorial as discussed below; however, the benefit most likely related to the avoidance of CPB.

3.2 Stroke

Postoperative strokes are the most disabling complication after CABG. Avoidance of aortic cannulation and aortic cross clamping decreases the risk of stroke and distal emboli. The incidence of postoperative stroke is favorable to OPCAB compared to on-pump CABG; however stroke has not been completely eliminated by OPCAB (Puskas et al., 2003, Cleveland et al., 2001, Sabik at al., 2002). The use of side-biting clamp for proximal anastomosis is potentially the cause of postoperative stroke. Calafiore reported that the stoke rate without using side-biting clamp was 0.2%, which was significantly lower than the stroke rate with side-biting clamp (1.2%) (Calafiore et al., 2002). All in-situ grafting using bilateral mammary arteries, gastroepiploic arteries and Y-composite grafting eliminates proximal aortic anastomoses. Using this aorta-non-touch surgery, theoretically no intraoperative stroke would occur and the postoperative risk of stroke should be minimal (Hirose et al., 2004). An investigation demonstrated that OPCAB significantly reduced the incidence of intraoperative stroke; however, the incidence of delayed strokes occurring more than 48 hours after OPCAB was similar to that after on-pump CABG (Nishiyama et al., 2009). These delayed strokes are not to be related to aortic manipulation during surgery, but could be related to a hypercoagulable state and/or postoperative atrial fibrillation.

3.3 Neurocongnitive dysfunction

Neurocongnitive disorder after CPB is a well known phenomenon, so called "pump head." Prolonged CPB time is a risk factor for postoperative neurocongnitive disorder, most likely related to non-pulsatile flow, hypothermia, low perfusion pressure, systemic inflammatory state, and most importantly micro-emboli from CPB. Studies of s100 protein, a marker of neurological damage, have shown lowers s100 protein after OPCAB compared to those after on-pump CABG; however, the incidence of clinical neurocongnitive manifestation was similar between OPCAB and on-pump CABG (Lloyd et al., 2000). The benefit of OPCAB in relation to neurocongnitive disorder remains controversial (Van Dijk et al., 2002, Browne et al., 1999, Marasco et al., 2008).

3.4 Inflammatory reaction

Contact between the blood and the CPB circuit triggers an inflammatory cascade. Cytokines, complements and coagulation-fibrinolytic system are activated by CPB, which inducing CPB-related inflammatory responses (Ngaage, 2003). This inflammatory response contributes to the increase in capillary permeability, fluid shift, and decrease in tissue perfusion. Systemic inflammatory response syndrome may cause multi-organ failure, including lung, brain, kidney and heart, which may promote patient mortality. Significant decrease in inflammatory markers has been observed in OPCAB compared to that in on-pump CABG (Ascione et al., 2000). Avoidance of CBP reduces the inflammatory state and contributes to early patient recovery (Raga, 2004). CPB-related inflammatory response could cause pulmonary edema resulting in hypoxia, brain edema resulting in neurocognitive disorder, renal hypoperfusion resulting in acute renal failure, and edema of the heart resulting in low cardiac output syndrome.

3.5 Blood transfusion

Perioperative anaemia among the patient undergoing CABG is common. Hemodilution may occur from the circuit and tubing of the CPB. The use of CPB activate fibrinolytic activity and reduce the actual number of platelet and function of the platelet, which aggregates perioperative blood loss anaemia (Khuri et al., 1992). Studies have shown that OPCAB has clear benefits in blood preservation. Postoperative blood loss and transfusion requirements are smaller in OPCAB than in on-pump CABG in almost all studies (Muneretto et al., 2003). Avoiding the need for transfusion is critical in caring for Jehovah's Witness patients.

3.6 Renal function

Hypoperfusion of the kidney during CABG may cause postoperative renal dysfunction. Risk factors for renal dysfunction are often observed in patients who undergo CABG, such as patients with diabetes, hypertension and peripheral vascular disease. Non-pulsatile flow and low perfusion pressure due to CPB contribute to hypoperfusion of the kidney, causing postoperative kidney injury (Laffey et al., 2002). The duration of CPB has been known to be directly related to the incidence of postoperative renal failure. The postoperative rise in creatinine after OPCAB is less frequently observed than that after on-pump CABG (Celik et al., 2005). A lower incidence of postoperative renal failure is observed after OPCAB (Calafiore et al., 2003). This renal protection with OPCAB would be most beneficial for patients showing moderate or severe preoperative renal dysfunction (Hirose et al., 2001).

3.7 Respiratory function

A randomized trial showed that OPCAB provides lower pulmonary compliance, better gas exchange after surgery than on-pump CABG (Staton et al., 2005). Clinically, intubation time after surgery as shorter after OPCAB than after on-pump CABG (Puskas et al., 2008).

3.8 Atrial fibrillation

Atrial fibrillation is the most common arrhythmia after cardiac surgery and occurs in 25-40 % of patients. The incidence of atrial fibrillation after OPCAB is known to be less than that for on-pump CABG (Ascione et al., 2000, Raga et al., 2004). Avoiding atrial cannulation and preserving the anterior epiaortic fat pad may contribute to lowering the incidence of postoperative atrial fibrillation (Cummings et al., 2004).

3.9 Patient recovery

Due to the benefits listed above, OPCAB provides overall decreased postoperative complications and mortality (Puskas et al., 2008, Reston et al., 2003, Legare et al., 2004). Postoperative hospitalization is shorter in OPCAB patients than that in on-pump CABG (Puskas et al., 2003, Cleveland et al., 2001, Van Dijk et al., 2001). Earlier patient recovery in OPCAB could be related to reduced inflammatory reaction compared to that after on-pump CABG. The benefits of early recovery following OPCAB are more strongly apparent in high-risk patients (Stamou et al., 2005, Puskas et al., 2009).

3.10 Cost

The cost effectiveness of OPCAB can be explained by the reduced utilization of the blood products, shorter intubation time, shorter ICU stay, shorter hospitalization, and reduced postoperative complications, as described above (Scott et al., 2009, Puskas et al., 2004).

4. Potential problems and disadvantages of OPCAB

In general, the disadvantage of OPCAB is associated with surgical technique. Despite advances in surgical instruments, exposure of the posterior wall could be potentially difficult, especially in a patient with poor ventricular function or when the surgeon has not had adequate training in OPCAB. Inadequate exposure of the target results in fewer number of distal anastomoses and incomplete revascularization. Table 2 summaries poor candidates for OPCAB.

Cardiogenic shock
Unable to maintain hemodynamics during anastomosis
ST changes or ventricular tachycardia during anastomosis
Redo surgery
Poor ventricular function, ischemic mitral regurgitation
Poor coronary target
Small, intramyocardial, and/or calcified coronary artery
Young healthy patient

Table 2. The patients that the benefit least from OPCAB

4.1 Myocardial protection

Postoperative cardiac enzyme release is lower after OPCAB than after on-pump CABG. (Van Dijk et al., 2001) However, in a patient in cardiogenic shock with a failing heart, placement on the CPB is unavoidable to prevent further end organ damage, and the role of OPCAB is limited because of hemodynamic instability. If the patient is experiencing global ischemia, pump failure and unstable hemodynamics, OPCAB should not be performed.

These patients need immediate placement on CPB to reestablish systemic circulation. Hemodynamic instability may occur during the positioning of the OPCAB especially doing anastomosis to the posterior wall of the heart. If pharmacological support is not adequate, IABP is helpful to maintain hemodynamic stability during OPCAB (Vohra & Dimitri, 2006). In patients with poor ventricular function, IAPB placement prior to surgery is recommended.

4.2 Redo cardiac surgery

Redo surgery requires extensive dissection of the scar tissue. Structural injury during redo-sternotomy will result in a high mortality and morbidity (Gillinov et al., 1999). Decompression of the heart by CPB is recommended for redo surgery (Hirose & Amano 2005).

4.3 Multivessel disease

In the early era of OPCAB, revascularization of the posterolateral wall was challenging. However, after improvement of the coronary stabilizer, anastomoses to the posterolateral vessels are no longer a contraindication (Hirose et al., 2003, Song et al. 2003). Similarly, with left main disease, is no longer a contraindication for OPCAB (Hirose, 2004). In case of left main disease, revascularization of the left anterior descending artery prior to the posterolateral branches is essential. IABP may be helpful to stabilize hemodynamics, while anastomoses, especially in a patient with poor ventricular function and left main disease.

4.4 Poor ventricular function

Although mutilvessel disease is no longer contraindication for OPCAB, incomplete revascularization has been observed more often in OPCAB than on-pump CABG. A large heart with poor ventricular function is difficult to manipulate and to expose the target vessel. Heart displacement without decompression of the heart is challenging in these patients with poor ventricular function and distended left ventricle.

4.5 Small and calcified target

The reasons for incomplete revascularization could be the quality of the target vessel, as an example a small, calcified, or intramyocardial coronary artery. Bypass to these small coronary arteries and/or calcified arteries is challenging, even under on-pump cardiac arrest. Tedious endarterectomy for calcified vessels should be performed under CPB. Extensive dissection of intramyocardial coronary artery under a beating heart carries risk of ventricular rupture and should be performed with a decompressed heart under CPB. Incomplete revascularization will negatively affect the patient long-term outcome (Scott et al., 2000, Synnergre et al., 2008). A hybrid procedure involving OPCAB and percutaneous intervention could be an option in these difficult OPCAB patients.

4.6 Emergent conversion to on-pump

In palatines with hemodynamic instability during anastomosis, emergent conversion to on-pump CABG is necessary. Conversion to on-pump surgery requires emergent arterial and venous cannulation, which may need to be done while CPR is in progress due to sudden ventricular arrhythmia or cardiac arrest. Emergent conversion from OPCAB to on-pump carries a ten-fold higher risk of operative mortality than elective OPCAB (Tabata et al.,

2006). One of the risk factors for emergent conversion is ischemic mitral regurgitation. Pre-existing ischemic mitral regurgitation may be accelerated during OPCAB due to displacement of the heart during anastomosis and due to distal ischemia.

4.7 Training

Cardiac motions during anastomosis are a major disturbance to the surgeon, and the OPCAB has a prominent learning curve. There is a direct correlation between the number of cases the surgeon has performed and the incidence of postoperative complications and graft patency. The surgeon with limited experience in OPCAB may produce a significant number of cardiac complications (Brown et al., 2001). Extensive training in performing OPCAB is necessary to improve patient outcomes.

4.8 Graft patency

Graft patency after OPCAB may be related to the surgeon's skill level. A previous study by Khan showed a decreased 3-months-graft patency rate in the OPCAB group compared to that in the on-pump group (Khan et al., 2004). However, the article was criticized because of the lack of the surgeon's adequate OPCAB experiences, lack of postoperative antiplatelet therapy with clopidogrel, and failure to use a suction device for stabilization of the heart (Dewey et al., 2004). A recent randomized trial by Puskas (Puskas et al., 2009), and the European study (Widimsky et al., 2004) independently confirmed similar 1-year graft patency rate between OPCAB and on-pump CABG.

5. Conclusion

Recent advances in surgical instruments and technique allows surgeons to perform OPCAB safely.

OPCAB for left main disease and multivessel revascularization is no longer a contraindication.
Except for patient undergoing redo CABG, hemodynamically compromised patients, and patient with poor target vessels, OPCAB can be performed by an experienced surgeon without increasing risks.
OPCAB requires a significant intensive training period.
OPCAB may expand the indications of CABG to patients with higher risks.
OPCAB contributes to shortening the length of stay and promotes an early recovery.

Table 3. Summary of the advantages and disadvantages of OPCAB

Although there is a steep learning curve for OPCAB techniques, OPCAB provides a favorable or at least equivalent postoperative outcome compared to on-pump CABG, with minimal contraindications. OPCAB will significantly reduce the risk of CPB-related complications. These benefits of OPCAB are more significant in high-risk patients, and there is a possibility to expand the indication of CABG.

6. References

Abu-Omar Y, Taggart DP. (2009) The present status of off-pump coronary artery bypass grafting. *Eur J Cardiothorac Surg*. Vol. 36, No. 2, 312-321.

Ascione R, Caputo M, Calori G, Lloyd CT, Underwood MJ, Angelini GD. (2000) Predictors of atrial fibrillation after conventional and beating heart coronary surgery: a prospective, randomized study. *Circulation*. Vol. 102, No. 13, 1530-1535.

Ascione R, Lloyd CT, Underwood MJ, Lotto AA, Pitsis AA, Angelini GD. (2000) Inflammatory response after coronary revascularization with or without cardiopulmonary bypass. *Ann Thorac Surg*. Vol. 69, No. 4, 1198-1204.

Brown PP, Mack MJ, Simon AW, et al. (2001) Comparing clinical outcomes in high-volume and low-volume off-pump coronary bypass operation programs. *Ann Thorac Surg*. Vol. 72, No. 3, S1009-S1015.

Browne SM, Halligan PW, Wade DT, Taggart DP. (1999) Cognitive performance after cardiac operation: implications of regression toward the mean. *J Thorac Cardiovasc Surg*. Vol. 117, No 3, 481-485.

Calafiore AM, Di Mauro M, Canosa C, Di Giammarco G, Iaco AL, Contini M. (2003) Myocardial revascularization with and without cardiopulmonary bypass: advantages, disadvantages and similarities. *Eur J Cardiothorac Surg*. Vol. 24, No. 6, 953-96.

Calafiore AM, Di Mauro M, Teodori G, et al. (2002) Impact of aortic manipulation on incidence of cerebrovascular accidents after surgical myocardial revascularization. *Ann Thorac Surg*. Vol. 73, No. 5, 1387-1393.

Celik JB, Gormus N, Topal A, Okesli S, Solak H. (2005) Effect of off-pump and on-pump coronary artery bypass grafting on renal function. *Ren Fail*. Vol. 27, No. 2, 183-188.

Cleveland JC, Shroyer LW, Chen AY, Peterson E, Grover FL. (2001) Off-pump coronary artery bypass grafting decreases risk-adjusted mortality and morbidity. *Ann Thorac Surg*. Vol. 72, No. 4, 1282-1289.

Cummings JE, Gill I, Akhrass R, Dery M, Biblo LA, Quan KJ. (2004) Preservation of the anterior fat pad paradoxically decreases the incidence of postoperative atrial fibrillation in humans. *J Am Coll Cardiol*. Vol. 43, No. 6, 994-1000.

Dewey TM, Magee MJ, Mack MJ. (2004) Off-pump versus on-pump coronary bypass surgery. *N Engl J Med*. Vol. 350, No. 17, 1791–1793.

Emmiler M, Kocogullari CU, Ela Y, Cekirdekci A. (2008) Influence of intracoronary shunt on myocardial damage: a prospective randomized study. *Eur J Cardiothorac Surg*. Vol 34, No 5,1000-1004.

Gillinov AM, Casselman FP, Lytle BW, et al. (1999) Injury to a patent left internal mammary artery graft at coronary artery reoperation. *Ann Thorac Surg*. Vol. 67, No. 2, 382-386.

Gunnert JF, Raumanns J, Opfermann UT, et al. (2008) Hemodynamic assessment using apical suction versus pericardial retraction in beating heart surgery. *Innovation*. Vol. 3, No.3, 125-130.

Hirose H, Amano A, Takahashi A, Nagano N. (2001) Coronary artery bypass grafting for patients with non-dialysis-dependent renal dysfunction (serum creatinine >/=2.0 mg/dl). *Euro J Cardiothoracic Surg*. Vol. 20, No. 3, 565-572.

Hirose H, Amano A, Takahashi A, Nagano N. (2003) Off-pump multivessel revascularization; efficacy of suction type of coronary stabilizer. *Jpn J Thorac Cardiovasc Surg*. Vol 51, No. 4, 130-137.

Hirose H, Amano A, Takahashi A. (2004) Aortic nontouch off-pump complete revascularization using 3 in situ arterial conduits: bilateral internal mammary arteries and gastroepiploic artery. *Heart Surgery Forum*. Vol. 7, No. 2, E122-125.

Hirose H, Amano A. (2005) Routine off-pump coronary artery bypass: reasons for on-pump conversion. *Innovations*. Vol. 1, No 1, 28-31.

Hirose H, Noguchi N, Inaba H, et al. (2010) The role of EuroSCORE in patients undergoing off-pump coronary artery bypass. *Interactive Cardiovasc Surg*. Vol. 10, No 5, 771-776.

Hirose H. (2004) Off-pump coronary artery bypass grafting for patients with left main disease. *Cardiology*. 101 (4), 194-198.

Khan NE, De Souza A, Mister R, et al. (2004) A randomized comparison of off-pump and on-pump multivessel coronary-artery bypass surgery. *N Engl J Med*. Vol. 350, No. 1, 21-28.

Khuri SF, Wolfe JA, Josa M, et al. (1992) Hematologic changes during and after cardiopulmonary bypass and their relationship to the bleeding time and nonsurgical blood loss. *J Thorac Cardiovasc Surg*. Vol. 104, No. 1, 94-107.

Kim K, Hyun Kang C, Lim C. (2005) Prediction of graft flow impairment by intraoperative transit time flow measurement in off-pump coronary artery bypass using arterial grafts. *Ann Thorac Surg*. Vol. 80, No. 2, 594–598.

Laffey JG, Boylan JF, Cheng DC. (2002) The systemic inflammatory response to cardiac surgery: implications for the anesthesiologist. *Anesthesiology*. Vol. 97, No. 1, 215-252.

Legare JF, Buth KJ, King S, et al. (2004) Coronary bypass surgery performed off-pump does not result in lower in-hospital morbidity than coronary artery bypass grafting performed on pump. *Circulation*. Vol. 109, No. 7, 887-892.

Lloyd CT, Ascione R, Underwood MJ, Gardner F, Black A, Angelini GD. (2000) Serum S-100 protein release and neuropsychologic outcome during coronary revascularization on the beating heart: a prospective randomized study. *J Thorac Cardiovasc Surg*. Vol. 119, No. 1, 148-154.

Marasco SF, Sharwood LN, Abramson MJ. (2008) No improvement in neurocongnitive outcomes after off-pump versus on-pump coronary revascularization: a meta-analysis. *Eur J Cardiothorac Surg*. Vol. 33, No. 6, 961-970.

Muneretto C, Bisleri G, Negri A, et al. (2003) Off-pump coronary artery bypass surgery technique for total arterial myocardial revascularization: a prospective randomized study. *Ann Thorac Surg*. Vol. 76, No. 3, 778-783.

Ngaage DL. (2003) Off-pump coronary artery bypass grafting: the myth, the logic and the science. *Eur J Cardio-thorac Surg*. Vol 24, No. 4, 557-570.

Nishiyama K, Horiguchi M, Shizuta S, et al. (2009) Temporal pattern of strokes after on-pump and off-pump coronary artery bypass graft surgery. *Ann Thorac Surg*. Vol. 87, No. 6, 1839-1844.

Puskas JD, Kilgo PD, Lattouf OM, et al. (2008) Off-pump coronary bypass provides reduced mortality and morbidity and equivalent 10-year survival. *Ann Thorac Surg*. Vol. 86, No. 4, 1139-1146.

Puskas JD, Thourani VH, Kilgo P, et al. (2009) Off-pump coronary artery bypass disproportionately benefits high-risk patients. *Ann Thorac Surg*. Vol. 88. No. 4, 1142-1147.

Puskas JD, Williams WH, Duke PG, et al. (2003) Off-pump coronary artery bypass grafting provides complete revascularization with reduced myocardial injury, transfusion requirements, and length of stay: A prospective randomized comparison of two hundred unselected patients undergoing off-pump versus conventional coronary artery bypass grafting. *J Thorac Cardiovasc Surg*. Vol. 125 No. 4, 797-808.

Puskas JD, Williams WH, Mahoney EM, et al. (2004) Off-pump vs conventional coronary artery bypass grafting: early and 1-year graft patency, cost, and quality-of-life outcomes: a randomized trial. *JAMA*. Vol. 29, No. 15, 1841-1849.

Quigley RL, Fried DW, Pym J, Highbloom RY. (2003) Off-pump coronary artery bypass surgery may produce a hypercoagulable patient. *Heart Surgery Forum*. Vol. 6, No. 2, 94-98.

Raja SG, Behranwala AA, Dunning J. (2004) Does off-pump coronary artery surgery reduce the incidence of postoperative atrial fibrillation? *Interact Cardiovasc Thorac Surg*. Vol. 3, No. 4, 647-52.

Raja SG. (2004) Decreased release of endothelin after OPCAB: implications of the evidence. *J Cardiothorac Vasc Anesth*. Vol. 18, No. 5, 25-29.

Reston JT, Tregear SJ, and Turkelson CM. (2003) Meta-analysis of short-term and mid-term outcomes following off-pump coronary artery bypass grafting. *Ann Thorac Surg*. Vol. 76, No. 5, 1510-1515.

Sabik JF, Gillinov AM, Blackstone EH, et al. (2002) Does off-pump coronary surgery reduce morbidity and mortality? *J Thorac Cardiovasc Surg*. Vol. 124, No. 4, 698-707.

Scott BH, Seifert FC, Grimson R, Glass PS. (2009) Resource utilization in on- and off-pump coronary artery surgery: factors influencing postoperative length of stay—an experience of 1,746 consecutive patients undergoing fast-track cardiac anesthesia. *J Cardiothorac Vasc Anesth*. Vol. 19, No. 1, 26-31.

Scott R, Blackstone EH, McCarthy PM, et al. (2000) Isolated bypass grafting of the left internal thoracic artery to the left anterior descending coronary artery: late consequences of incomplete revascularization. *J Thorac Cardiovasc Surg*. Vol. 120, No. 1, 173-184.

Song HK, Petersen RJ, Sharoni E, Guyton RA, Puskas JD. Safe evolution towards routine off-pump coronary artery bypass: negotiating the learning curve. Eur J Cardiothorac Surg. Vol. 24, No. 6, 947-952 (2003).

Stamou SC, Jablonski KA, Hill PC. (2005) Coronary revascularization without cardiopulmonary bypass versus the conventional approach in high-risk patients. *Ann Thorac Surg*. Vol. 79, No. 2, 552-557.

Staton GW, Williams WH, Mahoney EM, et al. (2005) Pulmonary outcomes of off-pump vs on-pump coronary artery bypass surgery in a randomized trial. *Chest*. Vol. 127, No. 3, 892-901.

Synnergren MJ, Ekroth R, Odén A, Rexius H, Wiklund L. (2008) Incomplete revascularization reduces survival benefit of coronary artery bypass grafting: role of off-pump surgery. *J Thorac Cardiovasc Surg*. Vol. 136, No. 1, 29-36.

Tabata M, Takanashi S, Horai T, Fukui T, Hosoda Y. (2006) Emergency conversion in off-pump coronary artery bypass grafting. Interact Cardiovasc Thorac Surg. Vol. 5, No. 5, 555-559.

Van Dijk D, Jansen EW, Hijman R, et al. (2002) Cognitive outcome after off-pump and on-pump coronary artery bypass graft surgery: a randomized trial. *JAMA*. Vol. 287 No.11, 1405-1412.

Van Dijk D, Nierich AP, Jansen EW, et al. (2001) Octopus Study Group. Early outcome after off-pump versus on-pump coronary bypass surgery: results from a randomized study. *Circulation*. Vol. 104, No. 15, 1761–1766.

Vohra HA, Dimitri WR. (2006) Elective intraaortic balloon counterpulsation in high-risk off-pump coronary artery bypass grafting. *J Card Surg*. Vol. 21, No.1, 1-5.

Widimsky P, Straka Z, Stros P, et al. (2004) One-year coronary bypass graft patency: a randomized comparison between off-pump and on-pump surgery angiographic results of the PRAGUE-4 trial. *Circulation*. Vol. 110, No. 22, 3418-3423.

4

Psychiatric Factors Which Impact Coronary Heart Disease and Influence Outcomes Post-Coronary Artery Bypass Grafting Surgery

James J. Mahoney, III[1,2,3], Emily A. Voelkel[1], Jenny A. Bannister[1], Raja R. Gopaldas[4] and Tam K. Dao[1,2]
[1]*University of Houston, Department of Educational Psychology,*
[2]*Baylor College of Medicine,*
[3]*Michael E. DeBakey Veteran Affairs Medical Center,*
[4]*University of Missouri – Columbia School of Medicine,*
United States

1. Introduction

1.1 Coronary Artery Bypass Grafting defined

It has been reported that over 13 million individuals in the United States have been diagnosed with Coronary Artery Disease (Morrow & Gersh, 2008), and it is the leading cause of death in the United States with more than 650,000 deaths in 2005 (Centers for Disease Control and Prevention, 2009). One of the most effective and common methods of treating Coronary Artery Disease is Coronary Artery Bypass Grafting surgery (Niles et al., 2001). Typically, those patients with severe narrowing of the left main coronary artery and/or those with disease in at least 3 coronary arteries are candidates for Coronary Artery Bypass Grafting Surgery.

1.2 Comorbidity with Coronary Artery Disease

There is also a high comorbidity between Peripheral Vascular Disease and Coronary Artery Disease (Brandt et al., 2004; Eagle et al., 1994; Hertzer et al., 1984). While several studies have reported short-term adverse outcomes in Coronary Artery Bypass Grafting patients that also have Peripheral Vascular Disease (Gersh et al., 1989; Grover et al., 1990; Higgins et al., 1992; Kunadian et al., 2007; Magovern et al., 1996; O'Connor et al., 1992; Rosenthal et al., 2003; Sutton-Tyrrell et al., 1998) the long-term outcomes have not been thoroughly investigated. To address this gap in the literature, Chu et al. (2008) conducted a study investigating the long-term impact of Coronary Artery Bypass Grafting surgery in patients who concurrently had Peripheral Vascular Disease. After comparing 370 Peripheral Vascular Disease and 794 non-Peripheral Vascular Disease patients, Chu and colleagues determined there were no significant group differences in 30 day mortality or major cardiac adverse events; however, patients with Peripheral Vascular Disease had a significantly worse 9 year survival rate (i.e., almost twice the risk of mortality) when compared to those without Peripheral Vascular Disease. While the short-term outcomes of this study are contradictory to previous studies, the long-term outcomes suggest that those with Peripheral Vascular Disease have poorer outcomes over time when compared to those without Peripheral Vascular Disease.

1.3 Variations of Coronary Artery Bypass Grafting Surgery

Typically Coronary Artery Bypass Grafting surgery is performed via Cardiopulmonary Bypass; however, there are several drawbacks associated with Cardiopulmonary Bypass which may lead to complications following or during surgery (Edmunds et al., 2003). As a result of these complications, a technique utilizing an Off-Pump Coronary Artery Bypass procedure was developed. The Off-Pump Coronary Artery Bypass technique has recently gained popularity and can also be performed without involving Cardiopulmonary Bypass (Benetti et al., 1995; Buffolo et al., 1996; Calafiore et al., 1996; Dewey et al., 2001; Guler et al., 2001; Guru et al., 2007;Magee et al., 2001; Puskas et al., 1998; Trehan et al., 2001). While Off-Pump Coronary Artery Bypass has gained notoriety, some surgeons have opted out of using the technique due to suspicions that Off-Pump Coronary Artery Bypass may compromise patient outcomes. To help clarify these suspicions, researchers have turned their focus to investigating the effectiveness of Off-Pump Coronary Artery Bypass for treating patients with Coronary Artery Disease. The results of such studies have often been counter indicative. Some studies suggest that Off-Pump Coronary Artery Bypass has similar outcomes to conventional Coronary Artery Bypass Grafting surgery with respect to length of hospital stay, morbidity, and neurological deficiencies (Halkos et al., 2008; Puskas et al., 1998; Puskas et al., 2001) as well as comparable graft patency and hospitalization costs (Puskas et al., 2004). Conversely, other studies have reported less favorable Off-Pump Coronary Artery Bypass patient outcomes (e.g., lower graft patency rates and less complete revascularization) when compared to Coronary Artery Bypass Grafting patient outcomes (Khan et al., 2004). Still several other studies report no difference in early mortality, morbidity and hospitalization costs between the two procedures (Bull et al., 2001; Cheng et al., 2005; Cheng et al., 2002; Marasco et al., 2008; Takagi et al., 2007). Clearly, the studies to date comparing the Off-Pump Coronary Artery Bypass and Coronary Artery Bypass Grafting procedures present an unclear picture of potential differential outcomes for patients. In order to further investigate the difference between these two methods, Chu and colleagues (2009a) conducted a study using a nationwide database of over 63,000 Coronary Artery Bypass Grafting and Off-Pump Coronary Artery Bypass patients. The results revealed that the Off-Pump Coronary Artery Bypass and Coronary Artery Bypass Grafting procedures had similar in-hospital mortality, post-operative stroke incidences, and routine discharge rates. However, Off-Pump Coronary Artery Bypass patients had comparatively longer hospital stays and higher hospital costs than Coronary Artery Bypass Grafting patients.

2. Coronary Artery Bypass Grafting and medical/demographic predictors

2.1 Coronary Artery Bypass Grafting and obesity

The accepted medical model for outcomes following Coronary Artery Bypass Grafting Surgery can be found in Figure 1. Falling second to Coronary Artery Disease, obesity is the second leading cause of death in the United States (Mokdad et al., 2000). It is well-known that patients categorized as obese are at unique risk for developing various cardiovascular diseases, including Coronary Artery Disease. Due to the general increased morbidity and reduced life expectancy of obese patients (Fontaine et al., 2003), many researchers have hypothesized that obesity should be linked to poorer outcomes post-Coronary Artery Bypass Grafting surgery. Yet, current research investigating the association between obesity (e.g., body mass index, BMI) and cardiac surgery outcomes has been contradictory. Some studies report no difference in short-term outcomes post-Coronary Artery Bypass Grafting between obese and non-obese patients (Engel et al., 2009; Engelman et al., 1999; Potapov et al., 2003; Rahmanian et al., 2007; Reeves et al., 2003; Schwann et al., 2003; Syrakas et al.,

2007). Others have found that morbid obesity independently predicts perioperative complications as well as operative mortality (Prabhakar et al., 2002). One study by Syrakas and colleagues (2007) even found that normal weight patients had a higher 30-day mortality rate than their obese peers post-surgery. In fact, overall, research seems to suggest that morbid obesity does not increase short-term mortality risk for Coronary Artery Bypass Grafting patients (Baslaim et al., 2008; Shirad et al., 2009; Syrakas et al., 2007). Since research regarding the association between obesity and cardiac surgery has included mostly short-term outcomes, Del Prete and associates (2010) investigated the independent effect of obesity on long-term survival in patients (472 obese and 691 non-obese) who had Coronary Artery Bypass Grafting surgery. Results revealed obese and non-obese patients had similar intraoperative characteristics (e.g., cardiopulmonary bypass time, aortic cross-clamp time, and number of vein and IMA grafts) and post-operative outcomes. Of particular interest was that the rates of mortality and major adverse cardiac events after 30 days were not significantly different between the two groups. Most interestingly, the researchers determined that obese Coronary Artery Bypass Grafting patients demonstrated long-term survival (9 years follow-up) similar to non-obese Coronary Artery Bypass Grafting patients. While these findings are counterintuitive, these results combined with results of studies examining short-term outcomes seem to indicate that obesity is not a significant risk for patients undergoing Coronary Artery Bypass Grafting surgery.

2.2 Coronary Artery Bypass Grafting and age

Due to improvements in medical care, the average life expectancy has increased significantly in recent years. Subsequently, there has been an increase in the number of geriatric patients with cardiac disease that need surgical intervention such as Coronary Artery Bypass Grafting surgery. In addition, this population also tends to have multiple comorbidities which may cause complications; however, Coronary Artery Bypass Grafting procedures in octogenarian patients (those over the age of 80), have demonstrated improved morbidity and mortality outcomes (Alexander et al., 2000; Kolh et al., 2001; Shigemitsu et al., 2001). However, while most of these Coronary Artery Bypass Grafting surgeries are technically successful, they may cause significant physiological adverse events, potentially deconditioning them substantially. Unfortunately, there has not been a wealth of literature investigating these physiological outcomes which may affect the health and well-being of these patients. As a result, Gopaldas et al. (2010) conducted a study investigating the disposition of octogerians following Coronary Artery Bypass Grafting surgery.

Gopaldas identified 5,731 patients over age 80 who underwent Coronary Artery Bypass Grafting surgery. It was discovered that the surgical mortality rate was 7%, and 21% of patients had a routine hospital discharge. Those that did not have a routine discharge had home health care (27%) or were transferred to another care facility (45%). In addition, several predictors of surgical mortality and nonroutine discharge were found: older age, females, a higher comorbidity index, and referral from the emergency room were all found to be independent predictors of these unfavorable outcomes. Thus, it is clear that while mortality rate in octogenarians is low, there are several circumstances that need to be considered to ensure more favorable outcomes following discharge.

2.3 Coronary Artery Bypass Grafting and gender

Women are particularly affected by heart disease, and coronary heart disease has consistently been reported as the leading cause of morbidity and mortality of women in most developed countries (Center for Disease Control and Prevention, 2010; Lloyd-Jones et al., 2010; Stoney et al., 2003). In 2006, 1 in 6 reported female deaths were due to Coronary Artery Disease (Januzzi et al., 2000), and research suggests that being female is related to poorer Coronary Artery Bypass Grafting outcomes (Blankstein et al., 2005; Culler et al., 2008; Kim et al., 2007; Sawatzky et al., 2009). Women have higher mortality rates, remain in the hospital longer (Dao, 2010b), experience a more difficult recovery (Sawatzky et al., 2009), and self-report being less satisfied with health status after Coronary Artery Bypass Grafting surgery (Sawatzky et al., 2009).

Dao and colleagues (2011c) conducted a study investigating gender differences and outcomes following Coronary Artery Bypass Grafting surgery. It was reported that being female and having an anxiety disorder diagnosis independently and collectively contributed to in-hospital length of stay and non-routine discharge following a Coronary Artery Bypass Grafting surgery. In addition, significant differences were found between groups in age, gender, race, median household income, medical comorbidities, and having an anxiety disorder diagnosis. Specifically, patients with non-routine discharges were more likely to be older, female, non-Caucasian, have more medical comorbidities, and have an anxiety disorder diagnosis.

2.4 Autonomic Nervous System dysregulation

As mentioned previously, the association between depression and cardiac events, particularly Coronary Artery Disease, has been validated consistently in research; yet, the mechanism behind this relationship is unclear. One proposed underlying factor in this relationship is altered autonomic nervous system (Autonomic Nervous System) activity. Altered Autonomic Nervous System activity has been suggested to contribute to elevated mortality risk (and poorer general outcomes) in patients with Coronary Artery Disease, and individuals with Major Depressive Disorder often have Autonomic Nervous System dysregulation (Barnes et al., 1983; Esler et al., 1982; Lake et al., 1982). In addition, research suggests that depressed individuals have higher baseline heart rates (Lake et al., 1982; Siever et al., 1985; Veith et al., 1994), increased heart rate response to stressors (Carney et al., 1988a; Guinjoan et al., 1995), and decreased heart rate variability (HRV) (Appelhans et al., 2006; Carney et al., 1988b; Dallack et al., 1990; Rechlin et al., 1994) when compared to similar peers. In particular, increased Heart Rate Variability has been associated with greater abilities to regulate stress, arousal, and attention, while decreased Heart Rate Variability has been associated with inadequate parasympathetic modulation and increased cardiac sympathetic modulation (Task Force of the European Society of Cardiology and the North American Society for Pacing and Electrophysiology, 1995). Most relevant to this chapter, studies suggest that Heart Rate Variability is lower in Coronary Artery Disease patients with comorbid depression than those with Coronary Artery Disease alone (Krittayaphong et al., 1997; Stein et al., 2000). Taken together, this literature suggests that depressed individuals may not only have an elevated initial heart rate and higher heart rate in reaction to stressors, but they may also have lower Heart Rate Variability that makes it more difficult to manage these other elevated heart rate situations.

Another factor not previously understood was whether patients with Autonomic Nervous System dysregulation also have increased mortality with these concurrent disorders. Dao and colleagues (2010a) proposed a study investigating three variables (heart rate, Heart Rate Variability, and plasma norepinephrine levels) in the following groups: 1) Patients with Coronary Artery Disease and depression, 2) Patients with Depression alone, 3) Patients with Coronary Artery Disease alone, and 4) Patients without neither Coronary Artery Disease nor depression. The focus of the study was to compare the association of heart rate, Heart

Rate Variability, and plasma norepinephrine levels with depression and Autonomic Nervous System activity in addition to their relationship to Coronary Artery Bypass Grafting outcomes. In addition, a second analysis was conducted investigating the 3 aforementioned variables in cardiac patients (Coronary Artery Disease and Depression versus Coronary Artery Disease alone) and surgery outcomes (length of hospital stay, routine versus non-routine discharge status) while controlling for other factors (medical factors such as diabetes and demographic factors such as age). It was hypothesized that patients with Coronary Artery Disease and Depression would have the greatest amount of Autonomic Nervous System dysregulation while the group without Coronary Artery Disease or depression would have the least Autonomic Nervous System dysregulation. In addition, it was hypothesized that the aforementioned variables would predict outcomes following Coronary Artery Bypass Grafting surgery. Analyses revealed that patients with Coronary Artery Disease and Depression had greater Autonomic Nervous System dysregulation when compared to those that had either Coronary Artery Disease or depression alone. Also, it was determined that depression, as well as elevated heart rate and depressed Heart Rate Variability, predicted increased length of hospital stay and non-routine discharge.

2.5 Diabetes

It has been found that systematic disease may increase the risks associated with Coronary Artery Bypass Grafting surgery. Several studies have reported that diabetes is a critical factor and mortality rates are two to three times higher than in non-diabetics (Johnson et al., 1982; Lawrie et al., 1986; Salomon et al., 1983). In addition, patients with diabetes tend to have more post-CABG surgery complications which reduce long-term survival.

3. Coronary Artery Bypass Grafting and psychological predictors

3.1 Depression and Post-Traumatic Stress Disorder

A proposed psychological model for outcomes following Coronary Artery Bypass Grafting Surgery is proposed in Figure 1. Research has demonstrated that medical and demographic factors such as age, gender, diabetes, etc. cannot fully explain the outcomes following Coronary Artery Bypass Grafting surgery (Blumenthal et al., 2003; Saur et al., 2001). Several studies have been published investigating the association between Coronary Artery Disease and psychological functioning, primarily depression (Bankier et al., 2004; Oxland et al., 2006). It has been reported that up to 60% of patients with Coronary Artery Disease have comorbid depression which has a significant impact on the outcomes of Coronary Artery Disease (Blumenthal et al., 2003; Connerney et al., 2001; Krannich et al., 2007; Tully et al., 2008). Those with depression have higher rates of mortality as well as an overall risk of major cardiac events (Blumenthal et al., 2003; Carney et al., 1988; Connerney et al., 2001). Specifically, depressive symptoms also significantly predict mortality 2 to 5 years after Coronary Artery Bypass Grafting surgery, independent of medical and operative factors (Blumenthal et al., 2003; Burg et al., 2003a; Burg et al., 2003b. Unlike depression, the impact of other psychological conditions, such as Post-traumatic Stress Disorder on outcomes after Coronary Artery Bypass Grafting surgery has received less attention in research.

The gap in the literature investigating the relationship between Post-traumatic Stress Disorder on outcomes after Coronary Artery Bypass Grafting surgery needs to be examined independently from depression for several reasons. Specifically, studies have demonstrated that both depression and Post-traumatic Stress Disorder involve increased secretion of corticotropin-releasing factor. However, patients with Post-traumatic Stress Disorder have hypocortisolemia due to the increased secretion, whereas severe depression is associated with hypercortisolemia, showing that the pathophysiology of the 2 disorders might be different (Lyons et al., 2001). In addition, the psychiatric comorbidities of Post-traumatic Stress Disorder and depression may potentially affect cardiac prognosis adversely. Thus, by treating only depression and not the Post-traumatic Stress Disorder, cardiac outcomes may be adversely affected.

Dao et al (2010c) proposed a study examining the effect of clinical depression, PTSD, and comorbid depression and PTSD on outcomes following Coronary Artery Bypass Grafting surgery. It was hypothesized that depression, PTSD, and comorbid depression and PTSD would independently contribute to an increased risk for mortality following Coronary Artery Bypass Grafting surgery. In addition, it was hypothesized that comorbid depression and PTSD will have the greatest effect on mortality rates and outcomes in general. It was determined that, depression, posttraumatic stress disorder, and comorbid depression and posttraumatic stress disorder are prevalent in patients undergoing Coronary Artery Bypass Grafting surgery. In addition, depression, posttraumatic stress disorder, and comorbid depression and posttraumatic stress disorder increased the risk of mortality following Coronary Artery Bypass Grafting surgery.

3.2 Geographic status

Another topic that has received limited focus in literature to date is the impact geographic status may have on Coronary Artery Bypass Grafting outcomes. While death rates due to heart disease have decreased in recent decades (Cooper et al., 2000), vulnerable populations (e.g., individuals in rural areas) persist (Barnett et al., 2000; Pearson et al., 1998). In fact, recent reports indicate that Coronary Artery Disease is 1.3 times more prevalent in rural areas than in urban areas (McCrone et al., 2007). Another recent survey revealed that Coronary Artery Disease was the second health priority for those residing in rural areas (Gamm et al., 2002). Given that individuals who reside in rural areas are more likely to experience circumstances and situations that could compromise their physical and mental health (Healthcare Cost Utilization Project, 2001), it makes sense that health concerns such as Coronary Artery Disease are such a persistent issue. These circumstances include poverty, physical inactivity, and alcohol abuse and dependence (Miller et al., 1987). Furthermore, the lack of rural health services and difficulties of traveling long distances to larger hospitals, increase the possibility that these rural residents will not receive the best preventative, medical, and psychological care (Wallace et al., 2006). Overall, the clear association between geographic status and Coronary Artery Disease leads to questions regarding whether geographic status may actually be a predictor of adverse outcomes following Coronary Artery Bypass Grafting surgery. Since depression is associated with adverse Coronary Artery Bypass Grafting outcomes (discussed previously), depressive symptomatology must also be taken into account in these investigations. This is particularly important because those who reside in rural areas experience the stressors mentioned above (poverty, alcohol abuse, etc.) and are likely to endorse some symptoms of depression as a result of these (or similar) situations.

In an attempt to address some of the above questions, Dao and colleagues (2010b) proposed a study investigating the relationships between depression, geographical status, and outcomes following Coronary Artery Bypass Grafting surgery. The primary focus was to determine the relationship between Coronary Artery Bypass Grafting outcomes, depression, and geographical status while controlling for medical and sociodemographic factors.

Secondarily, the study was designed to assess whether geographic status would serve as a moderating variable that would subsequently affect the relationship between depression and Coronary Artery Bypass Grafting surgery outcomes. The colleagues hypothesized that those living in the rural areas would have increased depression and that depression and geographical status would contribute to outcomes following Coronary Artery Bypass Grafting surgery (mortality and length of hospital stay). The results of the study indicated that rural patients were more likely than urban patients to have a concurrent depression diagnosis. In addition, both depression and living in rural areas combined were associated with less favorable outcomes (i.e., increased length of hospital stay) following Coronary Artery Bypass Grafting surgery. Similarly, those living in rural areas and having a depression diagnosis had an elevated probability of in-hospital mortality.

3.3 Anxiety as a moderator/mediator

Compared to depression and PTSD, there has been limited research on the influence of clinical anxiety in the relationship between psychological distress and outcomes following Coronary Artery Bypass Grafting surgery. The evidence that does exist suggests that anxiety in Coronary Artery Bypass Grafting patients contributes to post-surgery complications and elevated risk of sudden cardiac death (Rozanski et al., 1999; Stengrevics et al., 1996). In addition, it has been reported that up to 50% of patients undergoing Coronary Artery Bypass Grafting surgery have elevated anxiety scores (Januzzi et al., 2000; Rymaszewska et al; 2003; Krannich et al., 2007). Yet, there had been no previous evidence that those with anxiety would have better outcomes post-Coronary Artery Bypass Grafting surgery than those with depression and/or PTSD. In an effort to address this literature gap, Dao et al. (2011c) conducted a study investigating the relationship between anxiety and outcomes following Coronary Artery Bypass Grafting surgery. Results indicated that 27% of patients undergoing Coronary Artery Bypass Grafting surgery had a comorbid anxiety diagnosis, and patients who had non-routine discharge were more likely to have comorbid anxiety diagnoses compared to patients who had a routine discharge. Thus, for this study sample it was largely concluded that anxiety disorders are prevalent in patients who are undergoing a Coronary Artery Bypass Grafting surgery. Further, for this sample, anxiety was a significant independent predictor of both length of hospital stay and non-routine discharge for patients receiving Coronary Artery Bypass Grafting surgery.

It is expected that the number of octogenarians will increase from 6.9 million to 25 million by 2050 (Spencer, 1989). While there is a clear relationship between age and adverse Coronary Artery Bypass Grafting outcomes, the mechanism(s) underlying this relationship are not fully understood. There are two lines of evidence suggesting that psychosocial risk factors might mediate this relationship. Recent studies have suggested that Coronary Artery Bypass Grafting outcomes (e.g., mortality and patient disposition) cannot be fully explained by factors such as age, gender, and medical co-morbidities (Blumenthal et al., 2003). It has been reported that depression and anxiety can independently predict mortality and patient disposition following Coronary Artery Bypass Grafting surgery (Dao et al., 2010c). The second line of evidence has been shown in studies which have demonstrated the relationship between increased age with depression and anxiety disorders. The most common geriatric psychiatric disorders among the elderly are generalized anxiety disorder and depression (Beekmanet al., 1998). By simply looking at the relationship between age and Coronary Artery Bypass Grafting outcomes as linear, we may limit the understanding of potential critical mechanisms (i.e., mediators) influencing Coronary Artery Bypass Grafting outcomes.

Dao and colleagues (2011c) constructed a study to examine whether clinical levels of anxiety and depression act as a mediator between patient age and mortality and patient discharge status among octogenarian patients following Coronary Artery Bypass Grafting surgery. It was hypothesized that clinical anxiety and depression levels would mediate the relationship between increased age and Coronary Artery Bypass Grafting outcomes. This hypothesis was based on the established relationships between increased age and adverse Coronary Artery Bypass Grafting outcomes (Blumenthal et al., 2003), as well as the relationship between increased age and prevalence of anxiety and depression symptoms. Study results indicated that patients with an anxiety/depression diagnosis had a 6% higher postoperative mortality rate and had an 18% greater likelihood of having postoperative complications. In addition, it was found that an anxiety/depression diagnosis served as a partial mediator of the relationship between age and post-Coronary Artery Bypass Grafting outcomes for both postoperative mortality and discharge status.

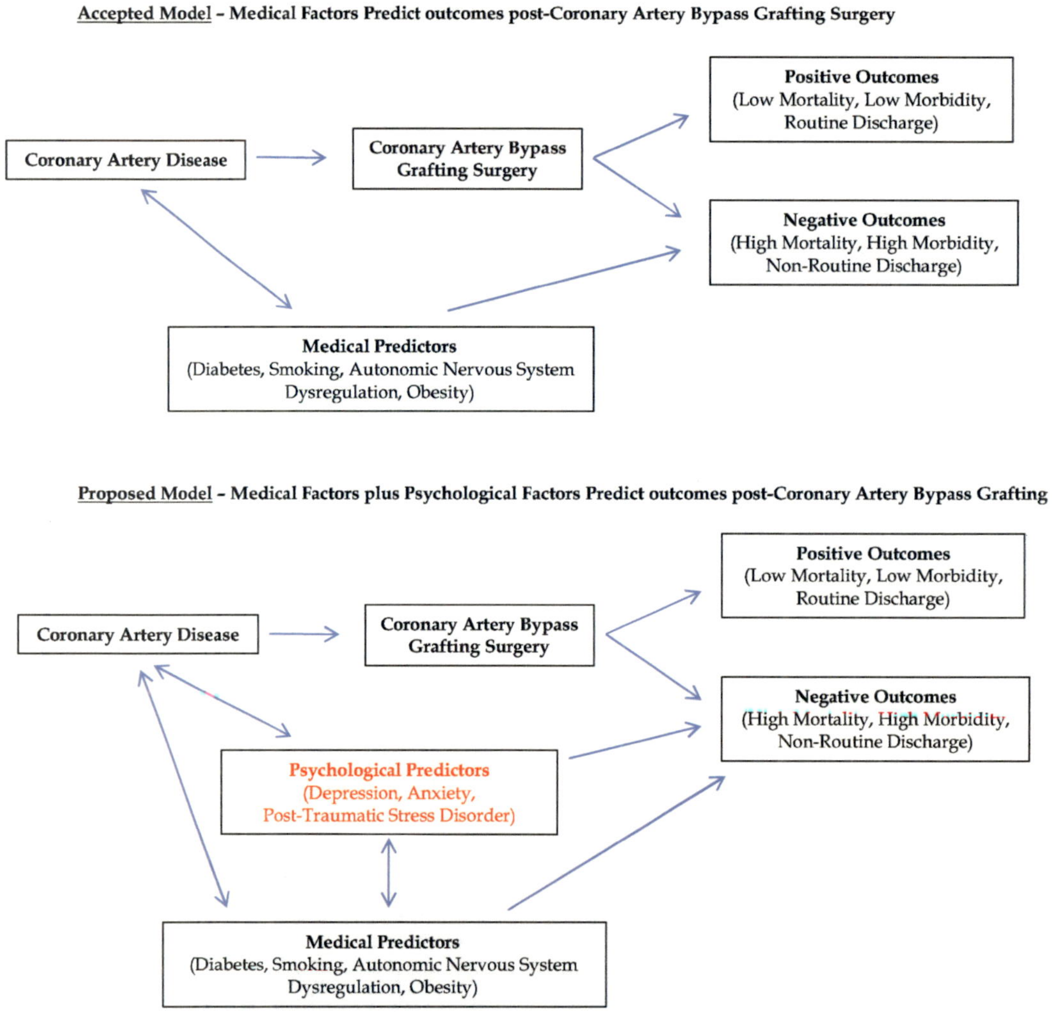

Fig. 1. Proposed Model of Psychological Factors Predicting Outcomes following Coronary Artery Bypass Grafting Surgery Versus the Traditional Medical Model

4. Treatments for comorbid psychological factors prior to Coronary Artery Bypass Grafting surgery

4.1 Treatment using Heart Rate Variability

Over the past several years, the relationship between emotional states and outcomes in cardiac patients has been the subject of increased scrutiny by researchers and clinicians (Doering et al., 2005). In particular, post-traumatic stress symptoms have been reported in up to 15 percent of Coronary Artery Bypass Grafting patients (Doerfler et al., 1994; Stoll et al., 2000). Similar to Coronary Artery Bypass Grafting patients with depression, higher levels of post-traumatic stress symptoms are related to increased mortality (Oxlad & Wade, 2006), lower health-related quality of life (Rothenhausler et al., 2010), and increased length of post-operative hospital stay (Oxlad et al., 2006). While several treatments for Post-Traumatic Stress Disorder have been proven to be effective, one of the primary drawbacks of these interventions is that they can be very lengthy and take weeks or months for treatment. Specifically, long term treatments are unrealistic and unfeasible given the sudden onset of Coronary Artery Bypass Grafting surgeries (Doerfler et al., 1994). Since there is evidence that patients suffering from Post-Traumatic Stress Disorder have an increased likelihood of mortality following Coronary Artery Bypass Grafting surgery (Dao et al., 2010a), in combination with length of treatment necessary for effective Post-Traumatic Stress Disorder care, there is a necessary need for an effective, short term treatment for improving outcomes following Coronary Artery Bypass Grafting surgery.

As mentioned earlier, Heart Rate Variability is a measure which examines the interplay between the parasympathetic and sympathetic influences on heart rate and represents the psychophysiological mechanism of emotion regulation (Appelhans & Luecken, 2006). In addition, increased Heart Rate Variability has been correlated with the increased capability of regulating stress, arousal, and attention (Bornstein et al., 2002). Recent research has demonstrated that the emotion regulation characteristics of patients with Post-Traumatic Stress Disorder have been associated with low Heart Rate Variability (Tan et al., 2010). Also, the physiological profile of a Coronary Artery Bypass Grafting patients with Post-Traumatic Stress Disorder may be complicated given purported research that low Heart Rate Variability is related to cardiovascular disease (van der Kolk, 2006). As previously discussed, it has been reported that patients with Coronary Artery Disease and a diagnosis of Post-Traumatic Stress Disorder have lower Heart Rate Variability than those patients with Coronary Artery Disease alone (Dao et al., 2010a; Krittayaphong et al., 1997; Stein et al., 2000). Since Post-Traumatic Stress Disorder and cardiovascular disease are associated with decreased Heart Rate Variability and Autonomic Nervous System dysregulation, Heart Rate Variability biofeedback training may reduce complications post-surgery. This has been supported by previous reports demonstrating that biofeedback training can increase Heart Rate Variability (Cohen et al., 2002; Tan et al., 2009). Other research has shown that Heart Rate Variability biofeedback training may be effective in reducing psychiatric symptoms associated with trauma (Karavidas et al., 2007; Zucker et al., 2009). Heart Rate Variability biofeedback training entails determining an individual's heart rate resonance frequency at baseline, calculating the optimal resonance frequency, and then providing specific breathing techniques to maximize his/her Heart Rate Variability (Lehrer et al., 2000).

Tan and colleagues (2010) reported that veterans with Post-Traumatic Stress Disorder exhibited significantly lower Heart Rate Variability compared to those without Post-Traumatic Stress Disorder. It was also discovered that those individuals receiving Heart Rate Variability biofeedback along with treatment as usual (TAU) had a significant reduction in Post-Traumatic Stress Disorder symptoms when compared to those receiving TAU alone (Tan et al.,

2010). Thus, evidence exists in support of the use of biofeedback as a potential, beneficial treatment for Post-Traumatic Stress Disorder. However, it remains unclear as to whether this treatment would be beneficial in reducing Post-Traumatic Stress Disorder symptoms in patients with Coronary Artery Disease or if it might improve outcomes post-Coronary Artery Bypass Grafting surgery. Incorporating Heart Rate Variability biofeedback training may result in Autonomic Nervous System regulation and subsequently improve outcomes post-surgery by reducing Post-Traumatic Stress Disorder symptoms.

Dao et al (2011b) proposed a study examining the efficacy of a Heart Rate Variability biofeedback treatment in 65 patients with Post-Traumatic Stress Disorder symptoms prior to Coronary Artery Bypass Grafting surgery. This study was designed to assess the impact of the Heart Rate Variability biofeedback intervention on Post-Traumatic Stress Disorder symptoms and in-hospital length of stay. It was hypothesized that symptoms associated with Post-Traumatic Stress Disorder would decrease following Heart Rate Variability biofeedback training and that their length of inpatient hospital duration would decrease following their Coronary Artery Bypass Grafting surgeries. The results from the study suggested that Heart Rate Variability biofeedback treatment can cause improvement in Post-Traumatic Stress Disorder symptoms in patients undergoing Coronary Artery Bypass Grafting surgery. It was also suggested that this treatment pre-surgery might improve patient quality of life and decrease the length of hospital stay.

4.2 Treatment using brief Cognitive Behavioral Therapy

While there have been some studies investigating the benefits of treating depression or anxiety in Coronary Artery Bypass Grafting patients postoperatively (Freedlandet al., 2009a; Freedlandet al., 2009b; Lie et al., 2007; Rollman et al., 2009), there has been little published investigating the impact of cognitive–behavioral approaches in treating depression or anxiety on Coronary Artery Bypass Grafting patients prior to surgery. Specifically, the SADHART (Sertraline Anti-Depressant Heart Attack Trial) study found a trend toward reduced cardiovascular mortality and morbidity when utilizing selective serotonin reuptake inhibitors. However, this trial had too small of a sample size and a too brief treatment duration to draw useful conclusions (Levin et al., 2005). Another study, the ENRICoronary Artery Disease (Enhancing Recovery in Coronary Heart Disease) trial found that cognitive behavioral therapy (CBT) after myocardial infarction had an effect on depression (Berkmanet al., 2003), but did not affect cardiac events such as nonfatal infarction, death from any cause, and cardiac death.

To further address questions stemming from the previous trials, Dao et al (2011a) proposed a study to examine the feasibility of a brief, tailored Cognitive Behavioral Therapy intervention entitled "Managing Anxiety and Depression using Education and Skills" (MADES), for treating patients with Coronary Artery Disease and symptoms of depression or anxiety prior to Coronary Artery Bypass Grafting surgery. The specific focus of this study was to assess the impact of this brief intervention on depression/anxiety symptoms and in-hospital length of stay. This study demonstrated that brief, tailored Cognitive Behavioral Therapy was not only feasible, but was successful in improving depressive/anxiety symptoms and quality of life while simultaneously reducing in-hospital length of stay.

5. Conclusion

5.1 What we still don't know

The studies reviewed in this chapter are important for several reasons (for a brief synopsis of each article, please refer to Table 1). First, these studies highlight the importance of psychological risk factors such as depression and anxiety in predicting adverse Coronary Artery Bypass Grafting outcomes. Second, the relations were more pronounced for certain groups of patients (e.g., rural versus non-rural and females versus males), which could help explain why females often seem to derive less functional benefit from Coronary Artery Bypass Grafting surgery than men. Third, while the treatment of presurgical and postsurgical depression and anxiety have not been extensively studied to date, the results thus far are somewhat promising. The aforementioned studies, however, do not fully explain the nature of psychological risk factors and outcomes following Coronary Artery Bypass Grafting surgery. In other words, are psychological risk factors such as depression and anxiety causal factors, directly related to adverse outcomes following Coronary Artery Bypass Grafting surgery? Or, are psychological risk factors risk markers, indirectly related to outcomes following Coronary Artery Bypass Grafting surgery through behavioral variables?

As pointed out by Rumsfeld and Ho (2005), the relations between psychological factors and adverse Coronary Artery Bypass Grafting outcomes may be mediated by behavioral mechanisms that are well documented in the literature to be associated with psychological symptoms. For instance, symptoms such as low energy or fatigue, loss of interest in activities, diminished ability to concentrate or indecisiveness, and psychomotor retardation are common in individuals diagnosed with depression. Thus, it is not surprising that these individuals are significantly less likely to adhere to prescribedmedications, follow lifestyle recommendations (e.g., exercising), practice self-management (e.g., monitor weight), and even follow up or receive recommended cardiac testing compared to those with no depression.

Overall, no studies to date have concurrently examined the physiological mechanisms (elevated plasma norepinephrine levels, cortisol, heart rate variability) and behavioral mechanisms (not following through with medication suggestions, lack of exercise, etc.) to determine which mechanisms (if any) are more responsible for adverse outcomes following Coronary Artery Bypass Grafting surgery.

Author	Year	Sample Size	Sample Characteristics	Primary Outcome	Result
Choi	2009	49,357	Pts who underwent CABG surgery	Compare outcomes of CABG surgery in VA versus non-VA hospitals	Pts who underwent CABG surgery at VA hospitals had significantly lower mortality rate than those at non-VA hospitals
Chu	2008	1,164	Pts who underwent CABG surgery	Compare outcomes of those with concurrent PVD with those that did not	PVD was a predictor of poor long-term survival among pts undergoing CABG surgery
Chu	2009	63,047	Pts who underwent on-pump CABG surgery or off-pump surgery	Compare outcomes of on-pump CABG surgery versus off-pump surgery	Off-pump did not produce lower mortality or stroke rates when compared to on-pump. Off-pump was associated with longer hospital stays and higher hospital costs

Table 1. Review of Research Reporting Predictors of Outcomes Following Coronary Artery Bypass Grafting Surgery

Author	Year	Sample Size	Sample Characteristics	Primary Outcome	Result
Dao	2010b	63,061	Pts who underwent CABG surgery	Compare outcomes and examine relationships between depression and geographic status following CABG surgery	Rural pts were more likely than urban pts to have a depression diagnosis Depression was a predictor of mortality and length of stay following CABG surgery Rural pts had increased lengths of hospital stays and increased mortality rates when compared to urban pts
Dao	2010c	62,665	Pts who underwent CABG surgery	Examine relationship between depression and PTSD on outcomes following CABG surgery	Depression and PTSD were prevalent in pts undergoing CABG surgery Depression and PTSD (and in combination) increased the risk of mortality as well as physical health risk factors following CABG surgery
Dao	2011a	100	Pts who were scheduled for CABG surgery	Examine the efficacy of a brief CBT for pts prior to CABG surgery	The intervention improved depressive and anxiety symptoms and quality of life and reduced length of hospital stay
Dao	2011b	65	Pts who underwent CABG surgery	Examine the efficacy of HRV biofeedback treatment for patients with PTSD prior to CABG surgery	HRV biofeedback training results in improvement in PTSD symptoms in patients undergoing CABG surgery, improves the quality of life, and decreases the length of hospital stay
Dao	2011c	17,885	Rural pts who underwent CABG surgery	Examine the effect of and anxiety and gender on outcomes following CABG surgery	Anxiety disorders are prevalent in rural patients who are undergoing a CABG operation Anxiety was a significant independent predictor of both length of hospital stay and non-routine discharge for patients receiving CABG surgery Females with an anxiety disorder seemed to have more aversive outcomes than males with an anxiety disorder

Table 1. Review of Research Reporting Predictors of Outcomes Following Coronary Artery Bypass Grafting Surgery (continuation)

Author	Year	Sample Size	Sample Characteristics	Primary Outcome	Result
Gopaldas	2009	5,731	Pts who were > 80 years of age that underwent CABG surgery	To examine outcomes and predictors of discharge status in pts> 80 years of age	27% were referred to home health care, 45% were transferred to another facility, 21% had normal discharge While those older than 80 years of age have acceptable mortality risk, these pts require further specialized care at discharge
Gopaldas	2010	614,177	Pts who underwent CABG surgery	Compare outcomes pre-work reform versus post-work reform	Work-hour reform did not affect mortality rates Work-hour reform was associated with increased morbidity
Mahoney	2011	51,266	Pts who were > 80 years of age that underwent CABG surgery	Investigate whether anxiety/depression mediates the relationship between age and outcomes following CABG surgery	Anxiety/depression diagnosis actsas a mediator through which age influences mortality and patient discharge status

Table 1. Review of Research Reporting Predictors of Outcomes Following Coronary Artery Bypass Grafting Surgery (continuation)

6. References

Alexander KP, Anstrom KJ, Muhlbaier LH, et al. Outcomes of cardiac surgery in patients 80 years: results from the National Cardiovascular Network. J Am CollCardiol 2000;35:731–8.

Appelhans BM, Luecken LJ: Heart rate variability as an index of regulated emotional responding. Review of General Psychology 2006, 10:229-240.

Bankier B, Januzzi JL, Littman AB: The high prevalence of psychiatric disorders in stable outpatients with coronary heart disease. Psychosom Med 2004, 66:645-650.

Barnes RF, Veith RC, Borson S, Verhey J, Raskind MA, Halter JB: High levels of plasma catecholamines in dexamethasone-resistant depressed patients. Am J Psychiat 1983, 140:1623-1625.

Barnett E, Halverson JA, Elmes GA, et al. Metropolitan and non-metropolitan trends in coronary heart disease mortality within Appalachia, 1980–1997. Ann Epidemiol. 2000;10(6):370-379.

Baslaim G, Bashore J, Alhoroub K. Impact of obesity on early outcomes after cardiac surgery: Experience in a Saudi Arabian center. Ann ThoracCardiovascSurg 2008;14:369.

Beekman A, Breemer M, Deeg D, et al. Anxiety disorder in later life: a report from the longitudinal aging study Amsterdam. International Journal of Geriatric Psychiatry. 1998; 13:717-726.

Benetti FJ, Ballester C, Sani G, Doonstra P, Grandjean J. Video assisted coronary bypass surgery. J Card Surg 1995;10:620–5.

Berkman LF, Blumenthal J, Burg M, Carney RM, Catellier D, Cowan MJ, Czajkowski SM, DeBusk R, Hosking J, Jaffe A, Kaufmann PG, Mitchell P, Norman J, Powell LH, Raczynski JM, Schneiderman N. Effects of treating depression and lo perceived social support on clinical events after myocardial infarction: the Enhancing Recovery in Coronary Heart Disease Patients (ENRICHD) Randomized Trial. JAMA 2003;289:3106-3116.

Blankstein R, Ward R, Arnsdorf M, Jones B, Lou Y, Pine M. Female gender is an independent predictor of operative mortality after coronary artery bypass graft surgery: contemporary analysis of 31 Midwestern hospitals. *Circulation* [serial online]. August 30, 2005;112(9 Suppl):I323-I327. Available from: MEDLINE, Ipswich, MA. Accessed January 31, 2011.

Blumenthal JA, Lett HS, Babyak MA, White W, Smith PK, Mark DB, Jones R, Matthew JP, Newman MF: Depression as a risk factor for mortality after coronary artery bypass surgery. Lancet 2003, 362:604-609.

Bornstein MH, Suess PE (2000) Physiological self-regulation and information processing in infancy: cardiac vagal tone and habituation. Child Dev 71: 273-87

Brandt M, Harder K, Walluscheck KP, Fraund S, Boning A, Cremer J. Coronary artery bypass surgery in diabetic patients. J Card Surg 2004;19:36 - 40.

Buffolo E, de Andrade CS, Branco JN, Teles CA, Aguiar LF, Gomes WJ. Coronary artery bypass grafting without cardiopulmonary bypass. Ann ThoracSurg 1996;61:63 –6.

Bull DA, Neumayer LA, Stringham JC, Meldrum P, Affleck DG, Karwande SV. Coronary artery bypass grafting with cardiopulmonary bypass versus off-pump cardiopulmonary bypass grafting: does eliminating the pump reduce morbidity and cost? Ann ThoracSurg 2001;71:170 –3; discussion 3–5.

Burg MM, Benedetto C, Rosenberg R, et al. Presurgical depression predicts medical morbidity 6 months after coronary artery bypass graft surgery. Psychosom Med. 2003a;65:111-8.

Burg MM, Benedetto C, Soufer R. Depressive symptoms and mortality two years after coronary artery bypass graft surgery (CABG) in men. Psychosom Med. 2003b;65:508-10.

Calafiore AM, Angelini GD, Bergsland J, Salerno TA. Minimally invasive coronary artery bypass grafting. Ann ThoracSurg 1996;62:1545– 8.

Carney RM, Rich MW, teVelde A, Saini J, Clark K, Freedland KE: Heart rate, heart rate variability and depression in patients with coronary artery disease. J Psychosom Res 1988a, 32:159-164.

Carney RM, Rich MW, Freedland KE, teVelde A, Saini J, Simeone C, Clark K: Major depressive disorder predicts cardiac events in patients with coronary artery disease. Psychosom Med 1988b 50:627-633.

Centers for Disease Control and Prevention (CDC).Web-based injury statistics query and reporting system (WISQARS).National Center for Injury Prevention and Control, CDC (producer). Available at: www.cdc.gov/ncipc/wisqar/default. htm. Accessed Dec 3, 2009.

Centers for Disease Control and Prevention. Profiling the leading causes of death in the united states. 2005. Available at: www.medicaid.alabama.gov/...807/Alabama_Top_Chronic_Disease.pdf.Accessed October 02, 2010.

Cheng DC, Bainbridge D, Martin JE, Novick RJ. Does off pump coronary artery bypass reduce mortality, morbidity, and resource utilization when compared with conventional coronary artery bypass? A meta-analysis of randomized trials. Anesthesiology 2005;102:188 -203.

Cheng W, Denton TA, Fontana GP, et al. Off-pump coronary surgery: effect on early mortality and stroke. J Thorac CardiovascSurg 2002;124:313–20.

Chu DC, Bakaeen FG, Dao TK, LeMaire SA, Coselli JS, Huh J. On-Pump Versus Off-Pump Coronary Artery Bypass Grafting in a Cohort of 63,000 Patients. (Ann ThoracSurg 2009a;87:1820–7)

Chu D, Bakaeen, FG, Wang, XL, Dao TK. The Impact of Peripheral Vascular Disease on Long-Term Survival After Coronary Artery Bypass Graft Surgery. Ann ThoracSurg 2008;86:1175- 80

Connerney I, Shapiro PA, McLaughlin JS, Bagiella E, Sloan RP: Relation between depression after coronary artery bypass surgery and 12-month outcome: A prospective study. Lancet 2001, 358:1766-1771.

Cooper R, Cutler J, Desvigne-Nickens P, et al. Trends and disparities in coronary heart disease, stroke, and other cardiovascular disease in the United States: findings of the national conference on cardiovascular disease prevention. Circulation. 2000;102:3137-3147. Available at: http://circ.ahajournals.org/cgi/reprint/102/25/3137. Accessed April 20, 2009.

Culler S, Simon A, Brown P, Kugelmass A, Reynolds M, Rask K. Sex differences in hospital risk-adjusted mortality rates for medicare beneficiaries undergoing CABG surgery. *Archives of Internal Medicine* [serial online]. November 24, 2008; 168(21):2317-2322. Available from: Academic Search Complete, Ipswich, MA. Accessed January 31, 2011.

Dallack GW, Roose SP: Perspectives on the relationship between cardiovascular disease and affective disorder. Clin Psychiat 1990, 51:4-9.

Dao TK, Youssef NA, Gopaldas RR, Armsworth M, Wear E, Papathopoulos KN. Randomized Controlled Trial of Brief Cognitive Behavioral Intervention for Depression and Anxiety Symptoms Preoperatively in Patients Undergoing Coronary Artery Bypass Graft Surgery. The Journal of Thoracic and Cardiovascular Surgery (2011a) in press.

Dao TK, Mahoney JJ. Huddleston C, Wear-Shum, E, Bannister JA, Voelkel EA, Gevirtz, R.Heart Rate Variability (HRV) Intervention for Post Traumatic Stress Disorder (PTSD) Symptoms Preoperatively in Patients Undergoing Coronary Artery Bypass Graft Surgery. (2011b)

Dao TK, Voelkel EA, Presley S, Doss B, Huddleston C, Gopaldas RR. Gender as a Moderator between having an Anxiety Disorder Diagnosis and Coronary Artery Bypass Grafting Surgery (CABG) Outcomes in Rural Patients. (2011c)

Dao TK, Youssef N, Gopaldas RR, et al. Autonomic cardiovascular dysregulation as a potential mechanism underlying depression and coronary artery bypass grafting surgery outcomes. J ThoracCardiovascSurg 2010a;5:1-9.

Dao T, Chu D, Springer J, Hiatt E, Nguyen Q. Depression and geographic status as predictors for coronary artery bypass surgery outcomes. *The Journal of Rural Health* [serial online].2010b;26(1):36-43. Available from: PsycINFO, Ipswich, MA. Accessed January 31, 2011.

Dao TK, Chu D, Springer J, et al. Clinical depression, posttraumatic stress disorder, and comorbid depression and posttraumatic stress disorder as risk factors for in-hospital mortality after coronary artery bypass grafting surgery. J Thorac Cardiovasc Surg 2010c;140:606-10.

Del Prete JC, Bakaeen FG, Dao TK, Huh J, LeMaire SA, Coselli JS, Chu D. The Impact of Obesity on Long-term Survival AfterCoronaryArtery Bypass Grafting. Journal of Surgical Research 163, 7–11 (2010)

Dewey TM, Magee MJ, Edgerton JR, Mathison M, Tennison D, Mack MJ. Off-pump bypass grafting is safe in patients with left main coronary disease. Ann ThoracSurg 2001;72: 788 –91; discussion 92.

Doerfler LA, Pbert L, DeCosimo D (1994) Symptoms of posttraumatic stress disorder following myocardial infarction and coronary artery bypass surgery. Gen Hosp Psychiatry 16: 193-9

Doering LV, Moser DK, Lemankiewicz W, Luper C, Khan S (2005) Depression, healing, and recovery from coronary artery bypass surgery. Am J Crit Care 14: 316-24

Eagle KA, Rihal CS, Foster ED, Mickel MC, Gersh BJ. Long-term survival in patients with coronary artery disease: importance of peripheral vascular disease. The Coronary Artery Surgery Study (CASS) Investigators. J Am CollCardiol 1994; 23:1091–5.

Edmunds LH Jr, Hessel EA 2nd, Colman RW, Menasche P, Hammon JW Jr. Extracorporeal circulation. In: Cohn LH, Edmunds LH, eds. Cardiac surgery in the adult. New York: McGraw-Hill, Medical Pub Division; 2003:315– 87.

Engel AM, McDonough S, Smith JM. Does an obese body mass index affect hospital outcomes after coronary artery bypass graft surgery? Ann ThoracSurg 2009;88:1793.

Engelman DT, Adams DH, Byrne JG, et al. Impact of body mass index and albumin on morbidity and mortality after cardiac surgery. J ThoracCardiovascSurg 1999;118:866.

Esler M, Turbott J, Schwarz R, Leonard P, Bobik A, Skews H, Jackman K: The peripheral kinetics of norepiniphrine in depressive illness. Arch Gen Psychiatry 1982, 39:285-300.

Fontaine KR, Redden DT, Wang C, et al. Years of life lost due to obesity. JAMA 2003;289: 187.

Freedland KE, Skala JA, Carney RM, Rubin EH, Lustman PJ, Davila-Roman VG, et al. Treatment of depression after coronary artery bypass surgery. Arch Gen Psychiatry 2009a;66:387-96.

Freedland KE, Skala JA, Carney RM, Rubin EH, Lustman PJ, Davila-Roman VG, et al. Treatment of depression after coronary artery bypass surgery: a randomized controlled trial. Arch Gen Psychiatry 2009b;66:387-96.

Gamm L, Hutchison L, Bellamy G, Dabney BJ. Rural healthy people 2010: identifying rural health priorities and models for practice. J Rural Health. 2002;18(1):9-14.

Gersh BJ, Califf RM, Loop FD, Akins CW, Pryor DB, Takaro TC.Coronary bypass surgery in chronic stable angina. Circulation 1989;79:I46 –59.

Gopaldas RR, Chu D, Dao TK, Huh J, LeMaire, SA, Coselli, JS, Bakaeen FG.Predictors of surgical mortality and discharge status after coronary artery bypass grafting in patients 80 years and older. The American Journal of Surgery (2009) 198, 633–638.

Grover FL, Hammermeister KE, Burchfiel C. Initial report of the Veterans Administration Preoperative Risk Assessment Study for Cardiac Surgery. Ann ThoracSurg 1990;50:12–26.

Guinjoan SM, Bernabó JL, Cardinali DP: Cardiovascular tests of autonomic function and sympathetic skin responses in patients with major depression. NeurolNeurosur Ps 1995, 58:299-302.

Güler M, Kirali K, Toker ME, et al. Different CABG methods in patients with chronic obstructive pulmonary disease. Ann ThoracSurg 2001;71:152–7.

Guru V, Glasgow KW, Fremes SE, Austin PC, Teoh K, Tu JV.The real-world outcomes of off-pump coronary artery bypass surgery in a public health care system. Can J Cardiol 2007;23:281– 6.

Halkos ME, Puskas JD, Lattouf OM, Kilgo P, Guyton RA, Thourani VH. Impact of preoperative neurologic events on outcomes after coronary artery bypass grafting. Ann ThoracSurg 2008;86:504 –10; discussion 10.

Healthcare Cost Utilization Project, Nationwide Inpatient Sample (NIS). Rockville, MD: Agency for Healthcare Research and Quality; 2001.

Hertzer NR, Beven EG, Young JR, et al. Coronary artery disease in peripheral vascular patients: a classification of 1000 coronary angiograms and results of surgical management. Ann Surg 1984;199:223–33.

Higgins TL, Estafanous FG, Loop FD, Beck GJ, Blum JM, Paranandi L. Stratification of morbidity and mortality outcome by preoperative risk factors in coronary artery bypass patients: a clinical severity score. JAMA 1992;267:2344 - 8.

Januzzi Jr. J, Stern T. The influence of anxiety and depression on outcomes of patients with coronary artery disease. *Archives of Internal Medicine* [serial online]. July 10, 2000;160(13):1913. Available from: Academic Search Complete, Ipswich, MA. Accessed January 31, 2011.

Johnson W, Pedraza P, Kayser K. Coronary artery surgery in diabetics: 261 consecutive patients followed 4 - 7 years. Am Heart J 1982; 104:823-827

Khan NE, De Souza A, Mister R, et al. A randomized comparison of off-pump and on-pump multivessel coronary-artery bypass surgery. N Engl J Med 2004;350:21 –8.

Kim C, Redberg R, Pavlic T, Eagle K. A systematic review of gender differences in mortality after coronary artery bypass graft surgery and percutaneous coronary interventions. *Clinical Cardiology* [serial online]. October 2007;30(10):491-495. Available from: MEDLINE, Ipswich, MA. Accessed January 31, 2011.

Kolh P, Kerzmann A, Lahaye L, et al. Cardiac surgery in octogenarians: peri-operative outcome and long-term results. Eur Heart J 2001; 22:1235–43.

Krannich JA, Weyers P, Lueger S, Herzog M, Bohrer T, Elert O: Presence of depression and anxiety before and after coronary artery bypass graft surgery and their relationship to age. BMC Psychiatry 2007, 7:1-6.

Krittayaphong R, Cascio WE, Light KC, Sheffield D, Golden RN, Finkel JB, Gleskas G, Koch GG, Sheps DS: Heart rate variability in patients with coronary artery disease: differences in patients with higher and lower depression scores. Psychosom Med 1997, 59:231-235.

Kunadian B, Dunning J, Millner RW. Modifiable risk factors remain significant causes of medium term mortality after first time coronary artery bypass grafting. J CardiothoracSurg 2007;2:51.

Lake CR, Pickar D, Ziegler MG, Lipper S, Slater S, Murphy DL: High plasma NE levels in patients with major affective disorder. Am J Psychiat 1982, 139:1315-1318.

Lawrie G, Morris GJ, Glaeser D. Influences of diabetes mellitus on the results of coronary artery bypass surgery. Follow-up of 212 diabetic patients ten to 15 years after surgery. JAMA 1986; 256: 2967-2971

Levin A. Depression, heart disease: links remains elusive. Psychiat News 2005;40:33-35.

Lie I, Arnesen H, Sandvik L, Hamilton G, Bunch EH. Effects of a home-based intervention program on anxiety and depression 6 months after coronary artery bypass grafting: a randomized controlled trial. J Psychosom Res 2007;62:411-8.

Lloyd-Jones D, Adams R, Wylie-Rosett J, et al. Heart disease and stroke statistics--2010 update: a report from the American Heart Association. *Circulation* [serial online]. February 23, 2010;121(7):e46-e215. Available from: MEDLINE, Ipswich, MA. Accessed January 31, 2011.

Lyons D, McLoughlin DM. Recent advances: psychiatry. BMJ. 2001;323: 1228-31.

Magee MJ, Dewey TM, Acuff T, et al. Influence of diabetes on mortality and morbidity: off-pump coronary artery bypass grafting versus coronary artery bypass grafting with cardiopulmonary bypass. Ann ThoracSurg 2001;72:776–80; discussion 80–1.

Magovern JA, Sakert T, Magovern GJ, et al. A model that predicts morbidity and mortality after coronary artery bypass graft surgery. J Am CollCardiol 1996;28:1147–53.

Mahoney JJ, Dao, TK, Voelkel EA, Bannister, JA, Gopaldas RR. Anxiety and Depressive Symptoms Mediate the Relationship between Age and Outcomes following Coronary Artery Bypass Grafting Surgery.Submitted to Journal of Cardio and Thoras Surg. (2011).

Marasco SF, Sharwood LN, Abramson MJ. No improvement in neurocognitive outcomes after off-pump versus on-pump coronary revascularisation: a meta-analysis. Eur JCardiothoracSurg 2008;33:961–70.

McCrone S, Cotton S, Jones L, Hawkins T, Constante J, Nuss M. Depression in a rural, free clinic providing Primary care: prevalence and predictive factors. Arch PsychiatrNurs. 2007;21(5):291-293.

Miller SS, Stokes CS, Clifford WB. A comparison of the rural-urban mortality differential for deaths from all causes, cardiovascular disease and cancer. J Rural Health. 1987;3(2):23-34.

Mokdad AH, Marks JS, Stroup DF, et al. Actual causes of death in the United States, 2000. JAMA 2004;291:1238.

Morrow DA, Gersh BJ.Chronic coronary artery disease. In: Libby P, Braunwald E, eds. Braunwald's heartdisease: atextbook of cardiovascular medicine. Philadelphia: Saunders/Elsevier; 2008:1353- 417.

Niles NW, McGrath PD, Malenka D, et al. Survival of patients with diabetes and multivessel coronary artery disease after surgical or percutaneous coronary revascularization: results of a large regional prospective study. Northern New England Cardiovascular Disease Study Group. J Am CollCardiol 2001;37:1008 –15.

O'Connor GT, Plume SK, Olmstead EM, et al. Multivariate prediction of in-hospital mortality associated with coronary artery bypass graft surgery. Northern New England Cardiovascular Disease Study Group. Circulation 1992; 85: 2110 –8.

Oxlad M, Stubberfield J, Stuklis R, Edwards J, Wade TD: Psychological risk factors for cardiac-related hospital readmission within 6 months of coronary artery bypass graft surgery. Psychosom Res 2006, 61:775-781.

Oxlad M, Stubberfield J, Stuklis R, Edwards J, Wade TD (2006) Psychological risk factors for increased post-operative length of hospital stay following coronary artery bypass graft surgery. J Behav Med 29: 179-90

Oxlad M, Wade TD (2006) Application of a chronic illness model as a means of understanding pre-operative psychological adjustment in coronary artery bypass graft patients. Br J Health Psychol 11: 401-19

Pearson TA, Lewis C. Rural epidemiology: insights from a rural population laboratory. Am J Epidemiol. 1998;148(10):949-957.

Potapov EV, Loebe M, Anker S, et al. Impact of body mass index on outcome in patients after coronary artery bypass grafting with and without valve surgery. Eur Heart J 2003; 24:1933.

Prabhakar G, Haan CK, Peterson ED, et al. The risks of moderate and extreme obesity for coronary artery bypass grafting outcomes: A study from the Society of Thoracic Surgeons' database. Ann ThoracSurg 2002;74:1125.

Puskas JD, Wright CE, Ronson RS, Brown WM 3rd, Gott JP, Guyton RA. Off-pump multivessel coronary bypass via sternotomy is safe and effective. Ann ThoracSurg 1998;66:1068–72.

Puskas JD, Thourani VH, Marshall JJ, et al. Clinical outcomes, angiographic patency, and resource utilization in 200 consecutive off-pump coronary bypass patients. Ann ThoracSurg 2001;71:1477- 83; discussion 83- 4.

Puskas JD, Williams WH, Mahoney EM, et al. Off-pump vs conventional coronary artery bypass grafting: early and 1-year graft patency, cost, and quality-of-life outcomes: a randomized trial. JAMA 2004;291:1841–9.

Rahmanian PB, Adams DH, Castillo JG, et al. Impact of body mass index on early outcome and late survival in patients undergoing coronary artery bypass grafting or valve surgery or both. Am J Cardiol 2007;100:1702.

Rechlin T: Are affective disorders associated with alterations of heart rate variability? Affective Disorders 1994, 32:1-5.

Reeves BC, Ascione R, Chamberlain MH, et al. Effect of body mass index on early outcomes in patients undergoing coronary artery bypass surgery. J Am CollCardiol 2003;42:668.

Rollman BL, Belnap BH, LeMenager MS, Mazumdar S, Houck PR, Counihan PJ, et al. Telephone-delivered collaborative care for treating post-CABG depression: a randomized controlled trial. JAMA 2009;302:2095-2103.

Rothenhausler HB, Stepan A, Hetterle R, Trantina-Yates A [The effects of coronary artery bypass graft surgery on health-related quality of life, cognitive performance, and emotional status outcomes: a prospective 6-month follow-up consultation-liaison psychiatry study]. FortschrNeurolPsychiatr 78: 343-54

Rosenthal GE, Vaughan Sarrazin M, Hannan EL. In-hospital mortality following coronary artery bypass graft surgery in Veterans Health Administration and private sector hospitals. Med Care 2003;41:522–35.

Rozanski A, Blumenthal J, Kaplan J. Impact of psychological factors on the pathogenesis of cardiovascular disease and implications for therapy. *Circulation* [serial online]. April 27, 1999; 99(16):2192-2217. Available from: MEDLINE, Ipswich, MA. Accessed January 31, 2011.

Rumsfeld JS, Ho M. Depression and cardiovascular disease. Circulation 2005;111:250-253.

Rymaszewska J, Kiejna A, Hadryś T. Depression and anxiety in coronary artery bypass grafting patients. *European Psychiatry* [serial online]. June 2003;18(4):155. Available from: Academic Search Complete, Ipswich, MA. Accessed January 31, 2011.

Sabik JF, Gillinov AM, Blackstone EH, et al. Does off-pump coronary surgery reduce morbidity and mortality? J ThoracCardiovascSurg 2002;124:698 –707.

Salomon, N, Page U, Okies, J et al. Diabetes mellitus and cornonaryarter bypass. Short term risk and long term prognosis. J ThoracCardiovascSurg 1983; 85:264-271

Saur C, Granger BB, Muhlbaier H, et al. Depressive symptoms and outcome of coronary artery bypass grafting. Am J Crit Care. 2001;10:4-10.

Sawatzky J, Naimark B. The coronary artery bypass graft surgery trajectory: Gender differences revisited. *European Journal of Cardiovascular Nursing* [serial online]. October 2009;8(4):302-308. Available from: Academic Search Complete, Ipswich, MA. Accessed January 31, 2011.

Schwann TA, Habib RH, Zacharias A, et al. Effects of body size on operative, intermediate, and long-term outcomes after coronary artery bypass operation. Ann ThoracSurg 2001;71:521.

Scott A. LeMaire, MD, Joseph S. Coselli, MD, and Joseph Huh, MD (Ann ThoracSurg 2008;86:1175– 80)

Shigemitsu O, Hadama T, Miyamoto S, et al. Early and long-term results of cardiovascular surgery in octogenarians. Ann ThoracCardiovascSurg 2001;7:223–31.

Shirzad M, Karimi A, Armadi SH, et al. Effects of body mass in dex on early outcome of coronary artery bypass surgery. Minerva Chir 2009;64:17.

Siever L, Davis K: Overview: Toward a dysregulation hypothesis of depression. Am J Psychiat 1985, 142:1017-1031.

Spencer G. Projections of the population of the United States, by age, sex, and race: 1988 to 2080. Current Population Reports Series P-25. Washington, DC: US Department of Commerce, Bureau of the Census; 1989:1-18.

Stein PE, Carney RM, Freedland KE, Skala JA, Kleiger RE, Rottman JN: Severe depression is associated with markedly reduced heart rate variability in patients with stable coronary heart disease. Psychosom Res 2000, 48:493-500.

Stengrevics S, Sirois C, Schwartz C, Friedman R. The prediction of cardiac surgery outcome based upon preoperative psychological factors. *Psychology & Health* [serial online]. June 1996;11(4):471-477. Available from: PsycINFO, Ipswich, MA. Accessed January 31, 2011.

Stoney C. Gender and cardiovascular disease: a psychobiological and integrative approach. *Current Directions in Psychological Science* (Wiley-Blackwell) [serial online]. August 2003;12(4):129. Available from: Academic Search Complete, Ipswich, MA. Accessed January 31, 2011.

Sutton-Tyrrell K, Rihal C, Sellers MA, et al. Long-term prognostic value of clinically evident noncoronary vascular disease in patients undergoing coronary revascularization in the Bypass Angioplasty Revascularization Investigation (BARI). Am J Cardiol 1998;81:375– 81.

Syrakas CA, Neumaier-Prauser P, Angelis I, et al. Is extreme obesity a risk factor for increased in-hospital mortality and post-operative morbidity after cardiac surgery? Results of 2251 obese patients with BMI of 30 to 50.ThoracCardiovascSurg 2007; 55:491.

Takagi H, Tanabashi T, Kawai N, Umemoto T. Off-pump surgery does not reduce stroke, compared with results of on-pump coronary artery bypass grafting: a meta-analysis of randomized clinical trials. J ThoracCardiovascSurg 2007; 134:1059 -60.

Tan G, Dao TK, Farmer L, Sutherland RJ, Gevirtz R (2010) Heart Rate Variability (HRV) and Posttraumatic Stress Disorder (PTSD): A Pilot Study. ApplPsychophysiol Biofeedback

Task Force of the European Society of Cardiology and the North American Society for Pacing and Electrophysiology. Circulation 1995, 93:1043-1065.

Trehan N, Mishra M, Sharma OP, Mishra A, Kasliwal RR. Further reduction in stroke after off-pump coronary artery bypass grafting: a 10-year experience. Ann ThoracSurg 2001;72:S1026 –32.

Tully PJ, Baker RA, Knight JL: Anxiety and depression as risk factors for mortality after coronary artery bypass surgery. Psychosom Res 2008, 64:285-290.

van der Kolk BA (2006) Clinical implications of neuroscience research in PTSD. Ann N Y AcadSci 1071: 277-93.

Veith RC, Lewis N, Linares OA, Barnes RF, Raskind MA, Villacres EC, Murburg MM, Ashleigh EA, Castillo S, Peskind ER, Pascualy M, Halter JB: Sympathetic nervous system activity in major depression. Arch Gen Psychiatry 1994, 51:411-422.

Wallace A, Weeks W, Wang S, Lee A, Kazis L. Rural and urban disparities in health-related quality of life among veterans with psychiatric disorders. Psychiatr Serv. 2006;57(6):851-856.

5

Surgical Ventricular Restoration for Ischemic Cardiomyopathy with Functional Mitral Regurgitation

Masanori Hirota, Shintaro Katahira, Joji Hoshino, Yasuhisa Fukada, Taichi Kondo, Takayuki Gyoten, Yuichi Notomi and Tadashi Isomura
Department of Cardiovascular Surgery, Hayama Heart Center, Kanagawa, Japan

1. Introduction

Ischemic cardiomyopathy (ICM) is defined as diffuse akinesis of the ventricle after myocardial ischemia[1)]. A subset of patients with ICM develop progressive heart failure as a consequence of adverse left ventricular (LV) remodeling, leading to a depressed ejection fraction, a dilated LV, a large akinetic region of the myocardium, an abnormal globular shape to the ventricular chamber, and functional mitral regurgitation (MR)[2-5)]. Although a dilated LV with poor cardiac function is a risk by itself, coexisting functional MR worsens the prognosis of ICM[6,7)]. Thus, for patients with ICM and functional MR, it is very important to repair the geometric changes of LV remodeling and to decrease the extent of functional MR.

For patients with ICM, surgical ventricular restoration (SVR) is an established treatment to reduce ventricular size and restore the elliptical shape of the LV[8-12)]. Anatomical restoration by SVR may decrease the severity of MR, through various mechanisms, including reduction of ventricular dimensions, lowering of end systolic volumes, and restoration of blood flow to the ischemic region of the mitral subvalvular apparatus[13,14)]. However, concomitant procedures for the mitral valve are required for further reduction of functional MR. In this chapter, our therapeutic strategy for patients with ICM is demonstrated, and we describe the details of the surgical techniques of SVR and mitral valve surgery.

2. Patients

Between May 2000 and May 2010, SVR was performed in 335 patients with ICM (n=199) and non-ischemic cardiomyopathy (n=136). Of the 199 patients with ICM, 88 had concomitant mitral valve surgery for functional MR.

These patients with ICM and functional MR included 77 males and 11 females, ranging in age from 32 to 83 years (mean, 61±10 years). The preoperative New York Heart Association (NYHA) functional class was class III for 55% (48/88) and class IV for 45% (40/88). Preoperative heart failure was medically controlled with inotropes in 34 patients (39%), and 2 of these patients (2%) required intra-aortic balloon pumping (IABP). Due to uncontrollable heart failure and worsening multiorgan failure, an emergent operation was performed in 12 patients (14%).

3. Materials and methods

3.1 Assessment of cardiac geometry and regional function of the LV

Two-dimensional echocardiography was used to evaluate cardiac geometry, including dimensions and LV volume, valvular morphology, and the subvalvular apparatus. As indices of LV volume, the LV end-systolic and end-diastolic volume indices (LVESVI and LVEDVI) were calculated.

Regional LV function was examined by cardiac magnetic resonance imaging (MRI)[15,16] and color kinesis echocardiography[17]. Regional LV strain was assessed by speckle-tracking echocardiography under normal and dobutamine-stress conditions[18].

a. Cardiac MRI

Cardiac MRI is a medical imaging technology for the non-invasive assessment of cardiac structure and function. Although it shows the precise myocardial anatomy in normal hearts, it is also useful for post-ischemic myocardial assessment[15,16]. To investigate LV wall motion, MRI images were obtained by cine acquisition. The depth and extension of the scarred LV wall were evaluated with 4 MRI projections. The 4-chamber view was used to assess the septum and lateral wall. The 2-chamber view (the vertical long-axis view) was useful for the anterior and posterior walls of the LV. The 3-chamber view (the LV outflow tract view) provided a detailed analysis of the mitral subvalvular apparatus. The short-axis view enabled a staged analysis of the septum and papillary muscles. Late gadolinium enhancement was also performed to investigate the irreversible myocardium of the LV wall[19].

b. Color kinesis echocardiography

Color kinesis is a non-invasive technology for the echocardiographic assessment of LV wall motion based on acoustic quantification[17]. This technique automatically detects endocardial motion in real time using integrated backscatter data to identify pixel transitions from blood to tissue during systole on a frame-by-frame basis. We have reported the usefulness of intra-operative color kinesis echocardiography under cardiopulmonary bypass (CPB) assist for patients with idiopathic dilated cardiomyopathy[20]. LV wall motion was observed by direct vision of the cardiac echogram (HP SONO 5500; Agilent Technologies, Palo Alto, CA, USA) under different preloads controlled by CPB (volume reduction test). The objective of this test was to assess the akinetic region of the LV wall for SVR.

c. Speckle-tracking echocardiography

Speckle-tracking echocardiography is a unique imaging technique that analyzes multidirectional components of LV deformation within an ultrasonic window by tracking interference patterns and natural acoustic reflections[21]. The tracking system is obtained by automatic measurement of the distance between 2 pixels of an LV segment during the cardiac cycle, independent of the angle of insonation[22,23].

Echocardiography was carried out using a Vivid 7 ultrasonography machine (GE Medical Systems, Milwaukee, WI, USA) with an M3S probe. Short-axis images from the mid-level (i.e., papillary muscle level) of the LV were obtained from the parasternal window to assess myocardial segmental viability and LV dyssynchrony. Caution was exercised to ensure short-axis images with circular cross-sections and minimal out-of-plane movement. Short-axis images were analyzed by the EchoPAC platform (2DS software package, version 7; GE Medical Systems), which uses a speckle-tracking technique to derive rotation and strain for selected regions of the myocardium[24)]. LV torsion is also calculated automatically from the LV basal and apical rotation data in the platform. For assessing segmental myocardial viability, the myocardial region obtained from the short-axis images of the midlevel LV was divided into four segments (septal, anterolateral, posterior, inferoseptal), and the circumferential strain profile was analyzed, which is closely related to myocardial viability[25,26)].

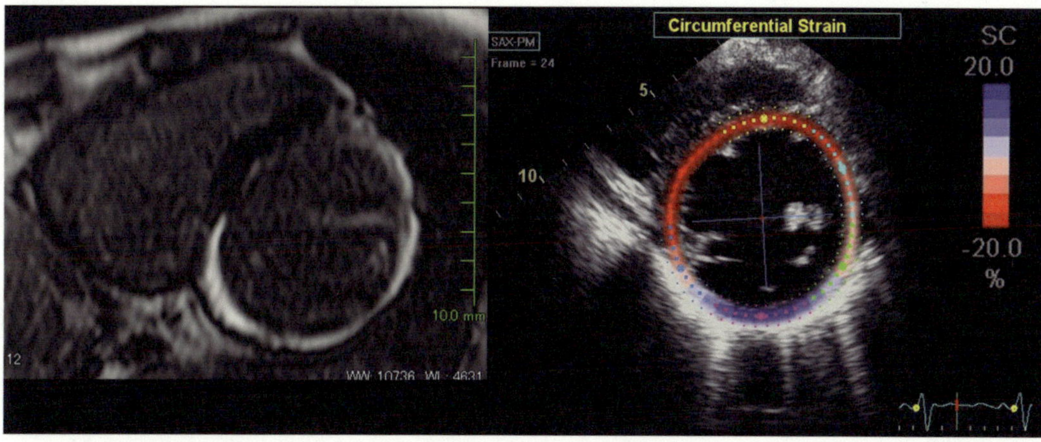

Fig. 1. Late gadolinium enhancement of cardiac magnetic resonance imaging (in the left panel) and two-dimensional speckle-tracking echocardiographic imaging (in the right panel) in a representative case with ischemic cardiomyopathy. Severe ischemic injury and a suggestion of fibrotic change (a tissue characteristic) are depicted in the lateral, posterior, and inferoseptal segments by late gadolinium enhancement, while end-systolic circumferential strain of speckle-tracking echocardiographic imaging detected nearly +20% lengthening at the posterior region only (shown as dark blue). Two-dimensional speckle-tracking echocardiography could identify such transmurally injured "dyskinetic scars" (a mechanodynamic myocardial property), which is critically important in ventricular restoration tactics.

d. Prediction of the non-functional akinetic region of the LV

Using these results, the exclusion area of non-functional myocardium for SVR was predicted preoperatively. A representative case with ICM is shown in **Fig. 1**. On the left side, late gadolinium enhancement of cardiac MRI demonstrated regional stains on the endocardium in the lateral, posterior, and infero-septal segments. On the right side, two-dimensional speckle-tracking echocardiography revealed LV torsion at the corresponding short-axis slice level seen on cardiac MRI. Severe ischemic injury and suggestions of fibrotic change (a tissue characteristic) were depicted by cardiac MRI, while end-systolic circumferential strain of speckle-tracking echocardiographic imaging detected nearly +20% lengthening at the posterior region only (shown as dark blue). Thus, two-dimensional speckle-tracking echocardiography could identify such transmurally injured "dyskinetic scars" (a mechanodynamic myocardial property), which are critically important in ventricular restoration tactics.

3.2 Technical details of our three SVR procedures for ICM

Surgical resection is the oldest and simplest technique for LV aneurysm following myocardial infarction. At the end of the 1970s, SVR with patchplasty had been reported for the posterior and anterior regions of the LV[27,28]. In 1980s, Dor and associates established a new surgical technique with a circular patch (endoventricular circular patch plasty; EVCCP) for antero-septo-apical aneurysms[29]. Around the same time, Cooley reported ventricular endoaneurysmorrhaphy with an elliptical patch to allow prompt recovery and restoration of ventricular function[30]. As Hutchins and coworkers suggested the importance of cardiac geometry after SVR, cardiac surgeons modified their technique to obtain a postoperative elliptical shape of the LV[31]. Recently, we have developed new techniques of septal anterior ventricular exclusion (SAVE) for the anterior wall of the LV and a posterior restoration procedure (PRP) for the posterior wall in patients with dilated cardiomyopathy[8,24]. We performed SVR with three different procedures (EVCPP, SAVE, and PRP) for patients with ICM, and the details of our modified techniques are described below.

a. Modified endoventricular circular patch plasty (EVCPP)

The presence of an antero-septo-apical akinetic region is a good indication for EVCPP, as reported by Dor and coworkers[29]. At first, coronary revascularization was completely performed under blood cardioplegic cardiac arrest. Valvular surgery, including mitral, tricuspid, and aortic valves, was completed prior to EVCPP. To obtain a better surgical field of the anterior LV wall, two 1-0 silk sutures were placed at the apex (**Fig. 2A**). The antero-apical LV wall was opened in the center of the akinetic region (**Fig. 2B**). When thrombus formation was detected in the LV trabeculation, it was entirely removed. The anatomical margin of the contractile myocardium around the scar, the so-called "contractility trail", was observed through the ventriculotomy. To prevent late ventricular tachycardia or fibrillation (VT/VF), cryoablation was performed on the viable LV myocardium along the junction. To plicate the circular defect of the LV muscle, 2-0 polypropylene purse-string suture (Prolene®; Ethicon, Somerville, NJ, USA) was placed around the entire circumference of the contractility trail (**Fig. 2C**). Then, a collagen-impregnated Dacron knitted fabric (MAQUET Cardiovascular LLC, Wayne, NJ, USA) (approximately 3×4 cm) was placed over the plicated defect of the myocardium and fixed with 2-0 polypropylene running suture after deaeration of the LV (**Fig. 2D**). Finally, two felt strips were placed along the ventriculotomy on each side, and the excluded external scar was folded to reinforce the suture line with 2-0 polypropylene horizontal mattress sutures with a large needle (Matsuda-ika Kogyo, Tokyo, Japan). The line was secured by double 2-0 polypropylene over-and-over sutures from both ends (**Fig. 2E**).

b. Septal anterior ventricular exclusion (SAVE)

The presence of a large antero-septal akinetic region is a good indication for SAVE or the Pacopexy technique developed by Isomura et al[8,12]. As for EVCPP, complete coronary revascularization was first preformed under blood cardioplegic arrest. Valvular surgery, including mitral, tricuspid, and aortic valves, was undertaken prior to SAVE. The aortic crossclamp was released to allow the heart to start beating, and perfusion pressure was

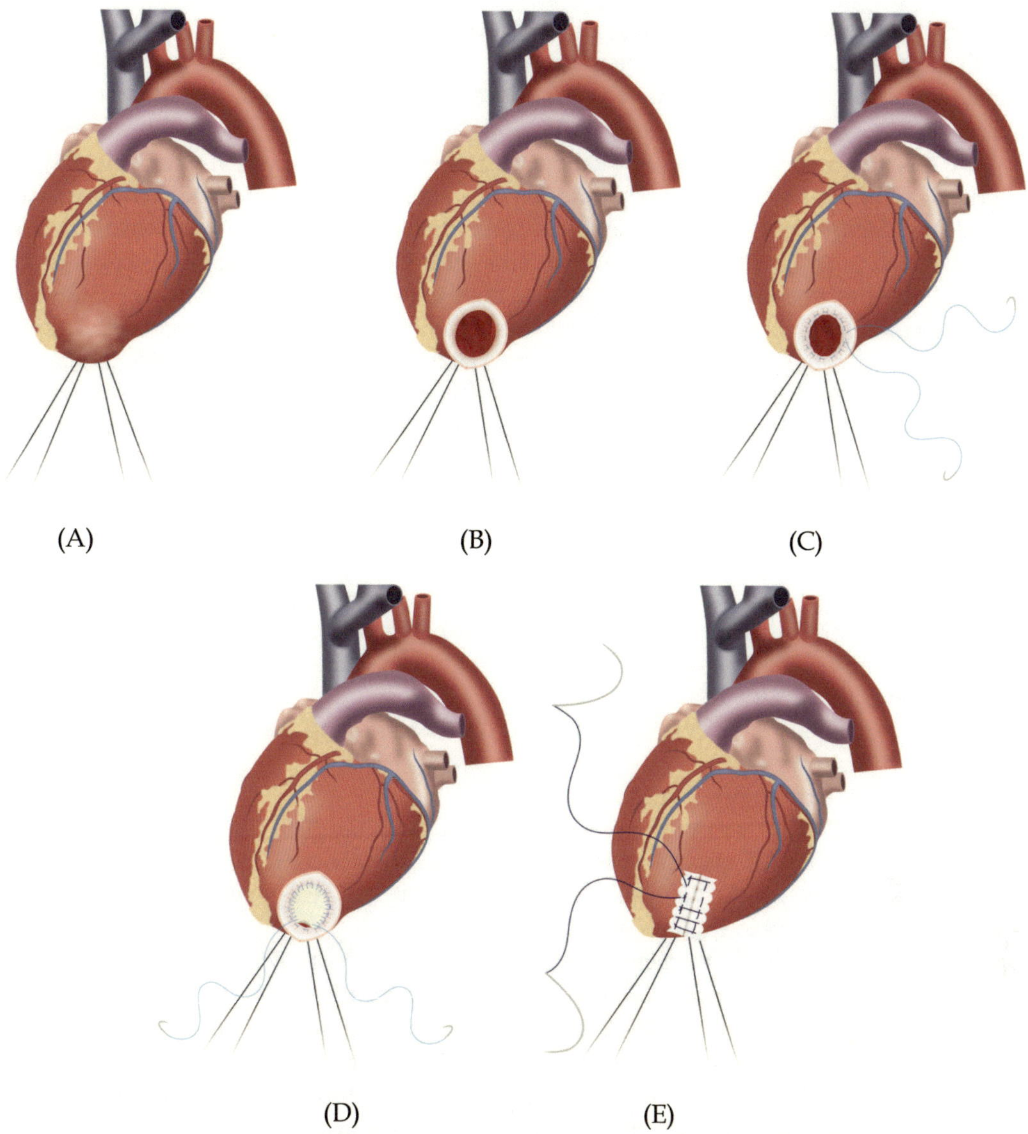

Fig. **2A**. The schema shows the heart with ICM including the antero-apical akinetic region. **2B.** The antero-apical LV wall is opened in the center of the region. The margin of the contractile myocardium around the scar, the so-called "contractility trail", is observed through the ventriculotomy. **2C.** To plicate the circular defect of the LV muscle, 2-0 polypropylene purse-string suture is placed around the entire circumference of the contractility trail. **2D.** A collagen-impregnated Dacron knitted fabric (approximate 3×4 cm) is placed over the plicated defect of the myocardium and fixed with 2-0 polypropylene running suture after deaeration of the LV. **2E.** Two felt strips are placed along the ventriculotomy on each side, and the excluded external scar is folded to reinforce the suture line with 2-0 polypropylene horizontal mattress sutures with a large needle. The line is secured by double 2-0 polypropylene over-and-over sutures from both ends.

kept >75 mmHg to ensure ongoing coronary perfusion. Thus, the SAVE operation was usually performed on the beating heart. During beating, the transitional zone between the scar and the viable myocardium was easily detected by direct manipulation of the LV muscle.

Two 1-0 silk sutures were placed at the apex to achieve a better surgical field (**Fig. 3A**). The anterior wall of the LV was opened along the left anterior descending artery from the apex toward the base (**Fig. 3B**). Cryoablation was performed on the viable LV myocardium along the incision to prevent late VT/VF. For patients with a dilated posterior wall between two papillary muscles, chordal cutting of the basal chordae and papillary muscle approximation was performed via this incision (see *Technical details of our mitral valve surgery*). Multiple 0 braided polyester horizontal mattress sutures (Ticron®; Tyco, Waltham, MA, USA) with pledgets were placed along the exclusion line of the septum, in a direction that proceeded from the apex to a septal site 1-2 cm below the aortic valve (**Fig. 3C**). A collagen-impregnated Dacron knitted fabric was trimmed to create an elliptical shape, approximately 3×8 cm, and placed along the site of the exclusion, with sutures placed 1 cm from the patch edge to leave a patch rim outside these sutures. The last two sutures were tied after deaeration of the LV (**Fig. 3D**). Finally, two felt strips were placed along the ventriculotomy on each side, and the excluded external scar was folded to reinforce the suture line with 2-0 polypropylene horizontal mattress sutures anchoring the allowance of Dacron fabric (**Fig. 3E**). The suture line was secured by double 2-0 polypropylene over-and-over sutures from both ends (**Fig. 3F**).

Some patients requiring SAVE were treated by overlapping cardiac volume reduction operations in this series[32)].

c. Posterior restoration procedure (PRP)

The posterior akinetic region of the LV was repaired with the PRP procedure developed by Isomura et al[24)]. One of the most important operative concepts was the postoperative elliptical shape of the LV. To achieve the elliptical shape, the LV apex and bilateral papillary muscles were preserved in this operation.

As for EVCPP and SAVE, complete coronary revascularization was first preformed under blood cardioplegic arrest. Valvular surgery, including mitral, tricuspid, and aortic valves, was undertaken prior to PRP. PRP was also performed in a beating heart as for the SAVE procedure. Two 1-0 silk sutures were placed at the apex. The akinetic region was opened 1 cm proximal from the apex on the posterior wall between bilateral papillary muscles (**Fig. 4A**). The incision was extended toward the base of the heart, reaching 1 cm above the mitral annulus (**Fig. 4B**). Cryoablation was performed on the viable LV myocardium along the incision to prevent late VT/VF, especially for the LV muscle between the end of the incision and the mitral annulus. Multiple 0 braided polyester horizontal mattress sutures with pledgets were placed along the exclusion line on the viable LV myocardium (**Fig. 3C**). As for the SAVE procedure, a collagen-impregnated Dacron knitted fabric was trimmed to create an elliptical shape and placed over the exclusion with a 1-cm allowance for LV closure. The last two sutures on the apex side were tied after deaeration of the LV (**Fig. 4D**). Finally, the LV was closed in a similar manner as in the SAVE procedure, and the bilateral papillary muscles were approximated during the PRP procedure (**Fig. 4E**). The line was secured by double 2-0 polypropylene over-and-over sutures from both ends (**Fig. 4F**).

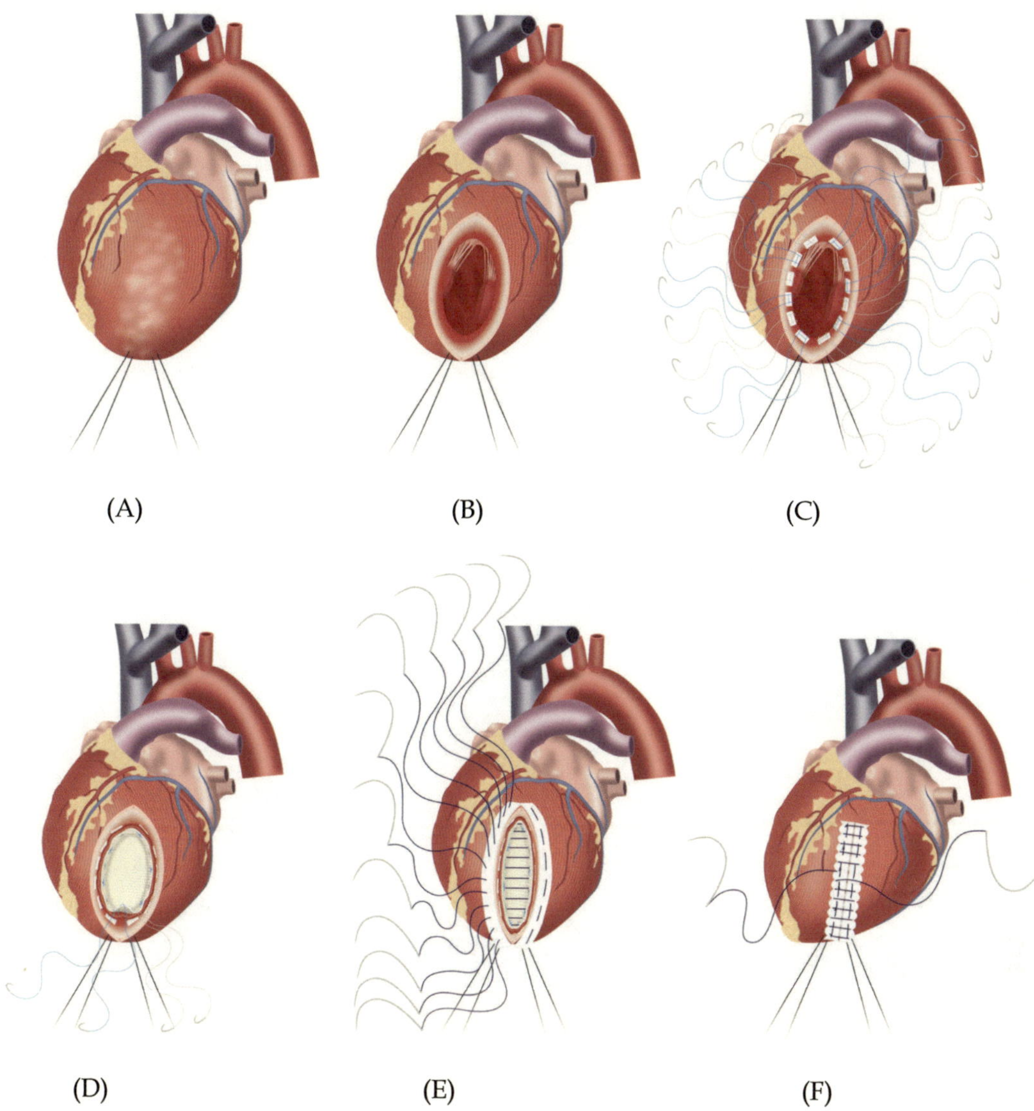

Fig. 3A. The schema shows the heart with ICM including a large antero-septal akinetic region. 3B. The antero-lateral LV wall is opened along the left descending artery from the apex toward the base. 3C. Multiple 0 braided polyester horizontal mattress sutures with pledgets are placed along the exclusion line of the septum, in a direction that proceeds from the apex to a septal site 1-2 cm below the aortic valve. 3D. A collagen-impregnated Dacron knitted fabric (approximate 3×4 cm) is placed over the plicated defect of the myocardium and fixed with 2-0 polypropylene running suture. The last two sutures on the apex side are tied after deaeration of the LV. 3E. Two felt strips are placed along the ventriculotomy on each side, and the excluded external scar is folded to reinforce the suture line with 2-0 polypropylene horizontal mattress sutures anchoring the allowance of Dacron fabric. 3F. The suture line is secured by double 2-0 polypropylene over-and-over sutures from both ends.

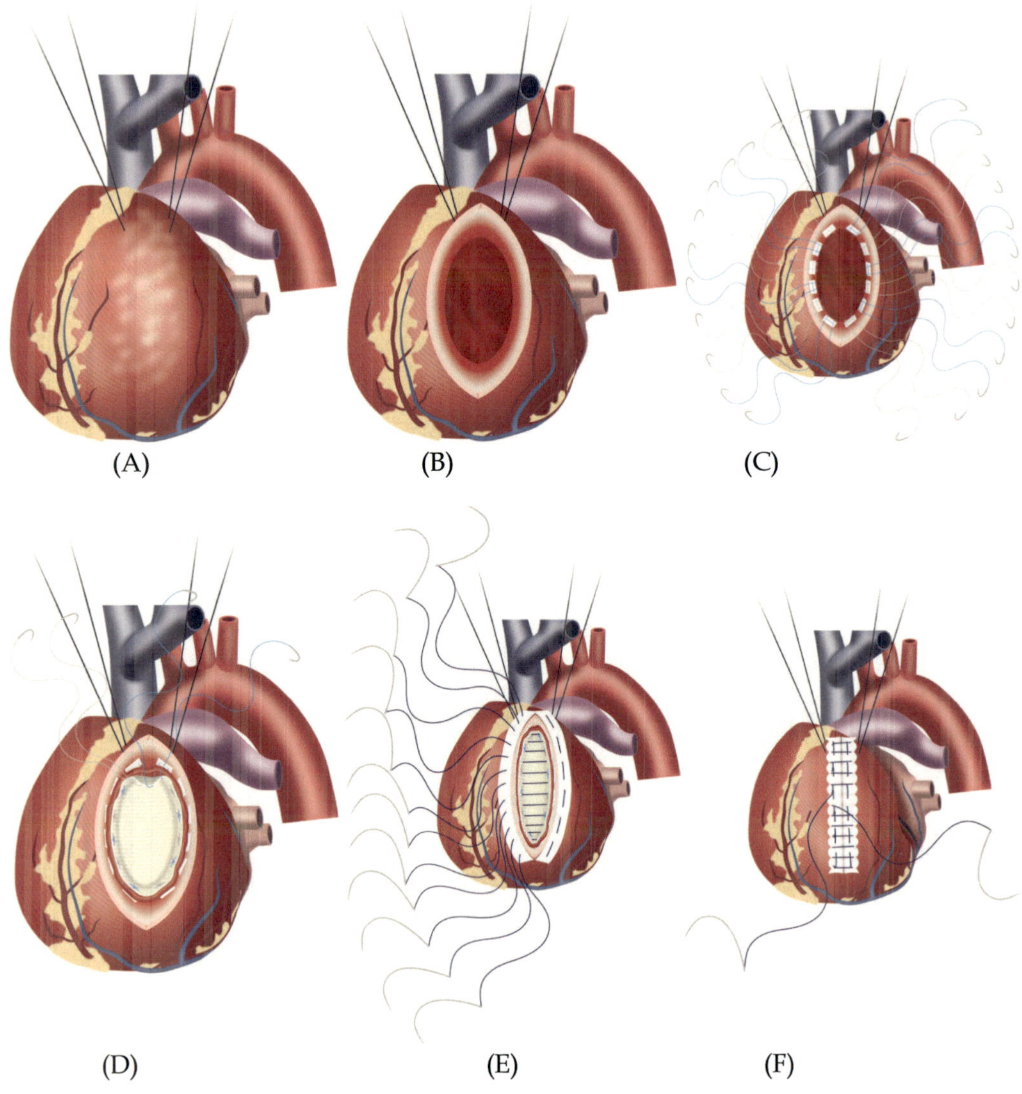

Fig. **4A**. The schema shows the heart with ICM including a posterior akinetic region. **4B.** The akinetic region is opened 1 cm proximal from the apex on the posterior wall between bilateral papillary muscles. The incision is extended toward the base of the heart, reaching 1 cm below the mitral annulus. **4C.** Multiple 0 braided polyester horizontal mattress sutures with pledgets are placed along the exclusion line of the septum, with a direction that proceeds from the apex to a septal site 1-2 cm below the aortic valve. **4D.** A collagen-impregnated Dacron knitted fabric is trimmed to create an elliptical shape and is placed over the exclusion with a 1-cm allowance for closure of the LV. The last two sutures on the apex side are tied after deaeration of the LV. **4E.** Two felt strips are placed along the ventriculotomy on each side, and the excluded external scar is folded to reinforce the suture line with 2-0 polypropylene horizontal mattress sutures anchoring the allowance of Dacron fabric. The bilateral papillary muscles are approximated during the PRP procedure. **4F.** The suture line is secured by double 2-0 polypropylene over-and-over sutures from both ends.

3.3 Anatomical relationships between the mitral leaflet and the subvalvular apparatus for ICM

The mitral valve consists of the anterior and posterior leaflets, annulus, and chordae, supported by two papillary muscles to regulate forward blood flow from the left atrium to the LV. Under normal conditions, both mitral leaflets create a deep coaptation zone at end-systole to prevent regurgitant blood flow. However, earlier experimental and clinical studies demonstrated that restricted diastolic opening of the mitral leaflets increased valve tethering, resulting in functional MR in hearts with LV dysfunction[33,34]. The mechanism of functional MR can be understood in terms of an altered force balance on the mitral leaflets in systole; i.e., a combination of increased tethering forces that restrain the leaflets from closing and result from an altered three-dimensional geometry of leaflet attachments associated with LV dilatation and decreased ventricular forces that act to close the mitral leaflets. As a consequence of geometric remodeling, laterally displaced papillary muscles were detected in dilated LVs with ICM[35]. Although annular dilation is also one of the primary causes of functional MR, understanding of the geometric imbalance between the LV dimensions and the subvalvular apparatus is important to repair functional MR in patients with ICM[36].

3.4 Mitral valve surgery for functional MR in patients with ICM

Earlier reports demonstrated that functional MR may result from dilation of the mitral annulus, laterally displaced papillary muscles, and enhanced tethering force of the valve leaflets in the hearts with dilated LV[33,35-37]. For these patients, functional MR was relieved by mitral valve plasty (MVP) including mitral annuloplasty (MAP) with an undersized flexible annuloplasty ring[38], chordal cutting of the basal chordae[39,40], papillary muscle approximation[41-44], and chordal translocation[45]. We usually repair functional MR using MAP with a semi-rigid ring, and/or chordal cutting, and/or papillary muscle approximation. Chordal cutting and papillary muscle approximation were indicated for patients with a severely dilated LV caused by broad myocardial infarction, who would be repaired by the SAVE procedure. Details of our techniques are described below.

3.5 Technical details of our mitral valve surgery

To perform MAP, the mitral valve was observed via the right-sided left atriotomy. When the MAZE procedure was required, radiofrequency ablation was performed prior to mitral valve surgery following Cox and associates[46]. The Cosgrove Valve Retractor System (Kapp Surgical Instrument, Inc. Cleveland, OH, USA) was used to obtain a wide surgical field around the mitral valve. First, 2-0 polyfilament braided vertical mattress sutures (Matsuda-ika Kogyo, Tokyo, Japan) were placed on the mitral annulus. The coaptation zone of the mitral valve was directly inspected by the water test to identify the valvular morphology. Basically, the etiology of functional MR with ICM involved tethering of the subvalvular apparatus caused by a dilated LV and annular dilatation. After identification of no organic changes of the mitral leaflet, a mitral annuloplasty ring was seated on the mitral annulus (**Fig. 5A**). An undersized semi-rigid ring (Carpenter-Edwards Physio Ring®; Edwards Life Science Corporation, Irvine, CA, USA) was used for patients with central MR, while a just-sized asymmetric rigid ring (Carpentier-McCarthy-Adams IMR ETlogix annuloplasty ring®; Edwards Life Science Corporation) was used for patients with asymmetric MR from the postero-median commissure. Chordal cutting was usually performed via the ventriculotomy during SVR, and thus the LA was closed with double 4-0 polypropylene over-and-over sutures.

For patients with a severely dilated LV requiring SAVE, chordal cutting was performed via the ventriculotomy during SVR. The basal chordae of the anterior and posterior mitral leaflets were completely cut with a pair of long scissors **(Fig. 5B)**. Before suturing for SVR, two 0 braided polyester horizontal mattress sutures with pledgets (Ticron®; Tyco, Waltham, MA, USA) were placed to plicate the posterior LV wall between bilateral papillary muscles **(Fig. 5C)**. They were then tied to approximate bilateral papillary muscles **(Fig. 5D)**. SVR followed mitral valve surgery.

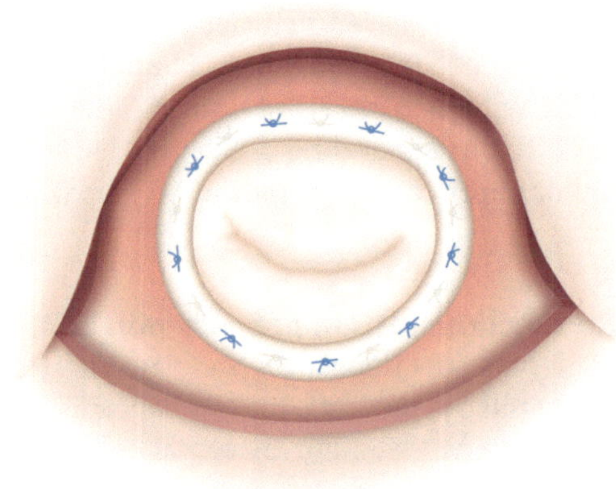

(A)

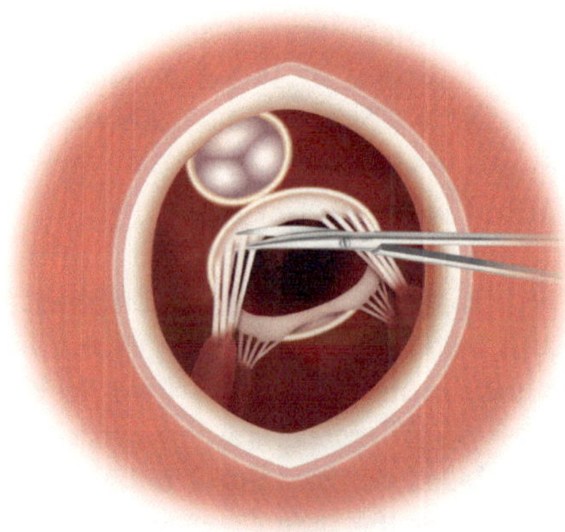

(B)

Fig. **5A**. The mitral valve is observed via the right-sided left atriotomy. After identification of no organic changes of the mitral leaflet, a mitral annuloplasty ring is seated on the mitral annulus. **5B.** For patients with a severely dilated LV requiring the SAVE procedure, the basal chordae of the anterior and posterior mitral leaflets are completely cut with a pair of long scissors via the ventriculotomy.

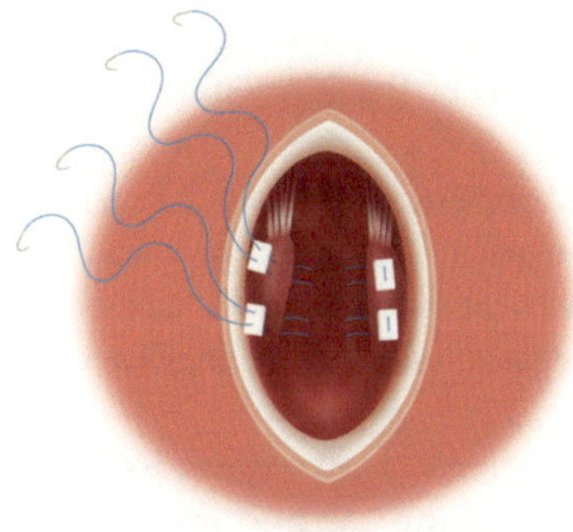

(C)

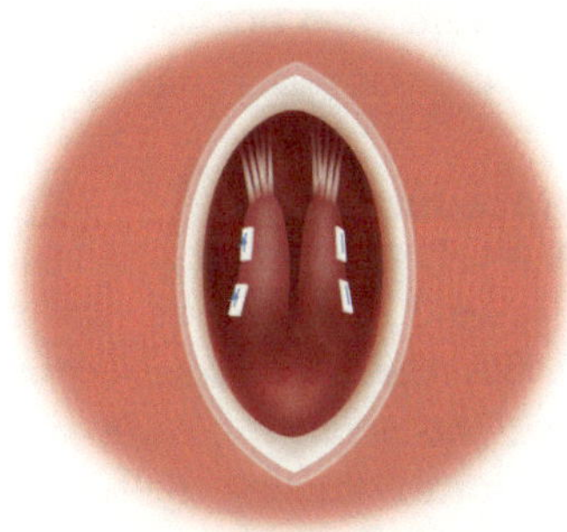

(D)

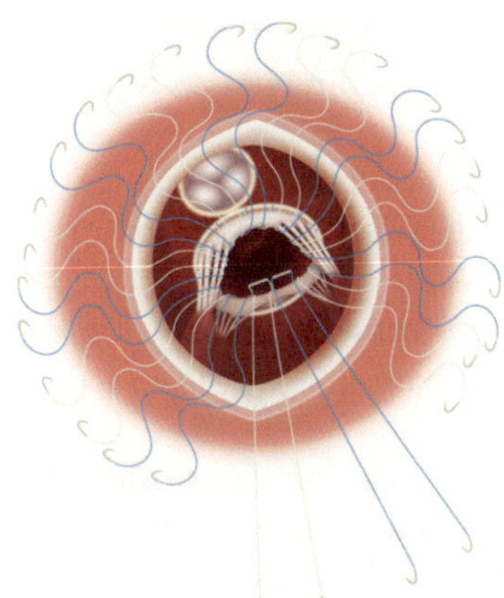

(E)

Fig. **5C**. Before suturing for PRP, two 0 braided polyester horizontal mattress sutures with pledgets are placed to plicate the posterior LV wall between bilateral papillary muscles. **5D.** Two sutures are tied to approximate bilateral papillary muscles. **5E.** MVR is performed via the ventriculotomy during SVR in a beating heart. The mitral leaflets are preserved as much as possible to prevent LV rupture, and 2-0 polyfilament braided vertical mattress sutures are placed on the mitral annulus from the LA toward the LV. These sutures are then anchored to the mitral leaflets.

For patients requiring PRP, the bilateral papillary muscles were surgically approximated during closure of the posterior wall of the LV. Thus, the posterior wall was approximated during the usual PRP procedure.

Although MVP is a standard operation for ICM with functional MR, mitral valve replacement (MVR) is indicated for a few limited cases. In the early period of this series, MVR via the ventriculotomy was performed to reduce aortic crossclamping time. Patients with ICM and MR caused by organic valvular changes were also treated by MVR, although they were excluded in this series.

MVR was performed via the ventriculotomy during SVR in a beating heart. The ascending aorta was declamped after closure of the LV, and the LV was opened in the akinetic region. The mitral leaflets were preserved as much as possible to prevent LV rupture, and 2-0 polyfilament braided vertical mattress sutures were placed on the mitral annulus from the LA toward the LV. These sutures were then anchored to the mitral leaflets. A prosthetic mitral valve was seated in the infravalvular position (**Fig. 5E**).

3.6 Overview of the operative procedure

a. Preparation for SVR and mitral valve surgery

Under general cardiac anesthesia and monitoring, the chest was entered via median sternotomy. CPB was installed via the ascending aorta with bicaval drainage under generalized heparinization. For patients requiring coronary artery bypass grafting (CABG), all anastomoses were completed prior to opening the LA. An LA vent tube was introduced via the right upper pulmonary vein (PV) to obtain a bloodless surgical field. When the MAZE procedure was required, left PV isolation was performed with a radiofrequency ablation system (AtriCure, Inc, West Chester, OH, USA). Under mild hypothermia, the ascending aorta was crossclamped. Antegrade tepid blood cardioplegia was delivered to obtain cardioplegic cardiac arrest. For maintenance, retrograde tepid blood cardioplegia was infused every 20 to 30 minutes.

b. MAP via the right-sided left atriotomy

MAP was performed via the right-sided left atriotomy. Details of the technique were described above. The LA was closed in two layers.

Aortic valve replacement was performed via the aortotomy prior to SVR, when it was required. Tricuspid valve surgery was also performed via the right atriotomy when it was necessary.

c. SVR and other mitral procedures via the ventriculotomy

After completion of MAP, the akinetic scar was opened to perform SVR and other mitral procedures via the LV. Selection of SVR depended on the location of the scar: the antero-septo-apical region for EVCCP, a broad antero-septal region for SAVE, and the posterior region for PRP. First, chordal cutting of both mitral leaflets was performed when it was indicated for patients requiring SAVE. Details of the technique were described above.

Secondly, papillary muscle approximation was performed for patients with a severely dilated LV requiring SAVE. The technical details were described above. For patients requiring PRP, the incision of the posterior wall was placed just between both papillary muscles, resulting in papillary muscle approximation by usual LV closure.

Finally, SVR was performed after completion of other mitral procedures. The details of the procedure were described above.

d. Supplemental procedures

For patients with LV dyssynchrony or the inevitable cases with transection of a previously implanted LV lead during SVR, an epicardial permanent LV lead was placed on the lateral wall for cardiac resynchronization therapy (CRT) or CRT defibrillator (CRT-D)[47]. For the extremely severe cases with out-of-date generators for CRT or CRT-D, a new generator was upgraded during the operation.

3.7 Statistical analysis

The results are expressed as means±SEM. An analysis was performed using the paired or unpaired Student's *t*-test to compare between before and after SVR, respectively. The criterion for statistical significance was set at a value of $P<0.05$.

4. Results

1. Operative procedures

In 88 patients with ICM and MR, SVR was performed with three different procedures: EVCPP in 25 patients (28%), SAVE in 50 patients (57%) and PRP in 13 patients (15%). Two cases with antero-septal scars repaired by an overlapping cardiac volume reduction operation had a SAVE procedure. Mitral valve surgery was performed with MAP in 78 patients (89%) and MVR in 10 patients (11%). Of a total of 78 patients repaired with MAP, an under-sized Carpentier-Edwards Physio Ring was used in 72 patients (92%), and a just-sized Carpentier-McCarthy-Adams IMR ETlogix annuloplasty ring was used in 6 patients (8%). Of a total of 46 cases repaired with SAVE plus MAP, chordal cutting was required in 10 patients (22%), and papillary muscle approximation was required in 16 patients (35%). In the early period of this series, 10 patients were treated by MVR with the Carpentier-Edwards pericardial bioprosthesis (Edwards Life Science Corporation). Detailed combinations of SVR and mitral valve surgery are summarized in **Table 1**.

		ICM with MR (n=88)			
			EVCPP (n=25)	SAVE (n=50)	PRP (n=13)
	Annuloplasty	78 (100%)	23	46	9
MVP (n=78)	Chordal cutting	10 (11%)	0	10	0
	Papillary muscle approximation	25 (28%)	0	16	9
MVR (n=10)		10	2	4	4

ICM, ischemic cardiomyopathy; MR, mitral regurgitation; EVCPP, endoventricular circular patch plasty; SAVE, septal anterior ventricular exclusion; PRP, posterior restoration procedure; MVP, mitral valve plasty; MVR, mitral valve replacement

Table 1. Surgical Ventricular Restoration and Mitral Valve Surgery.

Of the 88 patients with ICM and functional MR, concomitant procedures included CABG in 63 (72%), tricuspid valve surgery in 30 (34%), aortic valve surgery in 4 (5%), and the MAZE procedure in 7 (8%). The number of grafts for patients requiring CABG was 2.0±1.4/patient.

Tricuspid annuloplasty was performed with the Carpentier-Edwards classic annuloplasty ring (Edwards Life Science Corporation) in 13 patients, the Edwards MC3 annuloplasty ring (Edwards Life Science Corporation) in 9 patients, the Cosgrove-Edwards annuloplasty system (Edwards Life Science Corporation) in 3 patients, the St. Jude Medical Tailor flexible band (St. Jude Medical, Inc. St. Paul, MN, USA) in 2 patients, and the DeVega technique in 3 patients. Aortic valve replacement was performed with the Carpentier-Edwards pericardial bioprosthesis (Edwards Life Science Corporation) in 4 patients (5%). Intra- and post-operative CRT or CRT-D was required in 26 patients (30%).

2. Early surgical results

Aortic crossclamping and CPB times are shown in **Table 2**. IABP was preoperatively introduced in 2 patients (2%) requiring the SAVE procedure, and 20 patients (23%) required postoperative IABP (6 for EVCPP, 10 for SAVE, and 4 for PRP). Two patients repaired by the SAVE procedure required a left ventricular assist system and percutaneous cardiopulmonary support after the operation.

	ICM with MR (n=88)			
		EVCPP (n=25)	SAVE (n=50)	PRP (n=13)
ACC time (min)	71±10	72±10	66±35	97±42
CPB time (min)	149±29	134±29	158±68	154±36

ACC, aortic crossclamping; CPB, cardioplumonary bypass; ICM, ischemic cardiomyopathy; MR, mitral regurgitation; EVCPP, endoventricular circular patch plasty; SAVE, septal anterior ventricular exclusion; PRP, posterior restoration procedure

Table 2. ACC and CPB Time. (Hirota et al.)

Overall hospital mortality was 13% (11/88), with 9 patients in the SAVE group. Hospital mortalities of elective and emergent operations were 9% and 29%, respectively. The most frequent morbidity was non-sustained and sustained VT/VF (17/88; 19%). Details of hospital mortality and morbidity are shown in **Table 3**.

Geometric and hemodynamic parameters are summarized in **Table 4**. Both diastolic and systolic LV volumes (LVEDVI and LVESVI) were significantly decreased with each procedure ($p<0.05$). LVEDVI and LVESVI were the largest with SAVE (LVEDVI: EVCPP 166±46 ml/m^2, SAVE 185±53 ml/m^2, PRP 154±48 ml/m^2; LVESVI: EVCPP 129±44 ml/m^2, SAVE 149±49 ml/m^2, PRP 117±50 ml/m^2). As an index of the extent of volume reduction, the volume reduction rate (reduction volume by SVR/preoperative LV volume × 100 [%]) was calculated. The volume reduction rates of LVEDV and LVESV were similar (LVEDV: EVCPP 27%, SAVE 22%, PRP 26%; LVEDV: EVCPP 19%, SAVE 21%, PRP 26%). EF and peak pulmonary artery pressure were not significantly improved with any procedure. The severity of functional MR was less after each procedure. The majority of moderate or severe MR was improved to none or trivial MR (**Fig. 6**). NYHA functional class also improved with each procedure, and of all surviving patients in classes III and IV, 78% improved to class I or II (**Fig. 7**).

	ICM with MR (n=88)	EVCPP (n=25)		SAVE (n=50)		PRP (n=13)	
		Elective	Emergent	Elective	Emergent	Elective	Emergent
Hospital Mortality	11 (13%)	2	0	5	4	0	0
LOS	8	1	0	4	3	0	0
Sepsis	1	0	0	1	0	0	0
Gastrointestinal complication	1	0	0	0	1	0	0
Ventricular tachycardia	1	1	0	0	0	0	0
Morbidity							
Ventricular tachycardia/fibrillation	17 (19%)	3	1	10	1	2	0
Postoperative hemorrhage	3	2	0	0	1	0	0
Cerebrovascular accident	1	0	0	1	0	0	0
Gastrointestinal complication	1	0	0	0	1	0	0

ICM, ischemic cardiomyopathy; MR, mitral regurgitation; EVCPP, endoventricular circular patch plasty; SAVE, septal anterior ventricular exclusion; PRP, posterior restoration procedure; LOS, low output syndrome

Table 3. Hospital Mortality and Morbidity.

	ICM with MR (n=88)		EVCPP (n=25)		SAVE (n=50)		PRP (n=13)	
	Operation		Operation		Operation		Operation	
	Before	After	Before	After	Before	After	Before	After
LVDd (mm)	69±9	62±9*	67±7	64±8*	69±10	62±9*	71±9	58±9*
LVEDVI (mm/m²)	172±51	130±44*	166±46	122±47*	185±53	145±42*	154±48	114±56*
Volume reduction rate (%)				27%		22%		26%
LVESVI (mm/m²)	140±50	104±42*	129±44	104±37*	149±49	118±40*	117±50	87±54*
Volume reduction rate(%)				19%		21%		26%
EF (%)	19±6	19±8	19±6	19±10	19±6	19±6	22±7	21±9
Peak PAP (mmHg)	39±17	36±14	44±18	32±12	39±16	37±15	33±18	31±11

ICM, ischemic cardiomyopathy; MR, mitral regurgitation; EVCPP, endoventricular circular patch plasty; SAVE, septal anterior ventricular exclusion; PRP, posterior restoration procedure; LVDd, left ventricular end-diastolic diameter; LVEDVI, left ventricular end-diastolic volume index; LVESVI, left ventricular end-systolic volume index; EF, ejection fraction; PAP, pulmonary artery pressure; Volume reduction rate is calculated as reduction volume/preoperative left ventricular volume × 100 [%] ; *$P<0.05$ vs. before, Values are expressed as means ± SEM.

Table 4. Geometric and Hemodynamic Parameters.

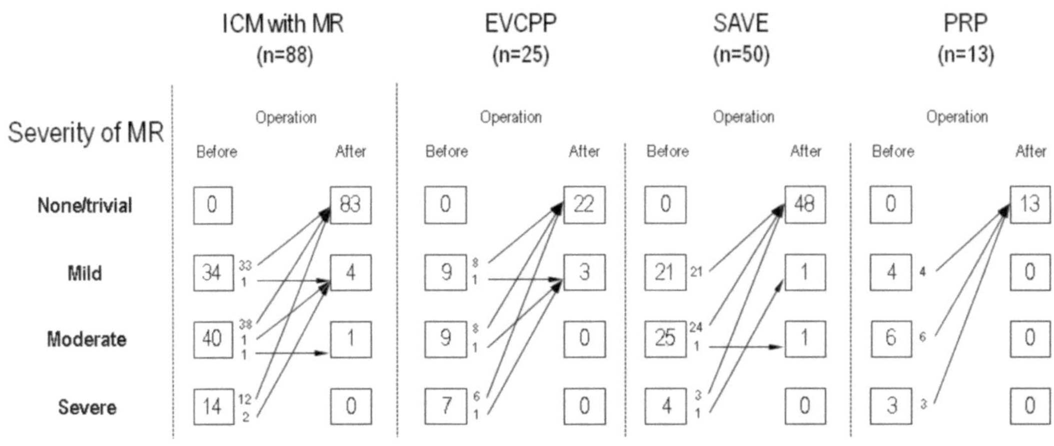

Fig. 6. The surgical effects on mitral regurgitation (MR) in patients with ischemic cardiomyopathy (ICM). In a total of 88 patients, the severity of MR was decreased after the operation. The similar effect was detected in three different procedures including endoventricular circular patch plasty (EVCCP), septal anterior ventricular exclusion (SAVE), and the posterior restoration procedure (PRP).

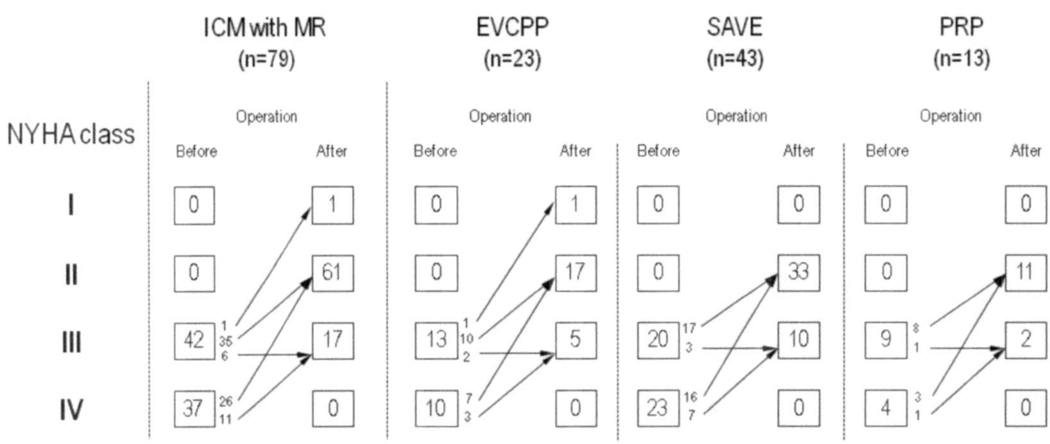

Fig. 7. The surgical effects on the New York Heart Association (NYHA) functional class in patients with ischemic cardiomyopathy (ICM) and mitral regurgitation (MR). In a total of 79 survived patients, the functional class was improved after the operation. The similar effect was detected in three different procedures including endoventricular circular patch plasty (EVCCP), septal anterior ventricular exclusion (SAVE), and the posterior restoration procedure (PRP).

3. Mid- to long-term surgical results

Mid- to long-term survival rates of elective operations were estimated by Kaplan-Meier analysis (**Fig. 8**). In this series, 1-year and 5-year overall survival rates were 84% (EVCPP 81%; SAVE 79%; PRP 100%) and 66% (EVCPP 50%; SAVE 66%; PRP 67%), respectively.

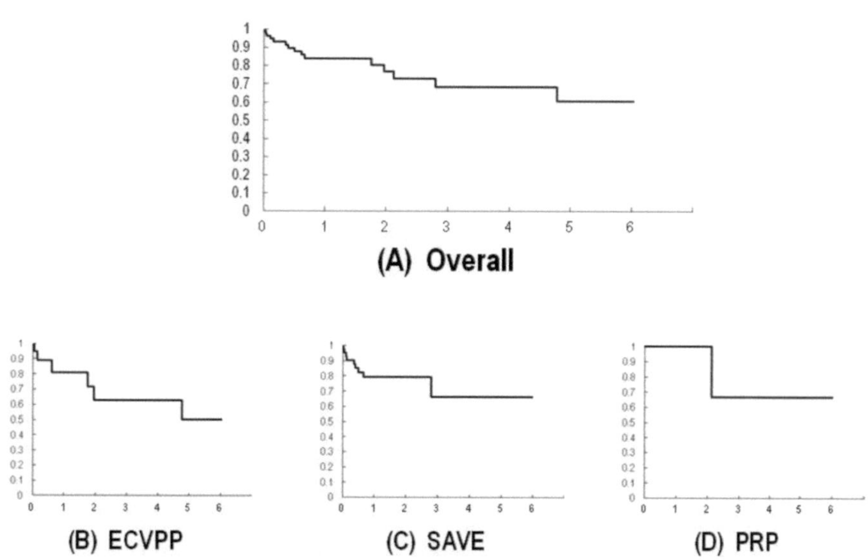

Fig. 8. Kaplan-Meier survival curves in patients with ischemic cardiomyopathy (ICM) and mitral regurgitation (MR). **(A)** In a total of 88 patients, overall survival repaired by the three different procedures including endoventricular circular patch plasty (EVCCP), septal anterior ventricular exclusion (SAVE), and the posterior restoration procedure (PRP). **(B)** Survival curve in patients repaired by EVCCP. **(C)** Survival curve in patients repaired by SAVE. **(D)** Survival curve in patients repaired by PRP.

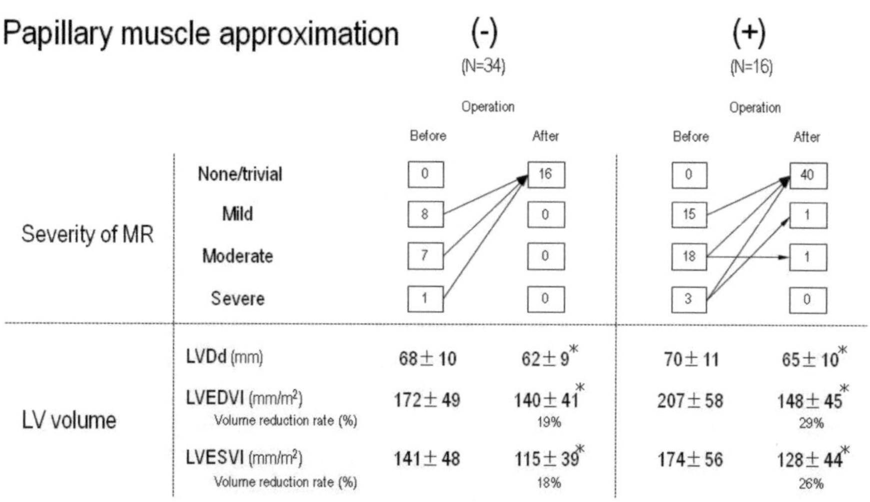

Fig. 9. The surgical effects of papillary muscle approximation on mitral regurgitation (MR) and left ventricular (LV) volume in patients repaired by the SAVE procedure and ring annuloplasty. In a total of 50 patients, the severity of MR was decreased irrespective of papillary muscle approximation. LV volumetric indices including LV end-diastolic diameter (LVDd), LV end-diastolic volume index (LVEDVI) and LV end-systolic volume index (LVESVI) were also decreased irrespective of papillary muscle approximation. However, the volume reduction rate was much smaller in patients repaired by concomitant papillary muscle approximation.

4. Effects of papillary muscle approximation in the SAVE procedure

Of the 50 patients treated with the SAVE procedure, 16 underwent papillary muscle approximation. To illustrate the effects of papillary muscle approximation, dimensional parameters and severity of MR are summarized in **Fig. 9**. Preoperative LVESVI was greater in patients repaired by SAVE and papillary muscle approximation than in patients repaired by SAVE alone (174±56 vs. 141±48 ml/m^2), but the difference was not significant. The volume reduction rate was also increased by additional papillary muscle approximation (26% vs. 19%). Irrespective of papillary muscle approximation, the severity of MR was improved after SAVE and mitral ring annuloplasty.

5. Discussion

We have reported the results of our surgical treatment of severe patients with ICM and functional MR and described the details of our surgical strategy. Three kinds of SVR technique effectively reduced LV dimension and changed the spherical shape of the LV into an elliptical shape. Concomitant mitral valve surgery decreased the severity of MR during SVR. This combined surgery would contribute to better surgical outcomes for these patients.

The final goal of SVR for ICM with functional MR is re-establishment of the geometric balance of the remodeled LV to increase the forward flow by obtaining concentric contraction and decreasing the extent of MR. We detected the akinetic region of the LV with various techniques and excluded it with three kinds of SVR based on the location of the region. Subsequently, the contractile myocardium was connected by the elliptical patch placed on the "contractility trail". Simultaneously, for patients with a dilated posterior LV wall between two papillary muscles, it was approximated during SVR to restore subvalvular geometry beneath the mitral valve. Although there is no gold standard technique for patients with ICM and functional MR, our combined surgery appears to achieve the final goal at this moment.

For patients with ischemic heart disease, SVR has yielded beneficial short-term effects on functional status, exercise performance, long-term results, and quality of life[48,49]. However, concomitant SVR is still controversial during CABG for these patients[48,49,50]. Recently, the Surgical Treatment for Ischemic Heart Failure (STICH) trial addressed this question and demonstrated that anatomical change by SVR was not associated with a greater improvement in symptoms or exercise tolerance or with a reduction in the rate of death or hospitalization for cardiac causes[50]. Patient selection issues and hemodynamic effects of LV volume reduction have been proposed to explain these contradictory results[50]. Thus, it would be very difficult to conclude anything about the efficacies associated with SVR, even though a large, multicenter, randomized trial such as STICH has been done. Especially for a small number of patients with ICM and functional MR, the same would be true.

More recently, we have suggested the effectiveness of SVR for patients with ICM[51]. According to our results, SVR is most effective when a >33% volume reduction rate achieves an LVESVI of <90 ml/m^2. No long-term benefits occur when SVR induces an LV volume reduction of <15%, leaving a residual LVESVI >90 ml/m^2. Although the results also contradict the STICH trial findings, long-term prognosis in ICM would be determined by the relationships between accurate methods for measuring ventricular volume and the extent of SVR volume reduction.

Due to the diverse patient population, it is very difficult to compare the surgical outcomes among clinical studies and trials. Although details of patients' background were

disregarded, the cumulative survival rate was assessed by a systematic review of the literature associated with SVR in ischemic heart disease[48]. According to the review, the weighted average early mortality (defined as in-hospital or 30-day mortality) was 6.9%, and the cumulative 1-year and 5-year survivals were 88.5% and 71.5%, respectively. Although our surgical outcome did not reach the cumulative value, the extent of LV dysfunction with coexisting MR secondary to ischemia was much more severe in our series. More than 50% of patients had a large antero-septal akinetic region of the LV requiring the SAVE procedure, and all of them were classified as NYHA functional class III and IV. In fact, the remodeled hearts presented with severe LV dysfunction (EF <20%) with a dilated LV (LVESVI > 140 ml/m^2). Moreover, more than half of the patients had concomitant severe MR (grade III and IV) in the present series. Earlier clinical reports demonstrated that the mortality risk is related to the degree of functional MR in patients with ICM[52,53]. Thus, our early and late surgical results would be acceptable in patients with such severe backgrounds.
Although SVR improved cardiac function and functional status for patients with ICM, it was reported that potential determinants of hospital mortality included preoperative advanced heart failure status, postoperative large LV volume (LVESVI > 60 ml/m^2, LVESV > 80 ml), coexisting MR, and need for mitral valve surgery[53,54]. Many potential risks were involved in this series, and baseline LVESV would be much larger in a patient population with ICM and functional MR. In the present series, preoperative LVESVI (140±50 ml/m^2) was larger than in other reports, and thus, postoperative LVESVI (104±42 ml/m^2) was not included in the smaller LV volume category with low mortality. Although more exclusions to reduce LVESV would result in better surgical results, we believe that excessive exclusions involving contractile myocardium should be avoided for such ICM patients with severely dilated LV accompanying MR. Accordingly, prediction of the exclusion area of non-functional scar or myocardium is very important to perform effective SVR for these patients.
As one of the additional surgical adjuncts, we performed papillary muscle approximation to reduce LV volume for patients with a severely dilated LV requiring the SAVE procedure. The SAVE procedure effectively excludes a broad akinetic region of the antero-septo-apical wall, and papillary muscle approximation shortens the posterior wall between both papillary muscles. Thus, these combined procedures achieve further reduction of the LVESV. Although the volume reduction rate was increased by papillary muscle approximation, the early surgical effect on functional MR was almost the same, irrespective of papillary muscle approximation. Although the long-term effect on the LV dimension has not been elucidated, it may contribute to prevention of MR due to re-dilation of the LV.

6. Conclusion

SVR for patients with ICM and functional MR requires various surgical combinations depending on the location of the akinetic region, ventricular size, and subvalvular morphology beneath the MV. The surgical strategy is very important to achieve better surgical outcomes for such high-risk patients.

7. References

[1] Kwan J, Shiota T, Agler DA, Popovic ZB, Qin JX, Gillinov MA, Stewart WJ, Cosgrove DM, McCarthy PM, Thomas JD; Realtime three-dimensional echocardiography study. Geometric differences of the mitral apparatus between ischemic and dilated

cardiomyopathy with significant mitral regurgitation: real-time three-dimensional echocardiography study. Circulation. 2003; 107: 1135-40

[2] Dor V, Di Donata M. Ventricular remodeling in coronary artery disease. Curr Opin Cardiol. 1997; 12: 533-7

[3] Gaudron P, Eilles C, Kugler I, Ertl G. Progressive left ventricular dysfunction and remodeling after myocardial infarction. Potential mechanisms and early predictors. Circulation. 1993; 87: 755-63

[4] Kaul S, Spotnitz WD, Glasfeen WP, Touchstone DA. Mechanism of ischemic mitral regurgitation: an experimental evaluation. Circulation. 1991; 84: 2167-80

[5] Lamas GA, Mitchell GF, Flaker GC, Smith SC Jr, Gersh BJ, Basta L, Moye L, Braunwald E, Pfeffer MA. Clinical significance of mitral regurgitation after myocardial infarction. Survival and Ventricular Enlargement Investigators. Circulation. 1997; 96: 827-33

[6] Enriquez-Sarano M, Schaff HV, Frye RL. Mitral regurgitation: what causes the leakage is fundamental to the outcome of valve repair. Circulation. 2003; 108: 253-6

[7] Di Mauro M, Di Giammarco G, Vitolla G, Contini M, laco AL, Bivona A, Weltert L, Calafiore AM. Impact of no-to-moderate mitral regurgitation on late results after isolated coronary artery bypass grafting in patients with ischemic cardiomyopathy. Ann Thorac Surg. 2006; 81: 2128-34

[8] Isomura T, Horii T, Suma H, Buckberg GD; RESTORE Group. Septal anterior ventricular exclusion operation (Pacopexy) for ischemic dilated cardiomyopathy: treatment form not disease. Eur J Cardiothorac Surg. 2006; 29 Suppl 1: S245-50

[9] Di Donato M, Sabatier M, Montiglio F, Maioi M, Toso A, Fantini F, Dor V. Outcome of left ventricular aneurysmectomy with patch repair in patients with severely depressed pump function. Am J Cardiol. 1995; 15: 557-61

[10] Dor V, Sabatier M, Di Donato M, Montiglio F, Toso A, Maioli M. Efficacy of endoventricular patch plasty in large postinfarction akinetic scar and severe left ventricular dysfunction: comparison with a series of large dyskinetic scars. J Thorac Cardiovasc Surg. 1998; 116: 50-9

[11] Di Donato M, Toso A, Maioli M, Sabatier M, Stanley AW Jr, Dor V; RESTORE group. Intermediate survival and predictors of death after surgical ventricular restoration. Semin Thorac Cardiovasc Surg. 2001; 13: 468-75

[12] Athanasuleas CL, Stanley AW Jr, Buckberg GD, Dor V, Di Donato M, Blaskstone EH. Surgical anterior ventricular endocardial restoration (SAVER) in the dilated remodeled ventricle after anterior myocardial infarction. RESTORE group. Reconstructive Endoventricular Surgery, returning Torsion Original Radius Elliptical Shape to the LV. J Am Coll Cardiol. 2001; 37: 1199-209

[13] Menicanti L, Di Donat M, Castelvecchio S, Santambrogio C, Montericcio V, Frigiola A, Buckberg G; RESTORE group. Functional ischemic mitral regurgitation in anterior ventricular remodeling: results of surgical ventricular restoration with and without mitral repair. Heart Fail Rev. 2004; 9: 317-27

[14] Kaza AK, Patel MR, Fiser SM, Long SM, Kern JA, Tribble CG, Kron IL. Ventricular reconstruction results in improved left ventricular function and amelioration of mitral insufficiency. Ann Surg. 2002; 235: 828-32

[15] Dor V, Civaia F, Alexandrescu C, Montiglio F. The post-myocardial infarction scarred ventricle and congestive heart failure: the preeminence of magnetic resonance imaging for preoperative, intraoperative, and postoperative assessment. J Thorac Cardiovasc Surg. 2008; 136: 1405-12

[16] Femandez-Golfin C, De Aqustin A, Manzano MC, Bustos A, Sanchez T, Perez de Isla L, Fuentes M, Macaya C, Zamorano J. Cardiac magnetic resonance determinants of functional mitral regurgitation in ischemic and non ischemic left ventricular dysfunction. Int J Cardiovasc Imaging. 2011; 27: 539-46

[17] Lang RM, Vignon P, Weinert L, Bednarz J, Korcarz C, Sandelski J, Koch R, Prater D, Mor-Avi V. Echocardiographic quantification of regional left ventricular wall motion with color kinesis. Circulation. 1996; 93: 1877-85

[18] Bansal M, Jeffiriess L, Leano R, Mundy J, Marwick TH. Assessment of myocardial viability at dobutamine echocardiography by deformation analysis using tissue velocity and speckle-tracking. JACC Cardiovasc Imaging. 2010; 3: 121-31

[19] Fieno DS, Kim RJ, Chen EL, Lomasney JW, Klocke FJ, Judd RM. Contrast-enhanced magnetic resonance imaging of myocardium at risk: distinction between reversible and irreversible injury throughout infarct healing. J Am Coll Cardiol. 2000; 36: 1985-91

[20] Isomura T, Suma H, Horii T, Sato T, Kikuchi N. Partial left ventriculectomy, ventriculoplasty or valvular surgery for idiopathic dilated cardiomyopathy - the role of intra-operative echocardiography. Eur J Cardiothorac Surg. 2000; 17: 239-45

[21] Geyer H, Caracciolo G, Abe H, Wilansky S, Careri S, Gentile F, Nesser HJ, Khandheria B, Narula J, Senqupta PP. Assessment of myocardial mechanics using speckle tracking echocardiography: fundamentals and clinical applications. J Am Soc Echocardiogr. 2010; 23: 351-69; quiz 453-5

[22] Reisner SA, Lysyansky P, Agmon Y, Mutlak D, Lessick J, Friedman Z. Global longitudinal strain: a novel index of left ventricular systolic function. J Am Soc Echocardiogr. 2004; 17: 630-3

[23] Leitman M, Lysyansky P, Sidenko S, Shir V, Peleq E, Binenbaum M, Kaluski E, Krakover R, Vered Z. Two-dimensional strain - a novel software for real-time quantitative echocardiographic assessment of myocardial function. J Am Soc Echocardiogr. 2004; 17: 1021-9

[24] Isomura T, Notomi Y, Hoshino J, Fukada Y, Katahira S, Kitamura A, Kondo T, Iwasaki T. Indication of posterior restoration and surgical results in patients with dilated cardiomyopathy. Eur J Cardiothorac Surg. 2010; 38: 171-5

[25] Becker M, Hoffmann R, Kuhl M. Analysis of myocardial deformation based on ultrasonic pixel tracking to determine transmurality in chronic myocardial infarction. Eur Heart J. 2006; 27: 2560-6

[26] Popovic Z, Benejam B, Bian C. Speckle-tracking echocardiography correctly identifies segmental left ventricular dysfunction induced by scarring in a rat model of myocardial infarction. Am J Physiol Heart Circ Physiol. 2007; 292: 2809-16

[27] Dagett, WM, Guyton RA, Mundth ED, Buckley MJ, McEnany MT, Gold HK, Leinbach RC, Austen WG. Surgery for post-myocardial infarct ventricular septal defect. Ann Gurg. 1977; 186: 260-71

[28] Levinsky L, Arani DT, Raza ST, Kohn R, Schimert G. Dacron patch enlargement of anterior wall of left ventricule after aneurysmectomy with concomitant infarctectomy. J Thorac Cardiovasc Surg. 1979; 77: 753-6

[29] Dor V, Saab M, Coste P, Kornaszewska M, Montigilo F. Left ventricular aneurysm: a new surgical approach. Thorac Cardiovasc Surg. 1989; 37: 11-9

[30] Cooley DA. Ventricular endoaneurysmorrhaphy: a simplified repair for extensive postinfarction aneurysm. J Card Surg. 1989; 4: 200-5

[31] Hutchins GM, Brawley RK. The influence of cardiac geometry on the results of ventricular aneurysm repair. Am J Pathol. 1980; 99: 221-30

[32] Matui Y, Fukada Y, Suto Y, Yamauchi H, Luo B, Miyama M, Sasaki S, Tanabe T, Yasuda K. Overlapping cardiac volume reduction operation. J Thorac Cardiovasc Surg. 2002; 124: 395-7

[33] Otsuji Y, Handschumacher MD, Schwammenthal E, Jiang L, Song JK, Guerrero JL, Vlahakes GJ, Levine RA. Insights from three-dimensional echocardiography into the mechanism of functional mitral regurgitation: direct in vivo demonstration of altered leaflet tethering geometry. Circulation. 1997; 96: 1999-2008

[34] Otsuji Y, Gilon D, Jiang L, He S, Leavitt M, Roy MJ, Birmingham MJ, Levine RA. Restricted diastolic opening of the mitral leaflets in patients with left ventricular dysfunction: evidence for increased valve tethering. J Am Coll Cardiol. 1998; 32: 398-404

[35] Kumanohoso T, Otsuji Y, Yoshifuku S, Matsukida K, Koriyama C, Kisanuki A, Minagoe S, Levine RA, Tei C. Mechanism of higher incidence of ischemic mitral regurgitation in patients with inferior myocardial infarction: quantitative analsis of left ventricular and mitral valve geometry in 103 patients with prior myocardial infarction. J Thorac Cardiovasc Surg. 2003; 125: 135-43

[36] Otsuji Y, Kumanohoso T, Yoshifuku S, Matsukida K, Koriyama C, Kisanuki A, Minagoe S, Levine RA, Tei C. Isolated annular dilation does not usually cause important functional mitral regurgitation: comparison between patients with lone atrial fibrillation and those with idiopathic or ischemic cardiomyopathy. J Am Coll Cardiol. 2002; 15: 1651-6

[37] Hueb AC, Jatene FB, Moreira LF, Pomerantzeff PM, Kallas E, de Oliveria SA. Ventricular remodeling and mitral valve modifications in dilated cardiomyopathy: new insights from anatomic study. J Thorac Cardiovasc Surg. 2002; 124: 1216-24

[38] Bolling SF, Pagani FD, Deeb GM, Bach DS. Intermediate-term outcome of mitral reconstruction in cardiomyopathy. J Thorac Cardiovasc Surg. 1998; 115: 381-8

[39] Messas E, Guerrero JL, Handschumacher MD, Conrad C, Chow CM, Sullivan S, Yoganathan AP, Levine RA. Chordal cutting: a new therapeutic approach for ischemic mitral regurgitation. Circulation. 2001; 104: 1958-63

[40] Borger MA, Murphy PM, Alam A, Fazel S, Maqanti M, Armstrong S, Rao V, David TE. Initial results of the chordal-cutting operation for ischemic mitral regurgitation. J Thorac Cardiovasc Surg. 2007; 133: 1483-92

[41] Nair RU, Williams SG, Nwafor KU, Hall AS, Tan LB. Left ventricular volume reduction without ventriculectomy. Ann Thorac Surg. 2001; 71: 2046-9

[42] Havss U, Tapia M, Baron F, Pouzet B, Shafy A. Papillary muscle sling: a new functional approach to mitral repair in patients with ischemic left ventricular dysfunction and functional mitral regurgitation. Ann Thorac Surg. 2003; 75: 809-11

[43] Matsui Y, Suto Y, Shimura S, Fukada Y, Naito Y, Yasuda K, Sasaki S. Impact of papillary muscles approximation on the adequacy of mitral coaptation in functional mitral regurgitation due to dilated cardiomyopathy. Ann Thorac Cardiovasc Surg. 2005; 11: 164-71

[44] Rama A, Prascheker L, Barreda E, Gandjbakhch I. Papillary muscle approximation for functional ischemic mitral regurgitation: Ann Thorac Surg. 2007; 84: 2130-1

[45] Masuyama S, Marui A, Shimamoto T, Nonaka M, Tsukiji M, Watanabe N, Ikeda T, Yoshida K, Komeda M. Chordal translocation for ischemic mitral regurgitation may ameliorate tethering of the posterior and anterior mitral leaflets. J Thorac Cardiovasc Surg. 2008; 136: 868-75

[46] Cox JL, Ad N, Palazzo T, Fitzpatrick S, Suyderhound JP, DeGroot KW, Pirovic EA, Lou HC, Duvall WZ, Kim YD. The Maze-III procedure combined with valve surgery. Semin Thorac Cardiovasc Surg. 2000; 12: 53-5

[47] Lindner O, Vogt J, Kammeier A, Wielepp P, Holzinger J, Baller D, Lamp B, Hansky B, Korfer R, Horstkotte D, Burchert W. Effect of cardiac resynchronization therapy on global and regional oxygen consumption and myocardial blood flow in patients with non-ischaemic and ischaemic cardiomyopathy. Eur Heart J. 2005; 26: 70-6

[48] Klein P, Bax JJ, Shaw LJ, Feringa HH, Versteegh MI, Dion RA, Klautz RJ. Early and late outcome of left ventricular reconstruction surgery in ischemic heart disease. Eur J Cardiothorac Surg. 2008; 34: 1149-57

[49] Athanasuleas CL, Buckberg GD, Stanley AW, siler W, Dor V, Di Donato M, Menicanti L, Almeida de, Oliveria S, Beyersdorf F, Kron IL, Suma H, Kouchoukos NT, Moore W, Oz MC, Fontan F, Scott ML, Accola KA; RESTORE group. J Am Coll Cardiol. 2004; 44: 1439-45

[50] Jones RH, Velazquez EJ, Michler RE, Sopko G, Oh JK, O'Connor CM, Hill JA, Menicanti L, Sadowski Z, Desvigne-Nickens P, Rouleau JL, Lee KL; STICH Hypothesis 2 Investigators. Coronary bypass surgery with or without surgical ventricular reconstruction. N Engl J Med. 2009; 360: 1705-17

[51] Isomura T, Hoshino J, Fukada Y, Kitamura A, Katahira S, Kondo T, Iwasaki T, Buckberg G; RESTORE Group. Volume reduction rate by surgical ventricular restoration determines late outcome in ischaemic cardiomyopathy. Eur J Heart Fail. 2011; 13: 423-31

[52] Grigioni F, Enriquez-Sarano M, Zehr KJ, Bailey KR, Tajik AJ. Ischemic mitral regurgitation: long-term outcome and prognostic implications with quantitative Doppler assessment. Circulation. 2001; 103: 1759-64

[53] Menicanti L, Castelvecchio S, Ranucci M, Frigiola A, Santambrogio C, de Vincentiis C, Brankovic J, Di Donato M. Surgical therapy for ischemic heart failure: single-center experience with surgical anterior ventricular restoration. J Thorac Cardiovasc Surg. 2007; 134: 433-41

[54] Witkowski TG, ten Brinke EA, Delgado V, Ng AC, Bertini M, Marsan NA, Ewe SH, Auger D, Yiu KH, Braun J, Klein P, Steendijk P, Versteegh MI, Klautz RJ, Bax JJ. Surgical ventricular restoration for patients with ischemic heart failure: determinants of two-year survival. Ann Thorac Surg: 2011; 91: 491-8

6

Morphological Predictors and Molecular Markers of Progressing Postoperative Remodeling of Left Ventricle in Patients with Ischemic Cardiomyopathy

Vladimir Shipulin[1], Vitaly Kazakov[1,2], Alexander Lezhnev[1], Boris Kozlov[1], Vadim Babokin[1], Sergey Gutor[2] and Irina Suhodolo[2]
[1]*Tomsk Institute of Cardiology, Tomsk,*
[2]*Siberian State Medical University, Tomsk,*
Russia

1. Introduction

1.1 Background

Coronary artery disease takes a leading role in the etiology of chronic heart insufficiency in 60% of the cases (Belenkov et al., 2002; Kalon et al., 1993; Oganov & Maslennikova, 2000; Simonsen, 2003). According to the data of different authors patients with coronary artery disease experience development of ischemic cariomyopathy preconditioned by diffuse, significantly pronounced atherosclerosis of coronary arteries manifesting as cardiomegaly termed as "heart remodeling" and symptoms of congestive heart failure in 10-35% of the cases (Belenkov et al., 2002; Mareev, 2002).

Postinfarction left ventricular remodeling is one of the most urgent challenges of modern cardiology and cardiac surgery. The heart remodeling process is a combination of changes in cavities' form and volume and in mass of postinfarction heart myocardium in response to significant inadequate hemodynamic conditions of its functioning not connected with sarcomeres elongation caused by their prior overstretching (Jackson, 2002; Maisch, 1996; Rosenberg & Nepomnyashchih, 2003). Among the patients with different cardiomyopathies these are the ones with ischemic cardiomyopathy who have the most unfavorable prognosis, which makes the problem of ischemic heart failure much more significant (Bellenger, 2000; Buckberg, 2005; Frazier, 2000).

Quite frequently the surgical intervention becomes the only treatment method for the patients with chronic heart insufficiency basing on deep changes of functional myocardium morphology. Different approaches to surgical ventricular reconstruction aimed at mechanical changes of the heart cavities sizes in combination with coronary artery bypass grafting (CABG) take the leading place in the complex treatment of this pathology. Nevertheless their outcomes show that in the late postoperative period repeated heart remodeling and CHF progressing i.e. return to the initial preoperative values of the heart cavities sizes and functional capacity of the heart takes place in a part of the operated patients (Batista, 1996; Dickstein, 1997; Dor, 1985; Gradinac, 1998; Menicanti & Di Donato,

2002; Menicanti & Di Donato, 2004; Moreira et al., 2001; Popovic et al., 1998; Popovic et al., 2001; Ratcliffe, 1998; Shah, 2003; Soo, 2005; Stolf, 1998).

The efforts to find clinical and instrumental prognostic criteria of unfavorable late outcomes of surgical treatment in patients with ICMP have not resulted in anything. According to publications, the following preoperative values have been associated with higher postoperative mortality and morbidity of the patients with ICMP: size of left ventricle (LV) (Yamaguchi, 2005), LV end-systolic volume index (LVESVI) (especially > 80 ml/m2 (Athanasuleas, 2004) and > 100 ml/m^2 (Yamaguchi, 2000)), LV ejection fraction (EF) (< 20% (Di Donato, 2001; Yamaguchi, 2005) or < 30%(Yamaguchi, 2000; Athanasuleas, 2004)), mitral regurgitation (Sartipy et al., 2006; Schroder, 2005), number of segments affected by dyssynergia (Di Donato, 1997), pulmonary hypertension >33mmHg (Di Donato, 1997), QRS>130ms (Yamaguchi, 2005), preoperative renal failure (Yamaguchi, 2005), time after previous myocardial infarction (Yamaguchi, 2005), age older than 75 years old (Athanasuleas, 2004). Nevertheless, there have not been any definite preoperative clinical predictors of postoperative LV remodeling offered.

Myocardium is a unique tissue consisting of highly differentiated cells - cardiomyocites which possess a number of morphological features in norm responding by a set of nonspecific structural changes to pathomorphism of cardiovascular diseases. In our opinion, the degree of revensability/irreversibility of advanced pathological processes in myocardium plays a key role in the success of reconstructive cardiac surgical interventions.

It has been 10-12 years since researchers started their first search for morphological predictors of postoperative heart remodeling in patients with cardiomyopathies, carrying out the analysis of the postoperative period course and evaluating morphofunctional condition of LV myocardium by the data of intraoperative biopsies (Gradinac, 1998; Moreira et al., 2001; Popovic et al., 2001; Stolf, 1998). However, the results of these solitary studies have been quite controversial (Moreira et al., 2001; Popovic et al., 2001). We have not found data about any attempts to search for morphological predictors of progressive postoperative LV remodeling in patients with ICMP. In the available Russian publications there are separate articles devoted to studies of morphofunctional condition of LV myocardium and myocardium of RA auricle in patients with coronary artery disease of different functional classes (Kuznetsov, 2003; Salikova et al., 2002). These works can hardly boast wide analysis of morphological parameters (Kuznetsov, 2003) and some authors only provide descriptive morphology without deep investigation of the mechanisms of possible pathogenesis of heart remodeling (Salikova et al., 2002).

At the same time, identification of morphological predictors of postoperative LV remodeling will not solve all the problems which cardiac surgeons face when choose the tactics for surgical intervention and think of the prognosis for each individual patient since pre- and postoperative morphological diagnostics of the pathological processes reversibility degree in ischemic myocardium in reality is limited very much by a definite degree of a risk associated with harvesting biopsies from heart walls which very often becomes a reason to refuse from this diagnostics. In the light of this, one of the perspective directions of scientific research is the finding of molecular predictors of postoperative heart remodeling in peripheral blood of patients together with tissue and cellular aspects of this phenomenon for the blood is always available for laboratory testing and monitoring of its content.

Until today, there have not been performed any complex fundamental scientific works devoted to the identification of tissue, cellular and molecular predictors of postoperative LV remodeling basing directly on real patients cases. The contemporary concept of CHF surgical treatment must be based on peculiarities of functional morphology of each individual patient's myocardium. Thorough patient selection basing on a complex clinical-morphological and biochemical analysis of the prognosis for surgical treatment outcome may improve the efficacy of a standard SVR procedure making a surgeon refuse from it in predeterminedly prospectless patients in favor of alternative methods of surgical treatment such as primary heart transplantation, implant of the devices preventing heart chambers dilatation, cardioresynchronizing therapy, etc.

The latter area has better perspective for the problem of organ transplantation is a very topical issue in modern medicine since the number of recipients exceeds significantly the number of donors. Cardiac support device (CSD) is a special device for suppression of heart chambers dilatation. Multi-centers randomized clinical trial for this device is being carried out at present and according to preliminary data its application is quite efficient for ischemic and dilated cardiomyopathies (Acorn cardiovascular, inc.™ Selected abstracts, 2000; Patel, 1997; Sabbah, 2001).

Objective of the study: The development of a diagnostic algorithm and justification of a modern concept of CHF surgical treatment basing on identification of morphological and blood markers of progressive postoperative LV remodeling in patients with ICMP.

2. Materials and methods

2.1 Design of the study. Object

One hundred and ninety five patients with ICMP and with previous myocardial infarctions have become the object of the study. All the patients were admitted to the cardiovascular surgery department at Tomsk Institute of Cardiology during the period from 2002 to 2009. Preoperative diagnostics included transthoracic EchoCG, Halter ECG monitoring, coronaroventriculography with manometry, SPECT imaging with 99mTc-technetril, MRI imaging of the heart with dye.

The clinical inclusion criteria for the patients enrolled into the study were the following parameters: LV end-diastolic volume index (LVEDVI) > 90 ml/m2, LVESVI > 70 ml/m2 , LV end-diastolic pressure (LVEDP) > 30 mmHg, EF LV < 40%, akinetic and dyskinetic areas of LV, angina II-IV CCS FC, heart failure (HF) II-IV NYHA, coronary artery disease from 1 - 10 years, lesions of coronary arteries – stenosis of more than 75% of LAD or of the trunk, or not less than 75% stenosis in at least two coronary arteries. The age of the patients included into the study was between 37 and 68 years (53.6±8.3), mean number of affected coronary arteries was 2.7±0.4. Lack of organic lesions of heart valves apart from ischemic mitral valve regurgitation was also a clinical criterion for patients' selection.

The reason for the development of ICMP in all the patients was an extensive transmural myocardial infarction. In 135 patients (69.2%) heart insufficiency appeared after their first myocardial infarction. All the patients in conditions of bypass and cardioplegia underwent surgical reconstruction of LV by V.Dor and L.Menicanti methods in different combinations with myocardial revascularization, reduction and reconstruction of LV volume and shape due to exclusion of its scarred septal, anterior and basal parts by endoventriculoplasty and by restoration of the mitral valve (MV) function.

Clinical characteristics		Value
Number of the patients		195 (100 %)
Men		177 (90.8 %)
Women		18 (9.2 %)
Mean age (years)		53.6±8.3
Number of previous MI	1	135 (69.2 %)
	2	39 (20.0 %)
	3	15 (7.7 %)
	4	6 (3.1 %)
Angina functional class (CSS)	Without angina	9 (4.6 %)
	I	15 (7.7 %)
	II	36 (18.5 %)
	III	132 (67.7 %)
	IV	3 (1.5 %)
NYHA functional class		2.86±0.40
Number of the coronary arteries with atherosclerotic lesions	1	72 (36.9 %)
	2	54 (27.7 %)
	3	69 (35.4 %)
LVEDVI (ml/m^2)		114.9±28.4
LVESVI (ml/m^2)		76.7±23.0
LV EF (%)		32.1±5.5
Degree of mitral regurgitation	0	36 (18.5 %)
	I	51 (26.2 %)
	II	63 (32.3 %)
	III	36 (18.4 %)
	IV	9 (4.6 %)
Hypertensive disease		126 (64.6 %)
Diabetes mellitus		30 (15.4 %)
Obesity		39 (20.0 %)
Peripheral atherosclerosis		33 (16.9 %)

Table 1. Initial clinical characteristics of the patients enrolled into the study

Intraoperative control of the remaining LV cavity was performed with the help of special devices (sizers) and satisfied a physiological norm for each patient (55-60 ml/m2). Reduction of LV cavity had to be combined with giving it elliptical shape, which was performed with the use of endovascular patch and retraction of papillary muscles. Interventions on mitral valve were performed in 51 patients (26.2 %). MV repair was made in 36 cases (18.5 %); MV prosthesis was placed in 12 cases (6.2 %). The spectrum of surgical interventions is shown in table 2.

Spectrum of surgical interventions	Absolute value (n = 195)	Relative value (%)
CABG+SVR	132	67.6
CABG+SVR+MV repair	39	20.0
CABG+SVR+MV prosthesis	12	6.2
SVR+TMLR	6	3.1
SVR+CABG+TMLR	6	3.1

Note: CABG - coronary artery bypass grafting; SVR - surgical ventricular reconstruction; MV repair - mitral valve repair; MV prosthesis - mitral valve prosthesis; TMLR - transmyocardial laser revascularization.

Table 2. The spectrum of surgical interventions carried out in the patients with ICMP enrolled into the study

Biopsy samples of RA auricle and LV were taken from the border area of endocardial scar and from the area of the myocardium without visual changes from all the patients (n=195, 100%) with ICMP. RA auricle biopsy was performed during the period of RA cannulation. LV biopsy samples were taken during surgical ventricular reconstruction from the transient zone on the border between scarred tissue and unchanged myocardium.

All the patients signed an informed consent form for the participation in the study; the study was approved by the local ethical committee of Tomsk Institute of Cardiology.

In order to find noninvasive molecular markers of postoperative LV remodeling blood samples were taken from 53 patients with ICMP (27.2%) to identify the content of natriuretic peptides and matrix metalloproteinases in blood plasma and serum correspondingly. In 37 patients antibodies titre to myocardial structures was identified in blood serum.

In the early postoperative period (1 month) control transthoracic EcoCG was made. In 12 months after the surgical treatment the patients were hospitalized again for clinical examination and control EchoCG.

In the late follow-up period repeated LV remodeling and HF progressing took place in a part of the patients which resulted in assignment of the patients into two groups: with positive (regressive remodeling - group I) and negative (progressing postoperative remodeling - group II) dynamics.

To achieve the objectives of identification tissue, cellular and molecular markers of postoperative LV remodeling we have used histological, electron-microscopic, morphometrical, biochemical and statistical methods of study.

To compare morphometrical parameters, as a control group we took autopsy samples of the identical sites of LV myocardium and myocardium of RA auricle from 25 cadavers of both sexes and of a comparable age died from an acute trauma with no signs of cardio-vascular pathology.

Seventeen healthy male and female volunteers of comparable age comprised a control group for the evaluation of the content of natriuretic peptide and matrix metalloproteinases in blood plasma and serum, respectively, as well as for identification of the antibodies titre to myocardial structures.

2.2 Histological study methods

Histological methods include preliminary treatment of the studied material necessary for its further microscopic evaluation. Preparation of histological samples was performed as follows (Krivolapov, 2006): the samples of myocardium were being fixed in 10% solution of

neutral formalin during 24 hours, and then they were washed in running water and dehydrated in the solution for histological treatment (dehydration and clearing) based on absolute isopropyl alcohol IsoPrep (BioVitrum, Saint Petersburg, Russia). After dehydration the myocardial samples were placed into homogenized paraffin media HISTOMIX® (BioVitrum, Saint Petersburg, Russia). Paraffin section of about 5-7mcm thick obtained with the use of a sliding microtome MC-2 were stained by hematoxylin and eosine and by Mallori method (stains and staining kits by BioOptica, Italy). The stained samples were place into synthetic monitoring media BioMount (BioOptica, Italy).
Histological samples were studied with a routine light and polarization microscopy on Axioskop 40 microscope (Carl Zeiss, Germany). Microimages of histological samples were taken with the Canon G10 camera (Japan).

2.3 Methods of electron-microscopic study

We took LV myocardium and RA auricle myocardium samples from 58 ICMP patients (50 men, 8 women) for electron-microscopy study. Myocardial samples of not more than 2mm^3 were fixed in 2.5% glutaric aldehyde solution on 0.2M cacodylate buffer with pH=7.2 with the temperature of +4 °C and postfixed in 1% OsO_4 solution in cold during 4 hours. The bioptates were then dehydrated in ethanol of rising concentration and placed into the mixture of epone and araldite. Semifine and ultrafine sections were prepared on ultratome LKB III (Sweden). The semifine sections were stained by 1% azure II solution and evaluated visually through a light microscope. The ultrafine sections were contrasted by lead citrate and uranyl acetate and studied in an electron microscope JEM-100 CX (Japan).

2.4 Morphological methods of study

For quantitative characteristic of the changes morphometrical methods were applied such as measurement of specific volume (SV) of edema, vessels, parenchyma and myocardial stroma by the point counting methods (Avtandilov, 1990; Glagolev & Chepulin, 1968). Measurement of parenchyma, stroma, vessels and edema SV was performed in 5-7 random microscopic fields of each section with the use of the software for graphic images procession (AxioVision by Carl Zeiss, ImageJ, Germany). One mm^3 of the tissue was considered as a unit volume for the study on the light-optical level (Avtandilov, 1990). Ocular micrometer MOB-1-16^x («ЛОМО», Saint Petersburg, Russia) was used to measure diameter of cardiomyocytes on longitudinal sections on the level of myocardial cells nuclei. For the quantitative characteristics of the interrelation among myocardial parenchyma, stroma of the organ and exchange link of microcirculatory bed the following morphometrical parameters were evaluated to reveal risk factors of postoperative heart remodeling: parenchyma-stromal ratio (PSR), trophic index (TI) and pericapillar diffusion zone (PcDZ); and for the quantitative characteristics of microvasculature and their capacity Kernogan index (KI) was calculated. PSR is a ratio between myocardial parenchyma SV and stromal SV; TI (the best index reflecting the condition of myocardial trophy) - is the ratio between capillary SV and parenchyma SV; PcDZ (the area of tissue supplied with blood by one capillar) - the ratio between the capillary diameter and their SV; KI (the index of carrying capacity of microcirculatory bed) - is the ratio between arterioles vascular wall and the radius of their lumens (Avtandilov, 1990).
Morphometry of the ultrastructures was performed on digitized negative photoplates with initial magnitude 4800–10000. We calculated SV of myofibrils, mitochondrias and granules

of atrial cardiomyocytes. One mcm^3 of tissue was taken as a unit volume for the study on a light-microscopic level (Avtandilov, 1990). Mitochondrial-myofibrillar ratio was evaluated as the ratio of mitochondrial SV to the SV of miofibrills.

Electron-microscopic study of myocardial microcirculatory bed allowed for evaluation of the ratio between open (functioning) and closed (not functioning) capillaries. For the open capillaries we performed quantitative evaluation of their lumen and active transport through endothelium with the help of micropinocytic vesicles. For that, we identified the number of pinocytic vesicles associated with a length unit of a luminal contour on an area unit of capillary lumen, as well as density of free pinocytic vesicles per a volume unit of endothelial cells cytoplasm.

2.5 Biochemical methods of study of blood plasma and serum of the ICMP patients

The content of natriuretic peptides (pro-ANP и NT-proBNP), matrix metalloproteinases (pro-MMP-1, MMP-3, MMP-9) and tissue inhibitor of metalloproteinase-1 (TIMP-1) in blood plasma and serum of the ICMP patients was identified by immunoenzyme method with standard kits by: pro-ANP and NT-proBNP - Biomedica (Austria); MMP-1 and MMP-9 - Quantikine® (R&D Systems, USA); MMP-3 and TIMP-1 - Biosource (Belgium). Evaluation of circulating antibodies to myocardium in blood serum had been performed in 37 patients with ICMP by the method based on the indirect immunofluorescence reaction («IMMCO Diagnostics» set, USA): we registered the presence of antifibrillar, antisarcolemmic and antinuclear antibodies by localization of fluorochrome on histological preparations by the method of fluorescent microscopy using the Axio Scope A1 microscope (Carl Zeiss, Germany). The concentration of the antibodies was expressed in titre.

2.6 Clinical and instrumental methods of study

Every patient underwent twelve-lead ECG study (Schiller AT-6 machine, Switzerland) before and after the surgery. The degree of cardiomegalia and the condition of pulmonary circulation was evaluated by radiographic methods of study. Each patient underwent EchoCG examination with color dopplerography on Acuson 128 XP/10 (Japan). To study global systolic function of LV the following parameters were evaluated: end-diastolic size of LV, end-systolic size of LV, LV stroke volume and their indexes, LV EF, thickness of ventricular septum and that of posterior LV wall. Contractility of 16 segments was evaluated by a 4-score system and the index of local contractility disturbance was calculated to study disturbances of local LV myocardial contractility. To study LV diastolic function we evaluated transmitral blood flow by dopplerography. We also assessed the sizes of left atrium, degree of mitral regurgitation, estimate pressure in pulmonary artery. All the patients underwent EchoCG study before the surgery and in the postoperative period. Using the obtained data of echocardiography we calculated an estimate indicator – the index of specific thickness of LV wall by the following formula: thickness of ventricular septum + thickness of LV posterior wall/end-diastolic LV size. To assess this indicator we used the following grading: with remodeling index <0.30 – maladaptive remodeling; with the index from 0.30 to 0.45 – adaptive remodeling; >0.45 – asymptomatic remodeling.

Coronary angiography and left ventriculargraphy were performed on Philips maximus C1250, Philips polydiagnost C20 angiographic units. Selective coronary angiography was performed by Judkins method (1967) with freezing monitoring images.

To calculate changes of ESVI expressed as a percentage we used the formula:

$$\Delta ESVI = (\text{preoperative ESVI / ESVI in a year after the surgery x } 100) - 100.$$

To study the values of central hemodynamics the patients were subjected to catheterization of heart chambers with measurements of LVEDP and pressure in the pulmonary artery.

2.7 Statistical analysis of the results

The results were statistically analyzed with the software package SSPS 11.5 for Windows. Normality of a distribution law of quantitative values was assessed by Shapiro-Wilk test. Parameters which obey the normal distribution law were described with the help of the mean value (M) and standard deviation (m); those which do not obey the normal distribution law - with the use of median (Me) and interquintile interval (Q_{25}–Q_{75}). Qualitative data were described by the frequency of occurrence or its percentage. If the distribution law was normal, Student t-test was used for the assessment of reliability of quantitative values differences in the compared groups; Mann-Whitney test - in the case of not normal distribution law. To evaluate reliability of quantitative data χ^2 criterion was used (or Fisher exact test in cases when χ^2 test was not possible). To find statistical dependences of linear character, to identify their strength and direction Pearson correlation coefficient (r) (among quantitative values obeying the law of normal distribution) and Spearsman correlation coefficient (for quantitative values not obeying the law of normal distribution and for qualitative values in the ordinal scale) were calculated. All statistical values were considered significant with $p<0.05$.

3. Results and discussion

3.1 Morphological predictors of postoperative LV remodeling in ICMP patients

During the study of morphofunctional condition of LV myocardium and myocardium of RA auricle in the patients with ICMP there was found that the density of vessels distribution was significantly decreased in comparison with that in the control group. Irrespectively of the blood vessels diameter the signs of hemodynamic disturbances were noticed everywhere: perivascular edema, venous plethora, desolation and spasm of arterioles and small arteries (fig. 1). Nuclei of endothelial cells in spasm arterioles were visually "extruded" into the vessels lumen. Microcirculatory link of vascular bed was plethoric; phenomena of erythrocyte stasis in capillaries, pericapillaries and arterioles were observed quite often. In separate capillaries we noticed rounding of endothelial cells manifesting as extrusion of endothelial cells nuclei into the capillaries lumen which, without any doubt, lowered their carrying capacity and the level of myocardial trophy.

In LV myocardium and in that of RA auricle of the ICMP patients stroma had enlarged volume and was edematous; its collagen fibers were curved and sometimes swollen. Mixed (lymphocytic-macrophage) infiltrate (> 14 per mm2 of tissue by Marburg classification (World Heart Federation Consensus Conferences Definition of Inflammatory Cardiomyopathy (Myocarditis), 1997) was found in some patients' LV myocardial stroma and RA auricle which was considered as myocarditis (fig. 2).

In the ICMP patients LV myocardial cardiomyocytes were, as a rule, hypertrophic and located either singly or in small foci surrounded by the areas of scarred tissue which had been formed at the sites of previous infarctions. It is worth mentioning a pronounced polymorphism of myocardial cells nuclei: their enlargement, changing shape and tinctoral properties. In the most cases the shape of cardiomyocytes was oval with fuzzy contours. Quite often the nuclei had the shapes of "eights", "bow", "spring", etc. Chromatin in such the nuclei was condensed and located mostly along the nuclei periphery. Oxyphilous inclusions looking like apoptotic bodies were noticed either close to some nuclei or inside them. Such cardiomyocytes had eosinophilic cytoplasm and irregular contours of the cells.

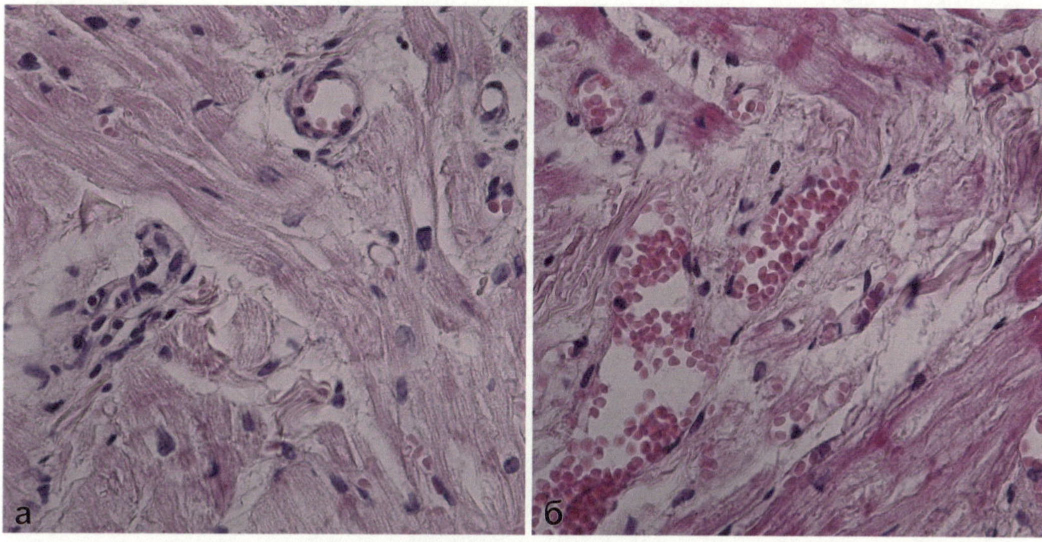

Fig. 1. LV myocardium of ICMP patients: a - perivascular edema; b -venous plethora. Stained with hematoxylin and eosin. X 450 (a) and 400 (b)

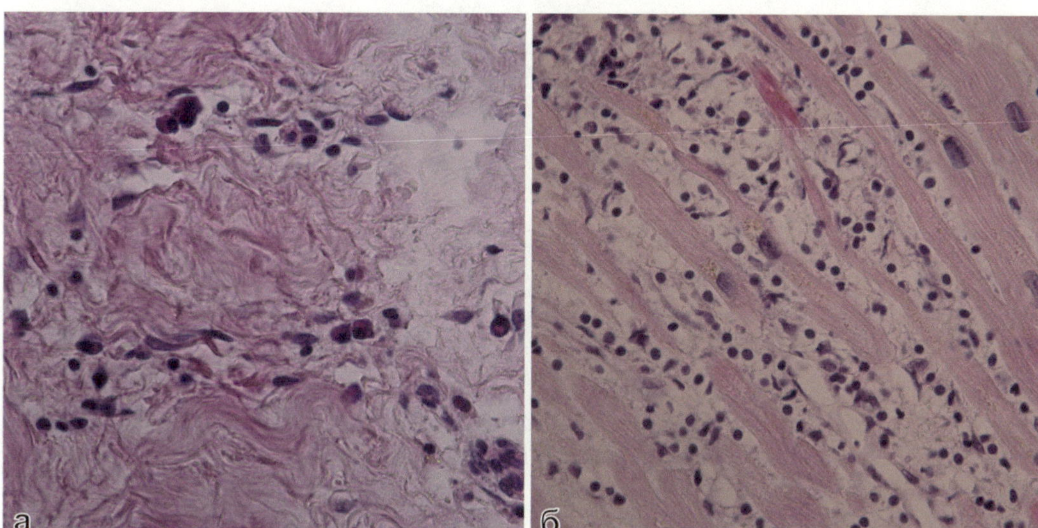

Fig. 2. LV myocardium of ICMP patients: a - mixed (lymphocytic-macrophage) focal infiltration; b - diffuse lymphocytic infiltration of myocardial stroma. Stained with hematoxylin and eosin. X 500 (a) and 300 (b)

Intracellular edema in cardiomyocytes of LV was noticed everywhere and its degree varied very much from cell to cell. In a polarized light on histological preparations stained with hematoxyline and eosine alongside with unchanged areas of cardiomyocytes' cytoplasm we observed damaged areas of sarcoplasm with predominantly subsegmental contractures, contracture lesions of the Ist, IInd and less often IIId degree which differed by the enhancement of luminescence of disdiaclasts with different degrees of isotropic discs shortening; we also noticed isolated areas of intracellular myocytolysis and primary clump disintegration of myofibrillas and cytolysis of cardiomyocytes. The described changes of mosaic nature were also noticed in RA auricle myocardium.
Study of morphofunctional condition of LV myocardium in patients with ICMP revealed very interesting peculiarities: cardiomyocytes organization disturbance in muscular fibers and disturbance of fibers orientation relative to each other, disintegration of myocardial cells on intercalated disks, elimination of cardiomyocytes along muscular fibers (fig. 3). Myocardium in these cases had not fibrous but cellular structure which resulted in its poor contractility (Anderson, 2005). Sometimes cardiac myocytes were star-shaped. Besides, on the longitudinal sections of LV myocardium of ICMP patients one could observe wave-shape deformation of cardiomyocytes along myocardial fibers.

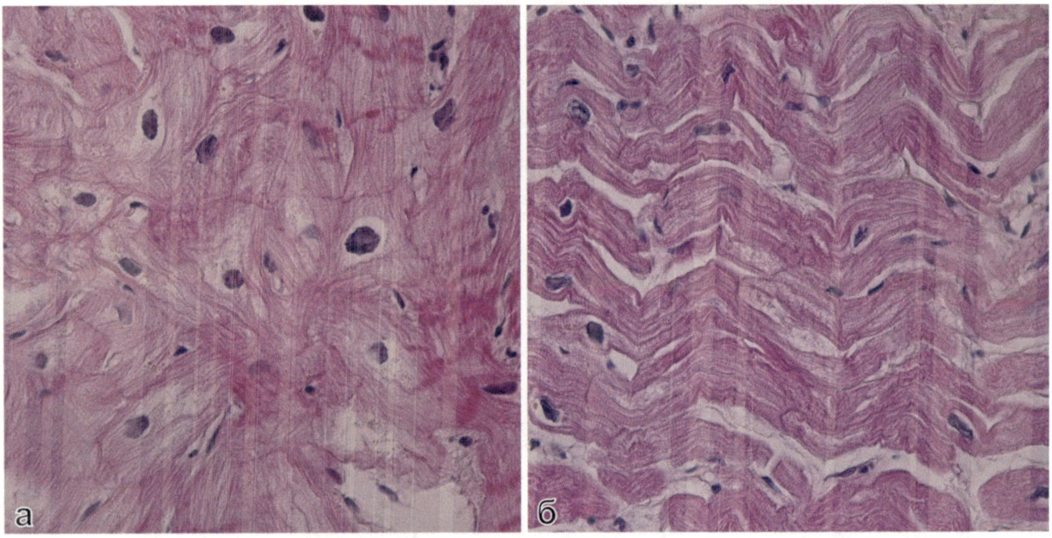

Fig. 3. LV myocardium of ICMP patients: a- disturbance of muscular fiber orientation, star-shaped cardiomyocytes; b- wave-shaped deformation of muscular fibers. Stained with hematoxylin and eosin. X 370 (a) and 330 (b)

During electron-microscopic study of myocardial cardiomyocytes of LV and RA auricle our attention was drawn to the polymorphism of ultrastructures of myocardial cells. Nuclei often having irregular scalloped shape with multiple intussusceptums and outgrowths of nuclear membrane were located in the center of the cells, but in some cardiomyocytes they were displaced into subsarcolemmic zone. Genetic material was observed mostly as euchromatin which took a central position. In some cardiomyocytes' nuclei, vice versa, heterochromatin prevailed and was situated mostly in juxtamembrane zone. Chromatin aggregation (compaction) was noticed quite often. Nuclear envelope was continuous throughout and had pores.

Perinuclear space was dilated; it was not filled with mitochondrias, granular reticulum and elements of Golgi organ but consisted mostly of rare matrix containing glycogen of β-shape and having round or elongated shape (monogranular glycogen) (fig. 4). Rosettes of α-glycogen were present in a very insignificant number in intermiofibrillar spaces.

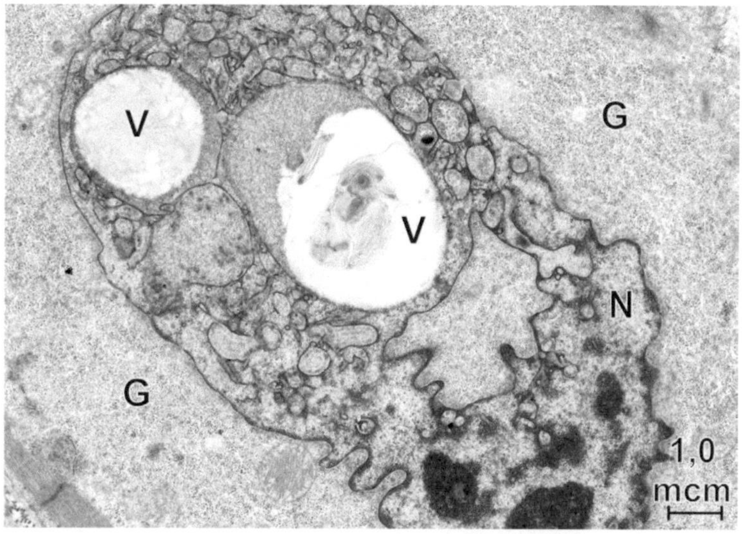

Fig. 4. A fragment of a left ventricular cardiomyocyte of an ICMP patient: vacuolization (V) of a nucleus (N) with its further desolation; dilatation of perinuclear space filled with β- glycogen (G)

Dispersed nucleoli, segregation of fibrillar and granular components of nucleolonema, ring-shaped nucleoli were noticed which evidenced suppression of rRNA biosynthesis (fig. 5).

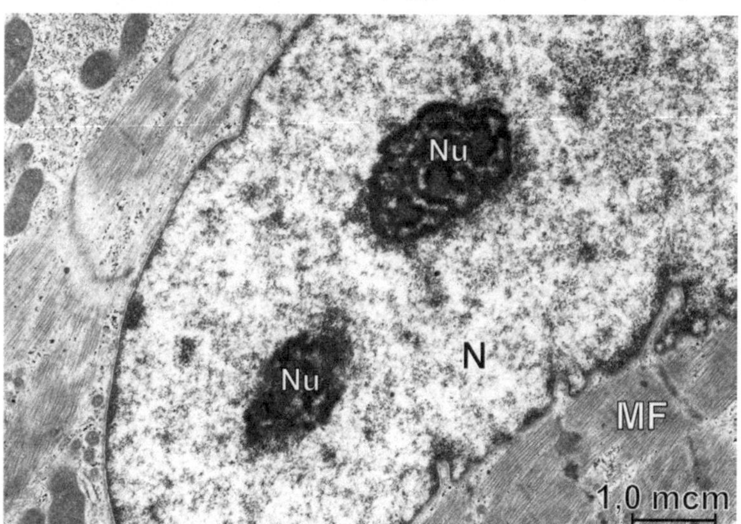

Fig. 5. A fragment of a left ventricular cardiomyocyte of an ICMP patient. Dispersion of nucleoles (Nu), segregation of granular and fibrillar components. N- a nucleus of a cardiomyocyte; MF – myofibrils

We also found wide variety of myofibril lesion forms in LV and RA auricle myocardial cardiomyocytes in ICMP patients such as: contracture lesions of myofibrils of the Ist, less often of the IInd and III^{d} degrees, isolated areas of primary clump of fibrillar disaggregation (fig. 6). The presence of contracture lesions of the III^{d} degree in a cell was associated with formation of sarcolemma festoons, contraction and deformation of a nucleus and mitochondrias due to overcontraction of myofibrils and with displacement of mitochondrias into the space between myofibrils and formation of compact assemblies.

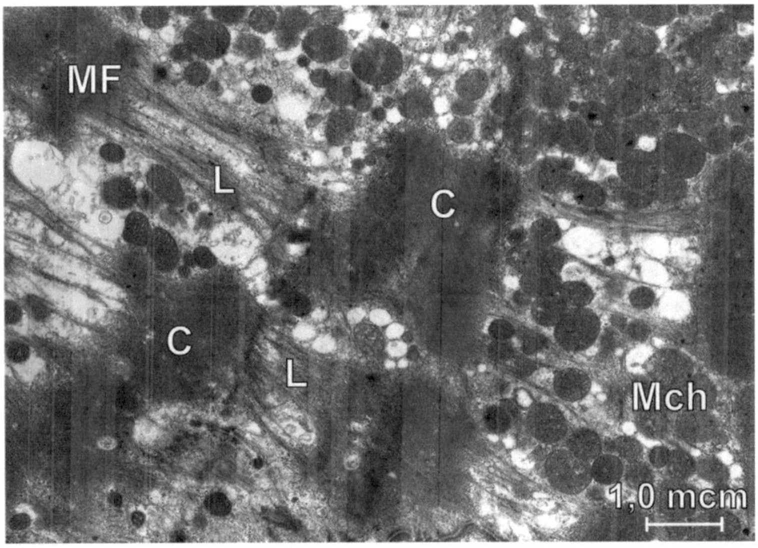

Fig. 6. Primary clump disintegration of LV myocardial cardiomyocite's myofibrils of an ICMP patient: alteration of the areas of mosaic lysis (L) and contractures (C) in isolated groups of myofibrillar (MF) sarcomeres; MCh- mitochondrias

In the most cardiomyocytes small-focal and diffuse lysis of myofibrillar bundles, myofibril "melting" were registered. I-disks with thin (actin) filaments in them were lysed to a greater extent. Myofibrils were becoming less dense, cavities appeared in some sarcomeres, total lysis of myofilaments within a sarcomere was noticed. Sarcomeres in the area of intercalated disks and in perinuclear zone were significantly destructed.

It was very seldom when foci of intracellular regeneration of ultrastructures were found in LV and RA auricle myocardial cardiomyocytes. The foci were evaluated by the accumulation of free ribosomes on the stumps of survived myofibrils contributing to the synthesis and neoformation of contractile proteins. As the newly formed myofilaments synthesized on polyribosomes and got matured they gathered into the bundles of myofibrils. But in the process of their neoformation their normal orientation is disturbed, they elongate excessively and it results in growing distance between Z-bands.

Apart from disturbance of normal orientation of the newly formed myofibrils we observed chaotic orientation of "mature" contractile proteins. Myofibrilar bundles and even individual myofilaments were oriented at different angles in relation to each other. Besides, wave-shaped deformation of a contractile apparatus of LV and RA auricle myocardial cardiomyocytes took place in the patients with ICMP. All these circumstances, with no doubt, made their contribution into desynchronization of contractile processes, thus preconditioning systolic dysfunction of myocardium (Anderson, 2005).

Polymorphism of mitochondrias attracted our attention. We observed large mitochondrias reaching a length of 2-3 sarcomeres in the space among myofibrils. On the contrary, more often we were observing small round mitochondrias located randomly or in clusters. Sometimes we saw mitochondrias with destructive and degenerative changes, with cleared matrix, destroyed and reduced cristas, few mitochondrias with electron-dense matrix in condition of vacuolization.

Cisterns and vacuoles of cytoplasmic reticulum and Golgi apparatus in LV and RA auricle myocardium cardiomyocytes were deduced and sometimes dilated in the samples of ICMP patients. Dilation of the cisterns was found mostly in perinuclear zone and less often in the space between fibrils (in the area of Z-bands) and mitochondrias.

Atrial cardiomyocytes contained electron-dense granules of atrial natriuretic peptide of various sizes.

Thus, electron-microscopic study revealed mixed, alterative and regenerative-plastic insufficiency of cardiomyocytes in both LV and RA auricle.

Electron-microscopic study of peculiarities of microvasculature functional morphology was performed for intraoperative samples of LV and RA auricle from 47 ICMP patients (44 men, 3 women). Hemocapillaries having a sufficient lumen for passage of blood cells or containing these cells in their lumen were considered open (functioning). Hemocapillaries with a minimal lumen between plasmalemmas of endothelial cells insufficient for blood cells circulation were considered closed (non-functioning).

In endothelial cells of myocardial capillaries a large number of micropinocytic vesicles of different diameters (from 30 to 120nm) was found; these vesicles were present in both closed and open capillaries. The content of small vesicles was electron-optically low dense. On the contrary, large vesicles were electron-optically transparent. The number of micropinocytic vesicles in endotheliocytes in different capillaries was variable and their number in closed capillaries was very insignificant.

In cytoplasm of endothelial cells unexpanded canaliculi of granular and granular endoplasmic reticulum were observed as well as multiple crests and dints on a luminal surface of the cells.

Electron-microscopic study of microvasculatory link of LV and RA auricle myocardial vascular bed one could notice a bulging endotheliocytes into the capillaries lumen, reduction of their lumen and their decreased capacity. Rounding of endotheliocytes, probably, has adaptive meaning and is directed toward slowing blood flow in capillaries and more efficient use of blood mass in transcapillar exchange (Kawamura et al., 1974).

Matrix of endothelial cells cytoplasm in one and the same capillary is vividly cleared in one cells evidencing swelling of cytoplasm and in other cells it becomes electron-optically dense. If an endothelial cell matrix was cleared, we could visualize mostly singular small size micropinocytic vesicles situated predominantly on free and basal edges of cytoplasm. In cytoplasm of dark endotheliocytes larger pinocytic vesicles were present quite often (fig. 7).

Often one could see mitochondrias in capillary endotheliocytes of LV and RA auricle myocardium. Usually no changes in functional morphology of cellular energy apparatus were noticed, but sometimes we observed mitochondrias with cleared matrix, dilated intracristal spaces and destroyed crysts. Myelin-like structures were found in some mitochondrias.

In clear endotheliocytes were swallow and chromatin was loose. In osmium dark cells nuclei remained unchanged. Chromatin aggregation and pyknotic nuclei were noticed eventually. In nuclei of singular endotheliocytes we noticed the lost connection between heterochromatin and nuclear membrain. Heterochromatin was displaced deeper into the nuclei of endothelial cells and was present there as ring-shaped structures.

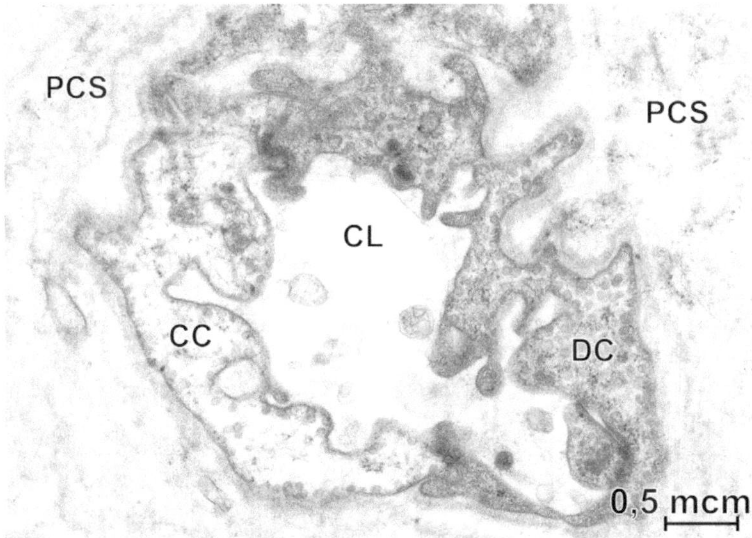

Fig. 7. A capillary from LV myocardium of an ICMP patient: Capillary lumen (CL) is limited by an endothelial cell with osmium dark matrix (a dark cell - DC) and by an endothelial cell with cleared matrix (a clear cell - CC). PCS – pericapillar space

Sometimes large lipid inclusions were noticed in cytoplasm of endothelial cells of capillaries in both LV and RV auricle myocardium; large vacuoles – only in singular cardiomyocytes. Glycogen granules were eventually found in insignificant amount.

Subendocardial capillary zone as a rule was not changed. Sometimes on longitudinal sections one could see isolated local dilations. Basal membrane was uninterrupted throughout and in most cases had the same thickness with only rare local thickened parts. Noncellular element of a basal layer was thickened locally and loose, occasionally thinned and interrupted.

The space between basal capillary membrane and cardiomyocytes (adventitious layer) was, as a rule, dilated and filled mostly with fibrous component of a loose connective tissue (with the prevalence of collagen fibers) and less often – with electron-transparent amorphous substance of low electron density (with separate fibrous structures like collagen fibers). In the latter case pericapillar space was sharply cleared; areas of a substance with low electron-optical density identical to that of plasma in a capillary lumen were found. The contours of these areas were not clear.

Cytoplasmic crest of pericytes were close to cytoplasm adjusting immediately to it. There were no any pronounced changes of functional morphology in pericytes found.

Pericapillar edema was registered in almost all the patients with ICMP, its degree varied significantly.

Thus, a thorough analysis of functional morphology of microvasculature in ICMP patients revealed specific changes of endothelial capillaries situated in foci of chronic ischemia.

Early postoperative mortality during 30 days after the surgery in the group of ICMP patients was 7.7% (n=15). First year postoperative mortality comprised 9.2% (n=18). Mean period of the control follow-up comprised 369±147 days. Only 153 (78.5 %) patients took part in the further study since 33 patients (16.9%) died in the early and mid-term postoperative period and communication with 9 patients (4.6%) was lost. During control examination (in a year after the surgery) clinical and echocardiography evaluation of the surgical treatment outcomes was performed.

In January 2009 all the patients who had underwent reexamination (n=153) were interviewed over the telephone. Mean follow-up period was 4.24 years, maximal follow-up period - 6 years. We managed to acquire information about all the patients who had had control examination. By the time of the interview there had been 108 alive patients of all included into the study. Mortality in the group during all the follow-up period comprised 29.4% (n=45), 27.5% (n=42) died from cardiac diseases.

Echocardiography was used as an instrumental method of the evaluation of heart cavities sizes and for the calculation of their indexed values. Despite obvious benefits of this method of study, it has low reproducibility of results, which varies within 20% from obtained values (Geidel, 2005; Gelsomino, 2008).

With an artificially introduced efficacy endpoint (ΔESVI - delta ESVI- postoperatively less than 20% from preoperative values) we managed to divide the initially homogeneous group of the patients into two subgroups, different by the character of clinical course of HF after surgical treatment. To calculate ΔESVI parameter we used the following formula:

$$\Delta ESVI = (\text{postoperative ESVI} / \text{preoperative ESVI} \times 100) - 100$$

To evaluate changes of LV ESVI 20% interval in comparison with preoperative values was used: changes > 20% into positive or negative side were considered sufficient to take these changes as true. The patients in which LV ESVI was <80% from preoperative values were assigned to group I. In these patients the process of LV remodeling was stopped and reversed by surgical intervention i.e. reverse (regressive) remodeling type. The calculated value of ΔESVI was < minus 20%.

The patients in which ESVI was > 80% from preoperative values were assigned to group II of the study. In these patients the course of HF remained unchanged due to the complex surgical treatment of ICMP: remodeling process was either resistant to the exposure or went on progressing after surgical treatment, i.e. had progressing remodeling type. The calculated value of ΔESVI was > minus 20%.

The distribution of the patients between the groups basing on the ΔESVI value was the following: the 1st group consisted of 97 patients (63.4%) with the reverse remodeling type (i.e. with positive dynamics of the late postoperative period); the 2nd group consisted of 56 patients (36.6%) with progressing remodeling type (i.e. with negative dynamics of the late postoperative period).

Analysis of the control EchoCG data showed that in the early postoperative period in all the patients end-diastolic and end-systolic heart volumes decreased: LV EDVI from (114.9±28.4) ml/m^2 to (98.0±25.3) ml/m^2, LV ESVI from (83.9 ±21.6) ml/m^2 to (64.3±21.0) ml/m^2; and LV EF significantly increased from (32.1±5.5) % to (36.7±8.9) %.The values of echocardiography study performed during control follow-up period are shown in Table 3.

Performed comparison of EchoCG data in the group of the patients with reverse LV remodeling showed that LV EF was significantly higher and the values of LVESVI and LVEDVI - significantly lower.

It should be noted that the great majority of the patients continued medical treatment recommended at the time of their dismissal from the hospital after the surgery. The groups with reverse and progressing types of remodeling were comparable in respect to the frequency of taking of different drug groups and their mean dosages.

Value	Before the surgery (n=153)	In a year after surgical intervention		
		All the pts (n=153)	Group I (n=97)	Group II (n=56)
FC NYHA	2.6±0.5*	2.3±0.3*	2.1±0.2**	3.0±0.2**
LV EDVI (ml/m²)	114.9±28.4*	98.0±25.3*	84.4±13.7**	102.6±14.6**
LV ESVI (ml/m²)	83.9±21.6*	64.3±21.0*	50.4±11.6**	71.9±17.3**
LV EF (%)	32.1±5.5*	36.7±8.9*	43.0±3.7**	33.0±5.1**

Note * – significance of the differences between the groups of the patients before surgical intervention and in a year after the surgery; ** – significance of the differences between the groups of the patients with reverse and progressive LV remodeling ($p < 0.05$).

Table 3. The values of HF functional class and the data of EchoCG study in the patients with ICMP in the control follow-up period

Among 153 patients included into the study and examined in a year after surgical treatment mean value of ΔESVI was minus 24.0: maximum value – 36.8, minimum – minus 64.7.
It is obvious that SVR results in higher values of ΔESVI in comparison with isolated CABG providing more significant decrease of LVESVI in a year after the surgery. To avoid statistical and methodological mistakes in the analysis of correlation relationships, the patients with maximum and minimum values of ΔESVI and the patients with hypercorrection associated with diastolic LV dysfunction with postoperative EDVI less than 60ml/m² were excluded from the further study. One hundred and thirty eight patients out from 153 were included into the further analysis: 90 patients with reverse remodeling (group I) and 48 patients with progressive remodeling (group II).
Screening analysis of correlation relationships between clinical data and ΔESVI with the use of Spearman test showed moderate reverse correlation relationship with the age of a patient (Table 4). This correlation relationship was also proved during detailed analysis; an absolute p value was 0.0001. Thus, taking into account that the smallest (negative) values of ΔESVI are optimal for a favorable clinical course, older patients with ICMP are prone to the development of progressive remodeling in postoperative period.
Initial clinical data characterizing the degree of coronary artery disease and heart failure did not demonstrate any correlation with the values of ΔESVI after surgical treatment.

Parameters	Value			R value	p<0.05
	ME	max	min		
Age	54.3	43	68	0.600	S
Number of MI	1	1	4	-0.097	NS
Hypertonic disease	3	0	3	-0.060	NS
Angina FC	III	I	IV	-0.244	NS
NYHA FC	3	2	4	0.127	NS
Men				-0.166	NS
Women				-0.166	NS
Diabetes mellitus				-0.088	NS
Obesity				-0.147	NS

Note: NS – statistically insignificant difference; S – statistically significant difference.

Table 4. Correlation relationships of clinical signs with the degree of LVESVI changes after surgical treatment of the patients with ICMP.

Analysis of preoperative EchoCG data and the values calculated on their basis revealed correlation relationship with ΔESVI shown in Table 5.

Mixed lymphocytic-macrophage infiltrate in LV myocardium of the IInd group patients was found in 42 out of 48 ICMP patients (87.5%) and in only 24 out of 90 patients (26.7 %) with reverse remodeling ($p<0.01$). In LV myocardium, as a rule, fibrosis was moderate (degree II according to Marburg classification) in the I[st] group of patients; in the IInd group of patients with ICM in the most cases it was severe (unfavorable, or the III[d] degree fibrosis) and in rare cases - moderate.

In 8 out of 24 patients from group I (33.3%) and in 33 out of 42 patients from group II (78.6) infiltration had diffuse nature ($p<0.01$), in the rest of the cases - focal and even less often - confluent.

Besides, in 18 patients (37.5%) with repeated LV dilatation and in 13 patients (14.4%) with favorable late outcomes of surgical treatment the infiltrate of a similar nature was found in myocardium of RA auricle ($p<0.01$). As a rule, fibrosis in RA auricle myocardium was I-II degrees lower by Marburg classification than that in LV myocardium.

Parameters	Values			R value	p<0.05
	ME	max	min		
Mitral regurgitation (degree)	2	4	0	-0.149	NS
Tricuspid regurgitation (degree)	0	3	0	-0.120	NS
Mean pressure in RV(mm Hg)	40	60	30	-0.025	NS
LV ESV (ml)	142	266	65	0.294	S
LV EDV(ml)	245.5	395.0	104.0	0.199	NS
LV ESVI (ml/m^2)	75.5	133.6	45.6	0.843	S
LV EDVI (ml/m^2)	111.1	190.0	71.2	-0.215	NS
LV EF M-mode (%)	34	40	20	-0.131	NS
LV EF B-mode (%)	32	38	19	-0.213	NS
Cardiac index (l/min/m^2)	2.2	5.0	1.6	-0.099	NS
Thickness of ventricular septum (mm)	10.5	15.0	6.0	-0.055	NS
Index of relative LV wall thickness	0.307	0.222	0.410	-0.026	NS

Note: NS - statistically insignificant difference; S - statistically significant difference.

Table 5. Correlation relationships of EchoCG parameters with the degree of LV dilatation in the patients with ICMP after combined surgical treatment.

It should be mentioned that there was no a case of cellular inflammatory infiltrate found in myocardial stroma in the autopsy material of the similar sites of LV myocardium and RA auricle myocardium taken from 25 cadavers which were the relative control group.

Statistical analysis of the obtained morphometrical data did not reveal any significant differences of the values of specific volume of edema and vessels among the patients with progressive and regressive remodeling. The specific volume of parenchyma was significantly higher and stroma specific volume - lower in both LV myocardium and in myocardium of RA auricle of the I[st] group patients. Morphometrical parameters of mean value of capillary diameter and diameter of LV and RA auricle myocardial cardiomyocytes did not differ significantly among the patients with different late outcomes of surgical treatment. Specific volume of capillaries in the aforementioned heart parts was significantly higher in the patients with reverse remodeling (group I). All the morphometrical parameters mentioned above differed statistically significantly from those of the control study group.

Parenchymo-stromal ratio reflecting quantitative relationships between parenchyma and stroma of cardiac muscular tissue was significantly lower in LV myocardium and in myocardium of RA auricle in 48 ICMP patients with unfavorable late outcomes of surgical treatment (Table 6).

Patients	Myocardium	PSR	TI	PcDZ (mcm)	KI
Group I (n=90)	RA	2.17±0.31*	0.042±0.016*	245.6±27.9*	1.61±0.37*
	LV	2.18±0.27**	0.027±0.011**	385.5±51.3**	1.55±0.32**
Group II (n=48)	RA	1.85±0.38*	0.024±0.008*	481.2±61.7*	1.84±0.30*
	LV	1.65±0.31**	0.008±0.003**	1315.7±88.2**	1.85±0.21**
Control group(n=25)	RA	5.96±0.14	0.086±0.006	81.0±1.7	1.13±0.10
	LV	9.48±0.20	0.087±0.003	66.1±2.6	1.15±0.08

Note: *, ** – significance of morphometrical values differences between the patient groups with positive and negative dynamics of late postoperative follow-up period for RA auricle and LV myocardium respectively ($p<0.05$).

Table 6. Morphometrical parameters of LV and RA auricle myocardium in ICMP patients with different late outcomes of surgical treatment, Van-der-Waerden test (M±m)

Trophic index of these parts of myocardium which better reflects the condition of cardiac muscular tissue and is assessed as a ratio between capillary specific volume and specific volume of cardiomyocytes, was statistically lower in patients with progressive remodeling; according to the data of intraoperative biopsies of LV myocardium the condition of myocardial trophy in these patients was 8-12 times lower in comparison with that of the control study group.

Pericapillar diffusion zone (the value reflecting load on capillary bed) and Kernogan index (the value showing carrying capacity of microvasculature – the bigger index is the less is carrying capacity of arterioles and the worse are the values of tissue trophy) of LV and RA auricle myocardium were statistically higher in the patients of group II. Values of PcDZ in ICMP patients with unfavorable late outcomes of surgical treatment assessed as a ratio of capillary diameter to their specific volume, 15-20 times exceeded those of the IInd group patients.

There was no significant difference between the groups concerning cardiomyocytes diameter in both LV and RA auricle myocardium found.

As a result of the complex clinical-morphological study we were granted the patent "The prognostic method for postoperative heart remodeling in patients with ischemic cardiomyopathy" #2310372 of 20.11.2007 by the Federal Intellectual Property, Patent and Trademark Service. The method was based on the evaluation of morphofunctional condition of LV myocardial samples on histological preparations stained with hematoxylin-eosin and by Mallory with the help of light microscopy. With simultaneous presence of pathomorphological picture of myocarditis and values of parenchyma-stromal ratio < 1.7, trophic index < 0.010, pericapillar diffusion zone > 1000 mcm and Kernogan index > 1.6 postoperative heart remodeling and progressive chronic heart failure can be predicted.

The offered prediction method of postoperative heart remodeling based on complex evaluation of myocardial morphology in preoperative period or during surgical intervention allows to avoid unfavorable late outcomes of surgical treatment. Clinical cases are the best proof of reliability of the patented prognostic method:

Clinical case 1. Patient N., 56 years old

Diagnosis: CAD. *Obliterating atherosclerotic stenosis of coronary arteries. Postinfarction cardiac sclerosis. LV aneurism. HF of III functional class by NYHA.*

CAD history - 5 years.

Preoperative examination

EchoCG: LV EDVI - 102.4 ml/m^2; LV ESVI - 68.2 ml/m^2; LV EF - 34 %. Mild mitral regurgitation.

Surgery: SVR by Menicanti, CABG. Intraoperative biopsy of LV myocardium taken for histological study.

During histological study of intraoperative samples of LV myocardium pathomorphological signs of myocarditis were found: presence of diffuse-macrophage inflammatory infiltration of myocardial stroma, the 3^d degree fibrosis (severe or unfavorable by Marburg classification of myocarditis).

Picture 8 shows a microimage of a histological preparation of LV from the patient N of 56 years old.

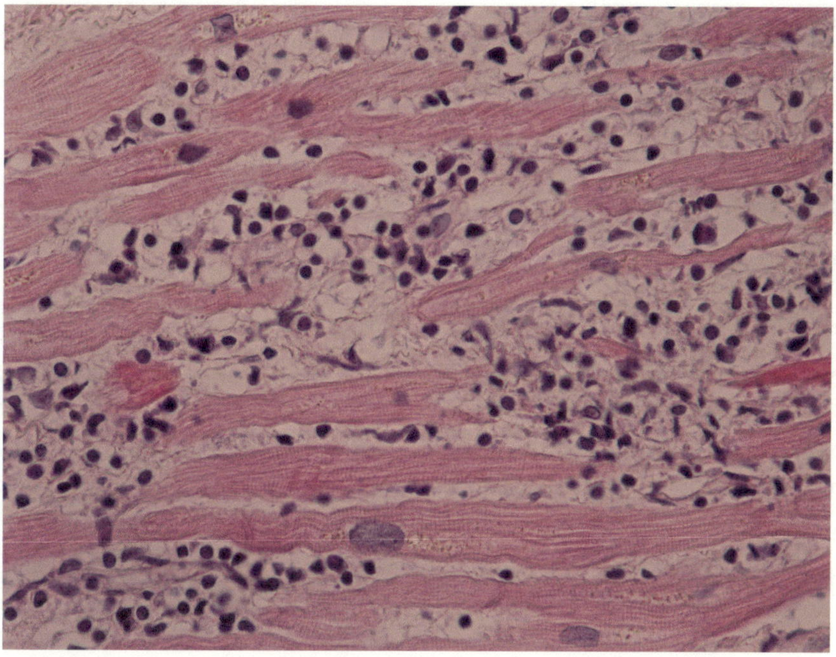

Fig. 8. Intraoperative biopsy sample of LV myocardium. Patient N, 56 year old. Diffuse-macrophage inflammatory infiltration of myocardial stroma. Severe (unfavorable) fibrosis. Stained with hematoxylin and eosin. X 300.

Morphometrical values of LV myocardium: parenchyma-stromal ratio - 1.04; trophic index - 0.0097; pericapillar diffusion zone - 1375.0 mcm; Kernogan index - 1.74; diameter of cardiomyocytes - 20.6 mcm. Thus, the morphological study revealed prognostic criteria associated with unfavorable late outcomes of surgical treatment.

Hospitalization in a year after the surgery.

CHF II FC. LV EDVI - 96.6 ml/m^2; LV ESVI - 62.2 ml/m^2, LV EF - 36%. Mild mitral regurgitation. Pre- and postoperative EchoCG images are shown in Figure 9.

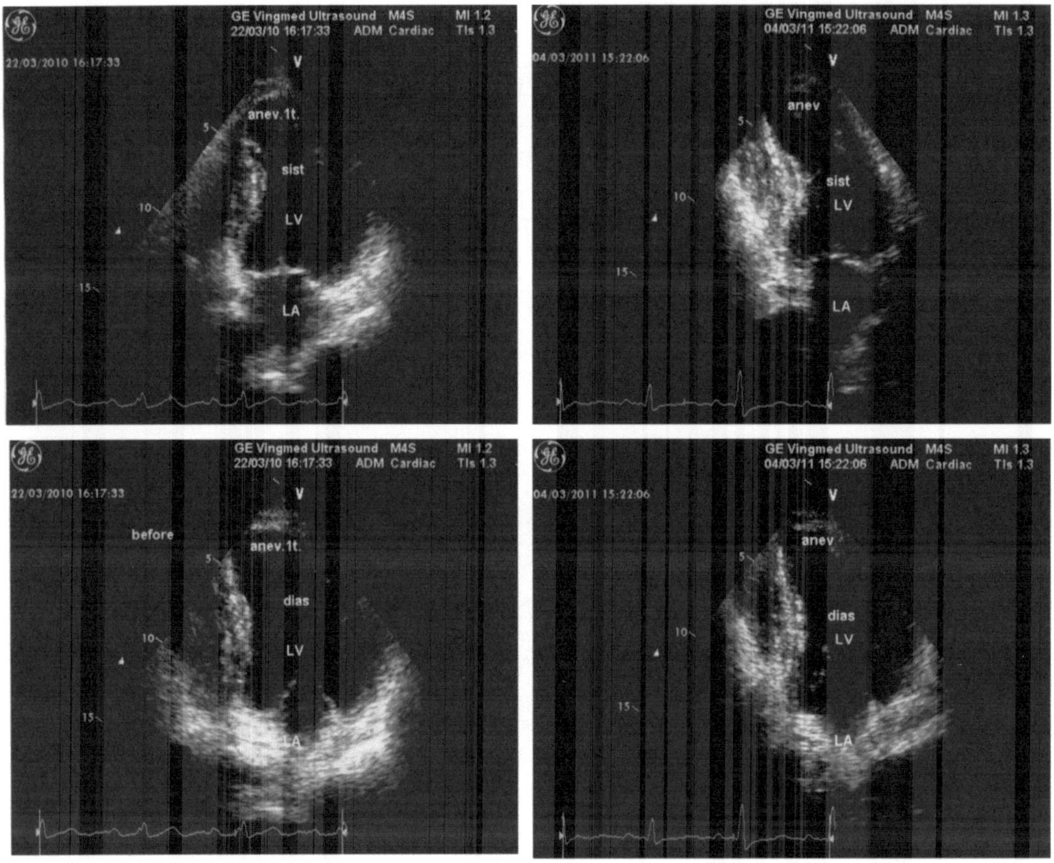

Fig. 9. Pre- and postoperative EchoCG images of the 56 year old patient N. Notice repeated postoperative LV remodeling and progression of chronic HF.

Clinical case 2. Patient B. 53 year old.

Diagnosis: CAD. *Obliterating atherosclerotic stenosis of coronary arteries. Postinfarction cardiosclerosis. LV aneurism. HF FC III by NYHA.*

Six year CAD history.

Preoperative examination

EchoCG: LV EDVI - 98.7 ml/m^2; LV ESVI - 61.3 ml/m^2; LV EF - 37 %. Mild mitral regurgitation.

Surgery: SVR by Menicanti, CABG. Intraoperative biopsy of myocardium taken for histological study.

Histological study of intraoperative samples of LV and RA auricle myocardium did not reveal any signs of inflammatory infiltration of myocardium. In Figure 10 one can see a microimage of the histological sample of LV myocardium from the 53 year old patient B.

Morphometrical values of LV myocardium: parenchyma-stromal ratio – 2.83; trophic index – 0.0417; pericapillar diffusion zone – 311.2 mcm; Kernogan index – 1.21; diameter of cardiomyocytes - 28.7 mcm. Thus, combination of the prognostic criteria for the progression of heart failure was not found, postoperative heart remodeling in the late follow-up period is not predicted.

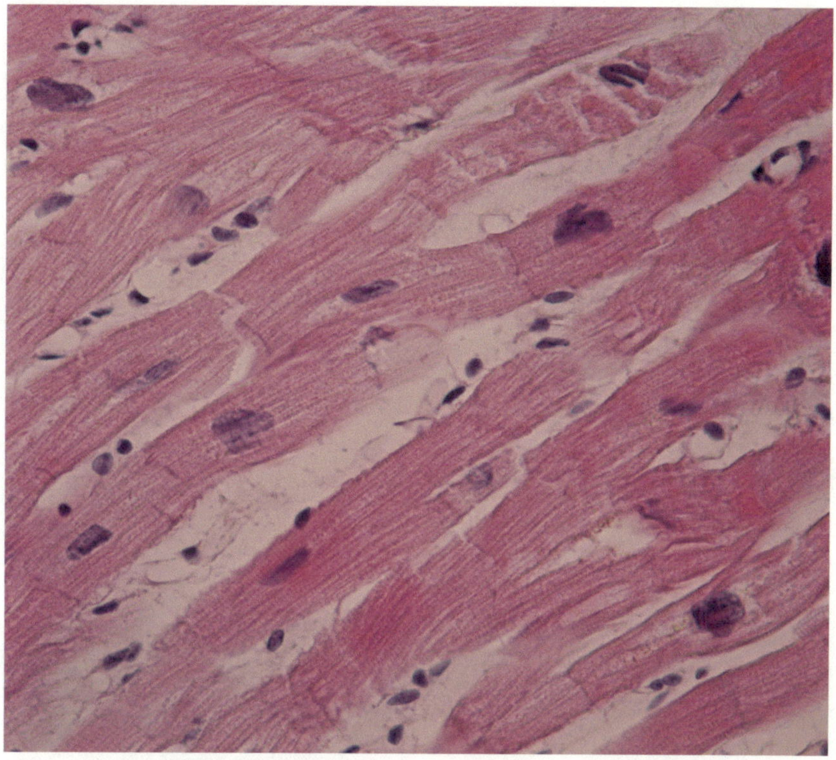

Fig. 10. A microimage of the histological sample of LV myocardium from the 53 year old patient B. No stromal inflammatory infiltration and fibrosis. Stained with hematoxylin and eosin. X 350.

Hospitalization in a year after the surgery.

CHF I FC. LV EDVI - 62.5 ml/m^2; LV ESVI - 33.8 ml/m^2, LV EF - 46%. Mild mitral regurgitation. Pre- and postoperative EchoCG images are shown in Figure 11.

Clinical examples support our conclusions about improper use of a mean value of LV myocardial cells diameter as a predictor of postoperative heart remodeling for ICMP patients: in a patient with the LV cardiomyocytes diameter > 28mcm signs of progressive HF were not found, however with the diameter of cardiac muscular cells <21mcm repeated heart remodeling was registered in the late postoperative follow-up period (as it was described by Moreira et al for the patients with dilated CMP (2001)).

Out from 58 ICMP patients whose myocardium was studied by electron-microscopy, 47 were included into the further analysis (43 men and 4 women): 34 with the reverse remodeling (group Ia) and 13 with the progressive remodeling (group IIa).

Morphometrical analysis of the specific volumes of LV and RA auricle myocardial cardiomyocytes ultrastructures confirmed our hypothesis about reduction of myocardial cells contractile apparatus as HF progressing as a result of exhaustion of compensatory adaptation processes: myofibrillar SV of cardiomyocytes significantly decreases. As myofibrillar SV decreases in cardiomyocytes, specific rate of mitochondrias grows, mitochondrial-myofibrillar ratio increases.

SV of natriuretic peptide of RA auricle cardiomyocytes insignificantly grows as chronic HF progressing. Nuclear SV does not change significantly.

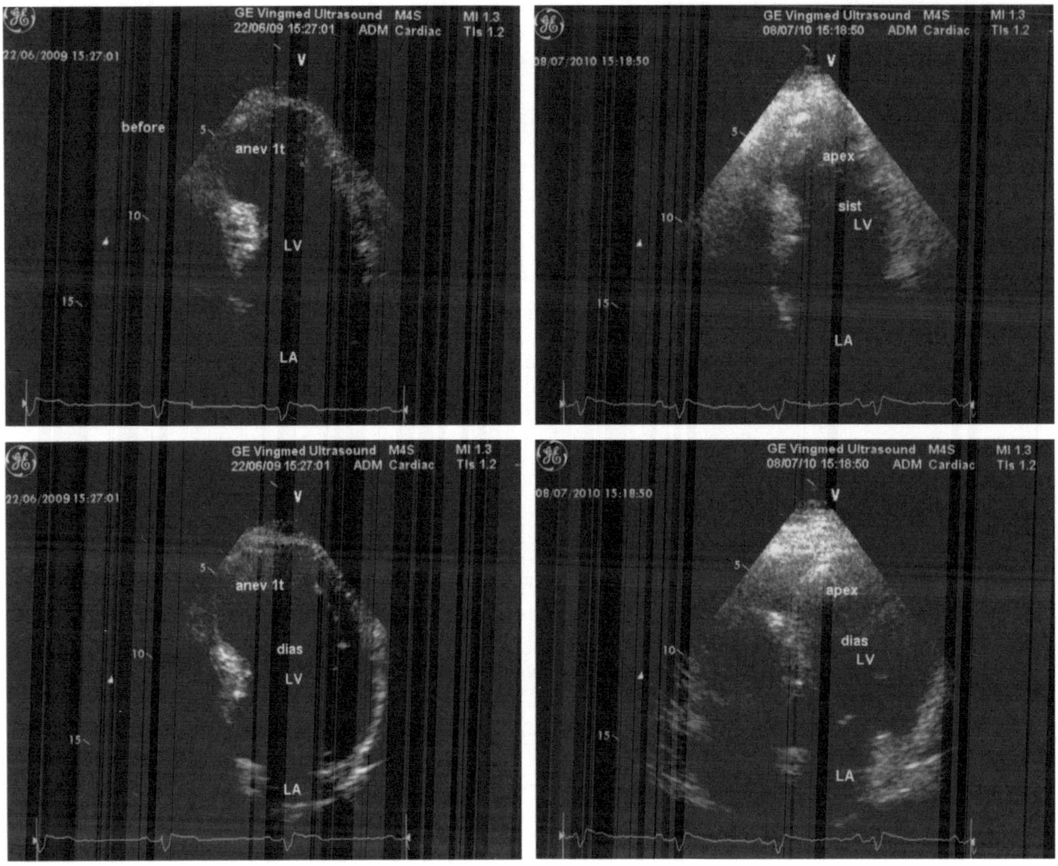

Fig. 11. Pre- and postoperative EchoCG images of the 53 year old patient B. Repeated postoperative LV remodeling and progressing chronic HF were not noticed.

Out from 47 ICMP patients whose myocardium was taken for the investigation of functional morphology of microcirculatory link of the LV and RA auricle vascular bed at an ultrasonic level, 39 patients were included into the further analysis (37 men and 2 women): 33 with the reverse remodeling (group Ib) and 6 with the progressive remodeling (group IIb).

Morphometrical values of functional morphology of microvasculature of the LV and RA auricle myocardium of ICMP patients are presented in Table 7.

The rate of open capillaries in myocardium of LV and RA auricle myocardium in ICMP patients with reverse remodeling type was significantly higher than that in the patients of Group II (73.0% vs 56.4% respectively). A similar value for RA auricle myocardium did not differ significantly among the patients with different late outcomes of surgical treatment. Luminal area of the open capillaries in ICMP patients with the reverse and progressive remodeling types as well as the number of pinocytic vesicles connected with a luminal contour of endotheliocytes per a unit of capillary luminal area were identical for both LV myocardium and myocardium of RA auricle.

Density of free pinocytic vesicles in capillary endotheliocytes of LV myocardium has become another value of functional morphology of microvasculature which differed significantly in ICMP patients with different late outcomes of surgical treatment: 0.0796 mcm^3/mcm^3 in the group of patients with positive postoperative dynamics versus

0.0678 mcm³/mcm³ in the group of ICMP patients with progressing chronic HF in the late follow-up period. All in all morphofunctional condition of microvasculature in ICMP patients with the reverse type of heart remodeling looks favorable in comparison with ICMP patients from group II.

Patients	Myocardium	Open capillary Rate (%)	Luminal area of open capillaries (mcm²)	Density of free pinocytic vesicles in endotheliocytes (mcm³/mcm³)	Number of pinocytic vesicles per 1 mcm²
Group Ib (n=33)	RA	82.0	10.5±1.9	0.0547±0.0079	5.7±0.6
	LV	73.0*	10.5±1.4	0.0796±0.0113*	6.8±0.7
Group IIb (n=6)	RA	82.8	10.4±2.1	0.0539±0.0092	5.5±0.8
	LV	56.4*	10.5±1.8	0.0678±0.0127*	6.3±0.9

Note: * – significance of morphological values differences between the groups of patients with positive and negative dynamics in the late follow-up period ($p<0.05$).

Table 7. Morphometrical values of functional morphology of the LV and RA auricle myocardial microvasulature of ICMP patients with different outcomes of surgical treatment, Van-der-Waerden test (M±m)

To make sure of diagnostic reliability of intraoperative myocardial biopsies we studied LV and RA autopsy material of 9 ICMP patients (7 men and 2 women) died at different periods after surgical intervention whose intraoperative myocardial samples we had taken during surgical intervention. We have not found any false-positive or false-negative results of diagnostics of pathomorphological myocarditis signs according to intraoperative biopsy samples (with the control on the autopsies material). Morphometric values of autopsy and biopsy samples were also comparable. Intraoperative biopsy of myocardium should not be considered as an absolute true, but on the whole, without any doubt, it reflects functional morphology of cardiac muscular tissue. First of all it depends on the volume of the material obtained for morphological studies and on the possibility of a targeted harvesting of a necessary LV area.

3.2 Molecular markers of postoperative LV remodeling in patients with ICMP

Samples of peripheral blood from 53 ICMP patients were taken 1-2 days prior to the surgical intervention. The control group consisted of 17 healthy volunteers.

Analysis of the obtained data revealed that in ICMP patients the content of pro-ANP and NT-proBNP in blood plasma was significantly higher than that in the group of healthy volunteers ($p<0.001$). The study of the content of matrix metalloproteinase in blood serum showed that between the groups of ICMP patients and healthy volunteers there were no differences in the content of matrix metalloproteinases of types 1, 3, 9 and tissue inhibitor MMP-1 (TIMP-1). But only MMP-9 content in blood serum obeyed normal distribution law.

During evaluation of the detection rate of antimyocardial antibodies of difference specificity in the healthy volunteers group in 53% of the cases there were no found autoantibodies to the cardiac tissue; in 47% of the cases antibodies to fibrillar structures were detected, but in only 6% of them these antibodies were present in a titre exceeding acceptable values. In the group of patients with ICMP the distribution of antibodies titres to fibrillar structures was the following: in 46 % of the patients the antibodies were detected in titre 20, in 24.3 % – in titre 40, in 21.6 % – in titre 80, in 2.7 % the titre reached 160 and in only 5.4 % of the patients autoantibodies were not detected.

In determining antibodies to sarcolemmic structures it was found that in 53% of the cases these antibodies in healthy donors were absent. Antibodies to sarcolemmic structures were

not found in 10.8 % of ICMP patients, in 24.3 % – they were detected in titre 20, in 43.3 % – in titre 40, in 16.2 % – in titre 80, in 5.4 % – in titre 160.
Maximal detection rate of antibodies to nuclear structures in titre 80 in the control group was 11.8%, in 88.2% of the patients did not have these antibodies. The highest titre in ICMP patients where nuclear antibodies were found was equal to 80 (2.7%); in 5.4% of the cases antibodies to nuclear structures were detected in titre 40, in 32.4% - in titre 20, in 59.5% autoantibodies of this specificity were absent.
In a year after the surgical treatment all the patients included into the study were examined (n=53, 100%). In accordance with the aforementioned algorithm for the evaluation of late postoperative period 40 patients were assigned into group I (with positive dynamics of the late postoperative period), 13 patients – into group II (with negative dynamics of the late postoperative period). The levels of pro-ANP, NT-proBNP and pro-MMP-1, MMP-3, MMP-9, TIMP-1 in blood plasma and serum In the ICMP patients with different dynamics of the late postoperative period are shown in Table 8.

Value	Normality of distribution law		Significance of differences between the groups		Group I			Group II		
	Shapiro-Wilk	p	Mann-Whitney t- TEST		n=40			n=13		
Nonnormal distribution law			U	p	Q_{25}	Me	Q_{75}	Q_{25}	Me	Q_{75}
pro-ANP (nmol/l)	0.917	0.03	57	0.73	3.69	6.34	8.59	3.31	5.30	7.78
NT-proBNP (fmol/l)	0.729	<0.01	59	0.82	12.30	38.45	58.42	19.48	39.93	90.37
MMP-3 (ng/ml)	0.861	0.002	25	0.03*	5.16	5.70	7.05	6.25	7.11	8.49
TIMP-1 (ng/ml)	0.838	0.001	46	0.32	426.0	455.8	502.6	447.4	480.8	512.4
Normal distribution law			t	p	Mean	Std. Dev.		Mean	Std. Dev.	
MMP-9 (ng/ml)	0.954	0.26*	-2.255	0.03*	64.51	24.23		90.64	27.97	
MMP-1 (ng/ml)	0.948	0.19*	-0.651	0.52	6.10	3.72		7.25	4.28	

Note: * – statistically significant data.

Table 8. The content of natriuretic peptides and matrix meatlloproteinases in blood plasma and serum in ICMP patients with different dynamics of the late postoperative treatment

We managed to follow the late postoperative period of 32 (86.5%) out from 37 patients whose blood was tested for antimyocardial antibodies. Postoperative LV remodeling took place in only 5 patients which does not allow to reliably associate the activity of inflammatory response in myocardium with postoperative heart function.
Thus, evaluation of the content of MMP-3 and MMP-9 in blood serum at the preoperative stage let us "foresee" the outcome of possible surgical treatment since their content is significantly higher in the group of patients with postoperative heart remodeling. We made

an attempt to calculate sensitivity and specificity of molecular prognostic criteria of postoperative heart remodeling basing on the obtained material.
Test sensitivity (Se) may be identified as a probability of a positive outcome in the patients: Se=p(P/D). Calculation is performed as follows:

Se=(the number of positive outcomes in the group of patients P / number of the patients D) × 100 %.

Specificity (Sp) - is the probability of negative results of the test in healthy volunteers: Sp=p(N/H). Calculated as follows:

Sp=(the number of negative results among the healthy N / number of the healthy H) × 100 %.

A test with high specificity, as a rule, does not refer healthy people to the category of patients.

For MMP-3

Cut-off value = 7.7 ng/ml.

$$Se = (11/13) \times 100\ \% = 84.6\ \%.$$

$$Sp = (40/40) \times 100\ \% = 100.0\ \%.$$

For MMP-9

Cut-off value = 102.4 ng/ml.

$$Se = (7/13) \times 100\ \% = 53.8\ \%.$$

$$Sp = (40/40) \times 100\ \% = 100.0\ \%.$$

As for antibodies to myocardial structures, their titre is much higher in ICMP patients. This fact proves our hypothesis about the presence of inflammatory infiltrate in myocardial stroma as the key factor for unfavorable outcome of surgical treatment. Nowadays it is obvious that taking blood of the patients with massive postinfarction cardiac sclerosis at the preoperative stage for the evaluation of MMPs content and antibodies titre to myocardial structures in order to make prognosis for the late postoperative period is not only perspective but reasonable. Identification of the antimyocardial antibodies titre in blood serum preoperatively as well as in the dynamics of early and mid-term postoperative period will indirectly allow for monitoring of inflammatory process in myocardium and evaluation of the efficacy of a complex medical treatment avoiding repeated biopsies of myocardium.

4. Conclusion

Our clinical observations demonstrate progress of chronic HF in the late postoperative period and inefficiency of SVR in ICMP patients in 35% of the cases. These patients should be refused from the standard procedure of surgical restoration of normal left ventricular geometry in favor of alternative methods of surgical treatment - isolated bypass grafting for the patients with symptomatic CAD, cardiac resynchronization therapy for patients with QRS >120 msec and left bundle branch block, primary heart transplantation and implant of the devices preventing ventricular dilatation. Attempts to find clinical, instrumental or other markers of chronic HF progression have been made many times but the results are very modest. The age older than 55 years and high values of LV ESVI in preoperative period have been considered as risk factors of such interventions.
In our opinion the reason of unfavorable outcomes of surgical treatment lies in peculiarities of myocardial functional morphology of an each and every patient and depends on irreversibility of the far gone pathological changes in cardiac muscular tissue. Assessment of an initial morphofunctional condition of myocardium (at the moment of surgical treatment)

based on pre- and/or intraoperative LV biopsies taken for the detection of irreversible pathological changes in myocardium by a number of qualitative and quantitative histomorphometrical values taking into account the condition of tissue trophy to the full extent, should contribute into prevention of repeated heart remodeling and progression of chronic HF in the late postoperative period.

Cellular-stromal relationships on the background of chronic ischemia of myocardium precondition destructive processes of a heart muscular tissue remodeling which is reflected also in peripheral blood of ICMP patients: the content of MMPs and MMP-3 and MMP-9 in particular, which becomes molecular prognostic markers of the late postoperative period.

Basing on the obtained data we offer the following algorithm of surgical treatment of patients with ICMP: for the candidates for a complex surgical treatment older than 55 years old with preoperative LV ESVI >80 ml/m^2 it would be reasonable to widen indications for endomyocadial biopsy at the preoperative stage or to perform intraoperative biopsy of LV myocardium in order to identify prognostic criteria of the postoperative progressive heart remodeling and take blood samples for the detection of blood markers of HF progression. If the combination of unfavorable prognostic criteria takes place: the presence of diffuse inflammatory infiltration of myocardial stroma in combination with pronounced fibrosis, low TI (<0.010) and high values of KI (>1.5) and PcDZ (>1000 mcm) of LV myocardium as well as high concentrations of MMP-3 (>7.7 ng/ml) and MMP-9 (>102.4 ng/ml) in blood serum, the patient should be refused from a standard procedure of surgical reconstruction of normal left ventricular geometry in favor of alternative methods of surgical treatment (in the case of taking preoperative biopsy of myocardium) or surgeons should refuse from SVR in favor of a surgical procedure with less risk (in case of taking intraoperative biopsy of myocardium).

5. Study limitations

The success of reconstructive surgeries in patients with ICMP depends not so much on functional morphology of cardiomyocytes and the condition of myocardial trophy as on cellular-stromal interactions in cardiac muscular tissue with the background of chronic ischemia. In our opinion, identification of myocarditis etiology with the purpose of its etiotropic treatment is one of the key factors of prevention of heart failure progression in the late postoperative period in patients with ICMP. By far the correlation of the presence of myocardial inflammatory infiltration with activation of metalloproteinase system has not been fully understood. Probably, quantitative and, what is also important, qualitative content of myocardial stroma (collagen types, fibronectin, laminin, etc) determines "tolerance" of the tissue to progressive dilatation.

6. References

Acorn cardiovascular, inc.™ Selected abstracts. 2000.

Anderson, R.A. 2005. The anatomical arrangement of the myocardial cells making up the ventricular mass. *Eur. J. Cardio-thorac. Surg*, Vol. 28, 2005, pp. 517–525

Athanasuleas, C.L. 2004. Surgical ventricular restoration in the treatment of congestive heart failure due to postinfarction ventricular dilation. *J. Am Coll. Cardiol*, Vol. 44, 2004, pp. 1439–1445

Avtandilov, G. 1990. *Medical morphometry*, Medicine, Moscow

Batista, R.J. 1996. Partial left ventriculectomy to improve left ventricular function in end-stage heart disease. *J. Card. Surg*, Vol. 11, 1996, pp. 96–98

Belenkov, Yu. et al. 2002. Epidemiological study of heart failure: state of the art. *Heart failure Journal*. No. 2, 2002, pp. C. 57–58.

Bellenger, N.G. 2000. Comparison of left ventricular ejection fraction and volumes in heart failure by echocardiography, radionuclide ventriculography and cardiovascular magnetic resonance: are they interchangeable? *Eur. Heart J.*, Vol. 21, pp. 1387–1396

Buckberg, G.D. 2005. Questions and answers about the STICH trial: A different perspective. *J. Thorac. Cardiovasc. Surg*, Vol. 130, 2005, pp. 245–249

Di Donato, M. 1997. Akinetic versus dyskinetic postinfarction scar: relation to surgical outcome in patients undergoing endoventricular circular patch plasty repair. *J. Am. Coll. Cardiol*, Vol. 29, 1997, pp. 1569–1575

Di Donato, M. 2001. Intermediate survival and predictors of death after surgical ventricular restoration. *Semin. Thorac. Cardiovasc. Surg*. Vol. 13, 2001, pp. 468–475

Dickstein, M.L. 1997. Heart reduction surgery: an analysis of the impact on cardiac function. *J. Thorac. Cardiovasc. Surg.*, Vol. 113, 1997, pp. 1032–1040

Dor, V. 1985. Interest of physiological closure (circumferential plasty on contractile areas) of left ventricle after resection and endocardectomy for aneurysm of akinetic zone: comparison with classical technique about a series of 209 left ventricular resection [abstract]. *J. Cardiovasc. Surg.*, Vol. 26, 1985, pp. 73

Frazier, O.H. 2000. Partial left ventriculectomy: which patients can be expected to benefit? *Ann. Thorac. Surg*, Vol. 69, 2000, pp. 1836–1841

Geidel, S. 2005. Downsizing of the mitral valve and coronary revascularization in severe ischemic mitral regurgitation results in reverse left ventricular and left atrial remodeling. *Eur. J. Cardiothorac. Surg.*, Vol. 27, 2005, pp. 1011–1016

Gelsomino, S. 2008. Left ventricular reverse remodeling after undersized mitral ring annuloplasty in patients with ischemic regurgitation. *Ann. Thorac. Surg.*, Vol. 85, 2008, pp. 1319–1330

Glagolev, V. & Chepulin, Yu. 1968. *Ultrastructural basis of a heart muscle function disturbance*, Moscow

Gradinac, S. 1998. Partial left ventriculectomy for idiopathic dilated cardiomyopathy: early results and six month follow-up. *Ann. Thorac. Surg.*, Vol. 66, 1998, pp. 1963–1968

Jackson, B.M. 2002. Extension of borderzone myocardium in postinfarction dilated cardiomyopathy. J. *Am. Coll. Cardiol.* Vol. 40, 2002, pp. 1160–1167

Kalon, K.Ho.L. et al. 1993. The epidemiology of heart failure: the Framingham Study. *Journal of American College of Cardiology*, Vol. 22, Suppl. A, 1993, pp. 6A–13A

Kawamura, F. et al. 1974. Endothelium as a tissue. *Jap. J. Histol.* Vol. 34, 1974, pp. 76–79

Krivolapov, Yu. 2006. *Morphological diagnostics of lymphomas*, COSTA, Saint Petersburg

Kuznetsov, G. 2003. Clinical-morphological parallels of left ventricular remodeling associated with chronic heart failure. *Cardiology*, No. 12, 2003, pp. 19–22

Maisch, B. 1996. Ventricular remodeling. *Cardiology*, Vol. 87, Suppl. 1, 1996, pp. 2–10.

Mareev, V. 2002. Design of the study and patients characteristic in "FASON" trial. Heart Failure Journal. No. 2, 2002, pp 97–98

Menicanti, L. & Di Donato, M. 2002. The Dor procedure: What has changed after fifteen years of clinical practice? *J. Thorac. Cardiovasc. Surg*. Vol. 124, 2002, pp. 886–890

Menicanti, L. & Di Donato, M. 2004. Surgical left ventricle reconstruction, pathophysiologic insights, results and expectation from the STICH trial. *Eur. J. Cardiothorac. Surg*, Vol. 26, 2004, pp. 42–47

Moreira, L.F. 2001. Current perspectives of partial left ventriculectomy in the treatment of dilated cardiomyopathy. *Eur. J. Cardio-thorac. Surg.*, Vol. 19, 2001, pp. 54–60

Oganov, R. & Maslennikova, G. 2000. Cardiovascular diseases in Russian Federation in the second half of the XX century: tendencies, possible reasons, perspective. *Cardiology,* No. 6, 2000, pp. 4–8

Patel, H.J. 1997. Stabilization of chronic remodeling by asynchronous cardiomyoplasty in dilated cardiomyopathy: effects of conditioned muscle wrap. *Circulation,* Vol. 96, 1997, pp. 3665–3671

Popovic, Z. 1998. Effects of partial left ventriculectomy on left ventricular performance in patients with nonischemic dilated cardiomyopathy. *J. Am. Coll. Cardiol.* Vol. 32, 1998, pp. 1801–1808

Popovic, Z. 2001. Functional capacity late after partial left ventriculectomy: relation to ventricular geometry and performance. *Eur. J. Cardio-thorac. Surg.*, Vol. 19, 2001, pp. 61–67

Ratcliffe, M.B. 1998. The effect of ventricular volume reduction surgery in the dilated, poorly contractile left ventricle: a simple finite element analysis. *J. Thorac. Cardiovasc. Surg,* Vol. 116, 1998, pp. 566–577.

Rosenberg, V. 2003. Nepomnyashchih, L. Pathomorphological criteria of postinfarction heart remodeling. *Bulletin of experimental biological medicine,* Vol. 135, No. 1, 2003, pp. 110–114

Rosenberg, V. 2003. Postinfarction heart remodeling: variants of pathomorphological changes of right ventricle. *Bulletin of experimental biological medicine,* Vol. 136, No. 9, 2003, pp. 331-335

Sabbah, H.N. 2001. Prevention of progressive left ventricular dilation with the Acorn cardiac support device downregulates stretch response proteins and improves sarcoplasmic reticulum calcium cycling in dogs with chronic heart failure. *J. Am. Coll. Cardiol,* Vol. 37, 2001, pp. 474

Salikova, S. et al. 2002. Morphological aspects of heart remodeling with chronic heart failure. *Morphology,* Vol. 122, No. 5, 2002, pp. 60–62

Sartipy, U. et al. 2006. Risk factors for mortality and hospital re-admission after surgical ventricular restoration. *Eur. J. Cardiothorac Surg,* Vol. 30, 2006, pp. 762–769

Schroder, J.N. 2005. Impact of mitral valve regurgitation evaluated by intraoperative transesophageal echocardiography on long-term outcomes after coronary artery bypass grafting. *Circulation,* Vol. 112, 2005, pp. 1293–1298

Shah, P.J. 2003. Survival after myocardial revascularization for ischemic cardiomyopathy: A prospective ten-year follow-up study. *J. Thorac. Cardiovasc. Surg,* Vol. 5, 2003, pp. 1320–1327

Simonsen, M. 2003. «Slow adoption of new device technologies seen in Europe». *American Health Consultants / Cardiovascular Device Update,* October, 2003, pp. 6

Soo, E.N. 2005. Eight years survival after partial left ventriculectomy (Case report). *Eur. J. Cardio-thorac. Surg.*, Vol. 27, 2005, pp. 724–725

Stolf, N.A. 1998. Determinants of midterm outcome of partial left ventriculectomy in dilated Cardiomyopathy. *Ann. Thorac. Surg,* Vol. 66, 1998, pp. 1585–1591

Yamaguchi, A. 2005. Left ventricular reconstruction benefits patients with dilated ischemic cardiomyopathy. *Ann. Thorac. Surg.* Vol. 79, 2005, pp. 456–461

Yamaguchi, H. 2000. Characteristics of myocardial 18F-fluorodeoxyglucose positron emission computed tomography in dilated cardiomyopathy and ischemic cardiomyopathy. *Ann. Nucl. Med.*, Vol. 14(1), 2000, pp. 33–38

7

Miniaturized Extracorporeal Circulation

Francesco Formica and Giovanni Paolini
Cardiac Surgery Clinic, University of Milano-Bicocca, San Gerardo Hospital, Monza, Italy

1. Introduction

Since the first cardiac surgical operations in the early '50s, the early and long-term outcomes have been dramatically improved also because of the refinement of technology regarding the extracorporeal circulation (ECC). It is recognized the ECC is associated with a systemic inflammatory response (SIRS), which is implicated in myocardial, renal, pulmonary and neurologic dysfunction. However, although the effects of ECC are very often subclinical, in some situations they can be responsible of worse outcome in the early post-operative period.
In the early 1990s, many surgeons started to perform coronary revascularization without the use of ECC with the aim of strongly reducing the subclinical and clinical effects of the SIRS. Over the past fifteen years, the "off-pump" coronary artery bypass grafting (OPCABG) has demonstrated to have good results by reducing postoperative morbidity and mortality. On the other hand, the OPCABG presents some drawbacks such as the significant learning curve of the surgeon, the high rate of incomplete revascularization in dilated and hypokinetic heart due to very difficult exposure of obtuse coronary marginal branches and the lesser quality of the coronary anastomosis.
Over the past 10 years, concepts of miniaturized extracorporeal circulation (MECC) were developed with the aim of reducing the side effects of the standard ECC, strengthening the advantages of ECC and eliminate the limitations of OPCABG. In other words, the MECC joins the best of ECC with the best of "off-pump" surgery.

2. Anatomy of the miniaturized extracorporeal circulation system

Different types of MECC circuits are on the market and although they can have some differences among them in terms of characteristics of blood pump, oxygenator membrane, length of tubing, arterial and venous filters, the principle key is substantially equal for each system: closed circuit without a venous cardiotomy reservoir.
The MECC circuit consists of a closed loop, which includes the oxygenator and the pump. The circuit has not any open venous reservoir. All components of MECC circuit are pre-treated with heparin according to different techniques available on the market. The heparin pre-treatment of the circuit minimizes the systemic heparinization dose requirements (usually half dose of conventional ECC: 150IU/Kg instead of 300IU/Kg) (Curtis et al. 2010; Formica et al. 2009, Puheler et al. 2009; Beghi et. 2006) and provides biocompatibility for blood cells (Koivisto et al. 2010; Remadi et al. 2007; Remadi et al. 2004; Fromes et al 2002;)

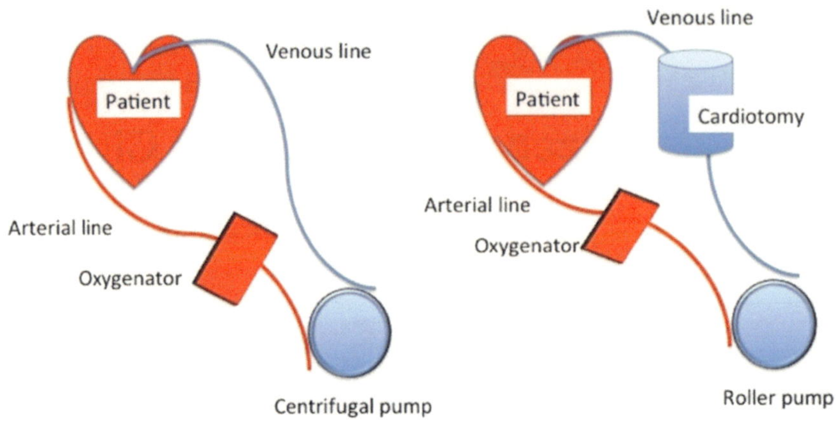

Fig. 1. Miniaturized extracorporeal circuit on the left and conventional extracorporeal circulation on the right

The tubing length is described to be shorter than conventional ECC in different published reports. Tubing length of about 100 cm is frequently reported as well as a smaller tubing section than conventional ECC tubing (3/8" size instead of 1/2" size) (Formica et al 2009; Mazzei et al 2007). These characteristics lead to a circuit prime volume smaller than standard ECC, ranging between 200-650 ml for the MECC against 1200-1600 ml for the standard ECC (Formica et al 2009, Stalder et al. 2007; Remady et al. 2006). The combination of short length tubing, heparin pre-treatment, small size tubing and absence of a venous reservoir, leads to a significant reduction of hemodilution with as well as a reduction in clotting factor consumption ad triggering of SIRS (Vohra et al 2009; Ohata et al. 2007; Wippermann et al. 2005; Fromes et al. 2002). The blood pump included in the circuit is usually a centrifugal pump. The centrifugal pump is a very versatile pump, which reduces the cells trauma on the erythrocytes, and the platelets with possible lower effects on hemolysis. Moreover the centrifugal pump can generate up to 900 mmHg of forward pressure and only 400 mmHg of negative pressure with less cavitation and lower microemboli formation. The oxygenator of the MECC circuit is one of the most important components of the circuit itself. Oxygenators have the oxygenation membrane of either microporous polypropylene (El-Essawi et al. 2010; Wippermann et al. 2005) or polymethylpentene (Anastasiadis et al. 2011; Puehler et al. 2010; Formica et al. 2009; Remady et al 2006;). In the latter case the membrane is considered as a diffusion membrane Usually the oxygenator has an integrated heat exchanger and one of the largest gas exchange surface areas, reaching about 2.4 m^2. In this way the oxygenator can give a full oxygenation also with high blood flow pump up to 7 L/min.

Many MECC circuits include an arterial filter between the oxygenator and the aortic cannula. The filter has a prime ranging between 150-200 ml but its presence is of extreme importance because strongly reduce the risk of cerebral and systemic embolization or air, thrombus and calcium. Moreover some MECC circuits include a venous bubble trap or some similar device with the aim of reducing the big air entrainment in the circuit that could be one of the causes of accidental blockage of the MECC circuit. These devices are located between the venous cannula and the blood centrifugal pump.

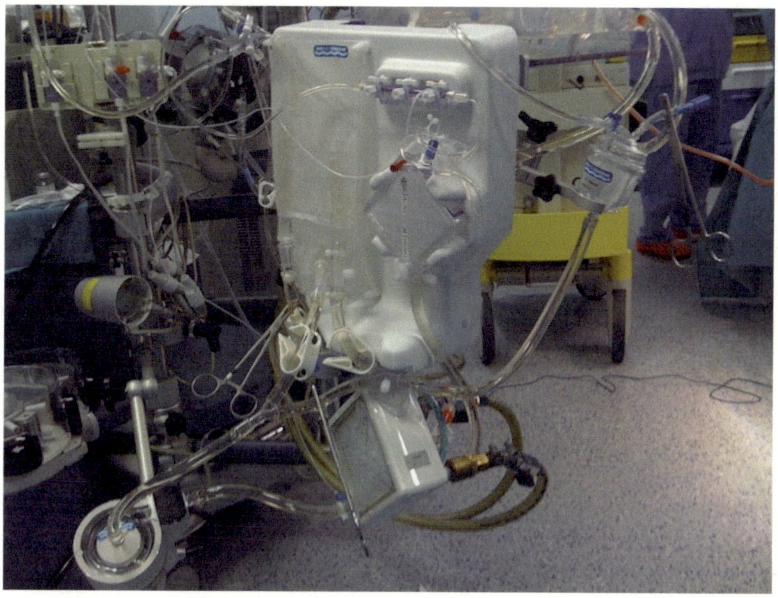

Fig. 2. MECC system.

Aortic and atrial cannulation are equal to conventional ECC. Usually an aortic vent is positioned in ascending aorta and a further vent is inserted in the pulmonary main trunk during aortic valve surgery.
A cell-saver device can be associated with the MECC with the aim to sucked all the pericardial and bloodshed.
The very strong difference between the MECC and the standard ECC circuit is the absence of a venous reservoir. In the MECC, the patient is the own venous reservoir and for this reason the straight collaboration among the cardiac surgeon, the anaesthesiologist and the perfusionist is extremely important to guarantee the best outcome. Use of vasodilator and vasoconstrictor drugs, Trendelemburg or anti-Trendelemburg position of the patient, reducing or increasing the centrifugal pump flow are all fundamental keys to manage a MECC system with the aim to avoiding malperfusion syndrome, systemic embolization, failure of the MECC and rapid conversion to standard ECC.

3. Systemic inflammatory response

The Systemic Inflammatory Response Syndrome (SIRS) is a complex plurifactorial syndrome often associated with the ECC. The SIRS to ECC is initiated by many aggressive factors including surgical trauma, blood contact with nonendothelial sufaces, cardioplegia, ischemia-reperfusion injury (Raja & Berg, 2007; Larmann & Theilmerr, 2004; Royston, 1997). Several blood elements such as neutrophils, monocytes, endothelial cells, platelets and complement proteins are involved in the SIRS. These blood components when activates, release of cytotoxic and vasoactive substances, produce inflammatory and inhibitory cytokine, express cell receptors interacting with specific cellular substance (Royston 1997). Therefore when SIRS is initiated, several inflammatory mediators, including anti-inflammatory and pro-inflammatory cytokines could be associated with a worse postoperative course.

3.1 Activated blood cells

3.1.1 Neutrophils

Neutrophils are strongly activated during ECC. When activated, the neutrophils are recruited to inflammation site by inflammatory cytokines (IL-1β, TNF-α, IL-8), complement proteins and adhesion molecules (Royston 1997). The activated neutrophils can contribute to myocardial damage by infiltrating the myocardium and worsening the mechanism of ischemia-reperfusion damage that initiates after aortic cross clamp removal (Paparella et al 2002). Moreover the neutrophils can infiltrate not only the myocardium but also the lungs and the brain (Lagan et al. 2008). Usually the neutrophils blood count and the total white blood cell count increase during ECC and over the first 48 hours after the operation (Fromes et al 2002)

3.1.2 Monocytes

Monocytes are activated during ECC and play a role in thrombin formation, but also they can produce a potent arsenal of pro-inflammatory cytokines (IL-1β, TNF-α, IL-6, IL-8, MCP-1 and CD40 ligand), reactive oxygen substances and prostaglandin (Borregaard & Cowland 1997). Monocytes also release different types of enzymes (elastase, collagenases, lipooxygenase), interferons, growth factors, matrix proteins. Moreover, monocytes produce nitric oxide (Paparella et al. 2002)

3.1.3 Endothelial cells

The vascular endothelium is actively involved during the pathologic processes of the SIRS by means of endothelial cells activation. During the SIRS the several endothelium control mechanisms of the vascular tone and permeability can modify. A large variety of agonist plays an important role in endothelial cells activation. Among them cytokines such as IL-1β, TNF-α, thrombin and complement C5 are the most important (Beghetti et al. 1998). In particular, IL-1β, TNF-α may induce the expression of P-Selectin and of E-Selectin by the endothelium. The P-Selectin is a glycoprotein that is stored in platelets and in the body of endothelial cells. P-Selectin participates in myocardial injury caused by myocardial ischemia-reperfusion mechanism (Robertson & Coopersmith 2006; Royston 1997). E-Selectin is minimally expressed on activated endothelium and for this reason this glycoprotein and its soluble form are considered a very strong marker of endothelial damage and activation (Asimakopoulous & Taylor 1998). Moreover E-Selectine is elevated in congestive heart failure (Chong et al. 2003). The activated endothelium induces also the expression of intercellular adhesion molecule-1 (ICAM-1) and vascular cell adhesion molecule-2 (VCAM-2). These two molecules bind monocytes and neutrophils to the endothelium (Asimakopoulous & Taylor 1998).

3.1.4 Platelets

Platelets are directly involved during the SIRS and several potent platelet agonists activate them. Thrombin is probably the most important of platelet agonist. Other platelet agonist activators are epinephrine, vasopressin, platelet-activating factor (PAF), serotonin and thromboxane A2 (Downing & Edmunds. 1992). Activation of platelets during and after ECC leads to platelet aggregation and aggregates with monocytes and neutrophils.

3.2 Other inflammation mediators

3.2.1 Cytokines

Cytokines are small pro-inflammatory peptides produced and released by tissue and blood cells. Cytokines influence hemodynamic mechanism and regulation and negatively affect

renal function and lung function (Royston 1997). Cytokines are strongly involved in myocardial stunning process and in multiorgan failure syndrome (Larmann & Theilmeier 2004) Important cytokines involved in the SIRS are the interleukin 1β (IL-1β), the interleukin 6 (IL-6), the tumor necrosis factor α (TNF-α), soluble CD 40 ligand (sCD40L).
IL-1β is produced mainly by monocytes. This cytokine derives from IL-1 by the action of the IL-1β converting enzyme. An increase of IL-1β was found after ECC with a peak concentration after 24 hours (Fromes et al 2002).
IL-6 is produced and released by the monocytes and endothelial cells following a stimulus by the IL-1 and TNF-α The IL-6 has the peak concentration few hours after the end of ECC and gradual decrease within the following 24 hours (Beghi et al 2006; Whipperman et al 2005; Fromes et al 2002). The IL-6 concentration increase also after major noncardiac operation and the peak concentration occur after 6-24 hours the end of operation.
TNF-α is a cytokine produced by neutrophils and monocytes. This cytokine stimulates the surrounding stromal and parenchymal cells to produce more cytokines and chemokines. A significant increase of TNF-α was shown after removal of the cross-clamp and a peak concentration is reached after 24 hours the end of ECC. The TNF-α has an inotropic negative effect and the myocardium is a major source after ischemia reperfusion injury.
sCD40L is produced by activated platelets and upregulates the expression of inflammatory adhesion receptors including E-selectin, VCAM-1, tissue factor and matrix mettalloproteinases (Nannizzi-Alaimo et al 2002). Furthermore, sCD40L was described has a major mediator of vascular inflammation (Antoniades et al 2009a). Plasma levels of CD40L increase within 1 hour on ECC and increased further to almost 4 fold hours after 2 hours. (Nannizzi-Alaimo et al 2002). High preoperative level of CD40L were associated with an high risk of postoperative atrial fibrillation in patients underwent off-pump myocardial revascularization (Antoniades et al 2009b)

3.2.2 Chemotactic proteins

Chemotactic proteins play an important role in inflammatory response to ECC. Monocyte chemotactic protein 1 (MCP-1) is implicated in transendothelian monocyte recruitment to inflammatory site (Luster 1998). Various stimuli in the heart cause the production and releasing of MCP-1, leading to recruitment of monocytes that causes a stress response in the heart. There is strong evidence that MCP-1 plays a role in atherosclerosis, myocarditis, ischemia/reperfusion injury and transplant rejection.

3.2.3 Mettalloproteinases

Metalloproteinases are proteolityc enzymes that have a role in degradation of proteins and collagens of extracellular matrix and vascular basement membrane. MMP-8 and MMP-13 increase at the end of ECC and 30 minutes later (Joffs et al. 2001). MMP-9 increases after the removal of aortic cross-clamp and the reaches the peak concentration after 24 hours

3.2.4 Oxidative stress

Oxidative stress describes an increased bioactivity of reactive oxidant substances (ROS) that can participate to endothelial and myocardial damage. The ROS are produced and released by neutrophils, monocytes and macrophages when they are activated. The ROS are a potent arsenal of cytotoxic mediators of acute inflammation response (Babior 2000). There are four enzymes that generate a various amount of ROS. They are represented by nicotamide adenine dinucleotide phosphate (NADPH), oxidase, superoxide dismutase and nitric oxide dismutase. When the aortic cross clamp is removed, myocardial ischemia is followed by reperfusion, which generates oxidative stress with production of reactive oxidants (O_2^-, H_2O_2, NO and HOCl) by the action of the four enzymes.

4. Clinical application of miniaturized extracorporeal circulation

Clinical experience with the MECC is rapidly increasing over the last 10 years. Several reports describe the application of MECC in isolated CABG operation; however some reports describe the use of this strategy during aortic valve replacement operation, mitral valve surgery, ascending aorta operation.

4.1 Miniaturized extracorporeal circulation and isolated CABG operation

Different studies have reported the use of MECC compared to conventional ECC strategy in isolated CABG to demonstrate a clinical superiority of the MECC versus ECC. Actually no clinical benefits of MECC were reported in terms of early mortality and in terms of neurological or renal impairment. The most important differences between MECC and standard ECC that were reported regard the impact of SIRS, the myocardial protection and hemodilution.

Many Authors have conducted randomized studies to compare MECC system with conventional ECC in patients undergoing isolated CABG operations. Fromes et al. (Fromes 2002) reported a series of 60 patients divided into two groups. They demonstrated that in both MECC and standard ECC groups the monocyte count drops following the initiation of bypass and then increases again during the next 24 hours. The drop in monocyte count was greater in standard ECC group probably as a consequent major hemodilution Moreover the MECC group had reduced release of IL-6, TNF-α, neutrophil elastase and S100B. No differences were found in IL-1β or β-thromboglobulin in both groups. In this study Fromes et al measured the release of cytokines at six interval points during and after extracorporeal circulation up to 24 hours postoperatively. Van Boven et al. (Van Boven et al. 2004) measured the levels of malondialdehyde (MDA) and allantoin/urate ratio in 184 patients divided in MECC and standard ECC. They can demonstrate a reduced release of MDA and allantoin/urate ratio in MECC patients. Moreover a significant blood transfusion rate was described in the MECC group. They found also reduced levels of oxidative stress in the MECC patients following the release of the aortic cross clamp. In a cohort of 400 patients, Remady et al. (Remady 2007) demonstrated a higher CRP levels in the standard ECC patients, at 24 and 48 hours, a less hemodilution and a reduced need for blood product transfusion in MECC patients, a higher evidence of focal neurological and renal impairment in standard ECC and a lower release of troponine in MECC groups. In another randomized trial, Skrabal et al (Skrabal et al. 2007) reported lower myocardial damage with lower levels of creatine-kinase MB and troponine T in patients operated on with MECC system. In a prospective randomized multicenter study (El-Essawi et al. 2010), comparing MECC system with conventional ECC, the Authors found statistical differences in need of total transfusion and blood product transfusion. Moreover a lower incidence rate of postoperative atrial fibrillation was detected in MECC group. In a big series of 1.053 patients operated on with the MECC system, Immer et al (Immer et al. 2007) reported a reduced troponine level release, a reduced postoperative release of IL-6 and also a low incidence of postoperative atrial fibrillation and an early extubation time. Similar results were already reported by others (Wiesenack 2004). In some prospective randomized trials comparing MECC and OPCAB, some Authors did not find dramatic difference between the two techniques. In particular Mazzei et al. (Mazzei et al. 2007) comparing 150 MECC patients with 150 OPCAB patients, found that the mortality and morbidity had not significant difference and the release of IL-6 and S-100 protein were similar in both groups as wel as the length of stay and the use of blood product. In a recent prospective randomized study (Formica et al.2009) we wanted to study the inflammatory response and the myocardial damage in two groups of patients operated either with MECC or with OPCAB technique. We can demonstrate that the releases of cardiac TNF-α and IL-6 from coronary sinus were similar in both groups during the operative period and that the hemoglobin levels were higher in MECC GROUP than in OPCAB after 24 hours. Moreover the production of blood lactate from coronary sinus did not reach statistical difference in both groups. Other Authors (Reber et al. 2010) have observed in a retrospective study that MECC system can guarantee a more complete revascularization compared to OPCAB. In a recent publication (Puelher et al 2011), the outcome of 2243 patients underwent CABG operation with MECC were reported. They found a 30-mortality of 2.3%, and a very low incidence of blood transfusion, need for inotropic support, renal substitute therapy, release of myocardial necrosis enzymes and neurological dysfunction. The rate of conversion from the MECC was extremely low (0.4%).

Other Autrhors (Anastasiadis et al 2011a) have reported better neurocognitive outcome in MECC system compared to conventional ECC on the day of discharge and at 3 months.

4.2 Miniaturized extracorporeal circulation and aortic valve replacement

The first application of MECC for aortic valve replacement (AVR) was reported by Remady et al (Remady et al. 2004). They applied the MECC system in 45 patients requiring isolated AVR or associated with CABG. The Authors reported a very low 30-day mortality and morbidity incidence rate and considered the MECC system a new cardiopulmonary concept safe and reliable in aortic valve surgery too. Since than few Authors reported the use of MECC for AVR. In a prospective randomized study Remady et al (Remady 2004) reported better clinical results with reduced myocardial damage, good preservation of renal function and better platelets count in MECC group compared than standard ECC group. In another prospective randomized study conducted on a total of 40 patients, Castiglioni et al (Castiglioni et al. 2007) reported better clinical data with lower hemodilution, lower intraoperative blood transfusion and lower postoperative bleeding in the MECC group compared to standard ECC. Furthermore they reported a lower release of troponine in MECC patients than standard ECC groups.

4.3 Miniaturized extracorporeal circulation and other surgical applications

At the best of our knowledge no other surgical application of MECC are schematically reported in the literature. Some reports (Anastasiadis et al 2011b; Palombo et al. 2004) described the use of MECC in elective thoracoabdominal aortic surgery. They described only 7 cases without any complications. We used the MECC system in few case of CABG associated with mitral valve annuloplasty and in 5 cases of kidney cancer and inferior vena cava metastathic thrombosis. In this operation, we used the MECC system to cool the patients during the isolation of renal tumor mass. The two surgical equips could work contemporaneously. Once the patients reaches the body temperature of 20 °C, the MECC system was converted in a standard ECC to drained all the blood and arrested the systemic circulation. Once the thrombus was from the inferior vena cava and the vessel was sutured, we restarted the systemic circulation and the standard ECC was converted in MECC system. We preferred to use this strategy to reduce the risk of bleeding from the abdomen, which is very high in such tumoral pathologies.

5. Conclusion

We did not find in the literature significant differences in terms of clinical results regarding post-operative mortality. One of the reasons is because the MECC strategy is widely applied in low risk populations and only few Authors describe the use of MECC in high-risk patients (Puehler 2011, Koivisto 2010). At the moment, most of the clinical benefits with the use of MECC were seen in the SIRS, hemodilution, platelet function protection.

The good amount of data described in favor of MECC could induce to apply this strategy in more cardiac surgical operations. However, the MECC system presents some limitations that create some concern about a wider use of this technique. One important limitation is high risk of air entrapment along the venous line that could suddenly stop the cardiopulmonary bypass. Another limitation is the need of learning curve because, as well as in the OPCAB, the MECC technique requires an experienced team (surgeon, anesthesiologist and perfusion) before to be applied routinely in all CABG patients and by all surgical staff.

We feel that the MECC technology gives better advantages than standard ECC and we feel that MECC could be applied to other surgical procedures. Of course more randomized, large, multicenter studies are mandatory to verify the safety of this technology in such cardiac complex surgical operation (aortic dissection, congenital disease).

6. Acknowledgment

The Authors thank Dr. Giorgia Pavan for her editing assistance during the preparation of the chapter and Dr. Silvia Mariani for her support about literature search.

7. References

Anastasiadis, K., Chalvatzoulis, O., Antonitsis, P., Deliopoulos, A., Argiriadou, H., Karapanagiotidis, G., Kambouroglou, D. & Papakonstantinou, C. (2011). Use of Minimized Extracorporeal Circulation System in Noncoronary and Valve Cardiac Surgical Procedures-A Case Series. *Artificial Organs*. 2011 (Epub ahead of print)

Anastasiadis, K., Chalvatzoulis, O., Antonitsis, P., Deliopoulos, A., Argiriadou, H., Karapanagiotidis, G., Kambouroglou, D. & Papakonstantinou C. (2011). Neurocognitive outcome after coronary artery bypass surgery using minimal versus conventional extracorporeal circulation: a randomised controlled pilot study. *Heart*. Vol 97, No 13 (July 2011) pp. 1082- 8.

Antoniades, C., Bakogiannis, C., Tousoulis, D., Antonopoulos, AS. & Stefanadis C. (2009)The CD40/CD40 ligand system: linking inflammation with atherothrombosis. *Journal of American College of Cardiology*. Vol. 54, No 8 (Agoust 2009) pp. 669-77.

Antoniades, C., Van-Assche, T., Shirodaria, C., Diesch, J., Antonopoulos, AS., Lee, J., Cunnington, C., Tousoulis, D., Stefanadis, C., Casadei, B., Taggart, D., Channon, KM. & Leeson P. (2009). Preoperative sCD40L levels predict risk of atrial fibrillation after off-pump coronary artery bypass graft surgery. *Circulation*. Vol. 120 No. Suppl 11 (September 2009) pp. S170-6.

Asimakopoulos ,G. & Taylor, KM. (1998). Effects of cardiopulmonary bypass on leukocyte and endothelial adhesion molecules. *Annals of Thoracic Surgery*. Vol. 66, No. 6 (December 1998) pp. 2135-44.

Babior, BM. (2000). Phagocytes and oxidative stress. *American Journal of Medicine*. Vol. 109, No 1 (July 2000) pp. 33-44.

Beghetti, M., Silkoff, PE., Caramori, M., Holtby, HM., Slutsky, AS., & Adatia, I. (1998). Decreased exhaled nitric oxide may be a marker of cardiopulmonary bypass-induced injury. *Annals of Thoracic Surgery*. Vol. 66, No 2 (Agoust 1998) pp. 532-4.

Beghi, C., Nicolini, F., Agostinelli, A., Borrello, B., Budillon, AM., Bacciottini, F., Friggeri, M., Costa, A., Belli, L., Battistelli, L. & Gherli T. (2006). Mini–Cardiopulmonary Bypass System: Results of a Prospective Randomized Study. *Annals of Thoracic Surgery*. Vol. 81, No 4 (April 2006), pp. 1396-400.

Borregaard ,N.& Cowland, JB. (1997) Granules of the human neutrophilic polymorphonuclear leukocyte. *Blood*. Vol 89, No 10 (May 1997), pp. 3503-21.

Castiglioni, A., Verzini, A., Pappalardo, F., Colangelo, N., Torracca, L., Zangrillo, A. & Alfieri, O. (2007). Minimally invasive closed circuit versus standard extracorporeal circulation for aortic valve replacement. *Annals of Thoracic Surgery*. Vol. 83, No 2 (Febraury 2007) pp. 586-91.

Chong, AY., Blann, AD. & Lip, GY. (2003) Assessment of endothelial damage and dysfunction: observations in relation to heart failure. *QJM. Monthly journal of the Association of Physicians* . Vol. 96, No 4 (April 2003) pp. 253-67.

Curtis, N., Vohra, HA., & Ohri SK. (2010). Mini extracorporeal circuit cardiopulmonary bypass system: a review *Perfusion*, Vol. 25, No. 3 (May 2010), pp. 115 124

Downing, SW. & Edmunds LH Jr. (1992) Release of vasoactive substances during cardiopulmonary bypass. *Annals of Thoracic Surgery* Vol. 54, No 6 (Decembre 1992) pp.1236-43.

El-Essawi, A., Hajek, T., Skorpil, J., Böning, A., Sabol, F., Hausmann, H., Ostrovsky, Y.& Harringer W. (2010) A prospective randomised multicentre clinical comparison of a minimised perfusion circuit versus conventional cardiopulmonary bypass. *European Journal of Cardiothoracic Surgery*. Vol 38, No 1 (July 2010) pp. 91-7.

Formica, F., Broccolo, F., Martino, A., Sciucchetti, JF., Giordano, V., Avalli, L., Radaelli, G., Ferro, O., Corti, F., Cocuzza, C.,& Paolini, G. (2009). Myocardial revascularization with miniaturized extracorporeal circulation versus off pump: Evaluation of systemic and myocardial inflammatory response in a prospective randomized study. *Journal of Thoracic and Cardiovascular Surgery* . Vol.137, No 5 (May 2009), pp.1206-12.

Fromes, Y., Gaillard, D., Ponzio, O., Chauffert, M., Gerhardt, MF., Deleuze, P. & Bical, OM. (2002) Reduction of the inflammatory response following coronary bypass grafting with total minimal extracorporeal circulation. *European Journal of Cardiothoracic Surgery*. Vol. 22, No 4 (October 2002), pp. 527-33.

Immer, FF., Ackermann, A., Gygax, E., Stalder, M., Englberger, L., Eckstein, FS., Tevaearai, HT., Schmidli, J. & Carrel, TP. (2007) Minimal extracorporeal circulation is a promising technique for coronary artery bypass grafting. *Annals of Thoracic Surgery*. Vol. 84, No 5 (November 2007) pp. 1515-20.

Joffs, C., Gunasinghe, HR., Multani, MM., Dorman, BH., Kratz, JM., Crumbley, AJ., Crawford, FA. & Spinale, FG. (2001) Cardiopulmonary bypass induces the synthesis and release of matrix metalloproteinases. *Annals of Thoracic Surgery* . Vol. 71, No. 5 (May 2001), pp 1518-23.

Koivisto, SP., Wistbacka, JO., Rimpiläinen, R., Nissinen, J., Loponen, P., Teittinen, K. & Biancari F., (2010). Miniaturized Versus conventional cardiopulmonary bypass in high-risk patients undergoing coronary artery bypass grafting. *Perfusion*. Vol. 25, No. 2 (March 2010), pp. 65-70.

Larmann, J. & Theilmeier, G. (2004). Inflammatory response to cardiac surgery: cardiopulmonary bypass versus non-cardiopulmonary bypass surgery. *Best Practice in Research and Clinical Anaesthesiology*. Vol 18, No 3 (September 2004) pp. 425-38.

Lagan, AL., Melley, DD., Evans, TW. & Quinlan, GJ. (2008) Pathogenesis of the systemic inflammatory syndrome and acute lung injury: role of iron mobilization and decompartmentalization. *American Journal of Physiology. Lung Cellular and Molecular Physiology*. Vol. 294, No 2 (Febraury 2008), pp. L161-74.

Mazzei, V., Nasso, G., Salamone, G., Castorino, F., Tommasini, A. & Anselmi A. (2007) Prospective randomized comparison of coronary bypass grafting with minimal extracorporeal circulation system (MECC) versus off-pump coronary surgery *Circulation*. Vol. 116, No 16 (October 2007) pp. 1761-7.

Nannizzi-Alaimo, L., Rubenstein, MH., Alves, VL., Leong, GY., Phillips, DR. & Gold, HK. (2002). Cardiopulmonary bypass induces release of soluble CD40 ligand. *Circulation*. Vol. 105, No 24 (June 2002), pp. 2849-54.

Ohata, T., Mitsuno, M., Yamamura, M., Tanaka, H., Kobayashi, Y., Ryomoto, M., Yoshioka, Y.& Miyamoto, Y. (2007) Minimal cardiopulmonary bypass attenuates neutrophil activation and cytokine release in coronary artery bypass grafting. *Journal of Artificial Organs*. Vol. 10 No 2 (October 2007;) pp. 92-5.

Palombo, D., Valenti, D., Gaggiano, A., Lupo, M. & Borin, P. (2004). Early experience with the minimal extracorporeal circulation system (MECC) during thoracoabdominal aortic aneurysm repair. *European Journal of Vascular and Endovascular Surgery* Vol. 27, No 3 (March 2004) pp. 324-6.

Paparella, D., Yau, TM., Young, E. (2002). Cardiopulmonary bypass induced inflammation: pathophysiology and treatment. An update. *European Journal of Cardiothoracic Surgery*. Vol. 21, No. 2 (Febraury 2002), pp. 232-44.

Puehler, T., Haneya, A., Philipp, A., Zausig, YA., Kobuch, R., Diez, C., Birnbaum, DE. & Schmid C. (2010). Minimized extracorporeal circulation system in coronary artery bypass surgery: a 10-year single-center experience with 2243 patients. *European Journal of Cardiothoracic Surgery*. Vol 39, No 4 (April 2011) pp. 459-64.

Puehler, T., Haneya, A., Philipp, A., Wiebe, K., Keyser, A., Rupprecht, L., Hirt, S., Kobuc ,R., Diez, C., Hilker & M., Schmid, C. (2009) Minimal Extracorporeal Circulation: An Alternative for On-Pump and Off-Pump Coronary Revascularization. *Annals of Thoracic Surgery*. Vol. 87, No 3 (March 2009), pp.766-72..

Raja, SG. & Berg, GA. (2007). Impact of off-pump coronary artery bypass surgery on systemic inflammation: current best available evidence. *Journal of Cardiac Surgery*. Vol. 22, No 5 (Sep-Oct 2007), pp. 445-55

Reber, D., Brouwer, R., Buchwald, D., Fritz, M., Germing, A., Lindstaedt, M., Klak, K. & Laczkovics, A. (2010). Beating-heart coronary artery bypass grafting with miniaturized cardiopulmonary bypass results in a more complete revascularization when compared to off-pump grafting. Artificial Organs. Vol. 34, No 3 (March 2010) pp. 179-84.

Remadi, JP., Rakotoarivelo, Z., Marticho, P.& Benamar A. (2006) Prospective randomized study comparing coronary artery bypass grafting with the new mini-extracorporeal circulation Jostra System or with a standard cardiopulmonary bypass *American Heart Journal*. Vol.151, No 151 (January 2006), pp. 198.e1-198.e7

Remadi, JP., Marticho, P., Butoi, I., Rakotoarivelo, Z., Trojette, F., Benamar, A., Beloucif, S., Foure, D. & Poulain, HJ. (2004). Clinical Experience With the Mini-Extracorporeal Circulation System: An Evolution or a Revolution? *Annals of Thoracic Surgery*. Vol. 77, No 6 (June 2004), pp. 2172-5;

Royston, D. (1997). The inflammatory response and extracorporeal circulation. *Journal of Cardiothoracic Vascular Anesthesia*. Vol. 11, No. 3 (May 1997) pp. 341-54.

Robertson, CM. & Coopersmith, CM. (2006).The systemic inflammatory response syndrome. *Microbes Infection*. Vol. 8, No 5 (April 2006) pp. 1382-9.

Skrabal, CA., Steinhoff, G. & Liebold, A. (2007). Minimizing cardiopulmonary bypass attenuates myocardial damage after cardiac surgery. *ASAIO Journal*. Vol. 53, No. 1 (January-Febrary 2007) pp. 32-5.

Stalder, M., Gygax, E., Immer, FF., Englberger, L., Tevaearai, H & Carrel TP. Minimized cardiopulmonary bypass combined with a smart suction device: the future of cardiopulmonary bypass? *Heart Surgery Forum*. Vol 10, No 3 (October 2007), pp. E235-8.

van Boven, WJ., Gerritsen, WB., Waanders, FG., Haas, FJ. & Aarts, LP. (2004). Mini extracorporeal circuit for coronary artery bypass grafting: initial clinical and biochemical results: a comparison with conventional and off-pump coronary artery bypass grafts concerning global oxidative stress and alveolar function. *Perfusion*. Vol. 19, No. 4 (July 2004) pp. 239-46.

Vohra, HA., Whistance, R., Modi, A. & Ohri SK. (2009). The inflammatory response to miniaturised extracorporeal circulation: a review of the literature. *Mediators of Inflammation*. Volume 2009, Article ID 707042, 7 pages.*European Journal of Cardiothoracic Surgery*. Vol 28, No 1 (July 2005) pp.127-32.

Wiesenack, C., Liebold, A., Philipp, A., Ritzka, M., Koppenberg, J., Birnbaum, DE. & Keyl, C. (2004). Four years' experience with a miniaturized extracorporeal circulation system and its influence on clinical outcome. *Artificial Organs*. Vol. 28, No 12 (December 2004), pp. 1082-8.

Wippermann, J., Albes, JM., Hartrumpf, M., Kaluza, M., Vollandt, R., Bruhin, R. & Wahlers, T. (2005). Comparison of minimally invasive closed circuit extracorporeal circulation with conventional cardiopulmonary bypass and with off-pump technique in CABG patients: selected parameters of coagulation and inflammatory system. European Journal of Cardiothoracic Surgery. Vol. 28, No 1 (July 2005) pp. 127-32.

8

Hypothermic Cardiac Arrest to Remove Right Atrial Thrombi Due to Abdominal Malignancies

Pier Luigi Stefano, Stefano Romagnoli,
Donata Villari and Giacomo Batignani
Università degli Studi di Firenze,
Italy

1. Introduction

The first use of hypothermia in cardiac surgery is attributed to Dr. John Lewis who performed an atrial septal defect closure on September 2, 1952 at the University of Minnesota (Gott, 2005).

Cardiopulmonary by-pass (CPB) and hypothermic cardio-circulatory arrest (HCCA) has been introduced for the first time in clinical practice for aortic arc substitution (Pierangeli et al., 1974). More recently the same technique has been proposed to remove atrial thrombi originated from renal carcinomas (Marshall et al., 1984), adrenal carcinomas (Shahinian et al., 1989), hepatocellular carcinoma (Hamazaki et al., 1995) and other abdominal malignancies such as caval leiomyosarcoma, uterine endometrial sarcoma or intravenous leiomyomatosis, ovarian or testicular tumors (Hassan et al.,, 2010; Vargas-Barron et al., 1990; Ariza et al., 1982; Kanda et al., 1991).

There is still a debate pro and cons the use of hypothermic arrest with some favours the normothermic (Lubahn et al., 2006; Stewart et al., 1991) and some others the hypothermic, because of the operative field appears better exposed and almost completely bloodless so the blood loss resulted much lower. Furthermore they claim a better visualization of some critical areas with an easier removal of the tumoural thrombus, that may invade the hepatic veins or the coronaric sinus, may either remain attached to the tricuspid valve or may have embolized into the pulmonary artery (Chiappini et al., 2002; Kalkat et al., 2008; Leo et al., 2010; Topcouglu et al., 2004). In all these occasions HCCA offers the possibility of a better tumoural cleaning with the possibility of R0 resection. The incomplete removal of this tumoural thrombi in fact is correlated to an early recurrence and a worst postoperative survival (Skinner et al., 1989). Furthermore the hepatic, renal and splacnic damage from warm ischemia due to the Pringle's manoeuvre and/or aortic/mesenteric cross-clamping (usually necessary when CPB is used without cardio-circulatory arrest) is reduced when the HCCA is instead used (Chiappini et al., 2002, Davlouros et al., 2005). This permits its use even in the setting of mild hepatic damage (Leo et al., 2010).

2. Kidney

Tumour thrombus extension in the inferior vena cava (IVC) occurs in 4 % to 10% of patients with renal cell carcinoma (RCC) (Marshall et al., 1988). The cephalic extension of tumour thrombus in RCC was first defined in 1987 by Neves and Zincke (Neves & Zincke, 1987) and classified in four levels (level I : thrombus at the level of the renal vein, level II : thrombus extending into the infra-hepatic IVC, level III : thrombus extending into the retro-hepatic IVC, level IV : intra-atrial thrombus (suprahepatic IVC involvement or right atrium thrombus). Libertino classification system (Moinzadeh & Libertino, 2004) distinguishes: renal vein only involvement, level I caval involvement (IVC below the diaphragm), level II caval involvement (IVC above the diaphragm) and level III involvement (when the thrombus reaches the atrium).

Recently an updated staging system by the American Joint Committee on Cancer (AJCC) and the "Union International Contre le Cancer" (UICC) was utilized and the current staging, according to the 2009 UICC/AJCC TNM staging classification system, designates renal vein involvement as pT3a Level III, when the thrombus involves the intra-hepatic portion of the IVC but below the diaphragm is designated as p T3b, while level IV when the thrombus extends above the diaphragm, as T3c. The thrombus may extend as far as the right atrium (IV level) in 1% of patients with RCC. Accurate information about the presence and complete extent of IVC involvement is essential for surgical planning. Routine CT scanning and abdominal ultrasonography are less reliable in delineating the cephalic extent of the thrombus. Contrast inferior venacavography is an accurate, but invasive, diagnostic tool and a single anterograde study may be insufficient in complete caval obstruction. Occasionally has been employed trans oesophageal echocardiography and trans-abdominal colour flow Doppler ultrasonography. MRI has become the preferred, non invasive, diagnostic study though its frequent inability to differentiate actual invasion of the vena cava wall which is generally associate with a poor prognosis. Contrast inferior venography is reserved for patients in whom MRI finings are equivocal or for whom MRI is contraindicated. Another option in this group of patients is multiplanar CT.

Renal arteriography is useful in the preoperative study because it may highlighted a distinct vascularisation of the thrombus (observed in 35% to 40% of the cases) allowing to perform a preoperative embolization of the kidney, causing the shrinkage of the thrombus and its more easily intra-operative removal.

The prognostic significance of venous involvement and tumour thrombus level remains highly controversial. According to the literature in the absence of metastasis, when adjusting for clinical and pathologic features, radical nephrectomy with total tumour thrombus excision in patients with RCC and level I to III vena caval involvement is associated with a cancer specific 5 -year survival rate between 47% and 68% (Staheler & Brkovic, 2000; Belis et al., 2000).

Some authors generally accepted that neoplastic extension in the IVC was not a prognostic determining factor (Libertino et al., 1987; Skinner et al., 1989; Ciancio et al., 2010). Some others, more recently, have shown that tumour thrombus level is an independent predictor of survival (Martı´nez-Salamanca et al., 2011).

RCC with vascular invasion into the IVC, direct invasion of the vein's wall appears to be an important prognostic factor and should be noted during tumour staging. With no peri-nephric fat or lymph nodal involvement, patients who undergo tumour excision with radical nephrectomy and IVC thrombectomy have an overall and cancer specific 5-year survival of 30% to 72% with an operative mortality of 2.7% to 13.5 %. When the thrombus locally invades the wall of the vena cava, aggressive resection of the vascular wall with reconstruction along with the attainment of negative surgical margins provides a survival benefit (Hatcher et al., 1991). Grafting or reconstitution sometimes is required only in those patients with not complete occlusion of IVC and collateral blood flow. In 1913, Berg first described nephrectomy and vena caval thrombectomy as primary surgical treatment of these patients (Berg, 1913). Usually, in level I and II disease the tumour thrombus can safely be excised by means of proximal and distal control of the IVC. In level III and IV disease the exposure and isolation of IVC requires liver mobilization with or without the use of CBP. Several techniques have been used during the years to remove large caval thrombi when distal caval control cannot be achieved below the liver such as cross-clamping of the supraceliac aorta (Cummings et al., 1979), occlusion of the intra pericardial vena cava with simultaneous occlusion of the "porta hepatis" and superior mesenteric artery (Skinner et al., 1989), use of an intraoperative venous (cava-atrial) shunt (Foster et al.,1988), and cardiopulmonary by pass alone (Novick & Cosgrove, 1980). The use of CBP alone is limited to the period during which the liver and the kidneys undergo warm ischemia. Skinner and co-workers reported an average warm ischemia of 14 minutes ranging from 8 to 20 minutes. Post operative complications occurred in 41% to 60% of the patients and included transient hyperbilirubinemia, renal dysfunction and respiratory failure (Skinner et al., 1989). When the thrombus extends above the diaphragm the use of CPB with deep HCCA have been used. Marshall et al., 1984 and Krane et al., 1984 first demonstrated the feasibility of this approach. The most common post operative complications related to this procedure are haemorrhage, coagulopathy, increased transient and/or permanent neurologic risk. Novick et al., 1990 in their experience reported up to 60 minutes of safe ischemia with direct visual inspection of the entire vena caval lumen in a bloodless field reducing risk of sudden massive intra-operative haemorrhage or distal pulmonary tumour Thrombo-embolization. Operative mortality rate reported was 4.7% (Novick et al., 1990). Heart surgery have been used more frequently to treat intra-cardiac extension of infra-diaphragmatic tumours and the safety of this procedure has increased. Chiappini and co-workers in their series of 13 patients reported no in-hospital deaths while 2 patients experienced postoperative complications such as respiratory failure and bleeding (Chiappini et al., 2002). On the other side, Ruel and co-workers in 2001 reported their experience in cavo-atrial thrombus excision in 6 patients affected by RCC without circulatory arrest (Ruel et al., 2001). During the last 10 years the traditional approach using CBP and HCCA was revisited. Deep hypothermic circulatory arrest was therefore not considered imperative and some studies reported that its avoidance may decrease morbidity and mortality. Shinghal et al., in 2003 reported in a single patient a novel technique by placing an aortic occlusive balloon in the abdominal aorta at the level of the diaphragm, limiting flow in the IVC and maintaining both cerebral and spinal cord perfusion during cardiopulmonary bypass (Shingai et al., 2003). In 2005 Ciancio & Soloway described a technique that can be safely used to approach RCC with a tumour thrombus extending into the supra-diaphragmatic IVC and right atrium through a trans-abdominal approach without sternotomy and/or cardiopulmonary bypass utilizing a complete liver mobilization and minimizing the vena caval cross–clamp time. The trans-abdominal incision exposes the intra-pericardial IVC and right atrium trans-diaphragmatically. (Ciancio & Soloway, 2005; Ciancio G, Shirodkar S et al.,2009). Step by step description of this technique based on orthotopic liver transplantation was reported in 2011 by the same author regarding a cohort of 56 patients with retro-hepatic extension of the thrombus and 12 patients with a supra-hepatic/intra atrial localizations. Mean operative time was 5h and 32 min. Five patients required CPB (7.3%). Three patients died in the immediate post operative period (4.4%) (Ciancio G, Gonzalez J,et al., 2011). In 2007 Chowdhury et al., reported their experience in a cohort of 6 patients with RCC and intra atrial tumour thrombus using mild hypothermic CPB and intermittent cross- clamping of the supra-celiac abdominal aorta (Chowdhury et al., 2007)

RCC with vascular invasion into the IVC remains a crucial challenge to the urologic oncologist. Complete excision of the tumour together with the thrombus and negative margins offers the best chance for patients survival. Surgical resection of these complex tumours requires multidisciplinary approach.

2.1 Adrenal

The use of CPB to remove the tumour thrombus from adrenocortical carcinoma (ACC) was first reported in 1976 (Scully et al., 1976) while the first procedure using HCCA was in 1989 (Shahian et al., 1989) but because of the poor prognosis of this tumour at this stage and the technical difficulties that has to be faced such as the invasion of surrounding organs and vascular control/reconstruction, radical surgical resection remains controversial. A recent review from France (Chiche et al., 2006) collected the outcome of 32 patients reported in literature with cavo-atrial invasion in whom a CPB was used in 26 including 6 under HCCA. Reported peri-operative mortality was 3/26 (11.5%) and took place in patients operated using CPB alone.

In their own series of ACC with tumour thrombi extending into the vena cava or in the right atrium, they reported the outcome of 15 patients treated by a combination of venous control ranging from cross clamping to hepatic vascular exclusion or normo/ipothermic cardio-pulmonary by-pass. The extension grade C (above the liver) was in 7 patients, including 4 with atrial thrombi and represents the 7% of the overall series. Of these patients 3 had HCCA and 1 (33.3%) died p.o. from multi-organ failure but the patient was cirrhotic with a portal thrombosis.

They concluded that CPB should always be used for tumours extending to the cavo-atrial junction or into the right atrium and additional HCCA provides a bloodless field that allow a precise dissection of the thrombus while reducing the blood loss.

2.2 Liver

Macroscopic vascular invasion (either portal or supra-hepatic) is a major complication of hepatocellular carcinoma (HCC). Major vascular invasion is the evolution of microscopic vascular invasion over the time so the liver tumour is of the large type at diagnosis and usually require major liver resection.

The natural history of HCC complicated with macroscopic vascular invasion of the portal vein, shows a median survival time of only 9 to 10 weeks (Okada et al., 1992).

Treatments with systemic chemotherapy, intra-arterial chemotherapy or radiofrequency ablation result in a dismal survival at 1 year ranging from 7% to 18% (Raul et al., 1994; Akashi et al., 1991; Poon et al., 2003). Hepatic resection remains the only option for these patients and a recent multicentric study showed that, resected patients lived longer, compared to those not treated surgically, with a five-year survival rate of 10% (Pawlik et al., 2005; Lin et al., 2007).

Liver tumour with extension to the hepatic veins represents instead a controversial issue and its extension in the right atrium (RA) via the inferior vena cava is more uncommon, with percentage of incidence reported of 2.9% by imaging techniques, 0.7% at operation, and 18.2% at autopsy in Japan (Yogita et al., 2000).

Therapeutics options at this stage are few and debatable because of the high risk for lung metastasis (Masaki et al., 1995) but, on the other hand, the risk of developing a "ball valve syndrome"(Hahne & Climie, 1962) or a pulmonary embolism is very high (Fujisaki et al.,1991). The overall survival time of these patients with cavo-atrial thrombi and who do not undergo operative treatment is reported to be very low: from 3 days to 2 months (Lin et al., 2007)

Liver resection and cavo-atrial thrombectomy remains, in this situation, the only effective therapeutic option with reported survival time ranging from 5 to 56 months (Miyazawa et al., 2005).

The firsts authors describing the removal of a tumoural thrombus in the RA from HCC on cirrhosis using CBP were Goto et al. in 1986 who removed only the thrombus. Fujisaki et al. in 1991 first removed the thrombus along with the primary tumour using CPB hepatic vascular exclusion while Hamazaki et al. in 1995 added the use of HCCA in a similar situation. Indeed, HCCA was first applied in liver surgery, in a young child to remove atrial thrombi from hepatoblastoma, which usually occurs on a normal liver parenchyma, in 1981 (Ein et al., 1981).

The majority of patients with HCC has a diseased liver because of the presence of hepatitis viruses infection and /or previous alcohol abuse. The presence of hepatic vein, vena cava and atrial thrombosis contraindicate liver transplantation and, liver resection with thrombectomy, is the only real therapeutic option in this setting (Wu et al., 2000). As previously stated, acute pulmonary embolism or congestive heart failure may complicate liver tumours involving hepatic vein with tumours thrombi in the inferior vena cava/right atrium. This latter situation represent an impending life-threatening condition that should be surgically treated as soon as possible (Novick et al., 1990).

Atrial thrombus removal may be achieved under normothermic CPB and total liver vascular exclusion. Tolerance of the cirrhotic liver to normothermic ischemia is reported as safe up to 33 minutes (Huguet et al., 1994) which is quite similar to the safety time reported to avoid neurological complications when using HCCA (McCullough et al., 1999).

Extracorporeal circulation with HCCA has been increasingly used to remove atrial thrombi due to retroperitoneal malignancies (Ogata et al., 2006) but its use in cirrhotic patients has been limited, for many years, because of the fear of post-operative liver failure and poor outcome. However, in more recent time, we have assisted to an increase number of reports where HCCA has been used to remove cavo-atrial thrombi due to HCC with no mortality and low morbidity, probably, lower than expected thus, we can assume that, a short lasting HCCA, has to be considered safe in a well compensated liver cirrhosis (Novick et al., 1990; Yogitaet al., 2000; Ohwada et al., 2008; Florman et al., 2009; Leo et al., 2010).

Since the vast majority of patients with HCC and atrial tumour thrombi has large type of HCC, a major liver resection is usually required and the possibility of postoperative liver failure raises accordingly, liver function tests and indocyanin green retention test, should be carried out in these patients in order to demonstrate the presence of a good functional reserve (Kawasaki et al., 1995). Furthermore we think that adding a sequential arterial and portal embolization of a hemi-liver could lessen the possibilities of post-operative liver failure when a major resection is planned (Ogata et al., 2006).

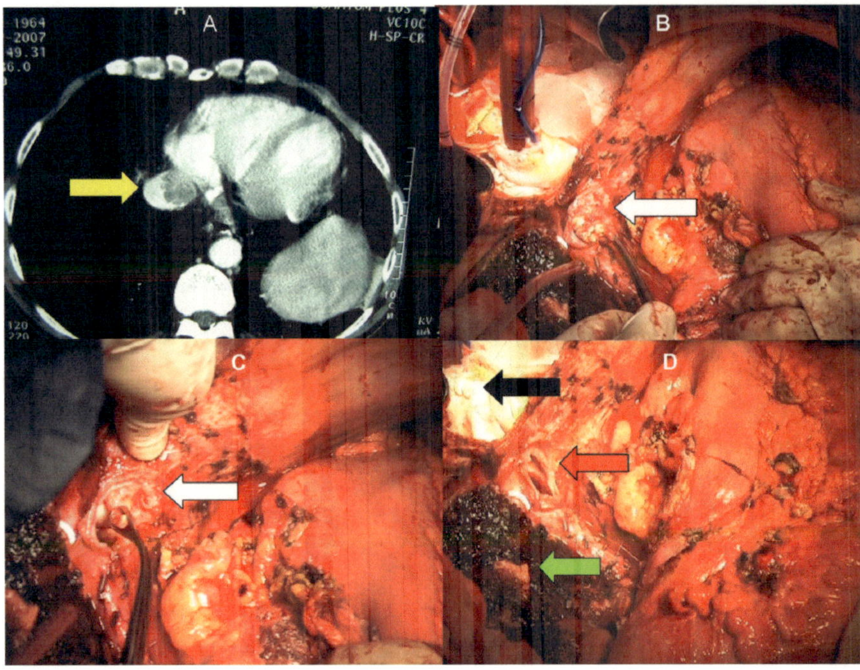

Fig. 1. A: Ct scan of a cavo-atrial tumour thrombus (yellow arrow). B and C: Extraction of the thrombus, after a left hemi-hepatectomy, from the sectioned left and middle hepatic vein ostium (white arrow) using a rings clamps to pull and an index finger, inserted from the atriotomy site, to push the thrombus downward. D: Cleaned ostium (red arrow), closed atriotomy (black arrow) and distal middle hepatic vein stump (green arrow) to be reconstructed. Please note the completely bloodless field of the procedure under hypothermic cardiocirculatory arrest.

2.3 Uterus

The uterus is seldom the site of origin of a cavo-atrial thrombi owing to two distinct tumours: the endometrial stromal sarcoma (ESS) and the "benign" intravenous leiomyomatosis (IVL). This latter situation differs from the other types of neoplastic thrombi because the endovascular material is represented mainly by myofibroblastic cells, growing into the vessel, rather than by a neoplastic thrombotic apposition.

2.3.1 Endometrial stromal sarcoma

ESS represents only the 0.2% of all uterine malignancies and it has been described to invade the great vessels rarely. In a recent review only 9 patients had a tumour thrombus reaching the right atrium, ventricle or the pulmonary artery that underwent radical resection by means of total abdominal hysterectomy and thrombectomy. Normothermic CPB was reported in 7 out the 9 patients with only 1 (14.3%) complication due to renal acute tubular necrosis. No perioperative deaths were reported (Renzulli et al., 2008).

2.3.2 Intravenous leyomiomatosis

IVL is an uncommon "benign" tumour of middle age parous women arising from either the uterine venous wall or uterine leiomyoma (Nam et al., 2002). It is known also as benign metastatic fibro-leiomyoma because pulmonary nodules (proliferating leiomycites) are often present. Although this tumour is usually confined to the pelvis, it sometime extends to the right cardiac cavities through the iliac vein and the vena cava (Wakiama et al., 2000) by means of intra-vascular proliferation and growth of fibro-myocites which results in an extension of the fibro-leiomyoma rather than in a thrombus formation conferring a typical consistency and resistance to traction to the endo-vascular proliferation (Galajda et al., 2010). IVL with cardiac extension is an exceedingly rare disease first reported in 1907 in an autopsy series (Durk, 1907). Since then a further 34 cases have been reported involving the right heart (Wakiyama et al., 2000). Patients often have a history of hysterectomy or leiomyoma resection and various lengths of intravascular proliferation up to 29 cm with a diagnosis performed up to 18 yrs after the primary surgery (Galajda et al., 2010).

Complete surgical removal of the uterus and IVL is the therapy of choice (Topcouglu et al., 2004) and it has been carried out for the first time in 1974 using CPB and HCCA (Mandelbaum et al., 1974).

We came across a similar case (Fig. 2) in whom we performed a total abdominal hysterectomy and IVL removal through a cavotomy and atriotomy under CPB and HCCA (Fig. 3). Due to the typical consistency of IVL and the usual absence of adhesions the complete heart and retro-hepatic vena cava cleaning was achieved by simple traction from the infra-renal cavotomy site (Fig. 3A) while the iliac portion was stacked and required separate iliac vein incision.

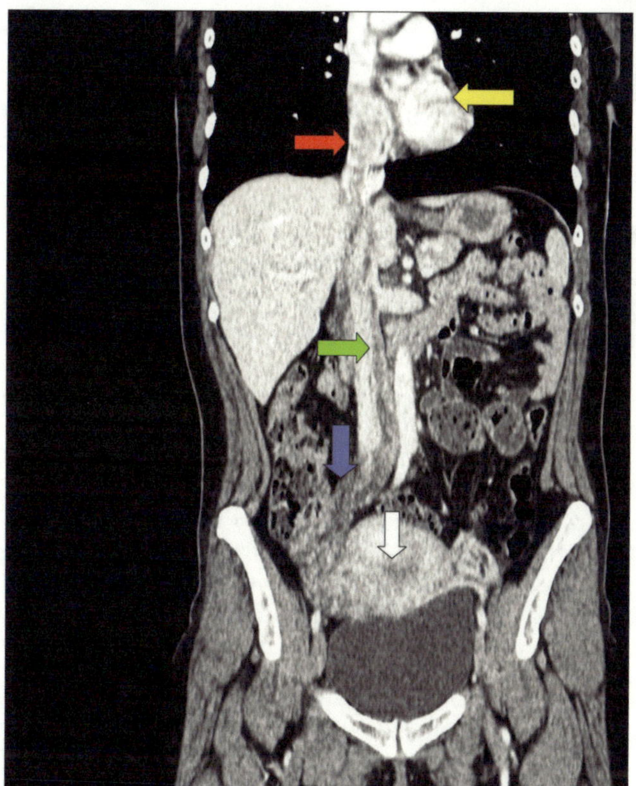

Fig. 2. Preoperative ct scan of intra-vascular leiomyomatosis arising from uterine leiomyoma (white arrow) extending to the right iliac vein (blue arrow), infra and retro-hepatic vena cava (green arrow), right atrium (red arrow) and to the rignt ventricle (yellow arrow).

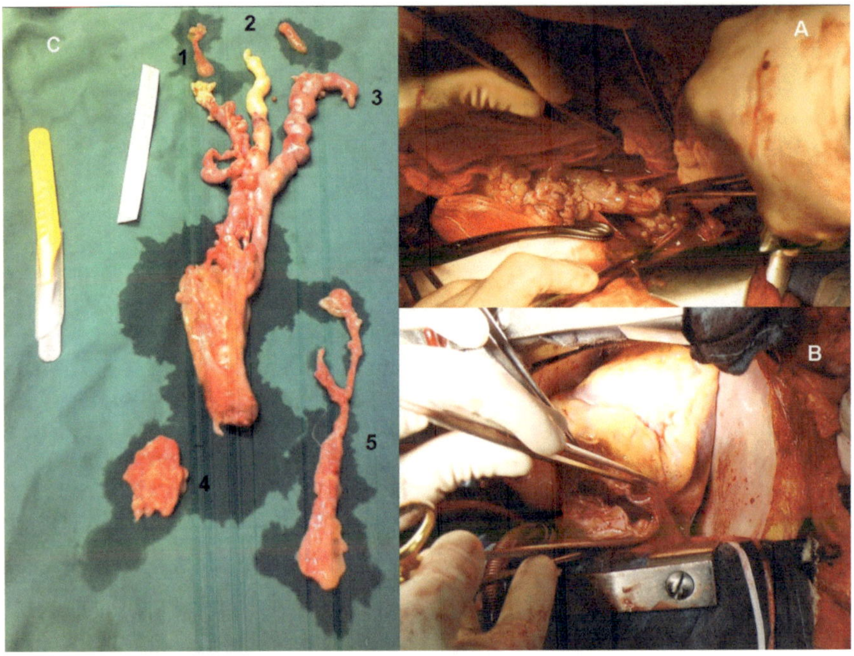

Fig. 3. Same Patient of figure 2. Operative view of the removal, through a cavotomy (A) and atriotomy (B), of intravascular leiomyomatosis. Operative specimen removed is shown in C: 1 and 2 are the right atrial extensions, 3 the right ventricular extension, 4 the caval iliac extensions and 5 right ovarian vein involvement.

2.4 Vena cava

Leiomysarcomas of the inferior vena cava (IVC) are rare malignant tumours originating from the smooth muscle cells of the media layer that typically show three growth patterns: extra-luminal, intra-luminal and both (Mingoli et al., 1996). They may be classified anatomically according to Chiappini et al., 2002, as for renal tumours, into four types: Type I infra-hepatic, type II retro-hepatic, type III supra-hepatic IVC and type IV the thrombus extends in the right atrium.

Patient with type IV was treated and reported by Hassan et al., 2010, using normothermic CPB and Pringle's manoeuvre to remove the atrial thrombus reporting mild hyperbilirubinemia and normal renal function. They discussed the possible advantages of the technique used, compared to HCCA which they thought to be associated with an extended CPB time, increased postoperative bleeding and coagulopathy, and increased neurological risk. On the other hand HCCA provides a bloodless surgical field with reduced risk of spreading/embolization, and fatal haemorrhage. Furthermore the advantages include reduced liver and kidney warm ischemia, reduced risk of incomplete excision, optimal visualization of the IVC/right atrial lumen minimizing the need for a too extensive retro-peritoneal dissection (Chiappini et al., 2002).

2.5 Others

Scattered case reports of ovarian haemangioma (Tamburino et al., 1992), testicular tumour (Kanda et al., 1991), embrional carcinoma of the testis (Paule et al., 1991), testicular teratoma (Moon et al., 1992) and even pancreatic cancer (Ozben et al., 2007) have been reported so far.

The problems when dealing with these situations are almost the same of those reported above and at the moment it is impossible to draw any conclusion due the scarcity of the cases.

3. Anesthetic management

In the following sections, an overview of the main technical features for the management of anaesthesia, extracorporeal circulation and hypothermic circulatory arrest for cavo-atrial thrombectomy are summarized.

3.1 Monitoring and anesthesia

Any operative procedure involving large vessels entail the risk of developing hemodynamic instability, mainly due to massive bleeding. Moreover, a number of specific conditions have to be taken into consideration, including coexisting multisystemic diseases, non-physiological conditions associated with CPB and deep HCCA. In light of these concerns, patients undergoing cavo-atrial thrombectomy require extensive monitoring to provide early warning of conditions that may lead to potentially life-threatening states.

3.1.1 Monitoring

An intraoperative electrocardiogram, using the five-leads technique, is the standard monitoring procedure always recommended during surgery and anesthesia. In this setting, it is useful for the diagnosis of both myocardial ischemia (D_{II} - V_5 identify 90% of ischemic episodes) and dysrhythmias.

Intravascular pressure measurements represent the standard technique during this type of surgery. Arterial pressure is usually measured by placing a catheter in a peripheral (radial, ulnar, brachial) or central (femoral) artery. Direct arterial pressure measurement allows monitoring during the pre-CPB stage and nonpulsatile ECC. Moreover, during the post-CPB/HCCA period, patients are usually hemodynamically unstable, and close surveillance of arterial blood pressure, other than with blood-gas analysis, is of primary importance.

A central venous line (internal jugular, subclavian) for pressure monitoring (central venous pressure [CVP]) is influenced by circulating blood volume, venous tone and capacitance, and right ventricular function; therefore, a number of pieces of information can be obtained from the CVP. A central venous catheter (3 lumens, 7-8.5 Fr) can be used for both pressure measurement and inotropic-vasoactive drug administration. Central venous lines can also be used for pulmonary artery catheter (PAC) positioning if the patient's comorbidities suggest the monitoring of pulmonary artery pressures, the measurement of cardiac output and mixed venous oxygen saturation. Central venous cannulation should be performed under ultrasound guidance because up to 30% of patients have some abnormalities of the jugular vein anatomy (Carid et al., 1988; Bevilacqua et al., 2005).

Hemodynamic monitoring is completed with transesophageal echocardiography, which has gained widespread use in cardiac operating rooms (where this intervention for cavo-atrial invasion is usually performed) because it provides a great deal of information about the heart's global performance during systole and diastole, the valve function and cardiac volume loads, as well as morphologic details on thrombotic cardiac invasion from the inferior vena cava.

Temperature monitoring. Assessment of accurate central temperature is of primary importance in this setting. The core temperature (vital organ temperature) can be measured by means of a PAC thermistor, nasopharyngeal probe (provides accurate measurement of brain temperature during CPB and HCCA), bladder probe (it may be inaccurate when renal blood flow and urine output are decreased), CPB arterial line (temperature of the heat exchanger), CPB venous line (reflects core temperature well during CPB, when no active cooling or warming is ongoing), or rectal probe (when the tip of the probe rests in stool, the measurement may be imprecise) (FIG. 4 & 5).

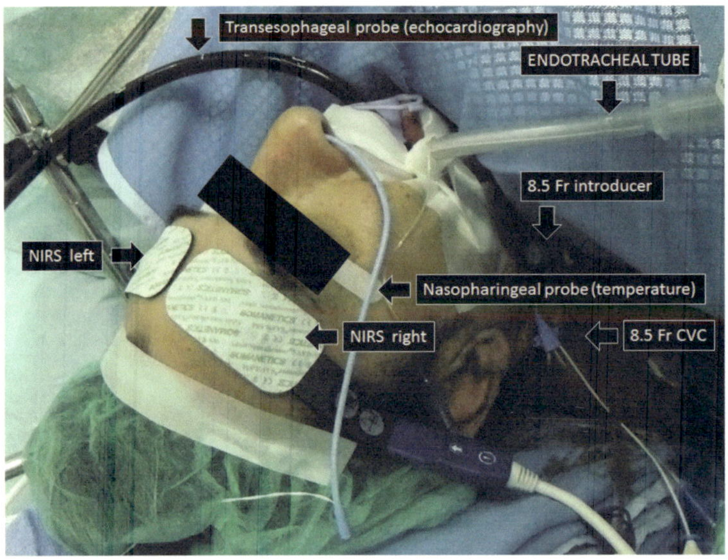

Fig. 4. Monitoring. (NIRS, near infrared spectroscopy; CVC, central venous catheter).

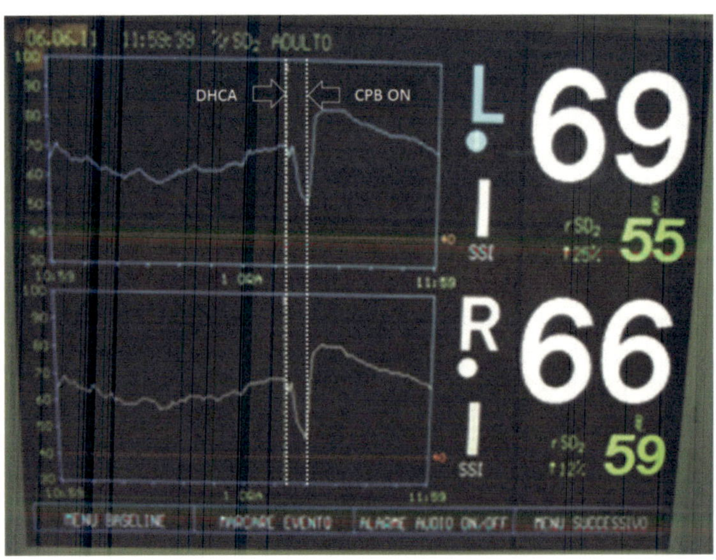

Fig. 5. Near infrared spectroscopy. (DHCA Deep Hypothermic Circulatory Arrest; CPB, cardiopulmonary bypass).

Renal function. Acute kidney injury (AKI) is one of the well-known complications occurring during CPB that has significant implications for both short- and long-term outcomes. The incidence of acute renal failure rages from 20 to 30% of patients (Kumar & Suneja, 2004). Pre-operative renal function is one of the most important factors related to post-CPB AKI. The major risk factors for AKI after CPB include advanced age, preexisting kidney disease, diabetes mellitus, chronic obstructive pulmonary disease, CPB duration, emergency surgery, female sex, left ventricle ejection fraction <40%, and hemodilution on CPB. Hemolysis always occurs during CPB, and serum hemoglobin levels rise; therefore, urine output should be maintained to avoid tubular damage. Diuretic therapies (mannitol is used routinely in CPB priming) are also useful for eliminating the hemodilution induced with the onset of CPB. As a consequence, urinary catheter positioning and urine output are the best monitoring systems for renal function evaluation.

3.1.2 Anesthesia

These patients usually require a smooth induction because wide modifications in vascular tone, myocardial contractility, and reductions in venous returns due to increased intra-thoracic pressures under mechanical ventilation may worsen the organ and tissue perfusion. Midazolam or etomidate, in association with an opioid (remifentanil, fentanyl), are useful drugs for anesthesia induction; propofol and/or sevoflurane or desflurane can be used for anesthesia maintenance, and a nondepolarizing muscle relaxant should be administered for the duration of the intervention (Table 1).

	Drug	**Induction dose**
Hypnotics	Propofol	1-1.5 mg/Kg
	Thiopental	3-4 mg/Kg
	Etomidate	0.2-0.3 mg/Kg
	Midazolam	0.1-0.2 mg/Kg
Opioids	Fentanyl	3-10 mcg/Kg
	Sufentanyl	0.5-1 mcg/Kg
	Remifentanil	0.1-0.75 mcg/Kg/min
Muscle relaxants	Cisatracurium	0.07- 0.1 mg/Kg
	Vecuronium	0.07- 0.1 mg/Kg
	Rocuronium	0.6 mg/Kg

Table 1. Hypnotics, opioids, and muscle relaxants (induction doses)

The choice of drug for anesthesia induction and maintenance depends on the patient's general conditions and, in particular, his/her heart, renal, and liver function. In addition, antibiotic prophylaxis should be administered at least 30 minutes before skin incision.

3.2 Cardiopulmonary bypass, deep hypothermic circulatory arrest and neuroprotection

3.2.1 Cardiopulmonary bypass

Cardiopulmonary bypass permits blood to bypass the heart and lungs (Fig. 6).

Venous blood is drained by gravity into an oxygenator (artificial lung), and a pump injects it, after oxygenation and removal of CO_2, into a great artery (aorta, subclavian, femoral artery). Adequate anticoagulation is necessary during the CPB period, and an activated clotting time longer than 420-480 seconds is usually considered safe (the optimal target of

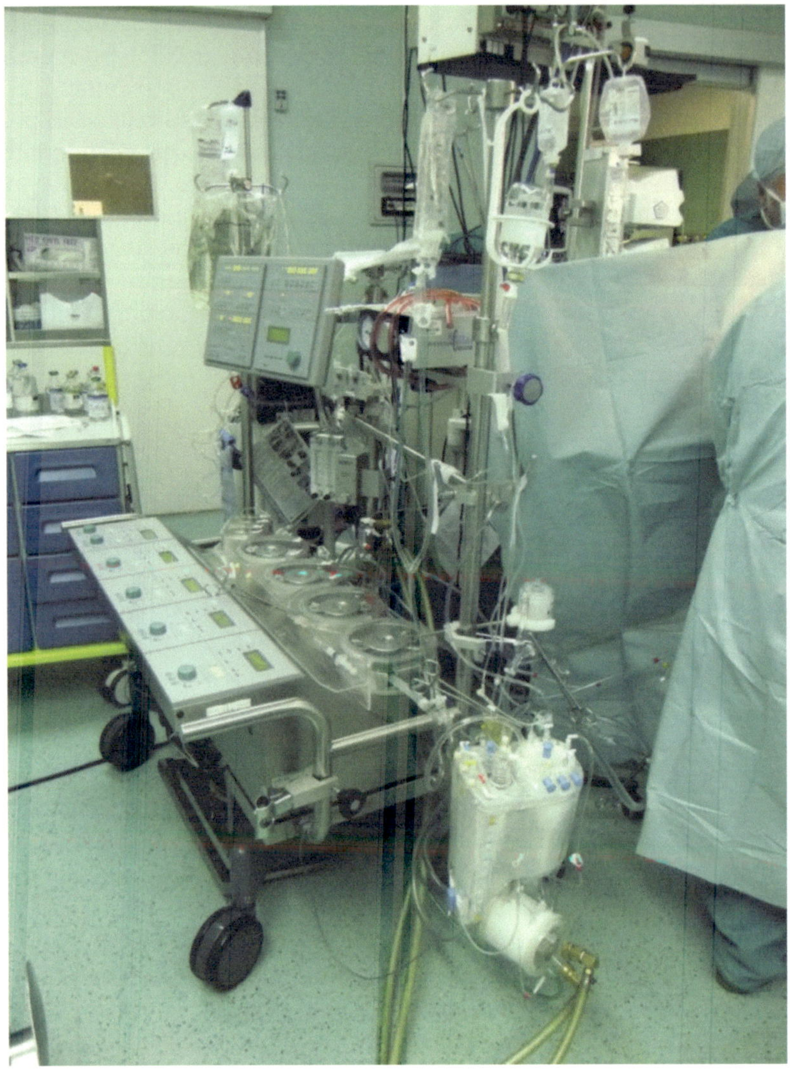

Fig. 6. Cardiopulmonary bypass.

ACT is still debated). Anticoagulation is obtained with heparin 300-400 U/kg, and supplemental doses of 5000 U can be administered if necessary. Use of heparin-coated circuits does not eliminate the need for heparin. The pump flow has to be set at values that guarantee an adequate oxygen delivery. "Normal" pump flow is considered to be 2.4 $l/min/m^2$, although recent studies have demonstrated that a redistribution of flow toward organs occurs during CPB in both normothermia and hypothermia (Slater et al., 2001). Muscle flow is significantly reduced during CPB, and if flow is reduced, splacnic, renal and cerebral flow decrease as well, in that order. During CPB, blood pressure depends on pump flow, total arterial impedance and haematocrit. During CPB, blood pressure is less important in determining global perfusion if pump flow is adequate, but minimal values of blood pressure may be significant in providing specific regional flows; therefore, during mild to moderate hypothermia (30-34°C), the blood pressure is generally maintained at approximately 70 mm Hg. During CPB and HCCA, the loss of flow auto regulation (<20°C and for several hours after HCCA) is still debated, but pressure levels as low as 30-40 mm Hg are considered safe values (Croughwell et al., 1992). Despite several techniques for cerebral protection have been developed, central nervous system dysfunction associated with cardiac surgery is very frequent, with an incidence that depends on the type of intervention (up to 65%) (Arrowsmith et al., 2000). Apart from ischemic events, cognitive dysfunction has been observed within the first postoperative week in more than 80% of patients undergoing coronary artery bypass grafting under CPB, and at five years after surgery, some degree of neuropsychological dysfunction can be observed in up to 35% of patients (Arrowsmith et al., 2000). A number of risk factors have been identified, and they can be divided into patient-related and technology-related factors. The patient-related factors are age>70 year old, cerebrovascular disease, aortic atherosclerosis, and diabetes mellitus; the technology-related factors are open chamber procedures, CPB duration >90 minutes, use of bubble rather than membrane oxygenators, and circulatory arrest. Apart from open chamber procedures, all the other risk factors have to be taken into consideration when cavo-atrial thrombectomy with CPB and HCCA is performed.

3.2.2 Deep hypothermic circulatory arrest

After CPB has been started, the temporary interruption of cerebral blood flow is a necessary condition to remove the thrombus from the vena cava and, in such cases, from the right atrium. Interruption of cerebral blood flow has been associated with a high incidence of neurologic injury because the brain is susceptible to ischemic injury within minutes of the onset of circulatory arrest as a result of its high metabolic rate and limited reserves (Harrington et al., 2003). The physiologic basis for hypothermia as a neuroprotective strategy is its ability to reduce the cerebral oxygen metabolic rate and the accumulation of toxic metabolites. In adults, a decrease in core temperature leads to a reduction in the cerebral metabolic rate that increases in ischemic tolerance from 2-3 minutes (normothermia) to 20-34 minutes (17°C) (Reich et al., 1999). However, the optimal level of hypothermia is still debated. Studies based on electroencephalographic monitoring have shown that a median nasopharyngeal temperature of 18°C allows electrocortical silence (Stecker et al., 2001). Today, based on the results of several studies, HCCA at 18°C is considered safe for durations of up to 40 minutes (Griepp, 2001). It has been also suggested that hypothermia provides neurological protection through mechanisms other than the cerebral metabolic rate. In the face of an incomplete understanding of the involved mechanisms, hypothermia remains the most efficacious intervention for preventing ischemic brain injuries. In addition to systemic hypothermia, topical cooling, obtained by packing the head with ice, can be used to prevent passive warming of the brain during circulatory arrest, but consensus on this adjunctive strategy is still lacking because re-warming during circulatory arrest could be negligible (Reich et al., 1999). After the targeted core temperature has been reached, the pump is turned off, allowing brain protection during surgery performed in a bloodless field. HCCA has several potential adverse consequences. Achieving the target temperature prolongs the duration of the CPB period, thus amplifying problems related to CPB (loss of pulsatile flow, injury to blood elements, risk of embolization, coagulation system derangements, etc.). Re-warming increases the cerebral metabolic rate and has the potential to make the brain vulnerable to ischemic injury. With the aim of limiting brain injuries, a short period (10 minutes) of hypothermic reperfusion is achieved before re-warming, and maintaining a temperature gradient of less than 10°C in the heat exchanger and avoiding complete re-warming are usually performed. Currently, there is no class of drug representing the standard of practice, but some drugs can be used as adjunctive strategies for cerebral protection. A number of drugs cause EEG burst suppression, resulting in a reduction in the cerebral metabolic rate by approximately 50%, but the most used of these drugs is thiopental at a dose of 5-8 mg/kg. The administration of thiopental results in EEG burst suppression for few minutes at normothermia. Thiopental and/or steroids are administered before circulatory arrest in some centres, without a clear demonstration of beneficial effects.

3.2.3 pH management during hypothermia

There is an inverse relationship between gas solubility and blood temperature. When blood temperature decreases, an apparent respiratory alkalosis occurs due to a decrease in $PaCO_2$ and an increase in pH. To compensate for this $PaCO_2$ reduction, CO_2 can be added to the oxygenator (pH-stat management) or the CPB gas sweep rate can be reduced. The technique of pH-stat management was commonly used until the mid-1980s, but there is more recent evidence that pH-stat management can increase the incidence of postoperative cognitive dysfunction when CPB lasts longer than 90 minutes (Murkin et al., 1995). It has been suspected that the increase in CO_2 should increase the cerebral blood flow during perfusion phases, uncoupling flow and metabolism. The most used α-stat (not temperature-correcting) requires that neutrality be maintained at only 37°C, and it permits hypothermic alkaline drift. Thus, additional CO_2 is not needed. Cellular trans-membrane pH gradients, protein functioning, and enzyme activity are more normal when the pH is allowed to drift into the alkaline range, in parallel with the temperature-dependent pKa of protein and the neutral pH of water. Moreover, a relatively alkaline pH is beneficial before the ischemic insult of circulatory arrest. Despite considerable laboratory and animal research into these mechanisms, substantial controversy remains over which strategy produces the best clinical outcomes (Duebener et al., 2002).

3.2.4 Coagulation management

Coagulation system management during and after CPB is based on the administration of heparin, followed by neutralization with protamine, and this approach has been unchanged for almost 50 years. Heparin binds to antithrombin-III (AT-III), potentiating the action of AT-III (more than 1000-fold) to inhibit thrombin and factor Xa most importantly (but also factors IXa, XIa, and XIIa). After central venous administration, heparin's effect peaks within 1 minute. The onset of CPB increases the circulating blood volume by approximately 1500 ml, reducing the heparin blood concentration; therefore, 5000 U of heparin are added to the CPB prime. Before CPB, heparin is administered at a dose of 300-400 U/kg to obtain ACT for 420-480 seconds, and successive supplemental doses are guided by monitoring the ACT. Some centres monitor blood heparin concentrations. ACT is prolonged by hypothermia and hemodilution. After CPB weaning is successfully achieved and a satisfactory spontaneous circulation is restored, heparin anticoagulation must be reversed with protamine administration. The most used protamine-heparin ratio is 0.6-1 mg/100 U. Protamine must always be administered slowly to prevent adverse hemodynamic effects. After protamine administration, ACT should return to a value no more than 10% above the basic value. If more prolonged, heparin residual activity is likely, and additional doses of protamine should be administered. During CPB, antifibrinolytic agents (ξ-aminocaproic acid or tranexamic acid) have beneficial effects in restoring coagulation equilibrium. Antifibrinolytics act as lysine analogues that bind to the lysine-binding sites of plasmin and plasminogen. ξ -aminocaproic acid can be administered at a dose of 100-150 mg/kg in bolus form, followed by 10-15 mg/kg/h or a 50 mg/kg bolus followed by 20-25 mg/kg/h. Tranexamic acid can be administered at a dose of 10-20 mg/kg followed by 1-2 mg/kg/h, although some centres prefer a 5 g bolus and repeat bolus to a total of 15 g. Post-bypass bleeding is common after CPB/HCCA. Evaluation of haemostasis and correct intervention are key factors for preventing indiscriminate use of transfusion medicine. After surgical haemostasis has been achieved, the first approach is the confirmation of adequate heparin neutralization (heparinase ACT, protamine titration test, thromboelastography-TEG). In addition, a test of platelet function should be available (TEG maximal amplitude, Platelet-Function-Analyzer-100). Finally, the fibrinolysis pathway must be explored (TEG lysis index). Packed red blood cells must be available at every moment of the intervention, and fresh frozen plasma and platelets should be prepared in case of established coagulation abnormalities (very frequent in this population of patients) to replace coagulation factors and platelets.

4. Conclusions

In conclusion we think that CPB with HCCA should be considered for atrial thrombi removal in patient affected by several abdominal malignancies such as renal, adrenal carcinomas, primary liver tumours also in presence of a well compensated liver cirrhosis, uterine endometrial stromal tumours and intravascular leiomyomatosis, vena cava leiomysarcoma and others, because it is simpler and safer compared to CPB alone. It permits the careful cleaning of the vena cava, right atrium, ventricle and even of the pulmonary artery in a bloodless field which entails in a lower recurrence rate. Mortality and morbidity seem to be the same when compared to CPB alone but further studies are necessary due to the small number of patients.

5. References

Akashi Y, Koreeda C, Enomoto S, et al. Prognosis of unresectable hepatocellular carcinoma: an evaluation based on multivariate analysis of 90 cases. Hepatology 1991;14:262-8.

Ariza A, Cerra C, Hahn IS, Shaw RK, Rigney B: Intravascular leiomyomatosis of the uterus. Conn Med 1982; 46: 700-3.

Arrowsmith JE, Grocott H, Reves, et al. Central nervous system complications of cardiac surgery. Br J Anaesth; 2000; 84:378-393.

Belis JA, Livinson ME, Pae WE. Complete radical nephrectomy and vena caval thrombectomy during circulatory arrest.J Urol 2000; Feb;163:434-6.

Berg AA. Malignant hypernephroma of the kidney, its clinical course and diagnosis, with a description of the author's method of radical operative cure. Surg Gynecol Obstet.1913;17:463-71.

Bevilacqua S, Romagnoli S, Ciappi F, et al. Transpharyngeal ultrasonography for cannulation of the internal jugular vein. Anesthesiology. 2005;102:873-4.

Carid JC, Hawkins IF Jr, Weichmann BN, et al. Sonographic guidance when using the right internal jugual vein fir central access. Am J Roentgenol 1988;171:1259-63.

Ciancio G, Manhoran M, Katkoori D, et al. Long term survival in patients undergoing radical nephrectomy and inferior vena ca thrombectomy: single centre experience. Eur Urol 2010; 57;667-672.

Ciancio G & Soloway MS :Renal cell carcinoma with tumour thrombus extending above diaphragm :avoiding cardiopulmonary bypass. Urology 2005; 66:266-270.

Ciancio G,Shirodkar S, Soloway MS et al: Techniques for avoidance of sternotomy and cardiopulmonary bypass during resection of extensive renal cell carcinoma with vena caval tumor thrombus extension above the diaphragm. J Card Surg 2009;24:657-60.

Ciancio G, Shiroddkar G, Soloway MS et al. Renal carcinomas with supradiaphragmatic tumor thrombus :avoiding sternotomy and cardiopulmonary bypass. Ann Thorac Surg 2010; 89: 505-10.

Ciancio G ,Gonzalez J, Shirodkar SP, et al.: Liver transplantation technique for the surgical management of RCC with tumour thrombus in the inferior vena cava :step by step description. Eur Urol 2011; 59;401-6.

Chowdhury UK, Mishra A K, Seth A, et al :Novel technique for tumour Thrombectomy for RCC with intra atrial tumour thrombus.Ann Thorac Surg 2007; 83:1.

Chiappini B, Savini C, Marinelli G, et al.: Cavoatrial tumor thrombus: Single-stage surgical approach with profound hypothermia and circulatory arrest, including a review of the literature. J Thorac Cardiovasc Surg 2002; 124: 684-8.

Chiche L, Dousset B, Kieffer E, et al.: Adrenocortical carcinoma extending into the inferior vena cava: Presentation of a 15-patient series and review of the literature. Surgery 2005; 139: 15-27.

Croughwell N, Smith LR, Quill T, et al.: The effect of temperature on cerebral metabolism and blood flow in adults during cardiopulmonary bypass. J Thorac Cardiovasc Surg. 1992;103:549-54.

Cummings KB ,Li WI, Ryan J A, et al.: Intraoperative management of renal cell carcinoma with supradiafragmatic caval extension of renal carcinoma.JUrol 1979;122:9.

Davlouros P, Manolis A, Apostolakis E: Renal tumour with cavoatrioventricular extension. Heart 2005; 91: 7-9.

Duebener LF, Hagino I, Sakamoto T et al.: Effects of pH management during deep hypothermic bypass on cerebral microcirculation: α-stat versus pH-stat. Circulation. 2002; 106(12 Suppl 1):I103-8.

Durck H: Ein kotinuierlich durch die untere. Hohlvene in das herz vorwschsendes leiomyom. Muchen Med Wochnschr 1907; 54: 1154-5.

Edmonds HL Jr, Ganzel BL, Austin EH 3rd.: Cerebral oximetry for cardiac and vascular surgery. Semin Cardiothorac Vasc Anesth. 2004;8:147-66.

Ein SH, Shandling B, Williams WG, et al.: Major hepatic tumor resection using profound hypothermia and circulation arrest. J Pediatr Surg. 1981;16:339-42.

Foster RS, Mahomed Y, Bihrle R, et al.: Use of a caval-atrial shunt for resection of a caval tumour thrombus in renal cell carcinoma. J Urol 1988;61:402.

Florman S, Weaver M, Primeaux P, et al.,: Aggressive resection of hepatocellular carcinoma with right atrial involvement. Am Surg. 2009;75:1104-8.

Fujisaki M, Kurihara E, Kikuchi K, et al.,: Hepatocellular carcinoma with tumor thrombus extending into the right atrium: report of a successful resection with the use of cardiopulmonary bypass. Surgery. 1991;109:214-9.

Galajda Z, Copotoiu C, Suciu H, Tint D, Glasz T, Deac R: The diagnosis, morphological particularities, and surgical technique in a case of intravascular leiomyoma extended to the right heart chambers. J Vasc Surg 2010; 51: 1000-2.

Goto H, Kaneko Y, Utoh J, et al., : Surgery of hepatoma with intracavitary cardiac extension. Heart and Vessels 1986; 2: 60-62.

Gott VL.: Lillehei, Lewis, and Wangensteen: The right mix for giant achievements in cardiac surgery. Ann Thorac Surg 2005; 79: S2210-3.

Griepp RB.: Cerebral protection during aortic arch surgery. J Thorac Cardiovasc Surg. 2003;125:S36–S38.

Hahne OH & Climie ARH: Right atria thrombi with ball-valve action. Am J Med 1962; 32: 942-6.

Hamazaki K, Yagi T, Katsuta K, et al., : Extracorporeal circulation and hypothermic perfusion for caval tumor thrombus complicating hepatocellular carcinoma: a case report. Hepatogastroenterology. 1995;42:282-5.

Harrington DH, Bonser M, Moss A, et al. Neuropsychometric outcome following aortic arch surgery: a prospective randomized trial of retrograde cerebral perfusion. J thorac cardiovasc surg 2003; 126:638-644.

Hassan M, Ciancio G, Shirodkar SP, et al.,: Surgical technique of removal of inferior vena cava leiomyosarcoma extending into the right atrium without deep hypothermic circulatory arrest. J Card Surg 2010; 25: 277-81.

Hatcher PA ,Anderson EE, Paulson DF ,et al : Surgical management and prognosis of renal cell carcinoma invading the vena cav,j Urol 1991; 145:20-4.

Huguet C, Gavelli A, Sakai H: Vascular exclusion technique in liver resection for hepatocellular carcinoma. J Hep Bil Pancr Surg 1994; 2: 123-127.

Kalkat MS, Abedin A, Rooney S, et al.,: Renal tumours with cavo-atrial extension: Surgical management and outcome. Interact Cardiovasc Thorac Surg 2008; 7: 981-5.

Kanda T, Miyamoto H, Hayakawa et al.,: A case of tumor thrombus in the right atrium after multimodal treatment of testicular tumor. Nippon Kyobu Geka Gakkai Zasshi 1991; 39: 1966-70.

Kawasaki S, Makuuchi M, Miyagawa S, et al.,: Results of hepatic resection for hepatocellular carcinoma. World J Surg 1995; 19: 31-4.

Krane RJ, White R ,et al :Removal of renal cell carcinoma extending into the right atrium using cardiopulmonary bypass, profound hypothermia and circulatory arrest. J Urol 1984; 131:945-7.

Kumar AB & Suneja M.: Cardiopulmonary Bypass–associated Acute Kidney Injury. Anesthesiology 2011; 114: 964–70

Leo F, Rapisarda F, Sefano PL, et al.,: Cavo-atril thrombectomy combined with left hemi-hepatectomy for vascular invasion from hepatocellular carcinoma on diseased liver under hypothermic cadio-circulatory arrest. Interact Cardivasc Thorac Surg 2010; 10: 473-5.

Libertino JA,Zinman L, Watkins E Jr.: Long term results of resection of renal cell cancer with extension into inferior vena cava.J Urol 1987;137;21-4.

Lin HH, Hsieh CB, Chu HC, et al., : Acute pulmonary embolism as the first manifestation of hepatocellular carcinoma complicated with tumor thrombi in the inferior vena cava: surgery or not? Dig Dis Sci. 2007;52:1554-7.

Lubahn J, Sagalowsky A, Rosenbaum D et al.: Contemporary techniques and safety of cardiovascular procedures in the surgical management of renal cell carcinoma with tumor thrombus. Thorac Cardiovasc Surg 2006; 131: 1289-95.

Mandelbaum I, Pauletto FJ, Nasser WK: Resection of a leiomyoma of the inferior vena cava that produced tricuspid valvular obstruction. J Thorac Cardiovasc Surg 1974; 67: 561-7.

McCullough JN, Zhang N, Reich DL, et al. Cerebral metabolic suppression during hypothermic circulatory arrest in humans. Ann Thorac Surg. 1999;67:1895-9.

Marshall FF, Reitz BA, Diamond DA: A new technique for the management of renal cell carcinoma involving the right atrium: Hypothermia and cardiac arrest. J Urol 1984; 131: 103-9.

Marshall FF, Dietrich DD, Baumgartner WA, et al. Surgical management of renal cell carcinoma with intracaval neoplastic extension above the hepatic veins. J Urol 1988;139:1166-72.

Martínez-Salamanca JI, Huang WC, et al., : Prognostic impact of the 2009 UICC/AJCC TNM staging system for renal cell carcinoma with venous extension. International Renal Cell Carcinoma-Venous Thrombus Consortium. Eur Urol 2011; 59:120-7.

Masaki N, Hayashi S, Maruyama T, et al.: Marked clinical improvement in patients with hepatocellular carcinoma by surgical removal of extended tumor mass in right atrium and pulmonary arteries. Cancer Chemother Pharmacol. 1994; 33 Suppl:S7-11.

Mingoli A, Cavallaro A, Sapienza P et al: International registry of inferior vena cava leiomyosarcoma: Analysis of a world series on 218 patients. Anticancer Res 1996; 16: 3201-5.

Miyazawa M, Torii T, Asano H, et al.: Does a surgery for hepatocellular carcinoma with tumor thrombus highly occupying in the right atrium have significance? A case report and review of the literature. Hepatogastroenterology. 2005; 52: 212-6.

Moinzadeh A Libertino JA Prognostic significance of tumour thrombus level in patients with renal cell carcinoma and venous thrombus extension. Is all T3b the same? J Urol 2004;171:598-601.

Moon TD, Fox LS; Varma DG: Testicular teratocarcinoma with intracaval metastases to the hearth. Urology 1992; 40: 368-70.

Murkin JM, Martzke JS, Buchan AM, et al. A randomized study of the influence of perfusion technique and pH management strategy in 316 patients undergoing coronary artery bypass surgery. II. Neurologic and cognitive outcomes. J Thorac Cardiovasc Surg. 1995;110:349-62.

Nam MS, Jeon MJ, Kim YT, Kim JW, Park KH, Hong YS: Pelvic leiomyomatosis with intracaval and intracardiac extension: a case report and review of the literature. Gynecologic Oncology 2003; 89: 175-80.

Neves RJ & Zincke H. Surgical treatment or renal cancer with vena cava extension. Br J Urol 1987;59:168:205-9

Novick AC, Cosgrove DM. Surgical approach for removal of renal cell carcinoma extending into the vena cava and the right atrium.J Urol 1980; 123: 947-50.

Novick AC, Kaye MC, Cosgrove DM, et al.: Experience with cardiopulmonary bypass and deep hypothermic circulatory arrest in the management of retroperitoneal tumors with large vena cava thrombi. Ann Surg. 1990; 212:472-7.

Ogata S, Belghiti J, Farges O, et al.: Sequential arterial and portal vein embolizations before right hepatectomy in patients with cirrhosis and hepatocellular carcinoma. Br J Surg 2006;93:1091-8.

Ohwada S, Takahashi T, Tsutsumi H, et al.: Hepatocellular carcinoma with a tumour thrombus extending to the tricuspid valve: report of a successful en bloc resection. Hepatogastroenterology. 2008; 55:903-6.

Okada S, Okazaki N, Nose H, et al.: Prognostic factors in patients with hepatocellular carcinoma receiving systemic chemotherapy. Hepatology 1992; 16:112-7.

Ozben B, Papila N, Tannikulu MA, et al.: Inferior vena cava tumor thrombus extending into the right atrium in a patient with pancreatic cancer. J Thromb Thrombolysis 2007; 24: 317-21.

Paule B, Brion N, Grunenwald D, et al.: Right atrial extension of an embryonal carcinoma of the testis. Cancer 1991; 66: 198-201.

Pawarode A, Voravud N, Sriuranpong V, et al.: Natural history of untreated primary hepatocellular carcinoma: a retrospective study of 157 patients. Am J Clin Oncol 1998; 21:386-91.

Pawlik TM, Poon RT, Abdalla EK, et al.: Hepatectomy for hepatocellular carcinoma with major portal or hepatic vein invasion: results of a multicenter study. Surgery. 2005;137:403-10.

Pierangeli A, Coli G, Mikus PM: Sostituzione dell'arco aortico in ipotermia profonda. Bull Scienze Med 1974; 2: 1-16.

Poon RT, Fan ST. Evaluation of the new AJCC/UICC staging system for hepatocellular carcinoma after hepatic resection in Chinese patients. Surg Oncol Clin N Am 2003;12:35-50

Renzulli P, Weimann R, Barras JP, et al: Low-grade endometrial stromal sarcoma with inferior vena cava tumor thrombus and intracardiac extension: radical resection may improve recurrence free survival. Surg Oncol 2009; 18: 57-64.

Scully RE, Galbadini JJ, McNeely BU: Case records of the Massachusetts general hospital. Case 40-1976. N Eng J Med 1976; 295: 774-82.

Shahinian DM, Nieh PT, Libertino JA: Resection of cavo-atrial carcinoma using hypothermic circulatory arrest. Ann Thorac Surg 1989; 48: 421-2.

Slater JM, Orszulak TA, Cook DJ. Distribution and hierarchy or regional blood flow during hypothermic bardiopulmonary bypass. Ann Thorac Surg 2001; 72:532-547.

Stecker MM, Cheung AT, Pochettino A, et al. Deep hypothermic circulatory arrest: II. Changes in electroencephalogram and evoked potentials during rewarming. Ann Thorac Surg. 2001; 71(1):22-8.

Stewart JR, Carey JA, McDougal S et al.: Cavoatrial tumor thrombectomy using cardiopulmonary bypass without circulatory arrest. Ann Throrac Surg 1991; 51: 717-22.

Sripathi V, Muralidharan KV, Ramesh S, Muralinath S: Wilms' tumor with vena cava, atrial and middle hepatic vein tumor thrombus. Pediatr Surg Int 2000; 16: 447-8.

Yogita S, Tashiro S, Harada M, et al.: Hepatocellular carcinoma with extension into the right atrium: report of a successful liver resection by hepatic vascular exclusion using cardiopulmonary bypass, J Med Invest. 2000; 47:155-60.

Yao FS, Tseng CC, Ho CY, et al. Cerebral oxygen desaturation is associated with early postoperative neuropsychological dysfunction in patients undergoing cardiac surgery. J Cardiothorac Vasc Anesth. 2004;18:552-8.

Reich DL, Uysal S, Sliwinski M, Ergin MA, et al. Neuropsychologic outcome after deep hypothermic circulatory arrest in adults. J Thorac Cardiovasc Surg. 1999;117:156-163.

Raoul JL, Guyader D, Bretagne JF, et al. : Randomized controlled trial for hepatocellular carcinoma with portal vein thrombosis: intra-arterial iodine-131-iodized oil versus medical support. J Nucl Med 1994; 35:1782-7

Ruel M ,Bedard P, Morash CG et al : Resection of right atrial tumour thrombi without circulatory arrest. Ann Thorac Surg 71:733-734, 2001.

Shingai R, Vricella L et al: Cavoatrial tumour thrombus excision without circulatory arrest.Urology 62:138-140, 2003.

Staheler G & Brkovic D: The role of radical surgery for renal cell carcinoma with extension into the vena cava.J Urol 2000;163:1671-75

Skinner DG, Pritchett TR, Lieskovsky G, et al.: Vena caval involvement by renal cell carcinoma. Surgical resection provides meaningful long-term survival. Ann Surg 1989; 210: 387-92.

Tamburino C, Russo G, Incognito G, et al.: Intracardiac extension of a calcified ovarian hemangioma: a case report. Angiology 1992; 43: 249-52.

Topcuoglu MS, Yaliniz H, Poyrazoglu H, et al.: Intravenous leiomyomatosis extending into the right ventricle after subtotal hysterectomy. Ann Thorac Surg 2004; 78: 330-2.

Wakiyama H, Sugimoto T, Ataka K, et al.: Intravenous leiomyomatosis extending into the right ventricular cavity : one-stage radical operation using cardiopulmonary by-pass-a case report. Angiology 2000; 51: 505-9.

Wu CC, Hseih S, Ho WM, et al.: Surgical treatment for recurrent hepatocellular carcinoma with tumour thrombi in right atrium: using cardiopulmonary bypass and deep hypothermic circulatory arrest. J Surg Oncol. 2000;74:227-31.

Vargas-Barron J, Keirns C, Barragan-Garcia R, et al.: Intracardiac extension of malignant uterine tumor. Echocardiographic detection and successful surgical resection. J Thorac Cardiovasc Surg 1990; 99: 1099-103.

Part 2

Pediatric Cardiac Surgery

Restoration of Transposed Great Arteries With or Without Subpulmonary Obstruction to Nature

Ing-Sh Chiu and Chi-Ren Hung
Department of Surgery, National Taiwan University Hospital and National Taiwan University, College of Medicine, Taipei, Taiwan

Surgical correction on transposition of the great arteries was proposed by many in the past half-century, and was claimed as the anatomical correction; but the treatment of choice was ever changing. The current technique usually included Lecompte maneuver to bring the pulmonary bifurcation in front of the aorta. Although the ventriculoarterial connection was corrected, it is not "normal" yet---------.

1. Introduction

Looking back into the evolution of surgical treatments on transposed great arteries (TGA), is full of fascinating and challenging stories. Many pondered the best option to correct this tricky, yet not the most complex congenital heart disease. Some operations that had been replaced by another were later revived. Senning once had been replaced by Mustard as the treatment of choice (Senning, 1959; Mustard, 1964), but was revived because autologous tissue was utilized, although it was more difficult (Quaegebeur, 1977). As people learned the functional implications of the ventricles, both atrial redirection procedures were replaced by the arterial switch operation (ASO) (Jatene et al., 1975; Lecompte et al., 1981; Castaneda et al., 1984). ASO was attempted initially, without transferring the larger right coronary artery, by Mustard (Mustard et al., 1954). Nikaidoh described aortic translocation, which in essence is an ASO including the arterial valve (Nikaidoh, 1984). In the past, few practiced this procedure because of its demanding techniques and potentially worse outcome. However, aortic translocation has recently gained popularity as an alternative to the Rastelli operation and Reparation l'etage ventriculaire (REV) as the treatment for TGA with a left ventricular outflow obstruction (Rastelli, 1969; Yeh et al., 2007; Emani et al., 2009). ASO has become the procedure of choice for TGA (Prêtre et al., 2001; Losay et al., 2002). However, TGA is considered to be a mere reversal of the great arteries anteroposteriorly (Shaher, 1964; Van Mierop, 1971); nonexistence of the normal spiral relationship of the great arteries in TGA has not been widely appreciated. Thus posterior pulmonary bifurcation is mobilised anteriorly to the aorta (the so-called Lecompte maneuver) in an effort simply to reverse transposed great arteries (Lecompte et al., 1981). We proposed an arterial Senning operation 13 years ago, to restore the spiral flow of nature in TGA (Chiu et al., 2000b; Chiu et al., 2002b, Chiu et al., 2010). The role of this operation is still uncertain and it requires continued refinement and development. The thinking process and evolving technique behind how we conceived our currrent technique was published (Chiu et al., 2001). Briefly, mobilization of the pulmonary arteries high above its original site to avoid compression the high take off coronary artey will result in supravalvular pulmonary stenosis (PS), similarly, Lecompte maneuver mobilized pulmonary arteries away from its original position. To avoid the complications of unnecessary mobilization, an *in situ* transfer technique and the common wall concept to redirect the coronary arteries should also be applied to the pulmonary arteries (Chiu et al., 2000b; Chiu et al., 2001). Tissue deficiency of the pulmonary outflow tract in cyanotic cardiac defects could be recruited from the larger aorta to compensate for the smaller main pulmonary artery (MPA); or vice versa, from the big MPA to a small aorta. We called this the Robin Hood approach or, in the current vernacular, a redistributive approach (Chiu et al., 2009). In this review, we describe an innovative technique to reconstruct the great arteries in spiral fashion, which is the natural relationship of aorta and pulmonary artery. The structural and functional studies underlying the basics of natural spiral great arteries we published in the last two decades will be presented. We emphasize the surgical principles of nature and even distribution, using autologous tissues. Anatomical features will be discussed first, then the technique of the above two redistributive approaches in TGA and finally their three-dimensional CT follow-up results.

2. Anatomical features

Transposition of the great arteries is the consequence of distal fusion between the dorsal protrusion of the aortic sac and the outflow cushions during embryogenesis (Figure 1) (Van Praagh, 2010). The conal septum and great arteries remain straight and parallel instead of being torsaded around each other. As a consequence, the aorta emerges from the right ventricle and the MPA from the left ventricle.

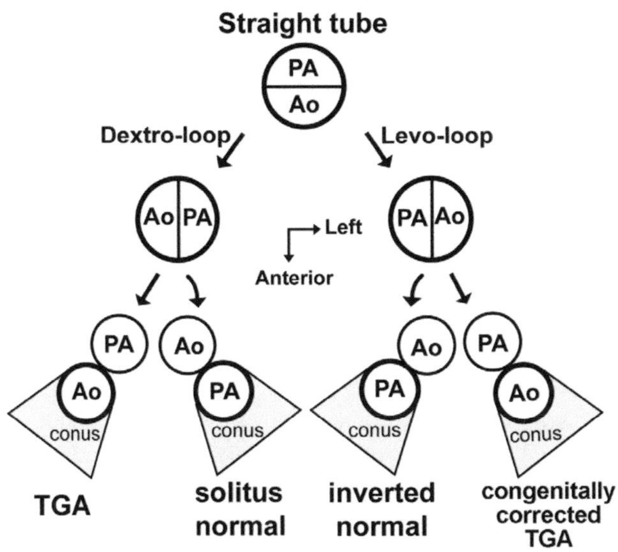

Fig. 1. There are only two ways in which conotruncal rotation can be done correctly as in: (1) solitus normally related great arteries and (2) inversus normally related great arteries; in contrast to many other ways that it can be done wrong.

2.1 Outlet septum

The ventricular outflows are in parallel when there is a side-by-side great arteries. When the aortic root is directly anterior or even left anterior, the outlet septum is no longer in parallel, it is vertical to the rest of the ventricular septum (Chiu et al., 1984). It is often asked that since the outflow tract was not switched and did a spiral ASO offer any help by just restoring the spiral arterial trunks without altering outflow tracts below the valves? Although the ventricular outflow was not switched in spiral ASO, the facing commissure of the old aorta was mobilized along with a topmost outflow below it and fixed it to the direction of future MPA (Figure 1, solitus normal). In other words, by our technique the top portion of the right ventricular outflow just below the facing commissure is rotated toward the direction of future MPA (Chiu et al., 2000b; Chiu et al., 2002b; Chiu et al., 2010). As just clarified, when the aorta is left-sided with usual atrial arrangement, there CAN be spiraling of the outflow tracts; the outlet septum is vertical to the rest of the ventricular septum in the setting with a directly anterior or left anterior old aortic root (Chiu et al., 1984; Anderson & Weinberg, 2005), thus a slight rotation like our technique is adequate for spiral correction at the ventricular outlet in that group. Wheras in side-by-side gruop, Lecompte maneuver is usually not performed by all, the ventricular outflows are in parallel as they are. When the aortic root is right anterior to MPA, we fix the facing commissure to the right anterior aspect of old MPA (Chiu et al., 2000b). The result is as the inverted normal in Figure 1. We did not fix the facing commissure of the new MPA to directly anterior aspect of new aortic root or leave the new MPA alone without fixation, as in conventional ASO, which corrects the ventriculo-arterial discordance without modifying the outflows. *Restoring the natural curvature of both great vessels is the key to avoiding obstruction at the ventricular outflows, instead of just reverse them anteroposteriorly.*

2.2 Coronary artery

Embryologically, the coronary arteries (CA) develop after septation of the aortopulmonary trunk and pierce the aortic sinus at the nearest site after aortopulmonary rotation. We found that the pattern of the CA is dependent on aortopulmonary rotation, thus proposed a new categorization scheme based on the aortic root rotation (Chiu et al., 1995). In addition to the short-axis rotation, which is related to the juxtacommissural origin of the CA (JOCA) (Chiu et al., 1997), there is also a long-axis rotation, which is related to high takeoff of the CA (Chiu et al., 1996b). On the basis of these findings, we have also proposed appropriate diagnostic and surgical techniques to manage unusual CA patterns in TGA (Chiu et al., 1997; Chiu et al., 1996a). In short, for JOCA near the facing commissure, a superiorly based trapdoor (single-button technique) or lateral funnel (two-button technique), and near the nonfacing commissure, a medially based trapdoor, are vital for coronary redirection. The categorization of CA based on the aortopulmonary rotation can be applied to all congenital heart defects and normal hearts (Chiu et al., 2000a; Chiu et al., 2002a; Chiu et al., 2003; Chen et al., 2007; Huang et al., 2011; Chiu et al., 2011).

2.3 Pulmonary artery

Paillole et al. documented the existence of central pulmonary artery (PA) hypoplasia before surgery and its persistence until after ASO (Paillole et al., 1988). Central PA hypoplasia, which is frequently seen in TGA, is related to posterior inclination of the proximal MPA in this setting (Figure 2, Chen et al., 2007). We have demonstrated that the same pathogenesis would lead to smaller PA size after a Senning procedure than ASO with Lecompte maneuver. In addition, Lecompte with Pacifico's modification (direct connection between the distal MPA and the aortic sinus defect), which mobilized the proximal MPA toward anterior aspect farther than by the patch-repair of the sinus defect, could facilitate better PA growth after ASO (Pacifico et al., 1983; Imoto et al., 1995). Spiral ASO would be even better to block that pathogenesis than the above to permit PA growth (Chiu et al., 2010).

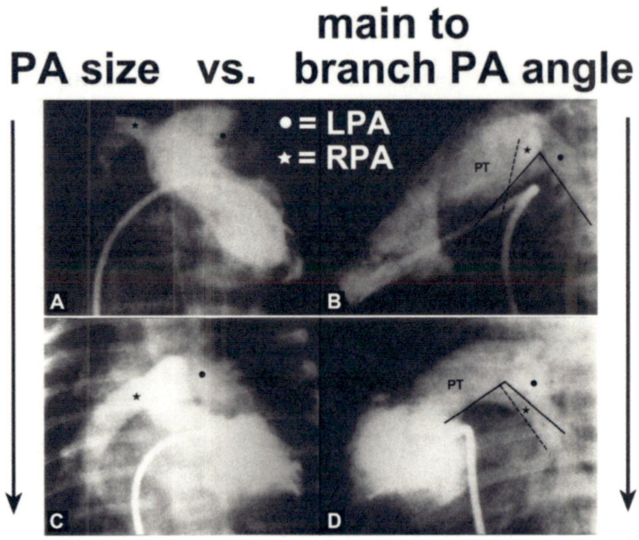

Fig. 2. Our studies on 101 angiograms showed the wider the main to branch PA angle, the better PA size. Narrow L/R PA angle resulted in bilateral PA hypoplasia in the upper panel. Thus wider angle facilitates bilateral PA growth before ASO. Any maneuver that did not correct this inborn error of ventriculoarterial discordance or make even narrower angle like Lecompte maneuver will compromise PA growth.

2.4 Aorta

The aortic arch is kept wide open by the presence of the MPA bifurcation below it (Chiu et al., 2000b; Chiu et al., 2002b). Neo-aortic kinking is the narrowing of the aortic arch window and may become slit-like, can also be called aortic neocoarctation (Figure 3, Chiu et al., 2010; Muster et al., 1987). One group reported an incidence of 0.54% (Serraf et al., 1995). A coarctation is not present and the arch is wide open before conventional ASO with Lecompte maneuver. A pressure gradient across it is rare, less seen than is supravalvular PS because of systemic-pressure in aorta.

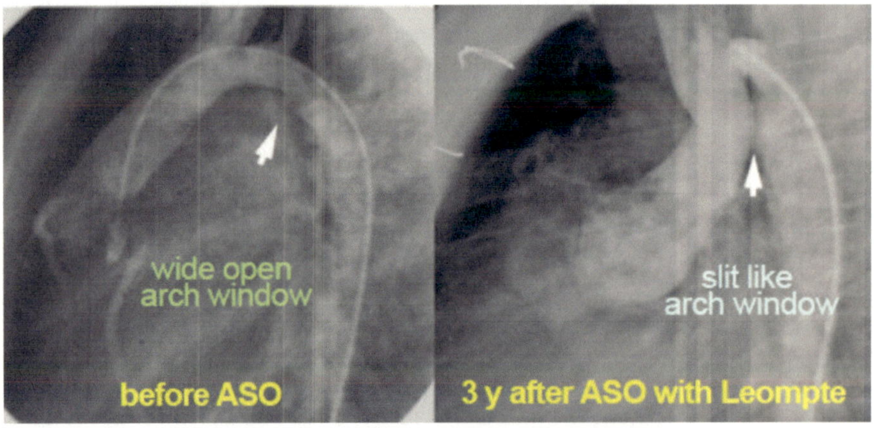

Fig. 3. After conventional arterial switch with Lecompte maneuver, a slit like arch window can be seen in the right panel, which was wide open before switch.

We have to take down the "Lecompte maneuver" in a patient eight years after conventional ASO to restore the spiral arterial trunks (Chen et al., 2010).

2.5 Bronchus

The aorta is not the only structure behind the MPA bifurcation after Lecompte maneuver, the left main bronchus (airway-pressure with cartilage) is also present. Bronchial compression or even atelectasis has been reported after Lecompte maneuver (Robotin et al., 1996; Toker et al., 2000), although in the majority of cases the bcronchial patency was not so severely compromised.

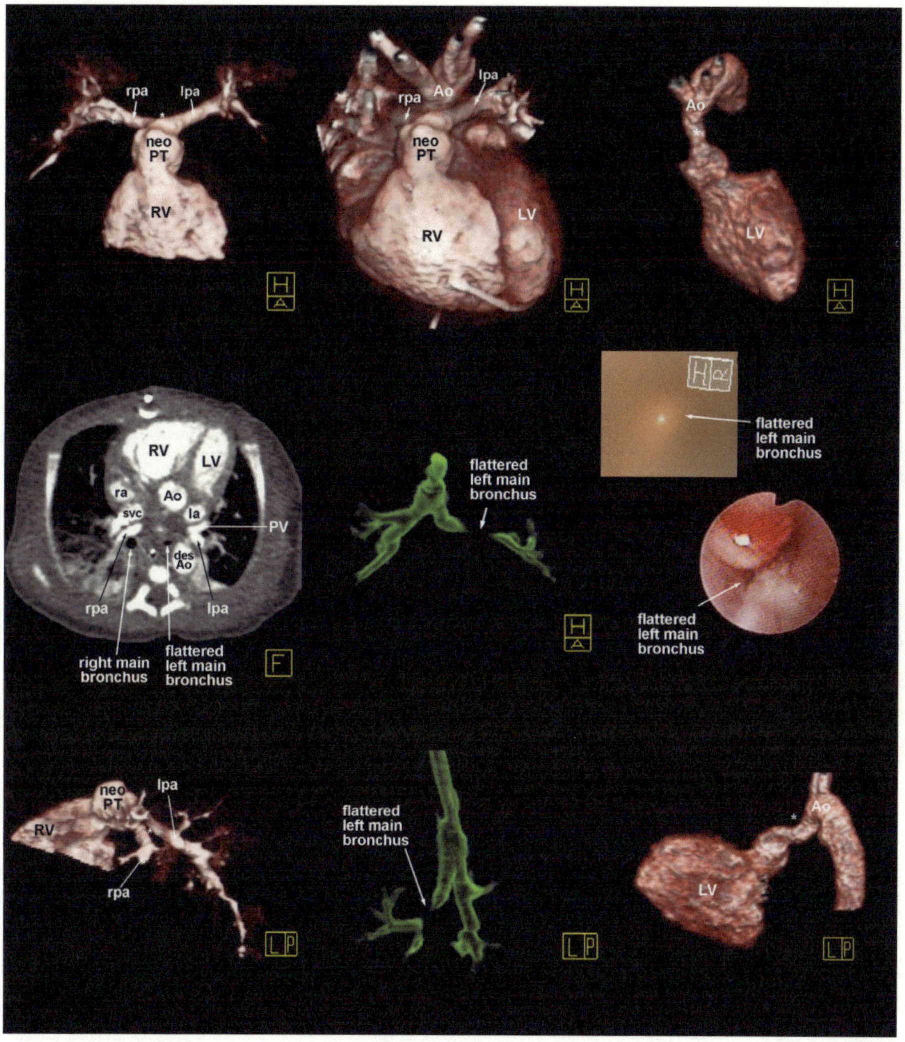

Fig. 4. After conventional ASO with Lecompte maneuver, not only supra-aortic stenosis occurs at the site posterior to the anteriorly mobilized pulmonary bifurcation (*), but also the left main brobchus, that is cartilage stented, is ccompreesed; its lumen becomes pin hole like on brochoscope, both virtual and real. In the right lower panel, the aortic arch window becomes slit-like at lesser curvature site.

3. Surgical management

3.1 Spiral ASO

(Chiu et al., 2000b; Chiu et al., 2002b; Chiu et al., 2010) Figure 5 and 6 showed the techniques that restored the heart to solitus normal in Figures 1, posterior MPA could remain undivided to avoid difficult posterior hemostasis and tamponade, and bilateral hilar dissection was not necessary. In-situ repair will lessen the chance of obstruction.

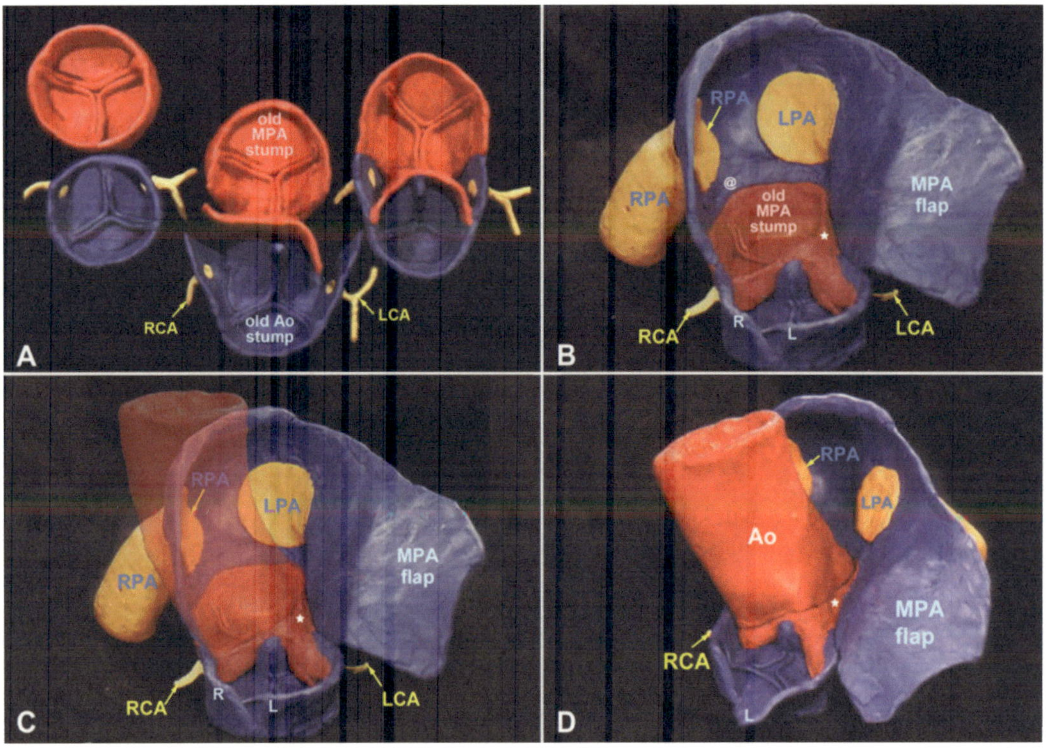

Fig. 5. Technical conceptions for spiral repair (B, C, D). (A) In-situ transfer and common wall were used to redirect the left ventricular output via the old MPA stump into right and left coronary artery (RCA and LCA) as reported (Murthy and Cherian, 1996). Semiflaps were fashioned on the facing sinuses of both great arteies, creating a common arterial trunk that was then septated. Red or blue color in B, C and D indicated the final result after ASO. (B) A big MPA flap was tailored from the MPA. A pericardial patch can be used to augment this flap if the MPA is not large enough. The distal MPA (blue clay) could be reattached to the old MPA stump (red clay), at the neoaortic anastomosis site (blue/red junction marked with @) or proximal to it on the posterior wall of old MPA stump (marked with an asterisk), or remain undivided (in that case blue/red junction indicated site of neoaortic anastomosis); thus, the troublesome posterior neoaortic

Fig. 5. (continued) anastomosis site bleeder can be drained into PAs. Nonfacing sinus was cut open for exposure during coronary transfer. (C) The transparent ascending aorta, with a left aortic lip (procured by oblique amputation of aorta, Chiu et al., 2000b), was rotated counterclockwise to sit on the neoaortic stump. The posterior cut-edge of MPA could be attached to the posterior neoaorta at this stage as leftward as possible.(D) The RPA orifice must be visible behind the aorta to ensure patency of RPA, not just probed with a Hegar dilator. A big enough MPA flap could be reattached to the neoaorta without pericardial patch. (Ao = Aorta, L or R = Left or Right portion of nonfacing sinus wall after cut back, LCA = Left Coronary Artery, LPA =Left Pulmonary Artery, RCA = Right Coronary Artery, RPA = Right Pulmonary Artery)

No-fault transfer of the coronary artery is the cornerstone of a successful ASO. Various techniques (Aubert et al., 1978; Yacoub and Randly Smith, 1978; Kurosawa et al., 1986; Quaegebeur et al., 1986; Brawn and Mee, 1988; Idriss et al., 1988; Bove et al., 1989; Takeuchi and Katogi, 1990; Mee, 1994; de Leval et al., 1994; Murthy & Cherian, 1996; Chiu et al., 1996a & 1997) have been proposed to achieve this goal: de Leval et al. (1994) pointed out that the key point is to take the aorta away from the coronary arteries and the MPA is brought to them, rather than moving the coronaries from the aorta and transferring the coronary scallops to the MPA or neoaorta. To implement this concept, *in situ* transfer technique, proposed by Aubert et al. (1978) and Takeuchi and Katogi (1990), was developed by Murthy and Cherian (1996). This principle is the key (Figure 5) we adopted to redirect the neoaortic outflow tract to the coronary arteries as *in situ* as possible by a common wall concept. In this way the coronary redirection can be achieved more securely than the conventional "coronary transfer".

In situ transfer and the common wall concept not only for the coronary arteries, but also for both great arteries are our guiding principle. We have designed two pedicled grafts, aortic lip and MPA flap, to achieve our goal. The purpose of these two flaps is described below. The aortic lip (Figures 2, 3A and 3B) is initially called left lip (Chiu et al., 2002b). In our first spiral arterial switch, we used a free flap taken from MPA to cover the left-sided portion of the neoaortic stump (Chiu et al., 2000b), to solve the size discrepancy when connecting small aorta to a very large, original MPA stump; the other effect is to act as the floor of the neopulmonic pathway. Since the nonfacing aortic sinus was cut back (Figure 5B and 5C) for exposure during coronary transfer, later we used an aortic pedicled graft including the nonfacing aortic sinus wall (Figure 6A and 6B) to achieve the above 2 purposes of the aortic lip. In addition, using the aortic lip taken from **anterior** sinus wall to cover the **left-sided** portion (Figure 6B and 6C, light blue arrow), we can achieve the effect of counterclockwise rotation of the ascending aorta. This, in turn, would give way to the RPA so that it can sling around the ascending aorta (Figure 6C, Hegar dilator in RPA). The fourth effect of the aortic lip might lessen the chance of coronary kinking by avoiding take-up the larger stump on neoaortic anastomosis, as noted by Quaegebeur et al. (1986).

The purposes of the MPA flap include: (1) accommodating the ascending aorta, (2) achieving a more leftward shift of RPA, and (3) attaching to the ascending aorta without pericardium. Thus, the spiral relationship of the great arteries is resumed by using the autologous pedicled flaps tailored from both arterial trunks, respectively.

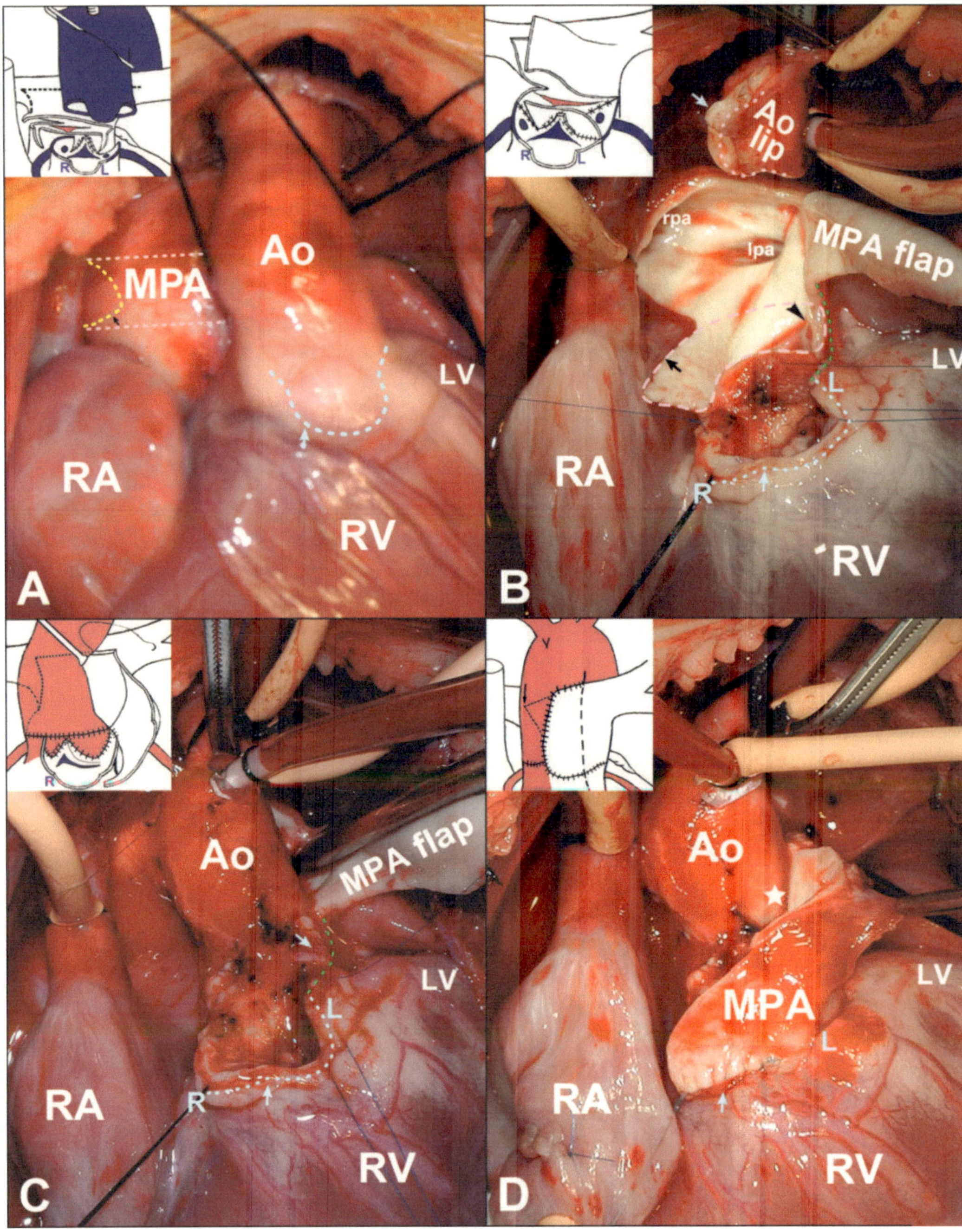

Fig. 6. Operative techniques for spiral ASO with neo-MPA in left anterior portion. Semilunar valves are all omitted for clear illustration in all insets. (A) The aorta is located left anterior to the MPA before ASO. The aortic lip will be taken from the anterior aortic sinus wall along the light blue line on the aorta, an excision that also facilitates exposure on coronary transfer. MPA flap will be incised along the pink dotted line on the anterior MPA, yellow line on the posterior MPA (black arrow) to accommodate the ascending aorta.

Fig. 6. (continued) Left posterior wall of MPA is not divided. Annulus near facing commissure in old aorta is fixed to left anterior wall of MPA (depicted by Y stitches in inset) before incising MPA. Two J-shaped incisions are made to fashion semiflaps on facing sinuses of both great arteries. (B) A big MPA flap can be tailored from the anterior wall of huge MPA, even to its posterior aspect (black arrow, see also inset). Coronary transfer was done, using the technique in Figure 5A. A big aortic lip, redundantly covering the distal aortic orifice in picture, was taken along with the distal aorta during aortic amputation. Pink dotted line along the cut edge of the aortic lip was concordant with the light blue dotted line along the nonfacing sinus wall, and almost the whole nonfacing sinus wall was excised; the light blue arrow indicated corresponding point of the aortic lip originally attached to the aortic sinus. Note the remaining sinus wall on the left (L) and right (R) portion of the remaining nonfacing sinus, and the light blue arrow indicated the same location through the whole Figure 6. One commissure of neoaortic valve is marked with black arrowhead. Neoaorta will sit on the pink dashed line. Aortic lip will cover the left-sided portion of neoaortic stump. (C) The distal aorta was sutured already above the neoaortic valve and coronary to LV outflow. Light blue arrow from anterior to left indicated counterclockwise rotation. Note the Hegar dilator in the RPA. After neoaortic connection and de-crossclamp, the rest of MPA cut-edge near RPA, which was shifted leftward, was attached to the posterior wall of the neoaorta (inset). Caudal edge of MPA flap can be attached at or proximal to cut edge of the old MPA stump and the aortic sinus 1 along the green dotted line (the tissue nearby is more clearly shown in B) and cut edge of the nonfacing sinus wall, which was stay-sutured and indicated here by light blue dots. (D) Attachment to form the floor of pulmonary pathway was finished. The adventitia of the aorta inside the pulmonary pathway (white asterisk) must be peeled off (Chiu et al., 2001; Chiu et al., 2010), because it will be the inner wall of future PA. Cephalic edge of anterior MPA flap can be attached to the outer wall of neoaorta directly (D inset) to roof the pulmonary pathway; ASO can be completed without any pericardial or prosthetic patch, and thus the procedure was named "arterial Senning". (L or R = Left or right portion of nonfacing sinus wall after excising the aortic lip, LV = Left Ventricle, RA = Right Atrium, RV = Right Ventricle, other Abbreviations see Figure 5)

It would be interesting to see the current status of this patient 7 years after such spiral ASO (Figure 7).

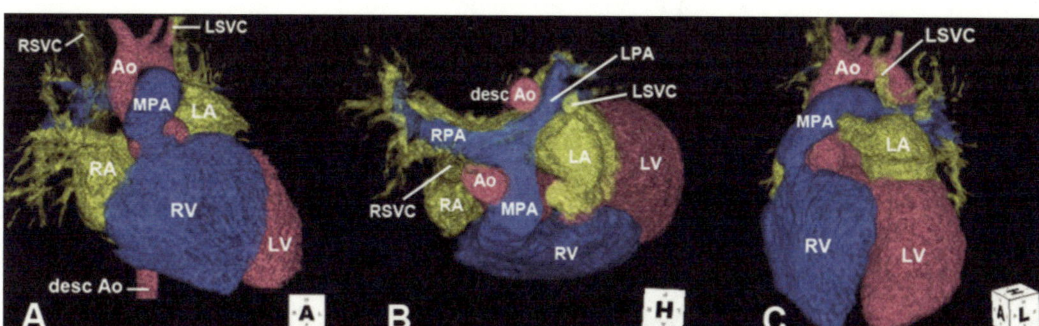

Fig. 7. Three-D CT reconstruction of the patient in Figure 6 seven years after ASO (A, B & C) showed the natural spiral relationship of the great arteries with harmonic growth of their branches. (desc = descending, LA = Left Atrium, R or L SVC = Right or Left Superior Vena Cava, other Abbreviations see Figure 5 & 6. Reproduced with permission from Chiu et al., 2010)

Between March 1998 and June 2011, spiral ASO was performed in 57 patients (38.3%), conventional nonspiral ASO with Lecompte maneuver in 92 patients (61.7%) at our hospital. The median age and weight at operation were 9 days and 3.3 kg. Cross-clamp time was significantly lower ($p < 0.011$) in the spiral than the nonspiral group (128 ± 36 vs 144 ± 37 minutes), because of the common wall technique in spiral ASO, wheras additional time for patch repair on defects in the sinuses of the new MPA was needed in conventional 2-vessel technique. The average follow-up was 6.9 ± 4.2 years (up to 13.5 years). Kaplan Meier survival was 94.1 ± 3.3% at 10 years and the reoperation-free rate 88.3 ± 4.5% for spiral repair. Both ratios were satisfactory and similar to those for the nonspiral group (89.6 ± 3.3% and 89.3 ± 4.1%, respectively). Signicant aortic regurgitatin in the nonspiral group (Chen et al., 2010) was not observed in the spiral group. The supravalvular PS and aortic neocoarctation that occurred in the nonspiral group (7.6% and 2.2 %, respectively) did not occur in the spiral group (0 %) (Chiu et al., 2010); these 2 complications are related to Lecompte maneuver and the unnatural relationship of the great arteries. Tiny aortopulmonary fenestration with a small left to right shunt occurred in 15 cases of spiral group (26.3%), but they closed spontaneously after a median follow up of 6 months by echo. TGA is not merely a reversal of the great arteries; nonexistence of the spiral function in TGA should be appreciated. Recognition of the spiral function and further modification might justify its future application.

3.2 Modified rastelli operation

In complete TGA with left ventricular outflow obstruction, a segment of the aorta is cut in transverse fashion and donated to the pulmonary circulation to establish the ventriculoarterial continuity (Figure 8).

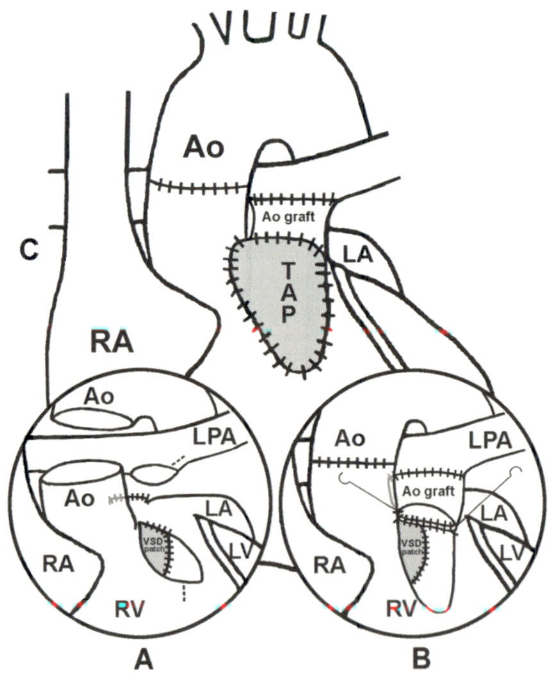

Fig. 8. Operative techniques for TGA with irreparable left ventricular outflow obstruction.

Fig. 8. (continued) The ascending aorta was amputated, and a curved segment (18 mm x 6 mm) was harvested (A) and then reconnected (B). The ventricular septal defect was rerouted to the systemic outflow with a patch. The MPA was divided and the proximal stump was closed. The aortic free graft was sutured to the distal MPA with the greater curvature on the left (B). The lengthened MPA was then connected directly to the cephalic margin of ventriculotomy. Finally, a piece of fresh pericardium was harvested and sutured to cover the right ventricular outflow tract (C). (TAP = TransAnnular Patch, other Abbreviations see Figures 5-7. Reproduced with permission from Chiu et al., 2009)

End to end anastomosis of the ascending aorta after excision of a segment shortened the distance between the right ventriculotomy and the PA, so that the aortic free graft could achieve its bridging effect comparable to the conventional conduit of double length without aortic shortening. This advantage of aortic shortening is also observed in patients undergoing Nikaidoh operation (Morell & Wearden, 2006). We agree with Metras and coworkers (Metras et al., 1997) that Lecompte maneuver to mobilize the pulmonary bifurcation anterior to the aorta is unnecessary. This is because if the pulmonary bifurcation is left *in situ* as it is originally by nature, the chance for developing supravalvular PS may decrease (Chiu et al., 2000b; Chiu et al., 2002b). Our direction for placement of a free graft of this curved aortic segment is opposite to that proposed by Metras (Metras et al., 1997). Follow-up CT showed satisfactory result (Figure 9).

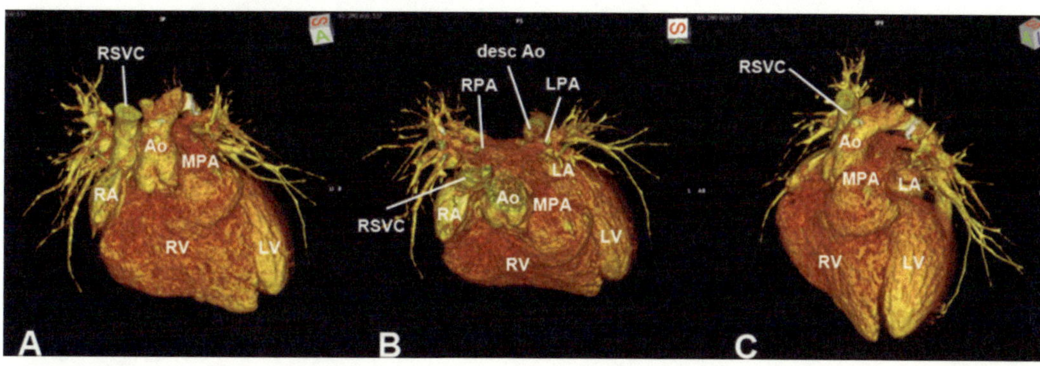

Fig. 9. Three-D CT reconstruction six years after Modified Rastelli operation; no stenosis was observed at the site of free graft. The natural spiral arterial trunks with harmonic growth of their branches were evident. Abbreviations see Figure 7.

A major complication of the Rastelli operation was related to the conduit itself; crossing the midline, conduit dysfunction or valve degeneration might lead to conduit failure early or late after surgery. Our technique of recruiting autologous arterial tissue will avoid these complications and help free the patients from reoperation.

4. Comment

The natural spiral relationship of the great arteries and their branches can grow on follow-up (Figure 7 and 9). We have demonstrated that the common wall between the great arteries could grow and become thinner on follow-up (Chiu et al., 2009). Spiral reconstruction in TGA is seldom performed, because the functional implications of spiral relationship of the great arteries remain unknown; thus, the Lecompte maneuver was used either in conventional ASO or Nikaidoh and Lecompte (REV) operation (Emani et al., 2009; Morell & Wearden, 2006;

Lecompte et al., 1982). Review of surgical treatment for TGA reveals that once the functional implications of two normal ventricles were well known, nobody selected the right ventricle as the systemic pumping chamber. The rationale of spiral reconstruction (Figure 10) at the great arterial and ventricular level includes (1) widening of arch window to avoid aortic neocoarctation (Figure 3), (2) widening of main to branch PA angle to facilitate PA growth (Figure 2, Chen et al., 2007), and (3) avoiding PA compression by the aorta posteriorly.

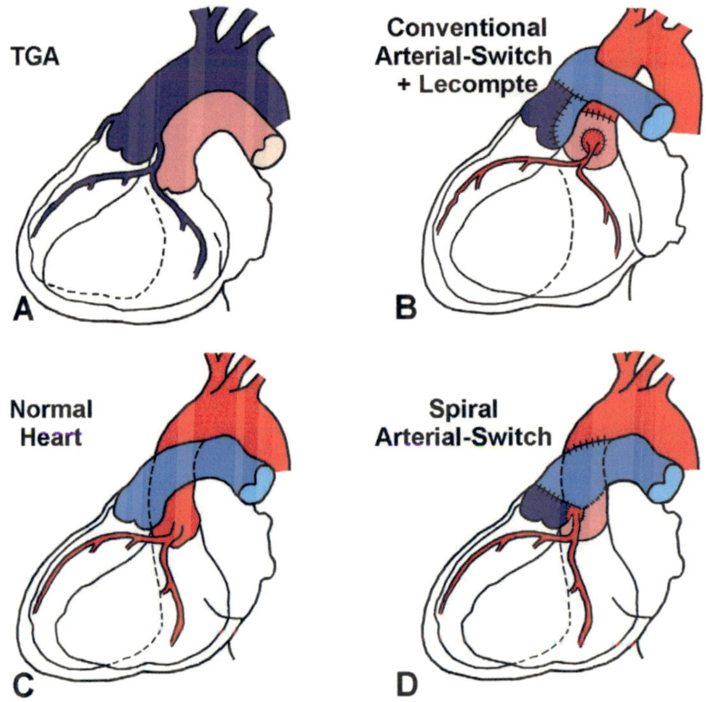

Fig. 10. Spiral relationship of the great arteries in normal heart (C) was not restored by conventional ASO with Lecompte maneuver (B) on TGA (A). With spiral ASO (D), pulmonary bifurcation is free from posterior compression by high-pressure aorta. Note that acute angulation of arch that is present after Lecompte maneuver (B) is absent in other three illustrations. Acute angulation from the main pulmonary artery to its branches is also present in A and B, but not in C and D, in which main to branch pulmonary artery angle is wider and smoother. Reprinted with permission from Elsevier (Eu J Cardiothorac Surg 2010;37:1239-45).

To facilitate PA growth, mobilise the posterior inclination of the proximal MPA and restore its 'normal' position (Figure 10C) to direct a natural and smooth blood flow into the PA in the neonatal period is the surgical principle. Thus widening this acute angle to both PA in spiral fashion (Figure 10D) is more helpful than the Lecompte maneuver with a huge patch (Figure 10B) for promoting PA growth (Norwood et al., 1988; Paillole et al., 1988; Lupinetti et al., 1992). The systemic high-pressure ascending aorta may compress the neo-MPA from its posterior end towards its anterior end. Insufficient dissection of the distal PAs was suggested to explain this flattened (oval-shaped) MPA in 1988 (Wernovsky et al., 1988), but a later study showed that the cross section of the MPA is still flattened 6 to 22 months after conventional ASO with hilar dissection and the Lecompte maneuver (Massin et al., 1998).

After the Lecompte maneuver, not only flattened anterior MPA (low-pressure), branch PA stenosis, and supravalvular PS at pulmonary bifurcation can occur as a consequence of posterior compression of MPA by the ascending aorta (Williams et al., 1997; Gutberlet et al., 2000); but also the aorta itself (systemic-pressure) may be compromised. Therfore, aortic neocaorctation was reported (Muster et al., 1987; Serraf et al., 1995).

Most interestingly, we used computational fluid dynamics on mathematic modeling to compare flow phenomena of the spiral and nonspiral models (Figure 11). The functional superiority of the spiral over the nonspiral model is demonstrated because the blood flow inside is more streamlined andthere is a smaller power loss ratio (Tang et al., 2001).

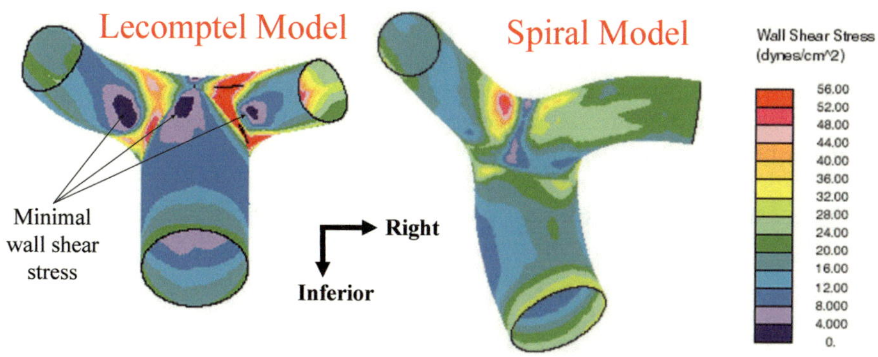

Fig. 11. The regions of minimal wall shear stress in purple color in the left panel are the site where supravalvular PS is prone to occur. On the contrary, there is no purple color in spiral model. Wall shear stress is more uniform and the blood flow is more in streamline.

Spiral reconstruction would be beneficial to reduce supravalvular PS (Figure 10), supra-aortic stenosis (Figure 4), and aortic neocoarctation (Figure 3 & 10). This is to say, the great arteries are normally in a spiral fashion, thus the MPA bifurcation avoids being compressed by the aorta, and the arch window is kept wide open by the adjacent pulmonary bifurcation.

Potential limitations of our proposal merit consideration. First, the number of cases studied is small. Second, this is aretrospective study, and longer-term follow-up is mandatory to ascertain the benefit or possible drawbacks of spiral ASO over non-spiral ASO. Subvalvular PS still occurred, but mainly related to infundibular hypertrophy, and not supravalvular as in the non-spiral group. Subvalvular PS was probably related to an unusual coronary artery traversing the infundibulum (Chiu et al., 2010), which may be associated with a thick subaortic muscle bundle that can produce subpulmonary narrowing after ASO (Kurosawa, 1991).

It might be questioned whether our technique will reproduce the old dire complicarions that was avoided by Lecompte maneuver such as compression on the transferred coronary arteries (Chiu et al., 2010, discussant). Acually secure coronary redirection like our method is more important than a mere absence of a near-by low-pressure vessel like pulmonary artery. The so-called complications are not seen in our series. Any method that redirect coronary safely can be done in combination with spiral arterial trunk reconstruction.

Our previous publications (Chiu et al., 2000b; Chiu et al., 2002b; Tang et al., 2001) were cited by Dr. Corno at the 86th annual meeting of American Association for Thoracic Surgery, in a symposium about the potential implications of the helical heart to congenital heart disease (Corno, 2006a; Corno, 2006b). In 2001, following we presented our spiral arteial switch at National Cardiovascular Center in Osaka, Japan, Dr. Hideki Uemura named our procedure as "arterial Senning". He is affiliated now with Royal Brompton Hospital in London, UK.

We are grateful to his thoughtful nomenclature for our procedure. We dare not call the spiral arterial switch this name by ourselves before his proposal.

5. Conclusions

The concept of *in situ* transfer and common wall technique should be applied to redirect not only the coronary arteries but also the PAs and the aorta in TGA. Thus, tamponade, coronary events, supravalvular PS, and aortic neocoarctation can be prevented and natural spiral flow can be restored. Study of TGA and its natural or secondary natural history provides a means to understand the functional implications of the normal cardiac anatomy. As said by Einstein: "All our science, measured against reality, is primitive and child-like and yet is the most precious thing we have." How to restore TGA as much as possible to resemble its natural and unique likeness, awaits further modification and continued effort to conceive more surgical options in the coming half-century. Those stick to the surgical principle of nature and even distribution using autologous tissues, although more difficult and technically demanding, will be revived again and again, as shown by examples such as Senning versus Mustard, arterial switch versus atrial redirection, Nikaidoh versus Rastelli, arterial Senning versus arterial Mustard----etc.

6. Acknowledgement

We are indebted to all our colleagues in Taiwan who contributed or help to earlier studies establishing the concepts of our ideas in congenitally malformed hearts. We are grateful to Miss Chang-Ying Lin for the preparation of Figures. This study was supported by a grant from the National Science Council in Taiwan (NSC97-2314-B-002-043-MY3).

7. References

Anderson, RH. & Weinberg, PM. The clinical anatomy of transposition. *Cardiol Young* 2005;15 (Suppl. 1):76-87, ISSN 1047-9511

Aubert, J., Pannetier, A., Couvelly, JP. & et al. (1978). Transposition of the great arteries: new technique for anatomical correction, *Br Heart J* 40:204-8 , ISSN 0007-0769

Bove, EL. (1989). Current technique of the arterial switch procedure for transposition of the great arteries. *J Card Surg* 4(3):193-9, ISSN 0886-0440

Brawn, WJ. & Mee, RB. (1988). Early results for anatomic correction of transposition of the great arteries and for double-outlet right ventricle with subpulmonary ventricular septal defect, *J Thorac Cardiovasc Surg* 95:230-8, ISSN 0022-5223

Castaneda, AR., Norwood, WI., Jonas, RA. & et al. (1984). Transposition of the great arteries and intact ventricular septum: anatomical repair in the neonate, *Ann Thorac Surg* 38:438-43, ISSN 0003-4975

Chen, MR., Wu, SJ., Chiu, IS. & et al. (2007). Morphologic substrates for first-branch pulmonary arterial hypoplasia in transposition of the great arteries, *Cardiology* 107:362-9, ISSN 0008-6312

Chen, SJ., Ling, MT., Lee, WJ. & et al. (2007). Coronary artery anatomy in children with congenital heart disease by computed tomography, *Int J Cardiol* 120:363-70, ISSN 0167-5273

Chen, YS., Chiu, IS., Huang, SC. & Chen, SJ. (2010). Valve-sparing procedure and de-Lecompte maneuver in patients with late aortic regurgitation and aortic aneurysm after arterial switch operation, *J Thorac Cardiovasc Surg* 140:1191-2, ISSN 0022-5223

Chiu, IS., Anderson, RH., Macartney, FJ. & et al. (1984). Morphologic features of an intact ventricular septum susceptible to subpulmonary obstruction in complete transposition, *Am J Cardiol* 53:1633-8, ISSN 0002-9149

Chiu, IS., Chu, SH., Wang, JK. & et al. (1995). Evolution of coronary artery pattern according to short-axis aortopulmonary rotation: A new categorization for complete transposition of the great arteries, *J Am Coll Cardiol* 26:250-8, ISSN 0735-1097

Chiu, IS., Chou, TF., Lin, SF. & et al. (1996). Utilization of the aortic flap above the facing commissure in arterial switch operations, *J Card Surg* 11:187-91, ISSN 0886-0440

Chiu, IS., Wang, JK., Wu, MH. & et al. (1996). Angiographic evidence of long-axis rotation in addition to short-axis aortopulmonary rotation: Its implication in transposition of the great arteries, *Cathet Cardiovasc Diagn* 39:21-30, ISSN 0098-6569

Chiu IS, Wu MH, Chang CI. & et al. (1997). Clinical implications of short-axis aortopulmonary rotation on juxtacommissural origin of the coronary artery in transposition of the great arteries and surgical strategy, *J Card Surg* 12:23-31, ISSN 0167-5273

Chiu, IS., Wu, CS., Wang, JK. & et al. (2000). Influence of aortopulmonary rotation on the anomalous coronary artery pattern in tetralogy of Fallot. Am J Cardiol 85:780-4, ISSN 0002-9149

Chiu, IS., Wu, SJ., Chen, MR. & et al. (2000). Modified arterial switch operation by spiral reconstruction of the great arteries in transposition, *Ann Thorac Surg* 69:1887-92, ISSN 0003-4975

Chiu, IS., Chen, SJ., Wu, SJ. & et al. (2001). Modified arterial switch operation by sharing the common wall between the great arteries.; *J Formos Med Assoc* 100:77-82, ISSN 0929-6646

Chiu, IS., Wu, SJ., Chen, MR. & et al. (2002). Anatomic relationship of the coronary orifice and truncal valve in truncus arteriosus and their surgical implication. *J Thorac Cardiovasc Surg* 123:350-2, ISSN 0022-5223

Chiu, IS., Wang, JK. & Wu, MH. (2002). Spiral arterial switch operation in transposition of the great arteries. *J Thorac Cardiovasc Surg* 124:1050-2, ISSN 0022-5223

Chiu, IS., Wu, SJ., Chen, SJ., Wang, JK., Wu, MH. & Lue, HC. (2003). Sequential diagnosis of coronary arterial anatomy in congenitally corrected transposition of the great arteries. *Ann Thorac Surg* 75:422-9, ISSN 0003-4975

Chiu, IS., Huang, SC., Wu, SJ. & et al. (2009). Surgical treatment of anomalies with discontinuity between the right ventricle and the pulmonary arteries without use of an extracardiac conduit. *Ann Thorac Surg* 87:1220-6, ISSN 0003-4975

Chiu, IS., Huang, SC., Chen, YS. & et al. (2010). Restoring the spiral flow of nature in transposed great arteries. *Eu J Cardiothorac Surg* 37:1239-45, ISSN 1010-7940

Chiu, IS., Chen, MR., Huang, SC. & et al. (2011). Restoration of Transposed Great Arteries to Nature, *World Journal for Pediatric and Congenital Heart Surgery*, 2:287-295, ISSN 2150-1351

Chiu, IS.; Chen, MR.; Anderson RH. & et al. (2011 submitted). How can we better understand the variations in coronary arterial anatomy?

Corno, AF., Kocica, MJ. & Torrent-Guasp F. (2006). The helical ventricular myocardial band of Torrent-Guasp potential implications in congenital heart defects. *Eu J Cardiothorac Surg* 29 (Suppl 1): S61-68, ISSN 1010-7940

Corno, AF. (2006). Potential implications of helical ventricular myocardial band to congenital heart disease, AATS/STS Congenital Heart Symposium, American Association for Thoracic Surgery, 86th Annual Meeting Philadelphia.

De Leval, MR., Francois, K., Bull, C. & et al. (1994). Analysis of a cluster of surgical failures. Application to a series of neonatal arterial switch operations. *J Thorac Cardiovasc Surg* 107:914-24, ISSN 0022-5223

Emani, SM., Beroukhim, R., Zurakowski, D. & et al. (2009). Outcomes after anatomic repair for d-transposition of the great arteries with left ventricular outflow tract obstruction. *Circulation 120*[suppl 1]:S53–S8, ISSN 0009-7322

Gutberlet, M., Boeckel, T., Hosten, N. & etal. (2000). Arterial switch procedure for d-transposition of the great arteries: quantitative midterm evaluation of hemodynamic changes with cine MR imaging and phase-shift velocity mapping-initial experience, *Radiology* 214:467-75

Huang, SC., Chiu, IS., Lee, ML. & et al. (2011). Coronary artery anatomy in anatomically corrected malposition of the great arteries and their surgical implications. *Eur J Cardiothorac Surg* 39:705-710, ISSN 1010-7940

Idriss, FS., Ilbawi, M N., DeLeon, S Y. & et al. (1988). Arterial switch in simple and complex transposition of the great arteries. *J Thorac Cardiovasc Surg* 95:29-36, ISSN 0022-5223

Imoto, Y., Kado, H. & Asou, T. (1995). Postoperative pulmonary stenosis after arterial switch operation, comparison in three methods of pulmonary reconstruction: modified Pacifico, autologous pericardial patch, and equine pericardial patch. *Jpn J Thorac Surg* 48: 433–8, ISSN 0021-5252

Jatene, AD., Fontes, VF., Paulista, PP. & et al. (1975). Successful anatomic correction of transposition of the great vessels. A preliminary report. *Arq Bras Cardiol* 28:461-4, ISSN 0066-782X

Kurosawa, H. Imai, Y. Takanashi, Y. & et al. (1986). Infundibular septum and coronary anatomy in Jatene operation. *J Thorac Cardiovasc Surg* 91(4):572-83, ISSN 0022-5223

Kurosawa, H., Imai, Y. & Kawada, M. (1991). Coronary arterial anatomy in regard to the arterial switch procedure, *Cardiol Young* 1:54-62, ISSN 1047-9511

Lecompte, Y., Zannini, L., Hazan, F. & et al. (1981). Anatomic correction of transposition of the great arteries. New technique without use of a prosthetic conduit. *J Thorac Cardiovasc Surg* 82:629-31, ISSN 0022-5223

Lecompte, Y., Neveux, JY., Leca, F. & et al. (1982). Reconstruction of the pulmonary outflow tract without prosthetic conduit. *J Thorac Cardiovasc Surg* 84:727-33, ISSN 0022-5223

Losay, J., Touchot, A., Serraf, A. & et al. (2001). Late outcome after arterial switch operation for transposition of the great arteries. *Circulation* 104:I121-6, ISSN 0009-7322

Lupinetti, FM., Bove, EL., Minich, LL. & et al. (1992). Intermediate-term survival and functional results after arterial repair for transposition of the great arteries. *J Thorac Cardiovasc Surg* 103: 421-7, ISSN 0022-5223

Massin, MM., Nitsch, GB., Däbritz, S. & et al. (1998). Growth of pulmonary artery after arterial switch operation for simple transposition of the great arteries, *Eur J Pediatr* 157:95-100, ISSN 0340-6199

Mee, R. (1994). The arterial switch operation, In: *Surgery for congenital heart defects,* Stark, J., & de Leval, M. eds., 2nd ed. 483-500, WB Saunders, Philadelphia.

Metras, D., Kreitmann, B., Riberi, A. & et al. (1997). Extending the concept of the autograft for complete repair of transposition of the great arteries with ventricular septal defect and left ventricular outflow tract obstruction: a report of ten cases of a modified procedure. *J Thorac Cardiovasc Surg* 114:746-53, ISSN 0022-5223

Morell, VO. & Wearden, PD. (2006). Nikaidoh operation for transposition of the great arteries with a ventricular septal defect and pulmonary stenosis. *Multimedia Manual of Cardiothoracic Surgery* doi:10.1510/mmcts..002337.

Murthy, KS. & Cherian, KM. (1996). A new technique of arterial switch operation with in situ coronary reallocation for transposition of great arteries. *J Thorac Cardiovasc Surg* 112:27-32, ISSN 0022-5223

Mustard, WT., Chute, AL., Keith, JD. & et al. (1954). A surgical approach to transposition of the great vessels with extracorporeal circuit. *Surgery* 36:31-51.

Mustard, WT. (1964). Successful two-stage correction of transposition of the great vessels. *Surgery* 55:469-72, ISSN 0039-6060

Muster, AJ., Berry, TE., Ilbawi, MN., DeLeon, SY. & Idriss, FS. (1987). Development of neo-coarctation in patients with transposed great arteries and hypoplastic aortic arch after Lecompte modification of anatomical correction. *J Thorac Cardiovasc Surg* 93:276-80, ISSN 0022-5223

Nikaidoh H. (1984). Aortic translocation and biventricular outflow tract. *J Thorac Cardiovasc Surg* 88:365-72, ISSN 0022-5223

Pacifico, AD., Stewart, RW. & Bargeron, LM Jr. (1983). Repair of transposition of the great arteries with ventricular septal defect by an arterial switch operation. *Circulation* 68(suppl II):II-49–II-55, ISSN 0009-7322

Paillole, C., Sidi, D. & Kachaner, J. (1988). Fate of pulmonary artery after anatomic correction of simple transposition of great arteries in newborn infants. *Circulation* 78: 870–6, ISSN 0009-7322

Prêtre, R., Tamisier, D., Bonhoeffer, P. & et al. (2001). Results of the arterial switch operation in neonates with transposed great arteries. *Lancet* 357:1826-30, ISSN 0140-6736

Quaegebeur, JM., Rohmer, J., Brom, AG. & et al. (1977). Revival of the Senning operation in the treatment of transposition of the great arteries. *Thorax* 32:517-24, ISSN 0040-6376

Quaegebeur, JM., Rohmer, J., Ottenkamp, J. & et al. (1986). The arterial switch operation. An eight-year experience. *J Thorac Cardiovasc Surg* 92:361-84, ISSN 0022-5223

Rastelli, GC. (1969). A new approach to "anatomic" repair of transposition of the great arteries. *Mayo Clin Proc* 44:1-12, ISSN 0025-6196

Robotin, MC., Bruniaux, J., Serraf, A. & et al. (1996). Unusual forms of tracheobronchial compression in infants with congenital heart disease. *J Thorac Cardiovasc Surg* 112:415-23, ISSN 0022-5223

Senning, A. (1959). Surgical correction of transposition of the great vessels. *Surgery* 45:966-80, ISSN 0039-6060

Serraf, A., Roux, D., Lacour-Gayet, F. & et al. (1995). Reoperation after the arterial switch operation for transposition of the great arteries. *J Thorac Cardiovasc Surg* 110:892-9, ISSN 0022-5223

Shaher, RM. (1964). Complete and inverted transposition of the great vessels. *Br Heart J* 26:51-66, ISSN 0007-0769

Takeuchi, S. & Katogi, T. (1990). New technique for the arterial switch operation in difficult situations. *Ann Thorac Surg* 50:1000-1, ISSN 0003-4975

Tang, T., Chiu, IS., Chen, HC. & et al. (2001). Comparison of pulmonary arterial flow phenomena in spiral and Lecompte models by computational fluid dynamics. *J Thorac Cardiovasc Surg* 122:529-34, ISSN 0022-5223

Toker, A., Tireli, E., Bostanci, K. & et al. (2000). Uncommon complication of arterial switch operation: tracheobronchial compression. *Ann Thorac Surg* 69:927-9, ISSN 0003-4975

Van Mierop, LH. (1971) Transposition of the great arteries. I. Clarification or further confusion? *Am J Cardiol* 28:735-8, ISSN 0002-9149

Van Praagh, R. (2010). Normally and abnormally related great arteries: What have we learned? *World Journal for Pediatric and Congenital Heart Surgery* October: 364-385, ISSN 2150-1351

Williams, WG., Quaegebeur, JM., Kirklin, JW. & et al. (1997). Outflow obstruction after the arterial switch operation: a multiinstitutional study, *J Thorac Cardiovasc Surg* 114:975-90, ISSN 0022-5223

Yacoub, MH. & Radley-Smith R. (1978). Anatomy of the coronary arteries in transposition of the great arteries and methods for their transfer in anatomical correction. *Thorax* 33:418-24, ISSN 0040-6376

Yeh, T Kr., Ramaciotti, C., Leonard, SR. & et al. (2007). The aortic translocation (Nikaidoh) procedure: midterm results superior to the Rastelli procedure. *J Thoracic Cardiovasc Surg* 133:461-9, ISSN 0022-5223

10

Gene Expression Profiling - A New Approach in the Study of Congenital Heart Disease

Mohamed T. Ghorbel, Gianni D. Angelini and Massimo Caputo
University of Bristol, UK

1. Introduction

Congenital heart defects (CHD) affect approximately 1% of live births. Some of them are associated with a significant morbidity and mortality and congenital heart diseases remain the first cause of death among infants in North America and Europe (Bruneau, 2008).
The major causes in CHD are thought to be chromosomal aberrations or mutations in genes regulating cardiac development during embryogenesis (Pierpont et al., 2007). However, from the epidemiological data, it seems that the environment can have a small "teratogenic" effect (Jenkins et al., 2007). For example, some substances (e.g. prenatal exposure to angiotensin converting-enzyme inhibitors, alcohol abuse and Rubella virus) can alter the function of certain genes during embryogenesis (Bruneau, 2008; Cooper et al., 2006). Though, these epidemiological studies have mostly suggested risk rather than pinpointing the underlying disease mechanisms.
During heart development complex interactions, among cells originating from different cell lineages, occur. In normal human heart development, a four-chambered heart ensure normal cardiac physiology with a right heart serving to the low-pressure pulmonary system and a left heart to the high pressure body circulation (Srivastava, 2004). A malformed cardiac growth results in abnormal hemodynamic characteristics because of volume or pressure overload leading to an adaptation process of the heart.
The completion of the Human Genome Project heralded the beginning of a new medical science era. The available genomic data will markedly improve our ability to diagnose and treat a great number of diseases including heart disease. Examining an individual's genomic profile or "molecular fingerprint" in a disease context now might help us to understand disease mechanisms and could found a new health care tailored to individual patient that take into account the predicted disease course and response to therapies of that patient. There's now a real opportunity to replace invasive diagnostic tests with genomic tests that can be carried out with no or little risk or stress to the patients (Bell, 2004; Collins et al., 2003).
The objective of this chapter is to provide an overview of gene expression profiling technology and the state of genomic research in congenital heart diseases, specifically with regard to the use of microarray approach.

2. Clinical overview of congenital heart diseases

Congenital heart defects, affecting most heart's parts (Figure 1), can be classified into three categories: cyanotic heart disease, left-sided obstruction defects and septation defects (Bruneau, 2008). In cyanotic heart disease, the mixing of oxygenated and deoxygenated blood results in the blue appearance of affected infants. Defects contributing to this condition include transposition of the great arteries (TGA), tetralogy of Fallot (TOF), tricuspid atresia, pulmonary atresia, Ebstein's anomaly of the tricuspid valve, double outlet right ventricle (DORV), persistent truncus arteriosus (PTA) and total anomalous pulmonary venous connection. The second main type of congenital heart disease, left-sided obstructive lesions, includes hypoplastic left heart syndrome (HLHS), mitral stenosis, aortic stenosis, aortic coarctation and interrupted aortic arch (IAA). The third type of congenital heart disease, septation defects, can affect septation of the atria (atrial septation defects, ASDs), septation of the ventricles (ventricular septal defects, VSDs) or formation of structures in the central part of the heart (atrioventricular septal defects, AVSDs). Other types of congenital defect that do not fit into the above three main categories are bicuspid aortic valve (BAV) and patent ductus arteriosus (PDA).

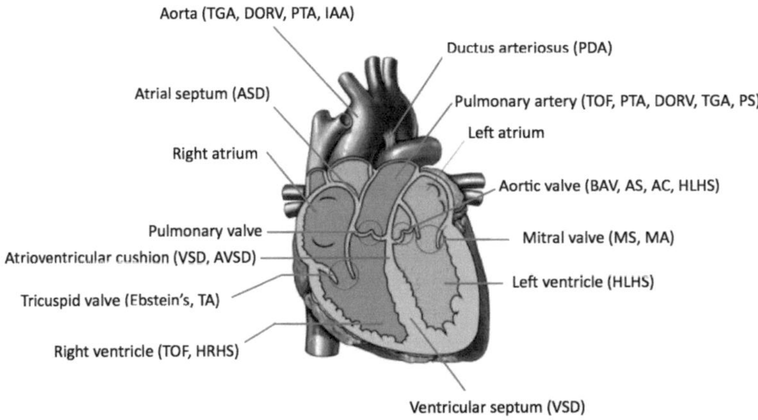

Fig. 1. Congenital heart defects. Diagram of heart illustrating the structures that are affected by congenital heart diseases. AC, aortic coarctation; AS, aortic stenosis; ASD, atrial septal defect; AVSD, atrioventricular septal defect; BAV, bicuspid aortic valve; DORV, double outlet right ventricle; Ebstein's, Ebstein's anomaly of the tricuspid valve; HLHS, hypoplastic left heart syndrome; HRHS, hypoplastic right heart; IAA, interrupted aortic arch; MA, mitral atresia; MS, mitral stenosis; PDA, patent ductus arteriosus; PS, pulmonary artery stenosis; PTA, persistent truncus arteriosus; TA, tricuspid atresia; TAPVR, total anomalous pulmonary venous return; TGA, transposition of the great arteries; TOF, tetralogy of Fallot; VSD, ventricular septal defect.

Depending on the severity of the congenital heart disease, mortality and morbidity varies but can be serious. The number of surgeries needed to correct many of the anatomical defects can weaken the affected children and considerably compromise their quality of life. Congenital heart surgery has made tremendous gains over the past 10 years; however, recovery and outcome statistics continue to point out the need for improvements in this increasingly younger patient population. Paediatric patients undergoing cardiac surgery continue to need mechanical assist devices, as well as prolonged inotropic support or an open chest despite a technically perfect repair. Moreover, perioperative myocardial damage with low cardiac output remains the most common cause of morbidity and death after repair of congenital lesions (Hammon, 1995). It is therefore essential to improve our understanding of the genetic mechanisms and pathways associated with the different congenital heart conditions and their response to the surgical stress of ischaemia and reperfusion injury and cardiopulmonary bypass.

3. Gene expression profiling

In the pre-human genome sequencing era, the possibility to identify a relevant set of causative genes for multigenic diseases such as cardiomyopathies was limited. Classical genetic approaches were developed to find single loci or genes with the power to cause Mendelian disorders. In this case, disorders can result from a single base change in the deoxyribonucleic acid (DNA) that leads to significant alteration in protein abundance or function. However in disorders resulting from multiple gene variants that collectively contribute to an individual's multigenic defect, new genomics approaches are needed. With the arrival of such genomics technologies, genes microarrays approach has emerged as a real opportunity allowing the performance of gene expression analysis of disease-relevant tissues. If DNA defines the inherent genetic make up of a person, it is the transcription of the DNA into RNA (that could be translated into protein) that integrates the dynamic interaction of an individual with the environment. Consequently, microarrays provide us with an opportunity to measure mRNA abundance that correlate with a particular disease state, clinical outcome, or therapeutic response, giving us an unprecedented opportunity to investigate the genomic contribution to cardiovascular diseases (Cook and Rosenzweig, 2002; Goldsmith and Dhanasekaran, 2004; Napoli et al., 2003).

3.1 Microarray technology

Expression profiling is the study of the expression level changes of large numbers of genes simultaneously. The concept of microarray technology is simple: specific DNA sequences, called "probes," are selected to "target" genes of interest. Microarrays refer to solid substrates of glass, plastic, or silicon containing hundreds or thousands of microscopic spots of DNA (Figure 2). Each of the DNA spots, apposed to the solid material, contains hundreds to thousands of identical probes. Each probe has a sequence of nucleotide bases that is complementary and unique to a single gene. Because of the technology's advances, it is common to use microarrays carrying the entire complement of the human genome in today's microarray experiments.

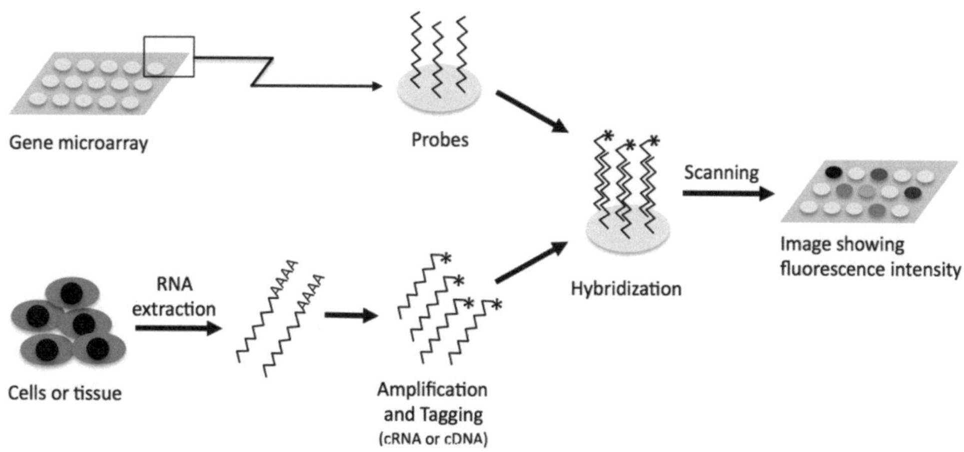

Fig. 2. Schematic of a microarray experiment. cDNA, complementary deoxyribonucleic acid; cRNA, complementary ribonucleic acid.

In a typical microarray experiment, RNA is extracted from a tissue or sample of interest. The small part of the RNA population that represents the transcribed genes, mRNA, is amplified, and fluorescent tags are attached to each molecule. The labelled mRNA is then incubated with the microarray allowing the tagged mRNA molecules to hybridize to the probes containing the specific complementary sequence of genes. Complementary mRNAs bind to probes on the array during hybridization. The microarray is then washed and placed in a scanner where a laser is directed onto each spot, causing the tags to fluoresce. The resulting fluorescence intensity is proportional to the number of tagged RNAs that have hybridized to the probes in each spot. The measured intensity represents the expression level or activity of that gene. Consequently, an expression profile can be generated for a particular tissue at different stages of health or disease.

The identified gene signatures are useful because they represent an initial step in identifying disease-associated genes, or "candidate genes". Furthermore, they represent a disease biomarker. The genes that comprise the genomic signature are associated with disease susceptibility or a particular treatment outcome. These candidate genes might substantially improve our understanding of disease biology and subsequently lead to identification of potential targets for new treatment strategies (King et al., 2005). The other great potential for transcriptomic information is to use the gene signatures as a disease biomarker. Gene expression data could offer a remarkable detailed patient phenotype that could be used to correctly classify patient populations as to their disease risk or response to therapies. In both cases, genomic data represent a means to distinguish between patients who are otherwise alike by classical clinical variables (Cook and Rosenzweig, 2002; Goldsmith and Dhanasekaran, 2004; Napoli et al., 2003). This is still a work in progress in cardiovascular medical research. But we can look to the cancer research field to see where the future lies.

3.2 Standardization

Experimental conditions can affect microarray technology in a way that leads to considerable variability and low reproducibility of the results. To make it possible to compare data obtained from different laboratories, efforts have been directed towards the definition of standards in gene expression studies (Stoeckert et al., 2002). These standards cover all experimental steps in microarray investigations and extend from sample selection and experimental design to the functional classification of altered genes. Complex statistical algorithms are increasingly used for data modeling and expression change identification. Additionally, comparative approaches have been proposed to evaluate the performance of various algorithms on gene expression data (Bolstad et al., 2003; Cope et al., 2004; Irizarry et al., 2006).

3.3 Experimental design

Microarray experiments should always be replicated. There are two types of replications: biological replication, where multiple homogeneous samples are used on multiple arrays, and technical replication, where RNA from the same sample is used on multiple arrays. If biological replication allows the estimation of both measurements and biological variability, technical replication allows only the estimation of measurement variability. Ideally, experimental design should include both types. Although there is no agreement about the optimum number of biological replicates, a minimum of 5 for each group is generally considered as a minimum.

RNA pooling is another crucial issue. Pooling RNA from biological replicates can reduce variability among arrays. Pooling can be necessary for samples of limited quantity. However the analysis of one single pool can be misleading because it prevents the estimation of biological variability and the presence of outlier samples which could change the results. An alternative approach is the multiple pooling, in which for example 25 samples can be divided into 5 pools of 5 samples, and each pool may be used on distinct microarray platforms. Many studies have used pooling. In contrast not many have used multiple pooling.

3.4 Data normalization

Because of variability of microarray data, each array must be brought into the same scale as others in order to compare 2 or more arrays. This normalization, performed by removing systematic variation between the arrays and rendering different experiments comparable, remains an issue that is not yet fully resolved. Although, many of the early microarray studies in the literature ignored this issue, a statistically rigorous approach is needed.
Early software allowed for array-to-array comparisons by using a scaling factor to normalize gene expression patterns across arrays. However, in general, these algorithms assume that intensity differences between arrays are linearly related (Schadt et al., 2000). Such linear relationship often does not hold true. An example of this approach is the global method that consists in re-scaling each chip data set by its total intensity.
A more advanced normalization approaches have been developed. The invariant set method is based on the assumption that there is a subset of unchanged genes between any two samples compared by microarray analysis so that their fluorescence values can be used to normalize the entire expression data set (Li and Wong, 2001). The LOcally WEighted Scatterplot Smoothing (LOWESS) is a widely used technique based on non-linear regression (Yang et al., 2002). The quantile normalization uses non-parametric procedure to normalize each chip (Bolstad et al., 2003). However, one of the best statistically robust normalization methods is the "Robust Multiarray Average" technique (RMA) (Irizarry et al., 2003). This method corrects microarray data for local background; it normalizes data on normal distribution and uses a linear model to estimate expression values on a log scale. It has been demonstrated that RMA performs better than other normalization technologies for Affymetrix data (Irizarry et al., 2003).

3.5 Identification of differentially expressed genes

The fold-change (FC) was the first used method to identify significantly deregulated genes. Although this simple technique can be efficient and effective for focusing on expanding sets of differentially expressed sequences, such an analysis does not take advantage of the full potential of genome-scale experiments to enhance our comprehension of cellular biology that would be provided by an inclusive analysis of the entire repertoire of transcripts in a cell as it goes through a biological process. Additionally, FC is now considered an inadequate statistical test since it does not incorporate variance and offers no associated levels of confidence. To compare groups of data, the parametric t-test and the analysis of variance (ANOVA) are more robust and commonly used. However, due to the small sample size in a microarray experiment, parametric methods are not recommended and should be substituted with a non-parametric moderated test.
Statistical analysis of microarray data faces an important challenge because testing the expression level of tens of thousands of transcripts (multiple testing) may produce hundreds of false positive. Therefore, multiple test corrections should be applied. Since the Bonferroni approach is too conservative in the case of large number of tests, a good alternative is the use of false discovery rate (FDR) (Benjamini and Hochberg, 1995). FDR, defined as the expected number of false positive in a list of genes, is at the present widely used for gene expression data analysis.

3.6 Data organization and presentation

In order to detect and extract patterns within microarray data, statistical algorithms can be applied. The basic assumption of many expression profiling' investigations is that knowing where and when a gene is expressed provides information about the function of the gene. Therefore, organizing genes on the basis of similarities in their expression profiles is a crucial starting point in the analysis (Bassett et al., 1999). However, similarity of gene expression profile does not guaranty similarity of function or mechanistic pathway, and it may occur entirely by chance. Nonetheless, clustering genes on the basis of their expression patterns is well accepted (Eisen et al., 1998). Typically, cluster analysis is applied when more than 3 experiments' data sets are available. It is generally performed in a two-way method (cluster analysis on genes and samples). Nowadays, cluster analysis is one of the most popular statistical techniques applied to large-scale microarray data.

Another method called discriminant analysis, that is different from the descriptive cluster analysis, belongs to the group of predictive algorithms. At the start of the analysis, the samples are divided into two or more classes. Then based on a training set, where the scientist knows *a priori* the source class of each sample, the algorithms predict the class of new samples using its expression profile.

The different cluster techniques can usefully organize tables of gene expression values. However the resulting organized but still large collection of numbers remains hard to assimilate. Therefore, powerful data visualization methods and tools have been developed. These approaches present clustering results in simple graphical displays such as dendrograms (Figure 3). Dendrograms represent relationships among genes by a tree whose branch lengths reflect the degree of mathematically defined similarity in expression between the genes (Alon et al., 1999). It is possible to make visual assimilation more intuitive by combining clustering methods with representation of each data point with a color that quantitatively and qualitatively reflects the original experimental observations (Eisen et al., 1998).

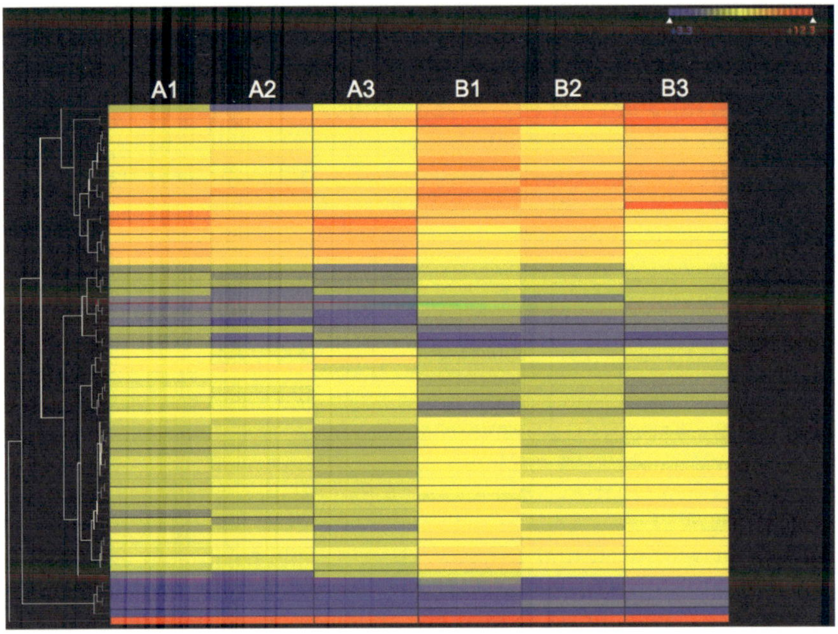

Fig. 3. Hierarchical clustering of two groups of three samples. Hierarchical groups are displayed on the heat map and dendrogram at the left side of the heat map.

3.7 Network and pathway analysis

More recently, new analysis methods have been developed to help interpreting microarray data within biological and physiopathological contexts. These approaches are gene interaction network analysis and pathway analysis. In gene interaction network analysis (Figure 4), automated text mining software is usually used to scan the scientific literature to identify gene-gene interactions. A human expert can improve the quality of these gene relationships. When a list of differentially expressed genes is presented to the program, a search system returns relevant interaction networks. In pathway analysis, the pathways, made-up of gene-gene interactions, are accepted by the scientific community and entered into the system by human experts. Because of the higher confidence, needed before a set of interacting genes is called a pathway, these databases are smaller but more accurate. It is however possible to identify new pathways based on gene network interactions if the interactions can be validated and accepted by the peer review community. Many bioinformatics programs are now available enabling in-depth analysis of any interrelated biological data, finding common regulators and associating pathway components with like-behaving biological entities and processes.

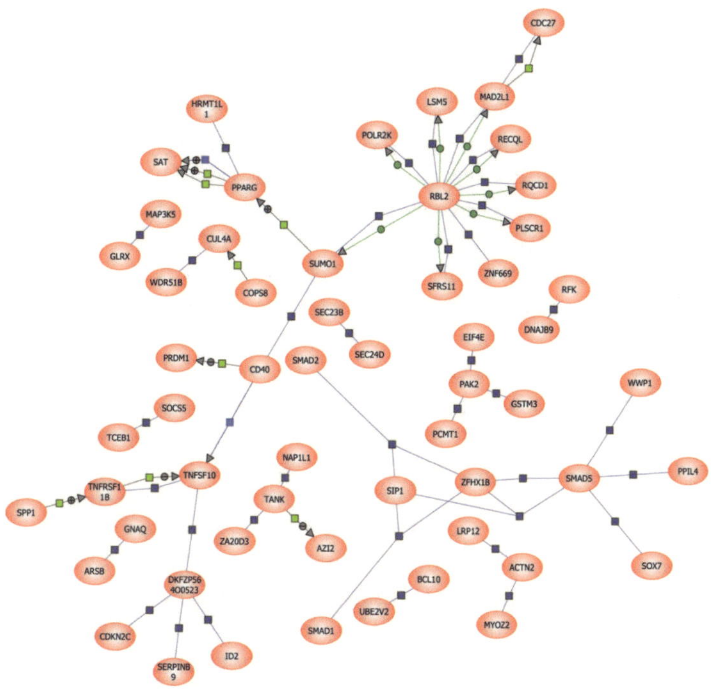

Fig. 4. Example of interaction network analysis (Ghorbel et al., 2010). The association between the network entities were based on available PubMed citations.

3.8 Data archiving

Successful interpretation of expression profiling investigations is likely to be dependent on the integration of experimental data with external information resources. Since the amount of data from multiple studies involving multiple cell types and tissues from multiple research groups is fast growing, data archiving is becoming an important issue. It is ideal if all gene expression data would be deposited in the public domain and are freely accessible.

Such endeavour would require a user-friendly and powerful database system and standardization of correction and normalization procedures to allow comparison of data sets from various projects (Granjeaud et al., 1999). Public data repositories have been developed at the European Bioinformatics Institute (ArrayExpress) and the National Center for Biotechnology Information (Gene Expression Omnibus), institutions that pursue these internationally recognized standards. Several scientific journals now request submission of microarray data into databases as a prerequisite for manuscript publication.

4. Exploring transcriptomic alterations in congenital heart diseases

The refinement of the human genome sequence and its associated annotation will soon have a great impact on the diagnosis and treatment of cardiovascular diseases when this information is coupled to the application of new technologies such as DNA microarrays. The latter provides a genomic approach to explore the genetic markers and molecular mechanisms leading to congenital heart disease and heart failure.

The first genome-wide gene expression study of congenitally malformed hearts in humans attempted to identify genes associated with dysdevelopment as well as genes involved in adaptation processes of the heart (Kaynak et al., 2003). The authors of this study, examined and compared genes dysregulated in defined congenitally malformed hearts with the molecular response to pressure overload leading to hypertrophy and the chamber-specific cardiac molecular portrait (Kaynak et al., 2003). By comparing the gene expression in atria and ventricle, this study found diverse previously unknown chamber-specific genes for muscle contraction, extracellular components, cell growth and differentiation, and energy metabolism (Kaynak et al., 2003). This is in addition to well-known chamber-specific genes, like atrial and ventricular myosin light chains. The comparison of Tetralogy of Fallot (TOF) and Right ventricular Hypertrophy (RVH), showed a distinct molecular portraits of TOF and RVH with genes of various functional classes (Kaynak et al., 2003) even though the right ventricular hypertrophy is part of TOF. Beside genes involved in cell cycle, a characteristic feature of the TOF signature is the upregulation of ribosomal proteins (Kaynak et al., 2003). Whereas a hypertrophy-specific gene expression pattern of genes mainly involved in stress response, cell proliferation, and metabolism was observed in RVH (Kaynak et al., 2003). In addition, to obtain a molecular portrait that is not influenced by biomechanical adaptation processes, RA samples of patients with ventricular septal defect (VSD), intact tricuspid valve, and normal RA pressure were studied (Kaynak et al., 2003). A VSD-specific molecular signature dominated by downregulated genes with respect to the other RA samples was shown (Kaynak et al., 2003). A thorough literature study of downregulated genes in VSD revealed that a major part is involved in cell proliferation and differentiation during embryogenesis as well as apoptosis (Kaynak et al., 2003). This investigation indicated distinct gene expression profiles associated with tetralogy of Fallot, ventricular septal defect, and right ventricular hypertrophy (Kaynak et al., 2003). Furthermore, the study design allowed the suggestion that alterations associated with primary genetic abnormalities can be distinguished from those associated with the adaptive response of the heart to the malformation (right ventricular pressure overload hypertrophy) (Kaynak et al., 2003).

The evidence for the developmentally regulated capacity of the immature heart to generate an adaptive response to reduced oxygen availability, although compelling, is derived largely from acute experimental interventions in animal models. Further, the reductionist approach of these studies, which typically address a single target, fails to capture the global complexity of the response. Nevertheless, the general observation that the human neonatal heart copes well with dramatic degrees of hypoxia and hypertrophy is in accordance with these experimental findings. To determine the molecular basis of this putatively adaptive response, Konstantinov et al. conducted microarray-based differential gene expression profiling on tissue samples acquired in patients of varying ages undergoing repair of right ventricular (RV) obstructive heart lesions, including TOF and focusing on potential age-related differences (Konstantinov et al., 2004). Their findings seem to confirm the existence of a protective reprogramming response that is most evident in the neonatal myocardium and is subject to the hemodynamic and metabolic stress imposed by structural congenital heart disease (Konstantinov et al., 2004). Indeed this study showed that neonatal myocardium has a unique pattern of gene expression dominated by genes with cardioprotective, antihypertrophic and antiproliferative properties reflecting a stress-induced protective program (Konstantinov et al., 2004).

Another investigation examined the differential gene expression profile during RVH in the developing heart with TOF congenital defect (Sharma et al., 2006). Using high-density DNA microarray, the authors showed that more than 200 myocardial genes are up- or downregulated in patients with TOF (Sharma et al., 2006). Among other genes, the expression of ECM proteins, such as collagens and fibronectin, was predominantly elevated, whereas MMP and TIMP expression either remained unchanged or decreased in TOF patients (Sharma et al., 2006). These results indicate for the myocardial fibrosis that may account for diminished function in patients with TOF (Sharma et al., 2006). They also provide further evidence that myocardial architecture in patients with TOF depict a complex and differential gene expression pattern with drastically increased expression level of ECM proteins (collagen Iα and III and fibronectin) mRNA and the VEGF/VEGF-R system (Sharma et al., 2006). The authors concluded that this up-regulation of genes involved in ECM homeostasis is associated with RVH and diminished cardiac function in TOF patients. Furthermore, the VEGF/VEGF-receptor (R) system could play an important role in enhanced myocardial angiogenesis that could be stunted due to limited vascular remodelling (Sharma et al., 2006).

In contrast to the previous investigation examining gene expression changes in cyanotic TOF in comparison to normal hearts (Sharma et al., 2006), we recently determined the global gene expression profiles associated with chronic hypoxia by comparing gene expression of cyanotic and acyanotic patients with TOF (Ghorbel et al., 2010). Our data showed that, overall, the transcriptional profile in the cyanotic group was characterized by increased expression level of genes with literature-validated apoptosis and growth/morphogenesis/remodeling properties. It also showed decreased expression levels of genes with cardiac function, cell survival, and cytoprotective properties (Ghorbel et al., 2010). The molecular signatures identified suggest a reprogramming response in the cyanotic myocardium activated by the chronic hypoxia imposed by the structural congenital heart disease (Ghorbel et al., 2010). The difference between the adaptive and injury-related responses would dictate the overall fate of heart cells.

In addition to investigating the gene expression profiling of the myocardium in response to congenital heart defect, other studies focused on gene expression alterations in response to surgery. One of these studies examined the gene expression profiles during intra-operative myocardial ischemia-reperfusion in corrective cardiac surgery of ventricular septal defect (Arab et al., 2007). It described the sequential changes in gene expression in the human ventricle during surgically imposed ischemia-reperfusion. The annotation of several genes exhibiting differential expression suggested that the elicited transcriptional response in this context is compensatory and adaptive. In silico functional clustering of several genes comprising this response revealed dominant up-regulation of transcripts encoding elements of pro-hypertrophic cellular growth factor pathways, involving multiple levels of regulation, including receptors, cognate signaling kinases, and programmatically linked transcription factors. The majority of genes up-regulated in response to cardioplegic arrest have literature-confirmed cytoprotective properties, including several that have been previously validated as endogenous mediators of ischemic preconditioning. This study provided evidence that myocardial ischemic stress associated with repair of VSD induces a net protective transcriptional response (Arab et al., 2007). It showed that reversible myocardial ischemia-reperfusion during cardiac surgery is associated with an immediate genomic response that predicts a net cardioprotective phenotype (Arab et al., 2007).

The molecular signatures identified with microarray technology can be interpreted as either mechanistically relevant to the congenital heart disease pathogenesis or as markers of disease progression. We believe that this approach can also be used to identify endogenous patterns of gene profiles that are activated in response to the primary disease-causing pathway and have the effect of generating a counteracting and highly adaptive pattern of gene activation, which serves to suppress aberrant disease-related molecular pathways.

5. Conclusion

Overall the information collected by gene expression profiling will help our understanding of disease mechanisms and provide insights useful for improving contemporary clinical treatment and prognosis of patients with congenital heart defects.

Congenital heart disease genomic research is still in its early stages with regard to the translation of studies' findings into clinical settings. However, inspection of other medical areas shows the potential of genomic medicine and where congenital heart medicine will be, possibly within the next few years. Microarrays are already being used in other fields to help clinicians better risk-stratify patients in addition to predict therapeutic responses and direct clinical and surgical decision making. Although considerable challenges remain, congenital heart disease genomic medicine promises to improve patient care and lower health care costs.

6. Acknowledgement

We are grateful to the Bristol NIHR BRU in Cardiovascular Medicine, The Garfield Weston Trust and the British Heart Foundation for their support.

7. References

Alon, U., Barkai, N., Notterman, D.A., Gish, K., Ybarra, S., Mack, D., and Levine, A.J. (1999). Broad patterns of gene expression revealed by clustering analysis of tumor and normal colon tissues probed by oligonucleotide arrays. Proc Natl Acad Sci U S A *96*, 6745-6750.

Arab, S., Konstantinov, I.E., Boscarino, C., Cukerman, E., Mori, A., Li, J., Liu, P.P., Redington, A.N., and Coles, J.G. (2007). Early gene expression profiles during intraoperative myocardial ischemia-reperfusion in cardiac surgery. J Thorac Cardiovasc Surg *134*, 74-81, 81 e71-72.

Bassett, D.E., Jr., Eisen, M.B., and Boguski, M.S. (1999). Gene expression informatics--it's all in your mine. Nat Genet *21*, 51-55.

Bell, J. (2004). Predicting disease using genomics. Nature *429*, 453-456.

Benjamini, Y., and Hochberg, Y. (1995). Controlling the false discovery rate - A parctical and powerful approach for multicomparison testing. J R Stat Soc *57*, 289-300.

Bolstad, B.M., Irizarry, R.A., Astrand, M., and Speed, T.P. (2003). A comparison of normalization methods for high density oligonucleotide array data based on variance and bias. Bioinformatics *19*, 185-193.

Bruneau, B.G. (2008). The developmental genetics of congenital heart disease. Nature *451*, 943-948.

Collins, F.S., Green, E.D., Guttmacher, A.E., and Guyer, M.S. (2003). A vision for the future of genomics research. Nature *422*, 835-847.

Cook, S.A., and Rosenzweig, A. (2002). DNA microarrays: implications for cardiovascular medicine. Circ Res *91*, 559-564.

Cooper, W.O., Hernandez-Diaz, S., Arbogast, P.G., Dudley, J.A., Dyer, S., Gideon, P.S., Hall, K., and Ray, W.A. (2006). Major congenital malformations after first-trimester exposure to ACE inhibitors. N Engl J Med *354*, 2443-2451.

Cope, L.M., Irizarry, R.A., Jaffee, H.A., Wu, Z., and Speed, T.P. (2004). A benchmark for Affymetrix GeneChip expression measures. Bioinformatics *20*, 323-331.

Eisen, M.B., Spellman, P.T., Brown, P.O., and Botstein, D. (1998). Cluster analysis and display of genome-wide expression patterns. Proc Natl Acad Sci U S A *95*, 14863-14868.

Ghorbel, M.T., Cherif, M., Jenkins, E., Mokhtari, A., Kenny, D., Angelini, G.D., and Caputo, M. (2010). Transcriptomic analysis of patients with tetralogy of Fallot reveals the effect of chronic hypoxia on myocardial gene expression. J Thorac Cardiovasc Surg *140*, 337-345 e326.

Goldsmith, Z.G., and Dhanasekaran, N. (2004). The microrevolution: applications and impacts of microarray technology on molecular biology and medicine (review). Int J Mol Med *13*, 483-495.

Granjeaud, S., Bertucci, F., and Jordan, B.R. (1999). Expression profiling: DNA arrays in many guises. BioEssays *21*, 781-790.

Hammon, J.W., Jr. (1995). Myocardial protection in the immature heart. Ann Thorac Surg *60*, 839-842.

Irizarry, R.A., Hobbs, B., Collin, F., Beazer-Barclay, Y.D., Antonellis, K.J., Scherf, U., and Speed, T.P. (2003). Exploration, normalization, and summaries of high density oligonucleotide array probe level data. Biostatistics *4*, 249-264.

Irizarry, R.A., Wu, Z., and Jaffee, H.A. (2006). Comparison of Affymetrix GeneChip expression measures. Bioinformatics *22*, 789-794.

Jenkins, K.J., Correa, A., Feinstein, J.A., Botto, L., Britt, A.E., Daniels, S.R., Elixson, M., Warnes, C.A., and Webb, C.L. (2007). Noninherited risk factors and congenital cardiovascular defects: current knowledge: a scientific statement from the American Heart Association Council on Cardiovascular Disease in the Young: endorsed by the American Academy of Pediatrics. Circulation *115*, 2995-3014.

Kaynak, B., von Heydebreck, A., Mebus, S., Seelow, D., Hennig, S., Vogel, J., Sperling, H.P., Pregla, R., Alexi-Meskishvili, V., Hetzer, R., *et al.* (2003). Genome-wide array analysis of normal and malformed human hearts. Circulation *107*, 2467-2474.

King, J.Y., Ferrara, R., Tabibiazar, R., Spin, J.M., Chen, M.M., Kuchinsky, A., Vailaya, A., Kincaid, R., Tsalenko, A., Deng, D.X., *et al.* (2005). Pathway analysis of coronary atherosclerosis. Physiol Genomics *23*, 103-118.

Konstantinov, I.E., Coles, J.G., Boscarino, C., Takahashi, M., Goncalves, J., Ritter, J., and Van Arsdell, G.S. (2004). Gene expression profiles in children undergoing cardiac surgery for right heart obstructive lesions. J Thorac Cardiovasc Surg *127*, 746-754.

Li, C., and Wong, W.H. (2001). Model-based analysis of oligonucleotide arrays: expression index computation and outlier detection. Proc Natl Acad Sci U S A *98*, 31-36.

Napoli, C., Lerman, L.O., Sica, V., Lerman, A., Tajana, G., and de Nigris, F. (2003). Microarray analysis: a novel research tool for cardiovascular scientists and physicians. Heart *89*, 597-604.

Pierpont, M.E., Basson, C.T., Benson, D.W., Jr., Gelb, B.D., Giglia, T.M., Goldmuntz, E., McGee, G., Sable, C.A., Srivastava, D., and Webb, C.L. (2007). Genetic basis for congenital heart defects: current knowledge: a scientific statement from the American Heart Association Congenital Cardiac Defects Committee, Council on Cardiovascular Disease in the Young: endorsed by the American Academy of Pediatrics. Circulation *115*, 3015-3038.

Schadt, E.E., Li, C., Su, C., and Wong, W.H. (2000). Analyzing high-density oligonucleotide gene expression array data. J Cell Biochem *80*, 192-202.

Sharma, H.S., Peters, T.H., Moorhouse, M.J., van der Spek, P.J., and Bogers, A.J. (2006). DNA microarray analysis for human congenital heart disease. Cell Biochem Biophys *44*, 1-9.

Srivastava, D. (2004). Heart disease: an ongoing genetic battle? Nature *429*, 819-822.

Stoeckert, C.J., Jr., Causton, H.C., and Ball, C.A. (2002). Microarray databases: standards and ontologies. Nat Genet *32 Suppl*, 469-473.

Yang, Y.H., Dudoit, S., Luu, P., Lin, D.M., Peng, V., Ngai, J., and Speed, T.P. (2002). Normalization for cDNA microarray data: a robust composite method addressing single and multiple slide systematic variation. Nucleic Acids Res *30*, e15.

11

B-Type Natriuretic Peptide (BNP) in Neonates, Infants and Children Undergoing Cardiac Surgery

Peter E. Oishi[1,2], Aida Field-Ridley[3],
Sanjeev A. Datar[1] and Jeffrey R. Fineman[1,2]
[1]University of California San Francisco, Pediatrics, Critical Care Medicine,
[2]Cardiovascular Research Institute, University of California San Francisco,
[3]Department of Pediatrics, University of California, Davis, Pediatrics, Critical Care Medicine,
USA

1. Introduction

In 1988 Sudoh and colleagues described a novel natriuretic peptide in porcine brain -- brain natriuretic peptide(Sudoh et al. 1988). In fact, the peptide is most abundant in the heart and thus it is now commonly termed B-type natriuretic peptide (BNP). Myocyte pressure and/or stretch results in the release of BNP, and BNP levels are easily quantified by several commercially available assays. Data from numerous studies have now firmly established a role for BNP as a biomarker for diagnosis, prognostication, and management of adults with cardiac disease, including those undergoing cardiac surgery(Silver et al. 2004; Mitchell and Webb 2011; Rodseth, Padayachee, and Biccard 2008; Fellahi et al. 2011). Unfortunately, far fewer data are available on the role of BNP in the management of neonates, infants, and children who require cardiac surgery. This chapter will provide a brief review of these data in order to understand the potential utility of BNP determinations in this population.

2. Natriuretic hormone system

Beginning with the observation by de Bold and colleagues that rats infused with atrial tissue extracts developed natriuresis and diuresis, much has been learned over the past three decades about the role of the natriuretic hormone system in the homeostatic control of fluid balance and vascular tone(de Bold et al. 1981). The natriuretic hormone system comprises several related peptides that activate specific receptors, particularly in the kidneys, myocardium, and vasculature, which use cyclic guanosine 3′,5′-monophosphate (cGMP) as a second messenger(Levin, Gardner, and Samson 1998). These peptides include atrial natriuretic peptide (ANP), BNP, C-type natriuretic peptide (CNP), dendroaspis natriuretic peptide (DNP), kaliuretic peptide, and urodilantin. The primary stimulus for their release is an increase in intravascular or cardiac volume, that causes increased atrial stretch, ventricular wall stress, vascular shear stress, intravascular volume, and/or intravascular sodium concentration(Levin, Gardner, and Samson 1998). The precise roles of individual natriuretic peptides depend upon their distribution and abundance within the cardiovascular system, as well as the specific stimulus for their release(Levin, Gardner, and Samson 1998).

3. B-Type natriuretic peptide (BNP)

BNP is predominantly produced in the cardiac ventricles. However under pathologic conditions, such as fluid overload, the cardiac atrium can also become a significant source of BNP(Sudoh et al. 1988; McGrath, de Bold, and de Bold 2005). Biosynthesis of BNP begins with a 134 amino acid precursor, preproBNP. Stimuli, such as myocyte stretch, trigger the cleavage of preproBNP forming proBNP, which is subsequently cleaved by a serine protease to the active C-terminal 32 amino acid hormone, BNP, and the inactive N-terminal proBNP (NT-proBNP). BNP binds to 3 known cell membrane receptors, termed natriuretic peptide receptors (NPR-A, NPR-B, and NPR-C). NPR-A and NPR-B are transmembrane receptors that activate particulate guanylate cyclase, which catalyzes the conversion of guanosine triphosphate to cGMP. The third receptor, NPR-C, is involved in clearance via endocytosis. Circulating BNP is also inactivated by cleavage by neutral endopeptidases found in vascular cells and renal tubules (Figure 1) (Yandle 1994; Silver et al. 2004). Animal studies suggest that approximately half of natriuretic peptide clearance is via the NPR-C receptor and half via endopeptidase degradation, but the relative contributions in the human are unclear.

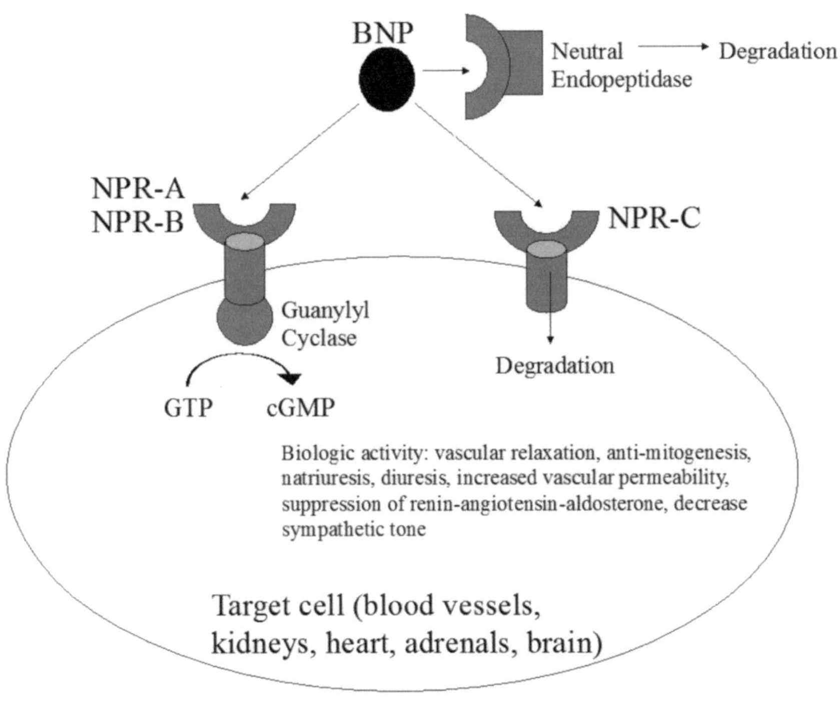

Fig. 1. A schematic of B-type natriuretic peptide (BNP) signaling. BNP binds to 3 natriuretic peptide receptors (NPR), types A, B, and C, on various target cells located in the vasculature, kidney, heart, adrenal glands, and brain. NPR-A and NPR-B are high-affinity receptors with an extracellular binding domain, a single membrane-spanning region, and an intracellular guanylylcyclase domain. Guanylylcyclase catalyzes the conversion of guanosine-5'-triphosphate (GTP) to guanosine-3',5'-cyclic monophosphate (cGMP). BNP is degraded by two mechanisms. Neutral endopeptidases degrade circulating BNP, and binding to NPR-C results in receptor internalization and degradation by endocytosis. NPR-C is then recycled to the cell membrance (not shown).

The mechanisms that mediate BNP release and metabolism in health and disease are incompletely understood. In addition, the effect of development on these mechanisms is unknown, but clearly may have great relevance in a pediatric population. Active BNP is stored in the atria in specific storage organelles(McGrath, de Bold, and de Bold 2005). Basal BNP levels result from continuous secretion from the atria. With acute myocardial distention, BNP release increases from this storage pool, in a manner independent of BNP synthesis. However, under acute, sub-acute and chronic conditions of increased cardiac volume or pressure loading, increases in circulating BNP are maintained due to ventricular re-expression of the fetal gene program (Zhang, Carreras, and de Bold 2003; Hama et al. 1995). In addition to volume and pressure loading, acute myocardial ischemia, α agonist stimulation, endothelin-1, and inflammatory mediators, such as tumor necrosis factor-α and interleukin-1β, result in rapid ventricular expression of BNP(Hama et al. 1995). The primary actions of BNP are vascular smooth muscle relaxation and anti-mitogenesis, mediated by cGMP, diuresis, caused by a shift of intravascular volume into the interstitium, and natriuresis, caused by antagonism of renin and aldosterone release(McGrath, de Bold, and de Bold 2005; Sudoh et al. 1988; Yandle 1994).
Of all the natriuretic peptides, BNP has emerged as the most useful biomarker for cardiac disease. Its major advantage over the other natriuretic peptides is the fact that it is produced predominantly in the ventricles, as opposed to the atrium (ANP) or the vascular endothelium (CNP)(Silver et al. 2004; Costello, Goodman, and Green 2006). Both active BNP and the inactive byproduct of its production, NT-proBNP, are used as biomarkers. BNP levels may be better suited to follow dynamic alterations in myocardial performance given the shorter circulating half-life of BNP compared to NT-proBNP (20 minutes vs. 60-120 minutes)(Costello, Goodman, and Green 2006). In addition, the kidneys excrete NT-proBNP, and thus renal function, independent of myocardial function, has a greater influence on NT-proBNP levels than BNP levels.
Limited data suggest that BNP levels are high at birth but fall during the first week of life, reaching levels below adult values by 2 weeks of age. Interestingly, although levels in boys tend to decrease with age, girls have an elevation during the second decade of life that is associated with puberty (Koch and Singer 2003; Yoshibayashi et al. 1995; Ationu and Carter 1993).

4. BNP in pediatric heart disease

In comparison to the adult experience, there are far fewer data regarding BNP in pediatric cardiac disease(Das 2010). Knirsch and colleagues measured BNP levels before and during treatment in 522 pediatric patients (age of 6.4±5.2 years, range of 14 days to 18 years) with congenital heart disease, cardiomyopathies, or pulmonary arterial hypertension(Knirsch et al. 2011). They found that BNP levels were elevated in each type of heart disease, and that levels fell in all groups with therapy.
As opposed to adults with congestive heart failure, BNP levels in infants and children with congenital heart disease are quite varied, and are dependent in part upon the age of the patient and the specific physiology associated with the cardiac defect. For example, Law and colleagues performed a study that included 42 neonates and 58 older children between the age of 7 days and 19 years presenting in an acute care setting with symptoms potentially attributable to heart disease. BNP levels were higher in both age groups in those patients with heart disease compared to those without heart disease, but the cut-off values differed. A BNP level of 170 pg/ml was 94% sensitive and 73% specific for heart disease in neonates,

whereas a lower level of 41 pg/ml was 87% sensitive and 70% specific for heart disease in the older patients(Law et al. 2009). Koch and colleagues found in a study of 288 pediatric patients (mean age of 6 years) with congenital cardiac defects that normal BNP levels did not exclude cardiac pathology such as the presence of structural defects or ventricular hypertrophy, but rather were associated with the extent of ventricular impairment(Koch, Zink, and Singer 2006). Conversely, Cantinotti and colleagues studied 152 neonates with congenital heart disease and 154 healthy neonatal controls, and found the BNP levels were higher in neonates with congenital heart disease than controls with a diagnostic accuracy defined by the area under the curve (on receiver operating characteristic analysis) of 0.935 for neonates with congenital heart disease between 4 and 30 days of age(Cantinotti et al. 2010). Thus, it appears that age modifies the diagnostic utility of BNP for cardiac disease in pediatric patients. In fact, in a separate study Koch and colleagues demonstrated age-dependent differences in the metabolic clearance of BNP and NT-proBNP(Koch, Rauh, et al. 2006).

A number of studies indicate that cardiopulmonary hemodynamics also modify the diagnostic utility of BNP in pediatric patients with congenital heart disease. For example, in a study of infants and children with ventricular septal defects, Suda and colleagues found that BNP levels correlated with the pulmonary-to-systemic blood flow (Qp:Qs) ratio and the mean pulmonary arterial pressure(Suda, Matsumura, and Matsumoto 2003). Koch and colleagues demonstrated similar correlations, in their study of 288 patients with various cardiac defects(Koch, Zink, and Singer 2006). They found that in patients with left-to-right shunts, BNP levels were increased and correlated with shunt volume, systolic right ventricular pressure, mean pulmonary artery pressure, and pulmonary vascular resistance(Koch, Zink, and Singer 2006). Likewise, Kunii and colleagues compared BNP levels between normal children (n=253), and children with ventricular septal defects (n=91), patent ductus arteriosus (n=29), and atrial septal defects (n=34). Like the studies of Suda and Koch, they found that BNP levels correlated with the Qp:Qs ratio, and also the left ventricular end-diastolic volume, and the right ventricular to left ventricular pressure ratio(Kunii et al. 2003). Mainwaring and colleagues also found a positive correlation between preoperative BNP levels and the Qp:Qs ratio in a study of 18 patients (2 months – 15.6 years of age) with ventricular septal defects(Mainwaring et al. 2007). Ozhan and colleagues found the same relationship between BNP and the Qp:Qs ratio in their study of 35 children (mean age 70±129 weeks) with ventricular or atrial septal defects. Receiver operating characteristic analysis found that a plasma BNP cutoff of ≥20 pg/ml was 69% sensitive and 79% specific for a Qp:Qs of greater than 1.5(Ozhan et al. 2007).

A number of studies of premature neonates found that BNP levels correlated with the degree of shunting across a patent ductus arteriosus and predicted hemodynamic significance as determined by echocardiography-based criteria(Choi et al. 2005; Flynn et al. 2005; Puddy et al. 2002; Sanjeev et al. 2005; Holmstrom and Omland 2002; da Graca et al. 2006). However, the precise cut-off value for BNP that was predictive varied widely. For example, Choi and colleagues reported that a BNP level of > 1110 pg/ml was 100% sensitive and 95% specific for the presence of a hemodynamically significant patent ductus arteriosus, while Sanjeev and colleagues reported a 92% sensitivity with a cut-off level of 70 pg/ml(Choi et al. 2005; Sanjeev et al. 2005).

Holmgren and colleagues studied 38 patients with single ventricular physiology. They found that BNP levels were higher in patients after first stage palliation (31.6 pg/ml) compared to patients after second and third stage palliation (6.7 and 9 pg/ml, respectively). In fact, BNP levels in patients after second and third stage palliation did not differ from normal control patients, but interestingly, BNP levels were higher in those patients with single ventricles of right ventricular morphology compared to left ventricular morphology(Holmgren et al. 2008). In contrast, Koch and colleagues studied 48 patients with d-transposition of the great arteries, after arterial switch procedure, or congenitally corrected transposition of the great arteries. They found no difference in BNP levels between patients with systemic ventricles of right ventricular morphology compared to left ventricular morphology(Koch, Zink, and Singer 2008). They did, however, find correlations between BNP and the severity of tricuspid regurgitation and decreasing exercise capacity. Likewise, Inuzuka and colleagues measured BNP levels in 51 patients (mean age 1.1 years) with single ventricular defects undergoing cardiac catheterization before second stage palliation. Mean BNP levels were 90.4 pg/ml. BNP levels above 100 pg/ml were associated with increased Qp:Qs, end-diastolic volume, AV valve regurgitation, and lower ventricular mass to end-diastolic volume ratio, all consistent with an inadequate adaptation to volume overload(Inuzuka et al. 2011). In addition, multivariate regression analysis demonstrated that the BNP concentration was independently predictive of death or the need for cardiac transplantation (with a hazard ratioof 3.05, CI: 1.06-8.83)(Inuzuka et al. 2011).

Thus, it is clear that BNP determinations can provide physiologically relevant information about individual patients, but that finding cut-off values that can be generalized for clinical use across the spectrum of congenital heart disease may not be possible. Indeed, in adult patients the primary utility of BNP determinations is in establishing the diagnosis of congestive heart failure in acute care settings(Maisel et al. 2002). In a pediatric population, the questions are more diverse. They might include, when to repair a left-to-right shunt, when to proceed with staged palliation of single ventricle defects, or when to refer for cardiac transplantation. However, even studies focused on pediatric heart failure have revealed a wide range of BNP values, again likely related at least in part to age and cardiopulmonary hemodynamics. For example, in a study of infants and children with biventricular hearts and chronic left ventricular dysfunction, Price and colleagues found that a BNP level of ≥300 pg/ml was predictive of death, hospitalization, or listing for cardiac transplant(Price et al. 2006). Shah and colleagues also found that increasing BNP was associated with heart failure in their study of 29 patients with single ventricular physiology, but with a ten-fold lower cut-off of 30 pg/ml (Shah, et al., 2009).

5. BNP as a biomarker following cardiac surgery

5.1 Early post-operative period

As a cardiac hormone with a relatively short circulating half life that is dynamically released in response to deranged myocardial performance, BNP appears perfectly suited for the perioperative management of pediatric patients undergoing cardiac surgery for repair or palliation of congenital cardiac defects.

A number of investigators have studied perioperative BNP levels in neonates, infants, and children undergoing cardiac surgery. Ationu and colleagues measured perioperative BNP levels in 9 children undergoing repair of congenital heart defects(Ationu et al. 1993). In that study, BNP levels decreased at 12 hours following surgery(Ationu et al. 1993). Most studies, however, have found increases in BNP and NT-proBNP levels after surgery. Costello and colleagues measured natriuretic peptide levels, including BNP, in 5 infants undergoing surgical repair of left-to-right shunts(Costello et al. 2004). As opposed to ANP and DNP, BNP concentrations increased after cardiopulmonary bypass. Sun and colleagues measured BNP levels before and after surgery in 27 infants and children undergoing biventricular repair and 27 patients undergoing palliation of univentricular congenital heart defects(Sun et al. 2005). Plasma BNP levels increased after bypass in patients with biventricular defects, but not in patients with univentricular defects(Sun et al. 2005). Costello and colleagues examined BNP levels before and following cardiac surgery in 25 infants and children with congenital heart disease undergoing complete or palliative repair with the use of cardiopulmonary bypass(Costello et al. 2004). BNP levels increased postoperatively, and remained elevated over the first postoperative day. The increase in BNP from baseline to 12 hours was associated with the cardiopulmonary bypass time.Koch and colleagues measured BNP levels in 65 pediatric patients (age 4 days - 17 years, mean age of 3.6), undergoing surgical repair of congenital cardiac defects preoperatively, and for one week after surgery(Koch, Kitzsteiner, et al. 2006). BNP levels increased after surgery (from a median of 31 pg/ml to 453 pg/ml) and remained elevated over the first week, with a bimodal pattern (initial peak at 1.3 days and a second peak at 5.1 days after surgery). Postoperative BNP levels correlated with cardiopulmonary bypass time and serum lactate concentrations on the first postoperative day.

Shih and colleagues conducted the first study demonstrating that BNP predicted outcome after cardiac surgery in children(Shih et al. 2006). BNP levels were determined before and after surgery in 51 patients. They found that BNP levels increased after surgery, peaking at 12 hours, and that BNP levels 12 hours following surgery were predictive of a requirement for mechanical ventilation beyond 48 hours and the presence of low cardiac output syndrome within the first 48 hours, postoperatively. Further, the study found that 12-hour BNP levels of 540 pg/ml had a sensitivity of 88.9% and a specificity of 82.5% for predicting the need for mechanical ventilation beyond 48 hours, and that a 12-hour BNP of 815 pg/ml had a sensitivity of 87.5% and a specificity of 90.2% for predicting the development of low cardiac output syndrome.

Similarly, Perez-Piaya and colleagues measured NT-proBNP levels in 68 patients (0-15 years of age) undergoing cardiac surgery(Perez-Piaya et al. 2011). They found that NT-proBNP levels increased postoperatively, peaking at 24 hours. Moreover, peak NT-proBNP levels correlated with risk adjustment congenital heart surgery-1 scores, length of cardiopulmonary bypass, inotropic score, duration of mechanical ventilation, and intensive care unit length of stay. In addition, preoperative NT-proBNP levels were independent predictors of intensive care unit length of stay. Gessler and colleagues also measured NT-proBNP levels before and after cardiac surgery in 40 children(Gessler et al. 2006). In their study, higher preoperative levels were noted in patients with a complicated postoperative course.

It is well known that neonates undergoing cardiac surgery and patients with single ventricular physiology represent high-risk groups. Hsu and colleagues examined BNP levels before and after surgery in 31 consecutive neonates undergoing repair or palliation of their cardiac defects(Hsu et al. 2007). BNP levels at all time points were markedly elevated, compared to published normal values. But interestingly, as opposed to the majority of studies of older patients, they found that 24-hour postoperative BNP levels were lower than preoperative BNP levels in most patients (75%). However, in those patients whose BNP levels increased after surgery outcomes were worse. In fact, an increase in post-operative BNP was associated with an increased incidence of low cardiac output syndrome (100% vs. 36 %), and fewer ventilator-free days (17 ± 13 days vs. 25 ± 3 days), and predicted the 6-month composite endpoint of death, an unplanned operation, or cardiac transplant (57% vs. 0%). Furthermore, an increase in BNP after surgery had a sensitivity of 100% and a specificity of 87% for predicting a poor postoperative outcome. Notably, neither arterial-venous oxygen saturation differences ($AVdO_2$) nor lactate levels (or their corresponding changes) were associated with postoperative outcomes in this study(Hsu et al. 2007).

In another neonatal study, Cannesson and colleagues measured perioperative BNP levels in 30 neonates undergoing the arterial switch operation (ASO) for d-transposition of the great arteries(Cannesson et al. 2007). Contrary to the findings of Hsu, BNP levels increased over the first 48 hours postoperatively. However, like the study by Hsu these investigators found that postoperative BNP levels predicted adverse clinical outcomes, including prolonged mechanical ventilation, prolonged stay in the intensive care unit, low cardiac output syndrome, and the need for inotropic support. These investigators found that a BNP level of >160 pg/ml, 6 hours postoperatively, predicted a complicated postoperative course with a sensitivity of 93% and a specificity of 67%. Similarly, Niedner and colleagues studied 102 neonates and non-neonatal controls undergoing surgical repair for various congenital cardiac defects(Niedner et al. 2010). They found that BNP levels increased after surgery, peaking at 12 hours. Levels at 24 hours were significantly higher in neonates than in non-neonates (median of 1506 vs 286 pg/ml). In addition, postoperative BNP levels correlated with the inotropic requirement, duration of mechanical ventilation, and intensive care unit and hospital length of stay. When comparing the various cardiac defects, these investigators found great variability between lesions and noted the significant impact of age, with postoperative elevations occurring earlier and to a much greater magnitude in neonates compared to older children. One might speculate that the differences between the neonatal studies of Hsu, Cannesson, and Niedner relate in part to differences between single and bi-ventricular physiology, and the impact of surgery on ventricular volume and pressure loading. Furthermore, these studies demonstrate that the potential clinical utility for BNP determinations as a part of management after cardiac surgery may depend upon analyzing patterns of change, as opposed to single time points. Moreover, relevant patterns of change may differ between cardiac defects and age groups.

In fact, Berry and colleagues studied 20 neonates, infants, and children undergoing various stages of palliation for cardiac defects with single ventricle physiology(Berry et al. 2007). They found that BNP levels were highest in neonates undergoing a Norwood procedure compared with patients undergoing bidirectional cavopulmonary anastomosis or a Fontan procedure. They also found that postoperative BNP levels were predictive of hospital length of stay and postoperative inotropic support.Likewise, Hsu and colleagues measured perioperative BNP levels in 36 infants and children undergoing bidirectional cavopulmonary anastomosis (n=25) or total cavopulmonary connection (n=11)(Hsu et al. 2008). Plasma BNP levels were measured before and at various time points after surgery. They found that BNP levels increased after surgery, peaking at 12 hours in most patients. In the bidirectional cavopulmonary anastomosis group, patients with a 12-hour BNP level of ≥500 pg/mL had a longer duration of mechanical ventilation, intensive care unit stay, and hospital stay. A 12-hour BNP level of ≥500 pg/mL had a sensitivity of 80% and a specificity of 80% for predicting an unplanned surgical or transcatheter cardiac intervention, including transplantation. In the total cavopulmonary connection group, preoperative BNP levels were highest in patients with total cavopulmonary connection failure compared with patients with a good outcome, whereas postoperative BNP levels were not predictive of outcome.Importantly, preoperative cardiac catheterization data did not correlate with these outcomes in either group.

5.2 BNP in patients requiring mechanical support after cardiac surgery

Chikovani and colleagues studied the potential utility of BNP levels in the assessment of native myocardial performance in ten neonates and infants being supported with

extracorporeal life support (ECLS) after cardiac surgery(Chikovani et al. 2007). In particular, alterations in BNP during weaning trials off of ECLS were determined and compared to other biochemical markers, including lactate and the $AVDO_2$.This study did not find associations between long-term outcome and alterations in lactate and the $AVDO_2$ during trials off ECLS. However, an increase in BNP during the final trial off ECLS had a sensitivity of 80% and a specificity of 100% for predicting the need for an unplanned operation or death within 3 months. A notable finding of this study was that BNP levels decreased during trials off of ECLS support (which were accomplished through the use of a bridge placed in the ECLS circuit, allowing mechanical support to be diverted away from the patient before the ECLS cannulae were removed) in patients who were successfully separated from ECLS after a trial. Since trials off ECLS were associated with increased cardiac filling (increased central venous pressures) in all patients, this study suggests that BNP levels may be regulated by additional mechanisms (other than just myocyte stretch). Furthermore, during trials off of ECLS, inotropic support, lactate levels and the $AVDO_2$ increased in all patients (both those who successfully separated from ECLS and those who did not), suggesting that BNP levels may capture myocardial performance in a unique manner.
In a similar earlier study, Huang and colleagues studied fifteen pediatric patients requiring ECLS for cardiogenic shock(Huang et al. 2006). Eleven of the fifteen patients developed shock after cardiac surgery. These investigators did not find an association between BNP levels during the course of ECLS and survival after ECLS. However, they did find that BNP levels on the first and fourth day following separation from ECLS were significantly higher in nonsurvivors than survivors(Huang et al. 2006).

5.3 Long-term outcomes

Koch and colleagues measured BNP levels in 130 children and adolescents (mean age of 16.1 years) with a history of surgically repaired tetralogy of Fallot, at a mean time of 13±6.5 years after repair. They also performed exercise testing and echocardiograms. BNP levels were increased above normal gender and age specific values in 60% of the patients, but were less than 200 pg/ml in all patients(Koch et al. 2010). BNP levels were higher in patients awaiting pulmonary valve replacement, and in those in NYHA class II compared to class I. Furthermore, BNP levels correlated with right ventricular dilatation and the severity of tricuspid and pulmonary valve regurgitation, and were inversely correlated with exercise time. In addition, BNP levels increased over time in patients awaiting pulmonary valve replacement and decreased after surgery. The authors suggested that BNP levels might aid in the long-term management of these patients, particularly in the timing of pulmonary valve replacement.
Pietrzak and Werner conducted a similar study, in which they measured NT-proBNP levels in 20 adolescents (10 to 17 years of age) during a follow-up period of 7 to 16 years after repair of tetralogy of Fallot(Pietrzak and Werner 2009). They found that NT-proBNP levels were higher in those patients than in age matched healthy controls. NT-proBNP levels were higher in patients who had undergone repair with a transannular patch compared to those who underwent repair without a transannular patch. Furthermore, NT-proBNP levels were increased in patients with: QRS prolongation during exercise testing, severe pulmonary regurgitation, and severe triscuspid regurgitation. Likewise, Dodge-Khatami and colleagues measured plasma NT-proBNP levels and obtained cardiac magnetic resonance imaging in

23 patients with repaired tetralogy of Fallot, severe pulmonary insufficiency, and increased right ventricular end-diastolic volume that were undergoing pulmonary valve replacement(Dodge-Khatami et al. 2006). Log-NT-proBNP levels were inversely correlated with right ventricular ejection fraction before and 6 months after surgery. NT-proBNP levels, right ventricular end-diastolic volume, and pulmonary insufficiency all decreased by 6 months after surgery.

These three studies differed from a study by Apitz and colleagues. These investigators measured BNP levels and recorded pressure-volume loops using conductance catheters in 16 adolescents (median age of 14.2 years) with a known history of right ventricular dilation (NYHA class I, and Ross class 0) secondary to pulmonary regurgitation after repair of tetralogy of Fallot(Apitz et al. 2009). Latent right ventricular dysfunction was defined as impaired contractility (calculated by the slope of the end-systolic pressure-volume relation) in response to a dobutamine infusion. Latent right ventricular dysfunction was identified in 5 patients, but no clear relationship with BNP levels could be observed. The difference between this study and those of Koch, Pietrzak, and Dodge-Khatami may relate to the severity of disease, suggesting that BNP may not be useful in detecting subclinical deterioration in this patient population.

In a small pilot study, Paul and colleagues measured BNP levels before and after surgical repair of ventricular septal defects in 14 patients who were less than 2 years of age(Paul et al. 2009). Mean BNP levels decreased by 94 pg/ml after repair. Longitudinal analysis found that there was a weak inverse correlation between the postoperative change in BNP and postoperative weight gain (weight z-score change per month).

Recently, Atz and colleagues described their findings in a study of 510 children (6-18 years of age), who were enrolled in the Pediatric Heart Network Fontan cross-sectional study(Atz et al. 2011). The patients had all undergone 3rd stage palliation of single ventricle cardiac defects with a Fontan procedure (median time from Fontan of 8.2 years). The distribution of BNP levels in these patients were highly skewed, but were generally within the normal range (median 13 pg/ml). However, logBNP levels were independently associated with a history of pre-Fontan systolic dysfunction, and post-Fontan complications, including thrombosis. LogBNP levels were higher in patients with atrial-to-pulmonary connections compared to extracardiac conduits. Furthermore, increased logBNP levels were associated with a lower level of physical functioning, chronotropic index during exercise, diastolic dysfunction, and greater ventricular mass measured by cardiac magnetic resonance imaging.

In a similar study, Koch and colleagues measured plasma BNP levels in 67 patients after a modified Fontan procedure(Koch et al. 2008). Although there was a wide range, BNP levels were normal in 81% of the patients, with a median value of 13 pg/ml. Levels were not different between patients with right or left ventricular morphology. BNP levels were higher in patients in NYHA class II compared to those in class I, and were positively correlated with the severity of AV valve regurgitation. Likewise, Man and colleagues measured plasma BNP levels and assessed ventricular function (by tissue Doppler assessments, acoustic quantification, and myocardial performance index) in 35 asymptomatic patients who had previously undergone a Fontan procedure(Man and Cheung 2007). Comparisons were made to 34 healthy controls. Although BNP levels were low in the Fontan group (median 21 pg/ml), they were higher than the control group. Moreover, BNP levels were inversely correlated with ventricular function, particularly diastolic function.

6. Conclusion

The essential relationship between BNP production by the cardiac ventricle and increased myocyte stretch is the foundation for the potential use of BNP as a biomarker in any condition in which abnormal ventricular loading conditions are primarily involved in the pathophysiology. To date, plasma BNP determinations have not attained the same clinical prominence in pediatric patients as in adults. The growing utilization of BNP determinations in the care of adult patients likely stems from the ability to make clinical decisions, indeed to titrate therapy, in response to BNP levels(Troughton et al. 2000). Thus, a widespread use of BNP in pediatric patients is restrained by the scarcity of data that supports BNP guided therapies. It is likely that this discrepancy between the adult and pediatric experience relates, in part, to the number of investigations. However, compared to adult CHF, pediatric cardiac diseases resulting in ventricular dysfunction and CHF are far more heterogeneous. In fact, coronary artery disease is the leading cause of CHF in adults, whereas pediatric CHF may result from a wide spectrum of congenital cardiac defects and various cardiomyopathies. Moreover, clinically relevant cutoff values for plasma BNP levels within these various disease processes are not well established or are completely unknown. Nonetheless, the ability to readily quantify plasma BNP levels is attractive as few markers are so directly related to the pathobiology of the cardiac ventricle. This is particularly true in the management of critically ill pediatric patients, where we often employ surrogate markers of disease severity, such as serum lactate levels, that reflect global processes as opposed to organ specific functioning.

Based on the studies outlined above, it is clear that BNP determinations can offer valuable clinical information to aid in the management of neonates, infants, and children undergoing surgical repair of cardiac defects. It is also clear, however, that the information is unlikely to come from single cut-off values that can be generalized across populations. Rather, a clinical utility for BNP determinations will likely come from an advanced understanding of expected perioperative patterns of change in BNP levels - patterns that will differ between age groups and specific cardiac defects. Furthermore, future studies must begin to evaluate the utility of guiding therapy in response to plasma BNP values. Fortunately, the ease of measuring BNP levels should facilitate these studies. For now the available data demonstrate that BNP has emerged as a novel biomarker with great potential.

7. References

Apitz, C., L. Sieverding, H. Latus, A. Uebing, S. Schoof, and M. Hofbeck. 2009. "Right ventricular dysfunction and B-type natriuretic peptide in asymptomatic patients after repair for tetralogy of Fallot." *Pediatric cardiology* no. 30 (7):898-904. doi: 10.1007/s00246-009-9453-y.

Ationu, A., and N. D. Carter. 1993. "Brain and atrial natriuretic peptide plasma concentrations in normal healthy children." *Br J Biomed Sci* no. 50 (2):92-5.

Ationu, A., D. R. Singer, A. Smith, M. Elliott, M. Burch, and N. D. Carter. 1993. "Studies of cardiopulmonary bypass in children: implications for the regulation of brain natriuretic peptide." *Cardiovasc Res* no. 27 (8):1538-41.

Atz, A. M., V. Zak, R. E. Breitbart, S. D. Colan, S. K. Pasquali, D. T. Hsu, M. Lu, L. Mahony, S. M. Paridon, M. D. Puchalski, T. Geva, and B. W. McCrindle. 2011. "Factors

Associated with Serum Brain Natriuretic Peptide Levels after the Fontan Procedure." *Congenital heart disease*. doi: 10.1111/j.1747-0803.2011.00496.x.

Berry, J. G., B. Askovich, R. E. Shaddy, J. A. Hawkins, and C. G. Cowley. 2007. "Prognostic Value of B-Type Natriuretic Peptide in Surgical Palliation of Children with Single-Ventricle Congenital Heart Disease." *Pediatr Cardiol.*

Cannesson, M., C. Bionda, B. Gostoli, O. Raisky, S. di Filippo, D. Bompard, C. Vedrinne, R. Rousson, J. Ninet, J. Neidecker, and J. J. Lehot. 2007. "Time course and prognostic value of plasma B-type natriuretic peptide concentration in neonates undergoing the arterial switch operation." *Anesth Analg* no. 104 (5):1059-65, tables of contents.

Cantinotti, M., S. Storti, A. Ripoli, L. Zyw, M. Crocetti, N. Assanta, B. Murzi, and A. Clerico. 2010. "Diagnostic accuracy of B-type natriuretic hormone for congenital heart disease in the first month of life." *Clinical chemistry and laboratory medicine : CCLM / FESCC* no. 48 (9):1333-8. doi: 10.1515/CCLM.2010.251.

Chikovani, O., J. Hsu, R. Keller, TR. Karl, A. Azakie, I. Adatia, P. Oishi, and JR. Fineman. 2007. "B-type natriuretic peptide levels predict outcomes for children on extracorporeal life support after cardiac surgery." *J Thorac Cardiovasc Surg*:In Press.

Choi, B. M., K. H. Lee, B. L. Eun, K. H. Yoo, Y. S. Hong, C. S. Son, and J. W. Lee. 2005. "Utility of rapid B-type natriuretic peptide assay for diagnosis of symptomatic patent ductus arteriosus in preterm infants." *Pediatrics* no. 115 (3):e255-61.

Costello, J. M., C. L. Backer, P. A. Checchia, C. Mavroudis, R. G. Seipelt, and D. M. Goodman. 2004. "Alterations in the natriuretic hormone system related to cardiopulmonary bypass in infants with congestive heart failure." *Pediatr Cardiol* no. 25 (4):347-53.

Costello, J. M., D. M. Goodman, and T. P. Green. 2006. "A review of the natriuretic hormone system's diagnostic and therapeutic potential in critically ill children." *Pediatr Crit Care Med* no. 7 (4):308-18.

da Graca, R. L., D. C. Hassinger, P. A. Flynn, C. P. Sison, M. Nesin, and P. A. Auld. 2006. "Longitudinal changes of brain-type natriuretic peptide in preterm neonates." *Pediatrics* no. 117 (6):2183-9.

Das, B. B. 2010. "Plasma B-type natriuretic peptides in children with cardiovascular diseases." *Pediatric cardiology* no. 31 (8):1135-45. doi: 10.1007/s00246-010-9758-x.

de Bold, A. J., H. B. Borenstein, A. T. Veress, and H. Sonnenberg. 1981. "A rapid and potent natriuretic response to intravenous injection of atrial myocardial extract in rats." *Life Sci* no. 28 (1):89-94.

Dodge-Khatami, A., E. V. Buchel, W. Knirsch, A. Kadner, V. Rousson, H. H. Dave, U. Bauersfeld, and R. Pretre. 2006. "Brain natriuretic peptide and magnetic resonance imaging in tetralogy with right ventricular dilatation." *The Annals of thoracic surgery* no. 82 (3):983-8. doi: 10.1016/j.athoracsur.2006.03.038.

Fellahi, J. L., G. Daccache, D. Rubes, M. Massetti, J. L. Gerard, and J. L. Hanouz. 2011. "Does preoperative B-type natriuretic peptide better predict adverse outcome and prolonged length of stay than the standard European System for Cardiac Operative Risk Evaluation after cardiac surgery?" *Journal of cardiothoracic and vascular anesthesia* no. 25 (2):256-62. doi: 10.1053/j.jvca.2010.05.009.

Flynn, P. A., R. L. da Graca, P. A. Auld, M. Nesin, and C. S. Kleinman. 2005. "The use of a bedside assay for plasma B-type natriuretic peptide as a biomarker in the management of patent ductus arteriosus in premature neonates." *J Pediatr* no. 147 (1):38-42.

Gessler, P., W. Knirsch, B. Schmitt, V. Rousson, and A. von Eckardstein. 2006. "Prognostic value of plasma N-terminal pro-brain natriuretic peptide in children with congenital heart defects and open-heart surgery." *J Pediatr* no. 148 (3):372-6.

Hama, N., H. Itoh, G. Shirakami, O. Nakagawa, S. Suga, Y. Ogawa, I. Masuda, K. Nakanishi, T. Yoshimasa, Y. Hashimoto, and et al. 1995. "Rapid ventricular induction of brain natriuretic peptide gene expression in experimental acute myocardial infarction." *Circulation* no. 92 (6):1558-64.

Holmgren, D., A. Westerlind, H. Berggren, P. A. Lundberg, and H. Wahlander. 2008. "Increased natriuretic peptide type B level after the second palliative step in children with univentricular hearts with right ventricular morphology but not left ventricular morphology." *Pediatric cardiology* no. 29 (4):786-92. doi: 10.1007/s00246-008-9201-8.

Holmstrom, H., and T. Omland. 2002. "Natriuretic peptides as markers of patent ductus arteriosus in preterm infants." *Clin Sci (Lond)* no. 103 (1):79-80.

Hsu, J. H., P. E. Oishi, R. L. Keller, O. Chikovani, T. R. Karl, A. Azakie, I. Adatia, and J. R. Fineman. 2008. "Perioperative B-type natriuretic peptide levels predict outcome after bidirectional cavopulmonary anastomosis and total cavopulmonary connection." *J Thorac Cardiovasc Surg* no. 135 (4):746-53.

Hsu, J., R. Keller, O. Chikovani, H. Cheng, SA. Hollander, TR. Karl, A. Azakie, I. Adatia, P. Oishi, and JR. Fineman. 2007. "B-type natriuretic peptide levels predict outcome after neonatal cardiac surgery." *J Thorac Cardiovasc Surg*:In Press.

Huang, S. C., E. T. Wu, W. J. Ko, L. P. Lai, J. Hsu, C. I. Chang, I. S. Chiu, S. S. Wang, M. H. Wu, F. Y. Lin, and Y. S. Chen. 2006. "Clinical implication of blood levels of B-type natriuretic peptide in pediatric patients on mechanical circulatory support." *Ann Thorac Surg* no. 81 (6):2267-72.

Inuzuka, R., S. Tatebe, S. Wakiguchi, H. Nakajima, H. Ohtsu, K. Dimopoulos, and H. Aotsuka. 2011. "B-type natriuretic peptide at the early stage of univentricular circulation reflects inadequate adaptation to volume overload." *International journal of cardiology*. doi: 10.1016/j.ijcard.2011.02.023.

Knirsch, W., E. Hausermann, M. Fasnacht, M. Hersberger, P. Gessler, and U. Bauersfeld. 2011. "Plasma B-type natriuretic peptide levels in children with heart disease." *Acta paediatrica*. doi: 10.1111/j.1651-2227.2011.02258.x.

Koch, A., T. Kitzsteiner, S. Zink, R. Cesnjevar, and H. Singer. 2006. "Impact of cardiac surgery on plasma levels of B-type natriuretic peptide in children with congenital heart disease." *Int J Cardiol*.

Koch, A. M., M. Rauh, S. Zink, and H. Singer. 2006. "Decreasing ratio of plasma N-terminal pro-B-type natriuretic peptide and B-type natriuretic peptide according to age." *Acta Paediatr* no. 95 (7):805-9.

Koch, A. M., S. Zink, M. Glockler, T. Seeliger, and S. Dittrich. 2010. "Plasma levels of B-type natriuretic peptide in patients with tetralogy of Fallot after surgical repair." *International journal of cardiology* no. 143 (2):130-4. doi: 10.1016/j.ijcard.2009.01.062.

Koch, A. M., S. Zink, and H. Singer. 2008. "B-type natriuretic peptide in patients with systemic right ventricle." *Cardiology* no. 110 (1):1-7. doi: 10.1159/000109399.

Koch, A. M., S. Zink, H. Singer, and S. Dittrich. 2008. "B-type natriuretic peptide levels in patients with functionally univentricular hearts after total cavopulmonary connection." *European journal of heart failure* no. 10 (1):60-2. doi: 10.1016/j.ejheart.2007.11.001.

Koch, A., and H. Singer. 2003. "Normal values of B type natriuretic peptide in infants, children, and adolescents." *Heart* no. 89 (8):875-8.

Koch, A., S. Zink, and H. Singer. 2006. "B-type natriuretic peptide in paediatric patients with congenital heart disease." *Eur Heart J* no. 27 (7):861-6.

Kunii, Y., M. Kamada, S. Ohtsuki, T. Araki, K. Kataoka, M. Kageyama, N. Nakagawa, and Y. Seino. 2003. "Plasma brain natriuretic peptide and the evaluation of volume overload in infants and children with congenital heart disease." *Acta Med Okayama* no. 57 (4):191-7.

Law, Y. M., A. W. Hoyer, M. D. Reller, and M. Silberbach. 2009. "Accuracy of plasma B-type natriuretic peptide to diagnose significant cardiovascular disease in children: the Better Not Pout Children! Study." *Journal of the American College of Cardiology* no. 54 (15):1467-75. doi: 10.1016/j.jacc.2009.06.020.

Levin, E. R., D. G. Gardner, and W. K. Samson. 1998. "Natriuretic peptides." *N Engl J Med* no. 339 (5):321-8.

Mainwaring, R. D., C. Parise, S. B. Wright, A. L. Juris, R. A. Achtel, and H. Fallah. 2007. "Brain natriuretic peptide levels before and after ventricular septal defect repair." *The Annals of thoracic surgery* no. 84 (6):2066-9. doi: 10.1016/j.athoracsur.2007.07.021.

Maisel, A. S., P. Krishnaswamy, R. M. Nowak, J. McCord, J. E. Hollander, P. Duc, T. Omland, A. B. Storrow, W. T. Abraham, A. H. Wu, P. Clopton, P. G. Steg, A. Westheim, C. W. Knudsen, A. Perez, R. Kazanegra, H. C. Herrmann, and P. A. McCullough. 2002. "Rapid measurement of B-type natriuretic peptide in the emergency diagnosis of heart failure." *N Engl J Med* no. 347 (3):161-7.

Man, B. L., and Y. F. Cheung. 2007. "Plasma brain natriuretic peptide and systemic ventricular function in asymptomatic patients late after the Fontan procedure." *Heart and vessels* no. 22 (6):398-403. doi: 10.1007/s00380-007-0993-x.

McGrath, M. F., M. L. de Bold, and A. J. de Bold. 2005. "The endocrine function of the heart." *Trends Endocrinol Metab* no. 16 (10):469-77.

Mitchell, J., and S. T. Webb. 2011. "Is brain natriuretic peptide a marker for adverse postoperative outcomes in patients undergoing cardiac surgery?" *Interactive cardiovascular and thoracic surgery* no. 12 (3):467-72. doi: 10.1510/icvts.2010.252601.

Niedner, M. F., J. L. Foley, R. H. Riffenburgh, D. P. Bichell, B. M. Peterson, and A. Rodarte. 2010. "B-type natriuretic peptide: perioperative patterns in congenital heart disease." *Congenital heart disease* no. 5 (3):243-55. doi: 10.1111/j.1747-0803.2010.00396.x.

Ozhan, H., S. Albayrak, H. Uzun, S. Ordu, A. Kaya, and M. Yazici. 2007. "Correlation of plasma B-type natriuretic peptide with shunt severity in patients with atrial or ventricular septal defect." *Pediatric cardiology* no. 28 (4):272-5. doi: 10.1007/s00246-006-0014-3.

Paul, M. A., C. L. Backer, H. J. Binns, C. Mavroudis, C. L. Webb, R. Yogev, and W. H. Franklin. 2009. "B-type natriuretic peptide and heart failure in patients with ventricular septal defect: a pilot study." *Pediatric cardiology* no. 30 (8):1094-7. doi: 10.1007/s00246-009-9503-5.

Perez-Piaya, M., E. Abarca, V. Soler, A. Coca, M. Cruz, F. Villagra, S. Giannivelli, and A. Asensio. 2011. "Levels of N-terminal-pro-brain natriuretic peptide in congenital heart disease surgery and its value as a predictive biomarker." *Interactive cardiovascular and thoracic surgery* no. 12 (3):461-6. doi: 10.1510/icvts.2010.245803.

Pietrzak, R., and B. Werner. 2009. "Usefulness of NT-proBNP in assessment of right ventricular function in children after tetralogy of Fallot correction - a preliminary study." *Kardiologia polska* no. 67 (4):378-83.

Price, J. F., A. K. Thomas, M. Grenier, B. W. Eidem, E. O'Brian Smith, S. W. Denfield, J. A. Towbin, and W. J. Dreyer. 2006. "B-type natriuretic peptide predicts adverse cardiovascular events in pediatric outpatients with chronic left ventricular systolic dysfunction." *Circulation* no. 114 (10):1063-9.

Puddy, V. F., C. Amirmansour, A. F. Williams, and D. R. Singer. 2002. "Plasma brain natriuretic peptide as a predictor of haemodynamically significant patent ductus arteriosus in preterm infants." *Clin Sci (Lond)* no. 103 (1):75-7.

Rodseth, R. N., L. Padayachee, and B. M. Biccard. 2008. "A meta-analysis of the utility of pre-operative brain natriuretic peptide in predicting early and intermediate-term mortality and major adverse cardiac events in vascular surgical patients." *Anaesthesia* no. 63 (11):1226-33. doi: 10.1111/j.1365-2044.2008.05574.x.

Sanjeev, S., M. Pettersen, J. Lua, R. Thomas, S. Shankaran, and T. L'Ecuyer. 2005. "Role of plasma B-type natriuretic peptide in screening for hemodynamically significant patent ductus arteriosus in preterm neonates." *J Perinatol* no. 25 (11):709-13.

Shah, A., A. M. Feraco, C. Harmon, T. Tacy, J. R. Fineman, and H. S. Bernstein. 2009. "Usefulness of various plasma biomarkers for diagnosis of heart failure in children with single ventricle physiology." *The American journal of cardiology* no. 104 (9):1280-4. doi: 10.1016/j.amjcard.2009.06.046.

Shih, C. Y., A. Sapru, P. Oishi, A. Azakie, T. R. Karl, C. Harmon, R. Asija, I. Adatia, and J. R. Fineman. 2006. "Alterations in plasma B-type natriuretic peptide levels after repair of congenital heart defects: a potential perioperative marker." *J Thorac Cardiovasc Surg* no. 131 (3):632-8.

Silver, M. A., A. Maisel, C. W. Yancy, P. A. McCullough, J. C. Burnett, Jr., G. S. Francis, M. R. Mehra, W. F. th Peacock, G. Fonarow, W. B. Gibler, D. A. Morrow, and J. Hollander. 2004. "BNP Consensus Panel 2004: A clinical approach for the diagnostic, prognostic, screening, treatment monitoring, and therapeutic roles of natriuretic peptides in cardiovascular diseases." *Congest Heart Fail* no. 10 (5 Suppl 3):1-30.

Suda, K., M. Matsumura, and M. Matsumoto. 2003. "Clinical implication of plasma natriuretic peptides in children with ventricular septal defect." *Pediatr Int* no. 45 (3):249-54.

Sudoh, T., K. Kangawa, N. Minamino, and H. Matsuo. 1988. "A new natriuretic peptide in porcine brain." *Nature* no. 332 (6159):78-81.

Sun, L. S., C. Dominguez, N. A. Mallavaram, and J. M. Quaegebeur. 2005. "Dysfunction of atrial and B-type natriuretic peptides in congenital univentricular defects." *J Thorac Cardiovasc Surg* no. 129 (5):1104-10.

Troughton, R. W., C. M. Frampton, T. G. Yandle, E. A. Espiner, M. G. Nicholls, and A. M. Richards. 2000. "Treatment of heart failure guided by plasma aminoterminal brain natriuretic peptide (N-BNP) concentrations." *Lancet* no. 355 (9210):1126-30.

Yandle, T. G. 1994. "Biochemistry of natriuretic peptides." *J Intern Med* no. 235 (6):561-76.

Yoshibayashi, M., T. Kamiya, Y. Saito, K. Nakao, K. Nishioka, S. Temma, H. Itoh, G. Shirakami, and H. Matsuo. 1995. "Plasma brain natriuretic peptide concentrations in healthy children from birth to adolescence: marked and rapid increase after birth." *Eur J Endocrinol* no. 133 (2):207-9.

Zhang, Y., D. Carreras, and A. J. de Bold. 2003. "Discoordinate re-expression of cardiac fetal genes in N(omega)-nitro-L-arginine methyl ester (L-NAME) hypertension." *Cardiovasc Res* no. 57 (1):158-67.

Part 3

Aortic Surgery

12

Cerbral Protection Strategies for Aortic Arch Surgery

Bradley G. Leshnower and Edward P. Chen
Division of Cardiothoracic Surgery,
Emory University School of Medicine,
USA

1. Introduction

Surgical therapy for aortic arch disease involves partial or complete replacement of the aortic arch with reimplantation of the great vessels while the cerebral blood flow is temporarily altered. Patients undergoing this mandatory period of circulatory arrest during arch replacement are at an increased risk for adverse neurologic outcomes, and strategies for cerebral protection must be implemented to achieve successful results. The optimal strategy for management of the circulation during aortic arch surgery remains controversial. Arch reconstruction has historically been associated with significant morbidity and mortality due to global ischemic end-organ damage occurring during the circulatory arrest period. As surgical techniques have evolved, survival has improved; however, neurologic dysfunction due to cerebral ischemia remains a significant concern.

Profound hypothermia was the initial method of cerebral protection utilized during the period of circulatory arrest. The first successful series of arch reconstructions using deep hypothermic circulatory arrest (DHCA) with body temperatures of 18°C was reported in 1975 (1). Further efforts to improve cerebral protection during arch reconstruction have led to the development of antegrade cerebral perfusion (ACP) and retrograde cerebral perfusion (RCP). Both techniques provide continuous blood flow to the brain and are used in conjunction with hypothermic circulatory arrest (HCA). The optimal method of cerebral perfusion (antegrade vs. retrograde) is a controversial topic and has yet to be determined. In the this chapter, the indications for aortic arch surgery will be delineated, and the various methods of cerebral protection strategies and their results will be reviewed.

2. Pathology/indications for aortic arch surgery

The most common indication for arch replacement is the presence of aneurysmal disease. The most common type of arch aneurysm is a degenerative aneurysm. The media of the aortic wall in degenerative aneurysms develops cellular necrosis which results in a loss of smooth muscle cells that are replaced by cystic spaces filled with mucoid material. Dr. Cooley coined the phrase cystic medial necrosis to describe this characteristic histologic pattern found in degenerative aneurysms (2). These aneurysms also have a significant reduction in elastin content due to a poorly understood increase in elastin fragmentation.

The second most common cause of arch aneurysms is atherosclerosis. The development of invasive atheromas is thought to destroy the elastin fibers and smooth muscle cells of the aortic media resulting in aneurysm formation.(3). Inherited genetic connective tissue disorders such as Marfan syndrome, Ehlers-Danlos and Loeys-Dietz syndrome are less common causes of arch aneurysms. Familial arch aneurysms are a subtype of heritable aneurysms which do not express a recognizable phenotype of a known connective tissue disorder, and do not have a specific gene or product which has been identified (3). Bicuspid aortic valve (BAV) disease is a congenital anomaly occurring in 0.9-2% of the population which is associated with an intrinsic aortopathy that leads to the development of proximal arch aneurysms. BAV aneurysms are thought to be due to an abnormal extracellular matrix of the aortic wall. Infection is a rare cause of (mycotic) arch aneurysms and requires replacement with aortic homograft.

The presence or absence of symptoms is the most important factor in the management of patients with arch aneurysms. Most patients with arch aneurysms are asymptomatic, and the aneurysm is discovered incidentally on radiographic imaging obtained for another purpose. Patients with symptomatic arch aneurysms typically experience chest or back pain. However, symptoms can also include compression or stretching of surrounding anatomic structures. Tracheal compression can cause stridor, esophageal compression may result in dysphagia, superior vena cava compression can cause plethora, and aneurysmal stretching of the recurrent laryngeal nerve produces hoarseness. The sudden onset of pain is considered an ominous warning sign of imminent rupture or dissection, and urgent surgery is indicated for all patients with symptomatic arch aneurysms (4). Operative therapy for asymptomatic arch aneurysms is performed for prophylactic replacement of the aorta in order to prevent rupture or dissection, and thereby improve patient survival. Total aortic arch replacement for an isolated arch aneurysm should be performed at sizes ≥ 5.5cm. Rapid expansion of the aneurysm at a rate ≥0.5cm/year is another indication for surgery. Concomitant proximal (hemi-) arch replacement is recommended at the time of ascending aortic replacement if the proximal arch is enlarged (4).

The other common indication for surgical intervention on the aortic arch is acute Type A aortic dissection. Surgical treatment of acute Type A aortic dissection requires resection of the primary tear, restoration of aortic valve competency, aortic replacement, and obliteration of the false lumen at the proximal and distal anastomoses. The distal extent of aortic replacement depends upon whether the arch is involved in the dissection. Arch involvement requires hemi-arch or total arch replacement under circulatory arrest using an open distal anastomosis. Total arch replacement in the setting of acute Type A aortic dissection is recommended when the arch is aneurysmal or there is extensive destruction or leakage (4). Nevertheless, it should be emphasized that total arch replacement significantly increases the risk of stroke and death during repair of an acute Type A dissection and should only be performed by experienced surgeons.

3. Cerebral protection strategies

3.1 Deep hypothermic circulatory arrest

In 1952, John Lewis used systemic hypothermia at 28°C and inflow occlusion to perform the first successful atrial septal defect repair in a 5 year old girl (5). Systemic hypothermia was gradually phased out with the introduction of the cardiopulmonary bypass machine, but was rediscovered and used by separate investigators in isolated reports of aortic arch replacement in the 1960's (6,7). Dr. Griepp reported the first successful series of total arch replacements in adults in 1975, using deep hypothermic circulatory arrest) at 18°C for cerebral protection (1).

The technique of DHCA for aortic arch replacement involves placing the patient on cardiopulmonary bypass and initiating systemic hypothermia to a core temperature of 18°C. Once this core temperature has been achieved, cardiopulmonary bypass is interrupted and the systemic circulation is arrested. The aortic arch is resected and reconstructed, deairing maneuvers are performed, and cardiopulmonary bypass is resumed. The exact mechanism of cerebral protection afforded by deep hypothermia is not completely understood, but its main beneficial effect is the suppression of cerebral metabolism. This is important because it enables an extension of the period of cerebral ischemic tolerance required for arch replacement.

Systemic hypothermia at 20°C has been shown to reduce the cerebral metabolic rate by 76% (8) (Table 1). It has also been postulated that there is an uncoupling of cerebral blood flow and cerebral metabolism at approximately 22°C, likely due to a loss of autoregulation in the cerebral vasculature. The ratio of cerebral blood flow to cerebral metabolism increases from 20:1 at normothermia, to 75:1 with deep hypothermia (9). Once the period of DHCA has been completed and cerebral reperfusion has been initiated, severe cerebral vasoconstriction occurs. There is also an accumulated cerebral oxygen debt from the ischemic period which must be "paid back", and therefore, normal levels of cerebral metabolism are maintained by increased oxygen extraction (10, 11, 12). During the period following DHCA, the brain is at high risk for both ongoing ischemic injury due to low cerebral blood flow, and reperfusion injury. There has also been experimental data to suggest that following DHCA, there is an increase in intracranial pressure due to cerebral edema which negatively impacts neurophysiologic recovery (13).

Temperature (°C)	Cerebral Metabolic Rate (% of baseline)	Safe Duration of HCA (min)
37	100	5
30	56 (52–60)	9 (8–10)
25	37 (33–42)	14 (12–15)
20	24 (21–29)	21 (17–24)
15	16 (13–20)	31 (25–38)
10	11 (8–14)	45 (36–62)

Calculations based on assumption that there is a 5-min tolerance for circulatory arrest at 37°C. Values in parenthesis are 95% confidence intervals. HCA = hypothermic circulatory arrest.

Table 1. From McCullough JN, Zhang N, Reich DL et al. Cerebral metabolic suppresion during hypothermic circulatory arrest in humans. Ann Thorac Surg 1999; 67:1895-1921.

Cerebral injury following procedures requiring circulatory arrest is manifested clinically as post-operative transient or permanent neurologic injury. Permanent neurologic dysfunction (PND) appears as a focal neurologic deficit or stroke, which is thought to be the result of embolic phenomena. The incidence of PND following arch reconstruction has been shown to be directly related to the site of arterial cannulation (14). Transient neurologic deficit (TND) is defined as postoperative confusion, delirium, obtundation, or transient focal deficits (resolution within 24 hours) with negative brain computed tomography or magnetic resonance imaging scans. TND is a reversible, diffuse, subtle injury which is an indicator of global cerebral injury due to inadequate cerebral protection. TND following arch reconstruction using DHCA alone has been shown to occur in approximately 25% of all cases, and a linear relationship has been demonstrated between the incidence of TND and the duration of DHCA (15, 16, 17).

In order to limit adverse neurologic outcomes, many investigations have focused upon determining a "safe" duration of DHCA. Based upon direct measurements of cerebral metabolism in adults, the safe period of DHCA has been estimated to be 30 minutes at 15°C, and 40 minutes at 10°C. Cellular anoxia occurs when these time periods are exceeded. (8). In a series of 656 patients undergoing arch surgery with DHCA alone, Svensson and colleagues reported a 10% mortality rate, and a 7% incidence of transient or permanent stroke. In a multivariate analysis, these authors demonstrated an increased risk of stroke following a period of DHCA > 40 minutes, and an increased mortality rate following a DHCA period >65 minutes (18). Griepp's group reported a 22% incidence of TND in 443 patients undergoing hemi-arch replacement with DHCA alone. In a multivariate analysis, these authors showed a DHCA time >30 minutes was an independent risk factor for TND (19). Using neuropsychologic tests, these investigators also demonstrated in a separate study that a DHCA duration > 25 minutes is a risk factor long-term deficits in neurocognitive function (20).

DHCA was the first successful cerebral protection strategy used in aortic arch surgery. Over the past three decades, aortic surgeons have improved their techniques for arch replacement and novel strategies for circulation management and cerebral protection have evolved. However, for short circulatory arrest times ≤ 30 minutes, there are still many surgeons who achieve excellent outcomes with DHCA alone as their sole method of cerebral protection during arch reconstruction. For more complex, extended arch reconstructions that require circulatory arrest times > 30 minutes, there is a consensus that DHCA alone is an inadequate cerebral protection strategy. In the current era, most experts in the field of aortic surgery use either antegrade or retrograde cerebral perfusion as an adjunctive method of cerebral protection in addtion to deep or moderate hypothermic circulatory arrest. (21).

3.2 Retrograde Cerebral Perfusion

Retrograde cerebral perfusion (RCP) was first described by Mills and Ochner as a method of treating a massive air embolus during cardiopulmonary bypass (22). RCP is employed by cannulating and snaring the superior vena cava, and infusing blood up the superior vena cava to perfuse the brain in a retrograde direction during the period of circulatory arrest. Flow rates are adjusted to achieve an SVC pressure of 20-25mm Hg. It is well recognized that RCP is a highly effective method of flushing embolic material from the cerebral circulation, and it maintains cerebral hypothermia by continuously bathing the brain in cold blood. There is a theoretical benefit that RCP can provide sufficient cerebral blood flow to support cerebral metabolism and remove toxic metabolites and waste products (9).

Although there was initial enthusiasm for RCP's ability to support cerebral metabolism, this hypothesis has subsequently been disproved. Multiple animal studies in different species have demonstrated minimal or no cerebral blood flow with the use of RCP (23, 24, 25). Although cerebral perfusion can be improved with higher retrograde perfusion pressures and occlusion of the inferior vena cava, there is a concomitant increase in cerebral edema with histologic evidence of cerebral injury (26).

Many groups adopted the use of RCP in conjunction with DHCA in the 1990's as their routine strategy for circulatory management during arch reconstruction with excellent outcomes. Bavaria and colleagues demonstrated a significant improvement over previous reported series of Type A aortic dissection repairs using DHCA and RCP. In their series of 104 patients, these investigators reported a 9% mortality rate and 5% stroke rate with a mean duration of DHCA+RCP of 42 minutes in 104 consecutive patients undergoing emergent repair of Type A aortic dissection (27). In a series of 479 patients undergoing arch surgery with DHCA for aneurysmal disease or dissection, Coselli compared the results using DHCA alone vs. DHCA+RCP. The subgroup who received DHCA+RCP had significantly reduced mortality (DHCA+RCP 3.4% vs. DHCA 14.8%, $p<0.001$) and stroke rates (DHCA+RCP 2.4% vs. DCHA 6.5%, $p<0.05$) (28).

Estrera and colleagues also reported excellent results with the use of DHCA+RCP in both elective and emergent arch repairs. These investigators reported a mortality rate of 10.4% and a 2.8% stroke rate in a series of 1107 patients in which 907 (82%) patients received DHCA+RCP. However, the incidence of TND was 15.5% with relatively short mean RCP times of 26 minutes (29). Although this is lower than the 25% incidence of TND associated with arch reconstruction using DHCA alone (17), it is still a significant incidence of inadequate cerebral protection. Other groups have also reported a significant incidence of TND with the use of DHCA+RCP (30, 31, 32). The high incidence of TND and the recent popularity of antegrade cerebral perfusion has led to decreased utilization of RCP by most aortic surgeons (21). Nevertheless, RCP remains an important adjunctive cerebral protection strategy to DHCA is still used by many high volume aortic centers with excellent outcomes (33, 34). It is a highly effective anti-embolic technique which is especially useful for arch reconstruction in patients with carrying a heavy atherosclerotic burden.

3.3 Antegrade Cerebral Perfusion

Debakey and Cooley were the first to successfully describe the use of antegrade cerebral perfusion (ACP) in the surgical repair of an arch aneurysm (35). In their initial report, cannulas were placed into the right femoral artery and both carotid arteries, and a separate pump from the main cardiopulmonary bypass machine was used to perfuse normothermic blood into the carotid arteries. Despite its initial success, this method was considered complex and cumbersome, and was subsequently abandoned in favor of DHCA + RCP. The use of ACP began to reappear in reports of arch reconstructions in the late 1980's. Bachet reported a 2.1% PND rate and a 4.3% TND rate with the use of ACP with "cold cerebroplegia" via bilateral carotid cannulation in a series of 54 patients (36). A year later, Kazui published excellent neurologic outcomes in a series of arch reconstructions by introducing catheters into the innominate and left common carotid arteries and providing ACP at a rate of 10mL/Kg/min during the period of DHCA. This perfusion rate was considered 50% of physiologic levels based upon experimental data, and has subsequently become the standard perfusion rate of ACP by most groups using this technique (37). During the 1990's most centers performing a significant volume of aortic arch surgery began using either ACP or RCP as an adjunctive form of cerebral protection in addition to DHCA.

It should be recognized that the utilization of ACP changes the paradigm of circulatory arrest. Circulatory arrest, as originally described, refers to the total arrest of the circulation and the absence of perfusion to all organs (except the heart via cardioplegia). The addition of ACP changes this concept from total body circulatory arrest to lower body circulatory arrest, as the brain, arms and the spinal cord (via collateral circulation) are being perfused. Therefore the legs and the abdominal visceral are the only truly ischemic organs during the circulatory arrest period with the use of ACP.

Different methods and nomenclature are used in the literature to describe ACP techniques. It is most commonly referred to as selective antegrade cerebral perfusion (SACP), because many surgeons introduce individual cathethers or cannulae into the orifices of the innominate and left common carotid arteries, thus selecting out the individual great vessels for cerebral perfusion. This is also referred to as bilateral selective antegrade cerebral perfusion (bSACP). Another modality is unilateral SACP (uSACP), which can refer to two different sites of cannulation. One method is to directly cannulate or sew a graft on to the base of the innominate artery to provide antegrade cerebral perfusion up the right common carotid artery. A different technique is to directly cannulate or sew a graft on to the right axillary artery. At the time of circulatory arrest, a clamp is placed across the base of the innominate artery, and blood is forced up the right common carotid. Both methods are considered uSACP.

The hypothesis of ACP is that antegrade cerebral blood flow is more physiologic than no blood flow (HCA) or retrograde blood flow (RCP), and should therefore provide superior cerebral protection. Data from experimental animal models of DHCA comparing ACP and RCP have confirmed this hypothesis. Hagl and colleagues showed in an acute porcine model that a strategy of DHCA+ACP compared to DHCA alone is associated with improved neurophysiologic recovery, lower intracranial pressure, less cerebral edema, and reduced tissue acidosis following the circulatory arrest period (38). In a porcine model of circulatory arrest and reperfusion, Filgueiras and colleagues showed that near normal cerebral metabolism was maintained with DHCA+ACP, based upon pH measurements and levels of cerebral metabolites. The pigs who underwent DHCA+RCP or DHCA alone demonstrated a significant drop in cerebral pH during the protocol (39). In a separate study using the same model, these same investigators demonstrated preserved cell structure upon histopathologic analysis with HCA+ACP compared to HCA+RCP (40)

The Mount Sinai group under Dr. Griepp has performed extensive laboratory work on the topic of ACP. These investigators determined that hypothermic SACP at 10°-15°C provides better cerebral protection than SACP at 20-25°C based upon post-op behavioral scores in a chronic porcine circulatory arrest model (41). They also showed that a short period of HCA prior to SACP initiation does not impact the level of cerebral protection compared to continuous SACP. This is important clinically because many surgeons will use a short period of HCA alone prior to initiating SACP to keep the field clean while they are performing arch resection in order to reduce the risk of atheroembolization (42). Ye and colleagues compared unilateral and bilateral SACP to determine whether there was any difference in cerebral perfusion and cerebral protection between the two techniques. Using magnetic resonance perfusion imaging, these investigators compared cerebral blood volume and regional cerebral perfusion patterns in pigs undergoing circulatory arrest with uSACP via the right axillary artery to a separate group undergoing bSACP via bilateral carotid artery cannulation. Both methods provided uniform blood distribution to both cerebral hemispheres and preserved normal morphology of the cerebral neurons (43).

Clinical studies have also supported DHCA+ACP as a superior method of cerebral protection compared to DHCA+RCP or DHCA alone. Using transcranial Doppler measurements during DHCA, Tanoue and colleagues demonstrated superior middle cerebral artery blood flow in patients undergoing DHCA+ACP compared to those undergoing DHCA+RCP (44). Neri and colleagues demonstrated that the cerebrovascular autoregulation function was preserved in the immediate postoperative period in patients undergoing DHCA+ACP. However, the autoregulatory function was significantly impaired in patients undergoing DHCA alone or DHCA+RCP. Based upon the higher incidence of TND in the DHCA and DHCA+RCP groups, this post-operative impairment in cerebral autoregulation was considered to be an expression of CNS injury (45).

Hagl reviewed the neurologic outcomes from the Mount Sinai experience of 717 patients undergoing arch replacement with the three different methods of cerebral protection. The incidence of stroke (PND) and TND was 5.7% and 30%. Due to significant differences in the circulatory arrest times, they were unable to determine whether the method of cerebral protection impacted the stroke rate. However, by using a multivariate analysis, the use of DHCA+ACP significantly reduced the incidence of TND compared to DHCA+RCP or DHCA alone (31). In a randomized controlled trials comparing ACP vs RCP for total arch replacements performed under DHCA, Okita and colleagues showed no difference in stroke between patients undergoing ACP vs RCP, however ACP significantly reduced the incidence of TND (ACP 13.3% vs. RCP 33.3%, p=0.05) (46). These results were also replicated in series of 48 patients undergoing arch reconstruction during type A aortic dissection repair. In this series, Apostolakis and colleagues reported no difference in mortality or PND between patients undergoing DHCA+ACP vs DHCA+RCP. However, the incidence of TND was significantly higher in the DHCA+RCP group (DHCA+RCP 43.5% vs. DHCA+ACP 16%, p=0.04) (47).

In the current era, ACP has become the preferred method of cerebral protection employed by most aortic surgeons at the time of arch reconstruction (21). The lessons learned from the majority of studies comparing the various methods of cerebral protection are: 1)an adjunct form of cerebral protection (ACP or RCP) is superior to DHCA alone and 2)the method of cerebral perfusion (ACP or RCP) has no impact upon the incidence of PND, however ACP significantly reduces the incidence of TND.

3.4 Moderate hypothermia

Since Griepp's initial report of the successful use of DHCA for cerebral protection during arch replacement, profound systemic hypothermia at a core temperature of 18°C has been the standard point of hypothermia at which most surgeons will initiate circulatory arrest. As discussed above, deep hypothermia affords excellent cerebral protection by suppressing cerebral metabolism. Studies in the field of transplantaiton have also demonstrated that hypothermia acts in a similar fashion in the preservation of organs (e.g. lungs, liver, heart, kidneys)(48). However, profound systemic hypothermia has been shown to have adverse effects in multiple organ systems including endothelial dysfunction, neuronal apoptosis, coagulopathy and renal failure (49, 50, 51, 52). The time required to cool and rewarm the body to 18°C leads to prolonged cardiopulmonary bypass which is detrimental to multiple organ system. Furthermore, deep hypothermia has been shown to be a strong risk factor for bleeding requiring re-exploration following arch reconstruction (16). Furthermore, despite the cerebral metabolic suppressive effects of profound hypothermia, a linear relationship has been demonstrated between the incidence of TND and the duration of DHCA alone (53).

In an attempt to avoid the morbidity associated with DHCA, reduce cardiopulmonary bypass times and improve neurologic outcomes there has been a strong initiative from many different high volume aortic centers to begin performing arch replacements under moderate hypothermia circulatory arrest with ACP. This technique still provides maximum cerebral protection because the brain is being perfused with antegrade "cold cerebroplegia" at temperatures ≤ 18°C for ACP. It is the abdominal viscera which are the organs placed at risk with the technique of MCHA+ACP. However there has yet to be a report of increased risk of mesenteric ischemia, liver or renal failure with the use of MHCA.

Bachet's initial description of arch reconstructions using "cold cerebroplegia" at 6°-12°C in 1991 was also remarkable for the fact that he performed all of his arch reconstructions under moderate hypothermic circulatory arrest at core temperatures between 25-28°C (36). Using this technique he reported excellent neurologic outcomes with an incidence of PND and TND of 2.1% and 4.3% respectively. Minatoya and colleagues evaluated outcomes of 229 patients who received arch reconstruction with HCA+bSACP at three different temperatures: 20°C (n=81), 25°C (n=81), and 28°C (n=67). 81% of all patients received total arch replacement. There were no significant differences between the three groups with regards to the incidence of mortality, PND or TND (54). The use of MHCA+ACP for arch reconstruction has also been reported by several groups in the setting of acute Type A aortic dissection with results equivalent to those achieved with DHCA (55, 56, 57).

At Emory, MHCA+uSACP is our preferred method of cerebral protection. All circulatory arrest cases are performed by cannulating an 8mm Dacron graft sewn to the right axillary artery. This is based upon a strong belief that axillary artery cannulation reduces the incidence of PND. This is supported by the important analysis by Svensson and colleagues who reviewed their stroke rates in 1336 circulatory arrest cases with different sites for arterial cannulation (ascending aorta, femoral, axillary, and innominate). They determined that cannulating a graft sewn to the right axillary artery resulted in the lowest incidence of PND (14). Although the mechanism of the protective effect of axillary cannulation is unknown, we have two hypotheses. The first is that axillary artery cannulation provides retrograde blood flow down the innominate artery, which may prevent atheroembolic disease from the ascending aorta. The second hypothesis relates to the differences in technique between uSACP and bSACP. In bSACP, there is a risk of cannulation-induced embolic injury from the introduction of cerebral perfusion catheters into the innominate and left common carotid arteries, especially in patients with atheromatous aortic arch disease. With uSACP, the innominate artery is occluded at the time of circulatory arrest and antegrade blood at 16°C is perfused at 10ml/kg/min through the right common carotid artery, right vertebral artery as well as through the left carotid system via intracranial and extracranial collaterals (58). This avoids manipulation of the ostia of the great vessels which are often covered with large, friable atherosclerotic plaques.

In our initial report using this technique, we reviewed 412 arch reconstruction cases (elective and emergent) performed under MHCA with uSACP at core temperature of 25.7°C at the initiation of circulatory arrest. Operative mortality was 7.0%, and the incidence of PND and TND were 3.6% and 5.1% respectively with no cases of paraplegia. There were four (1%) deaths due to mesenteric inschemia, and three of these four patients presented with an acute Type A aortic dissection with preoperative visceral malperfusion. There was a 4.6% incidence of renal failure requiring dialysis. In a multivariate analysis, moderate hypothermia was not found to be an independent risk factor for mortality, PND, TND or renal failure requiring dialysis (55). Since that initial report, our experience has grown and we have continued to perform arch reconstructions at more moderate levels of hypothermia. In our recent study, we compared the outcomes of 257 patients undergoing arch reconstruction at 24.3°C to 265 patients undergoing arch reconstruction using at 28.5 °C. Both groups had adjunctive uSACP. There was no difference in mortality, TND or renal failure requiring dialysis between the two groups. The Stroke rate, cardiopulmonary bypass, cross clamp, post op ventilator times and ICU and hospital lengths of stay were all reduced in the 28.5°C group (Table 2) (59). We feel that these results add to the growing body of literature which supports the strategy of moderate hypothermic circulatory arrest + uSACP as a highly effective cerebral protection strategy for aortic arch replacement (36, 54, 55, 56).

	Mild (>26°C) n=265	Moderate (22-26°C) n=257	P
Temperature (°C)	28.5 ±1.1	24.3 ± 1.3	<0.01
Mortality	5.8%	7.8%	0.37
Stroke	1.5%	4.7%	0.04
TND	3.9%	5.1%	0.49
Dialysis	3.9%	3.9%	0.61
CPB (min)	183 ± 57	209 ± 67	<0.01
Cross Clamp (min)	145 ± 55	162 ± 65	<0.01
HCA (min)	29 ± 14	34 ± 18	<0.01
Ventilator time (hours)	44 ± 101	69 ± 128	0.02
ICU Stay (hours)	102 ± 144	127 ± 149	0.06
Hospital stay (Days)	9.5 ± 7.8	10.8 ± 7.2	0.06

TND=Temporary Neurologic Dysfunction, HCA=Hypothermic Circulatory Arrest,*P<0.05

Table 2. Comparative Analysis of Perioperative Data and Outcomes between Patients undergoing Aortic Arch Reconstruction at Mild vs. Moderate levels of Hypothermia. From Leshnower BG, Thourani VH, Myung RJ, et al. Aortic Arch Reconstruction at 28°C: A Comparative Analysis of Outcomes using Mild vs Moderate Hypothermia. *Ann Thorac Surg* Submitted.

4. Conclusion

Overall outcomes of patients undergoing aortic arch surgery have significantly improved over the past 3 decades. Advancements in surgical technique, prosthetic grafts and most importantly cerebral protection strategies have all contributed to better results. Despite the evidence presented in the preceding paragraphs, the optimal method of cerebral protection for arch reconstruction remains a controversial topic. All of these data are observational or retrospective studies. Due to surgeon bias and the limited number of arch cases performed, it is unlikely that there will ever be a prospective, randomized, controlled trial to determine the "gold standard" method of cerebral protection.

As we have demonstrated, there are many different methods of cerebral protection which range from simple to complex. The arterial cannulation site, level of hypothermia, and the use of adjunctive cerebral perfusion are factors which have been shown to impact neurologic outcomes following arch reconstruction. It is highly likely that most cardiothoracic surgeons do 1-2 arch reconstructions/year (usually in the setting of Type A dissection) and are most comfortable using DHCA at 18°C with femoral cannulation as their sole method of cerebral protection (Personal communications). The cerebral protection conferred by deep hypothermia is undisputed, and for short circulatory arrest times (<30 minutes) the addition of RCP or ACP may not significantly impact neurologic outcomes. However it is generally agreed upon that for prolonged circulatory arrest times (>45) minutes, adjunctive ACP or RCP should be utilized. When using MHCA, ACP must be employed as it is the only adjunctive method reported with more moderate levels of hypothermia. Animal studies have demonstrated equivalent bilateral perfusion with the use of uSACP or bSACP, and clinical data has reported excellent neurologic outcomes with either method (43, 54, 55, 57). Surgeons should be familiar with the technical aspects of all of these different methods of cerebral protection. The arch pathology of each individual patient is different and may dictate the optimal method of cerebral protection on an individual case basis.

5. References

[1] Griepp RB, Stinson EB, Hollingsworth JF, Buehler D. Prosthetic replacement of the aortic arch. J Thorac Cardiovasc Surg 1975;70:1051-63.

[2] Chapman DW, Beazley HL, Peterson PK, Webb JA, Cooley DA. Annulo-aortic ectasia with cystic medial necrosis. Diagnosis and treatment. *Am J Cardiol* 1965;16(5):679-87.

[3] Coady MA, Rizzo JA, Hammond GL et al. Surgical intervention criteria for thoracic aortic aneurysms: A study of growth rates and complications. *Ann Thorac Surg* 67:1922-1926, 1999.

[4] Hiratzka LF, Bakris GL, Beckman JA et al. 2010 ACCF / AHA /AATS / ACR / ASA / SCA / SCAI / SIR / STS / SVM Guidelines for the Diagnosis and Management of Patients with Thoracic Aortic Disease: A Report of the American College of Cardiology Foundation/American Heart Association Task Force on Practice Guidelines, American Association for Thoracic Surgery, Amercian College of Radiology, American Stroke Association, Society of Cardiovascular Anesthesiologists, Society for Cardiovascular Angiography and Interventions, Society of Interventional Radiology, Society of Thoracic Surgeons, and Society for Vascular Medicine. *Circulation* 121:e266-e369, 2010.

[5] Lewis FJ, Taufic M. Closure of atrial septal defects with the aid of hypothermia: Experimental accomplishments and the report of one successful case. *Surgery* 1953; 33:52.

[6] Borst GH, Schaudig A, Rudolph W. Arteriovenous fistula of the aortic arch repair during deep hypothermia and circulatory arrest. *J Thorac Cardiovasc Surg* 1964;3:443.

[7] Lillehei CW, Todd DB, Levy MJ et al. Partial cardiopulmonary bypass, hypothermia and total circulatory arrest: a lifesaving technique for ruptured mycotic aneurysms, ruptured left ventricle and other complicated aortic pathology. *J Thorac Cardiovasc Surg* 1969;58:530.

[8] McCullough JN, Zhang N, Reich DL et al. Cerebral metabolic suppresion during hypothermic circulatory arrest in humans. Ann Thorac Surg 1999; 67:1895-1921.

[9] Harrington DK, Fragomeni F, Bonser RS. Cerebral Perfusion. *Ann Thorac Surg* 2007;83:S799-804.

[10] Spielvogel D, Mathur MN, Griepp RB. Aneurysms of the Aortic Arch Aneurysms. In: Cohn LH, ed. *Cardiac Surgery in the Adult.* New York, NY: McGraw Hill:1251-1276, 2008.

[11] Bonser R, Wong C, Harrington DK, et al. Failure of retrograde cerebral perfusion to attenuate metabolic changes associated with hypothermic circulatory arrest. *J Thorac Cardiovasc Surg* 2002;123:943-50.

[12] Mault J, Ohtake S, Klingensmith M, Heinle J, Greeley W, Ungerleider R. Cerebral metabolism and circulatory arrest: effects of duration and strategies for protection. *Ann Thorac Surg* 1993;1993:57-64.

[13] Hagl C, Khaladi N, Weisz DJ, et al. Impact of high intracranial pressure on neurophysiological recovery and behavior in a chronic porcine model of hypothermic circulatory arrest. *Eur J Cardiothorac Surg* 2002;22(4):510-6.

[14] Svensson LG, Blackstone EH, Rajeswaran J et al. Does the arterial cannulation site for circulatory arrest influence stroke risk? Ann Thorac Surg 2004; 78:1274-84.

[15] Ergin MA, Galla JD, Lansman SL, Quintana C, Bodian C, Griepp RB. Hypothermic circulatory arrest in operations on the thoracic aorta. Determinanats of operative mortality and neurologic outcome. J Thorac Cardiovasc Surg 1994; 107:788-97.

[16] Kamiya H, Hagl C, Kropivnitskaya I et al. The safety of moderate hypothermic lower body circulatory arrest with selective cerebral perfusion: a propensity score analysis. J Thorac Cardiovasc Surg 2007; 133:501-9.

[17] Ergin MA, Uysal S, Reich DL, Apaydin A, Lansman SL, McCullough JN, Griepp RB. Temporary neurologic dysfunction after deep hypothermic circulatory arrest: a clinical marker of long-term functional deficit. Ann Thorac Surg 1999; 67:1887-1894.

[18] Svensson LG, Crawford ES, Hess KR, et al. Deep hypothermia with circulatory arrest. Determinants of stroke and early mortality in 656 patients. *J Thorac Cardiovasc Surg*1993;106:19-31.

[19] Ehrlich MP, Ergin MA, McCullough JN, et al. Predictors of adverse outcome and transient neurologic dysfunction after ascending aorta/hemiarch replacement. *Ann Thorac Surg* 2000; 69:1755-63.

[20] Reich DL, Uysal S, Silwinski M, et al. Neuropsychologic outcome after deep hypothermic circulatory arrest in adults. *J Thorac Cardiovasc Surg* 1999;117(1):156-63.

[21] Griepp RB, Bonser R, Haverich A, et al. Panel Discussion: Session II-Aortic Arch from the Aortic Surgery Symposium X. *Ann Thorac Surg* 2007;83:S824-31.

[22] Mills NL, Ochsner JL. Massive air embolism during cardiopulmonary bypass: causes, preventions, and management. *J Thorac Cardiovasc Surg* 1980;80:708.

[23] Boeckxstans CJ, Fleming WJ. Retrograde cerebral perfusion does not protect the brain in non-human primates. *Ann Thorac Surg* 1995;60:319.

[24] Ye J, Yang L, Del Rigio MR, et al. Retrograde cerebral perfusion provides limited distribution of blood to the brain: a study in pigs. *J Thorac Cardiovasc Surg* 1997;114:660.

[25] Ehrlich MP, Hagl C, McCullough JN, et al. Retrograde cerebral perfusion provides negligibleflow through brain capillaries in the pig. *J Thorac Cardiovasc Surg* 122:331.

[26] Juvonen T, Zhang N, Wolfe D, et al. Retrograde cerebral perfusion enhances cerebral protection during prolonged hypothermic circulatory arrest: a study in a chronic porcine model. *Ann Thorac Surg* 1998;66(1):38-50.

[27] Bavaria JE, Pochettino A, Brinster DR, et al. New paradigms and improved results for the surgical treatment of acute type A dissection. *Ann Surg* 2001;234(3):336-42.

[28] Coselli JS, Lemaire SA. Experience with retrograde cerebral perfusion during proximal aortic surgery in 290 patients. *J Card Surg* 1997;12(2):322-5.

[29] Estrera Al, Miller III CC, Lee TY, Shah P, Safi HJ. Ascending and Transverse Aortic Arch Repair: The Impact of Retrograde Cerebral Perfusion. *Circulation* 2008;188:S160-S166.

[30] Okita Y, Takamoto S, Ando M, Morota T, Matsukawa R, Kawashima Y. Mortality and cerebral outcome in patients who underwent aortic arch operations using deep hypothermic circulatory arrest with retrograde cerebral perfusion: no relation of early death, stroke and delirium to the duration of circulatory arrest. *J Thorac Cardiovasc Surg* 1998; 115(1):129-38.

[31] Hagl C, Ergin MA, Galla JD et al. Neurologic outcome after ascending aorta-aortic arch operations: effect of brain protection technique in high-risk patients. *J Thorac Cardiovasc Surg* 2001; 121:1107-21.

[32] Moon MR, Sundt TM 3rd. Influence of retrograde cerebral perfusion during aortic arch procedures. *Ann Thorac Surg* 2002; 74(2):426-31.

[33] Milewski RK, Pacini D, Moser GW, et al. Retrograde and Antegrade Cerebral Perfusion: Results in Short Elective Arch Reconstructive Times. *Ann Thorac Surg* 2010;89:1448-57.

[34] Safi HJ, Miller III CC, Lee TY, Estrera AL. Repair of ascending and transverse aortic arch. *J Thoraci Cardiovasc Surg* 2011; 142:630-33.

[35] DeBakey ME, Crawford ES, Cooley DA, et al. Successful resection of fusiform aneurysm of the aortic arch with replacement homograft. *Surg Gynecol Obstet* 1957; 105:657.

[36] Bachet J, Guilmet D, Boudot B, et al. Cold cerebroplegia. A new technique of cerebral protection during operations on the transverse aortic arch. *J Thorac Cardovasc Surg* 1991;102(1):85-94.

[37] Kazui T, Inoue N, Yamada O, Komatsu S. Selective cerebral perfusion during operations for aneurysms of the aortic arch: a reassessment. *Ann Thorac Surg* 1992;53(1):109-14.

[38] Hagl C, Khaladj N, Peterss S, et al. Hypothermic circuloatory arrest with and without cold selective antegrade cerebral perfusion: impact on neurolocial recoveray and issue metabolism in an acute porcine model. *Eur J Cardiothorac Surg* 2004;26:73-80.

[39] Filgueiras CL, Winsborrow B, Ye J, et al. A 31p-magnetic resonance study of antegrade and regtrograde cerebral perfusion during aortic arch surgery in pigs. *J Thorac Cardovasc Surg* 1995;110(1):55-62.

[40] Filgueiras CL, Ryner L, Ye J, et al. Cerebral protection during moderate hypothermic circulatory arrest: histopathology and magnetic resonance spectroscopy of brain energetics and intracellular pH in pigs. *J Thorac Cardiovasc Surg.* 1996;112(4):1073-80.

[41] Strauch JT, Spielvogel D, Lauten A, et al. Optimal temperature for selective cerebral perfusion. *J Thorac Cardiovasc Surg* 2005;130(1):74-82.

[42] Strauch JT, Spielvogel D, Haldenwang PL, et al. Cerebral physiology and outcome after hypothermic circulatory arrest followed by selective cerebral perfusion. *Ann Thorac Surg* 2003;76(6):1972-81.

[43] Ye J, Dai G, Ryner LN, et al. Unilateral antegrade cerebral perfusion through the right axillary artery provides uniform flow distribution to both hemispheres of the brain: A magnetic resonance and histopathological study in pigs. *Circulation* 1999. 100 (19 Suppl):II309-15.

[44] Tanoue Y, Tominaga R, Ochiai Y et al. Comparative study of retrograde and selective cerebral perfusion with transcranial Doppler. *Ann Thorac Surg* 1999;67:672-675.

[45] Neri E, Sassi C Barabesi L, et al. Cerebral autoregulation after hypothermic circulatory arrest in operations on the aortic arch. *Ann Thorac Surg* 2004;77:72-79.

[46] Okita Y, Minatoya K, Tagusari O, Ando M, Nagatsuka K, Kitamura S. Prospective comparative study of brain protection in total aortic arch replacement: deep hypothermic circulatory arrest with retrograde cerebral perfusion or selective antegrade cerebral perfusion. Ann Thorac Surg 2001; 72:72-9.

[47] Apostolakis E, Koletsis EN, Dedeilias P et al. Antegrade versus retrograde cerebral perfusion in relation to postoperative complications following aortic surgery for acute aortic dissection type A. J Card Surg 2008; 23:480-7.

[48] Yuan X, Theruvath AJ, Ge X, et al. Machine perfusion or cold storage in organ transplantation: indication, mechanisms, and future perspectives. *Transplant International* 2010;23(6):561-70.

[49] Mora Mangano CT, Neville MJ, Hsu PH, Mignea I, King J, Miller, DC. Aprotinin, blood loss and renal dysfunction in deep hypothermic circulatory arrest. Circulation 2001; 104:276-81

[50] Cooper WA, Duarte IG, Thourani VH et al. Hypothermic circulatory arrest causes multi-system vascular endothelial dysfunction and apoptosis. Ann Thorac Surg 2000;69:696-702.

[51] Hagl C, Tatton NA, Khadalaj N et al. Involvement of apoptosis in neurological injury after hypothermic circulatory arrest: a new target for therapeutic intervention? Ann Thorac Surg 2001;72:1457-64.

[52] Augoustides JG, Pochettino A, Ochroch EA et al. Renal dysfunction after thoracic aortic surgery requiring deep hypothermic circulatory arrest: definition, incidence, and clinical predictors. J Cardiothorac Vasc Anesth 2006; 20: 673-7.

[53] Ergin MA, Griepp EB, Lansman SL, Galla JD, Levy M, Griepp RB. Hypothermic circulatory arrest and other methods of cerebral protection during operations on the thoracic aorta. J Card Surg 1994; 9:525-37.

[54] Minatoya K, Ogino H, Matsuda H et al. Evolving selective cerebral perfusion for aortic arch replacement: high flow rate with moderate hypothermic circulatory arrest. Ann Thorac Surg 2008; 861827-31.

[55] Leshnower BG, Myung RJ, Kilgo PD, et al. Moderate Hypothermia and Unilateral Selective Antegrade Cerebral Perfusion: A Contemporary Cerebral Protection Strategy for Aortic Arch Surgery. *Ann Thorac Surg* 2010;90(2):547-54.

[56] Khaladj N, Shrestha M, Meck S et al. Hypothermic circulatory arrest with selective antegrade cerebral perfusion in ascending aortic and aortic arch surgery: a risk factor analysis for adverse outcome in 501 patients. J Thorac Cardiovasc Surg 2008; 135: 908-14.

[57] DiEusanio M, Tan ME, Schepens MA, Dossche KM, DiBartolomeo R, Pierangeli A, Morshuis WJ. Surgery for acute type A using antegrade selective cerebral perfusion: experience with 122 patients. Ann Thorac Surg 2003; 75:514-9.

[58] Halkos ME, Kerendi F, Myung R, Kilgo P, Puskas JD, Chen EP. Selective antegrade cerebral perfusion via right axillary artery cannulation reduces morbidity and mortality after proximal aortic surgery. J Thorac Cardiovasc Surg 2009; 138:1081-9.

[59] Leshnower BG, Thourani VH, Myung RJ, et al. Aortic Arch Reconstruction at 28°C: A Comparative Analysis of Outcomes using Mild vs Moderate Hypothermia. *Ann Thorac Surg* Submitted.

13

Recent Advances in the Management of Acute Aortic Syndrome

Laszlo Göbölös[1,3*] et al.,
[1]*Department of Cardiothoracic Surgery, University Hospital Regensburg,*
[2]*Institute for Clinical Chemistry and Laboratory Medicine, University Hospital Regensburg,*
[3]*Department Cardiothoracic Surgery, Southampton General Hospital, Southampton University Hospital Trust,*
[1,2]*Germany*
[3]*United Kingdom*

1. Introduction

Type A acute aortic dissection is one of the most serious cardiovascular conditions and is associated with significant morbidity and mortality. A half century ago, Hirst et al published a milestone article describing the linearized mortality rate of one percent per hour after the onset of an ascending aortic dissection [1]. Hence, the importance of accurate, quick and reliable diagnosis, as the timing of procedure is vital for optimal management of this highly lethal condition. Despite improvements in the diagnostic modalities, surgical techniques and perioperative care, the overall mortality remains high, between 10% and 30% [2].

Due to its major role in systemic perfusion, the aorta and its main branches after dissection are often challenging when trying to prevent surgical morbidity and mortality. The complexity of aortic dissection presents not only a pure cardiovascular surgical task, but also consideration must be given to protection of the myocardium, cerebrum, peripheral tissues and organs. An early fatal result of aortic dissection is due to ischaemic injury to the brain or heart, although longer peripheral ischaemia can cause multiorgan failure resulting in extended hospital stay, increased morbidity and mortality. Alexis Carrel highlighted the risks of surgery in 1910 with the following short summary on aortic interventions: "The main danger of the aortic operation does not come from the heart or from the aorta itself, but from the central nervous system." Even a century later, we are still trying to optimize cerebral protection, despite having significantly wider range of diagnostic and therapeutic modalities.

Advances in our understanding of varying pathologies of aortic dissections have improved as have the technological developments in the modes of detection. These advances together with improved therapeutic options have raised expectations for better outcomes.

Maik Foltan[1], Peter Ugocsai[2], Andrea Thrum[1], Alois Philipp[1], Steven A. Livesey[3], Geoffrey M. Tsang[3] and Sunil K. Ohri[3]

2. Acute aortic syndrome

The term "acute aortic syndrome" (AAS) became widely accepted in the last decade. It involves not only aortic dissections, but intramural haematomas and penetrating atherosclerotic ulcers in the same anatomical location. This constellation of presentations have similar emergency status, diagnostic and therapeutic requirements. As a definition, AAS is an acute pathophysiological process involving the tunica media of aortic wall, which results in rupture or any further life-threatening complications.

2.1 Epidemiology

Population-based epidemiological studies suggest an incidence of AAS of about thirty cases per one million people per year. Eighty percent is represented by acute aortic dissections, 15% by intramural haematomas and 5% as penetrating ulcers. Seventy percent of the affected population is male with an average of 60 years [3]. A Swedish epidemiological study found the same incidence in an observational period between 1987 and 2002 among 4425 cases. In this study, the incidence of AAS has increased by 50% in men and 30% in women over study period. This may be related to enhanced diagnostics, although a further component could also be the increasing age of the population. Overall, 20% of affected patients died before reaching a medical facility, 30% during the hospital stay and further 20% over the following 10 years [4]. Both circadian and seasonal variations have been observed in the occurrence of AAS, with the peak frequency found between 0800hr and 0900hr, with an increased likelihood during the winter period. The most likely explanation is a link to the circadian variation in blood pressure [5, 6].

2.2 Pathophysiology

The mechanisms leading to AAS arise from many sources, although preexisting medial degeneration is proven to be an important risk factor for acute aortic dissection. Cystic medial necrosis is a hallmark of the histology, especially in aortic aneurysm patients. Microscopic features include decreased amount of vascular smooth-muscle cells, mucoid deposits and elastin deficiency [7]. However, over 80% of acute dissections occur in absence of a pre-existing aneurysm. The International Registry of Acute Aortic Dissection (IRAD) has collected an impressive amount of data for the demography of patients who present with AAS. The most commonly associated factors are:

- Hypertension
- Atherosclerosis
- Elderly
- Previous cardiovascular surgery, especially previous aortic aneurysm or dissection repair
- Connective tissue disorders (Marfan`s syndrome, Ehlers-Danlos` syndrome, Erdheim-Gsell`s syndrome)
- Infective involvement of the aortic tissue (Lues, Takayashu aortitis)
- Congenital causes (PDA ampulla, Sinus of Valsava aneurysm, bicuspid aortic valve)
- External factors (Trauma, cocaine abuse)

Improvements in the resolution of aortic imaging has led to the identification of pathological submodalities, i.e. intramural haematoma or penetrating atherosclerotic ulcer. Histological findings of these lesions generally demonstrate significant intimal atherosclerosis, which is not a constant finding in aortic dissection biopsies. Studies suggest that aortic dissection is an end process with a wide pathological spectrum, many of which facilitate weakening and/or increased stress of the aortic wall. The chain of pathological events might begin with a small superficial intimal rupture; atherosclerotic ulcers may provide a good millieu for development of such a tear. Alternatively, disruption of vasa vasorum might result in an intramural haematoma, which later ruptures into the aortic lumen or leads to dissection. However, it is likely that many aortic dissections develop without having a pre-stage of intramural haematoma or penetrating ulcer [8].

2.3 Presentation and diagnosis

Although the typical symptom is described as sharp, tearing, ripping chest pain, the presentation is diverse and about 10% do not complain of pain; sometimes the aortic pathology is an accidental clinical finding. In some patients shoulder or back pain occurs or just a husky voice, with or without shortness of breath and/or haemophthysis. Hypotension or shock is seen in 25% of patients, whereas hypertension can also be a presenting symptom, although more often found in type B dissections. Further findings, such as migrating pain, neurological deficits, acute abdomen, cardiac failure, myocardial ischaemia, aortic valve regurgitation are less common. Connective tissue diseases are characterized by additional specific symptoms, i.e. skeletal, pharyngeal or lens abnormalities and extreme laxity [3].

Early acute diagnosis can be vital, as an emergency surgery may be indicated. Blood pressure control is essential, and a goal of systolic ≤110 mmHg is recommended. The administration of β-blockers, sodium-nitroprusside, calcium-channel-blockers with analgesia is helpful, if indicated. In some advanced dissections resustitative measurements such as intubation and pericardiocentesis may be required.

	Transthoracic echocardiography	Transoesophageal echocardiography	Computed tomography	Magnetic resonance imaging
Aortic dissection	+	+++	+++	+++
Intramural haematoma	-	++	++	+++
Penetrating ulcer	-	+	+++	+++
Dissection entry	+	+++	++	++
Aortic regurgitation	+++	+++	-	+++
Pericardial effusion	+++	+++	++	++
Periaortic bleeding	-	+	+++	+++

Table 1. Efficacy of different imaging modalities in AAS.

In patients with suspected acute aortic dissection various investigations are performed on admission including blood tests, electrocardiography, chest radiography, echocardiography, computed tomography and magnetic resonance imaging. Some investigations, such as ECG, chest radiography and routine blood tests do not carry sufficient sensitivity and specificity to exclude or confirm the diagnosis of an acute aortic dissection. Biomarker assays are increasingly utilized in the diagnosis of AAS, i.e. elastin fragments, smooth-muscle myosin heavy-chain protein, D-dimers, but are not widely available and provide only supporting evidence. The definite diagnosis can only be established using an imaging modality [9]. Table 1. summarizes efficacy of different imaging modalities in AAS. Table 2. shows the diagnostic features of the imaging modalities currently available in a hospital setting.

	Transthoracic echocardiography	Transoesophageal echocardiography	Computed tomography	Magnetic resonance imaging
Availability	+++	++	+++	+
Speed	+++	+++	++	+
Portability	+++	+++	-	-
Tolerance	+++	+	++	++
Monitoring	+++	++	++	++

Table 2. Diagnostic features of imaging modalities in AAS.

2.4 Management of AAS

Currently, there are no randomized trials available to guide the management of AAS. The European Society of Cardiology has developed guidelines for diagnosis and management of aortic dissection based on a task force of international societies [10], although in most of decision making clinical pathways are usually based on case series or registries, systematic reviews, local experience, consensus based guidelines. Following initial stabilization of the patient, after diagnostic measurements and imaging, a treatment should be tailored to the pathological entity:

- *Type A dissection*

Over 50% mortality in the first 48 hours without surgical intervention, only 1-10% survives the first 5 weeks on conservative treatment. The perioperative mortality is 10-30%. Contraindications are quite limited as type A dissection is a highly lethal condition without surgical treatment, although age >80 years, ongoing coma with definitive extensive cerebral lesions (but not localized ischaemia or paraplegia!) or extensive abdominal necrosis may be contraindications for surgery. A subacute type A dissection, is a rare finding that requires an elective/semi-urgent operation as the patient has already successfully survived the high mortality period may now benefit from a well planned elective procedure [10].

- *Intramural haematoma*

Classical therapeutic indication as for type A dissection, although in an uncomplicated and non-progressing situation, without ongoing pain and periaortic bleeding, patients can undergo surgery on an urgent basis (within 24 hours) rather than as an emergency. Over the age of 80 years, accompanied by significant comorbidities, conservative therapy in an intensive care facility with the support of repeat imaging should be considered. If sudden progression occurs, a surgical intervention may be life saving. In this patient group 40% of intramural haematomas resolve after 4 years of follow up without mortality according to a small patient cohort study [11]. Another study demonstrated 34% regression of the disease, while 36% progressed into a dissection (12% acute type A dissection, 24% localized dissection) and 30% resulted in aneurysm formation over long term. They have also demonstrated, that a rupture or dissection is a very rare phenomenon with an aortic diameter of <60 mm at any location with an intramural haematoma [9]. These observations guide the clinical management of intramural haematomas, despite the lack of large multicentric studies, each patient requires a tailored individual management plan. As penetrating atherosclerotic ulcers are usually incidental operative or postmortem findings and are seldom discovered at imaging, there are no widely discussed clinical therapeutic strategies available.

- *Typ B dissection*

As this diagnosis generally requires conservative medical treatment in an intensive care setting, we only briefly discuss the indications for surgery. Medical treatment is associated with a mortality of 20%, compared to surgery, which has much higher mortality of 30%; medical therapy is therefore considered first. Classical operative indications are progressive organ malperfusion, ongoing pain with uncontrollable hypertension. In the last decade stent grafting of the affected region has become an alternative option as it can treat these problems at a low risk profile in most of the cases and without need for further cardiovascular surgery [12].

3. Surgical considerations and recent techniques for repair of type A dissections

3.1 Perfusion approaches in type A dissections

Cannulation of an extended type A dissection often represents a challenge for surgeons when either the subclavian or lower limb arteries are involved in the process. There are some alternative cannulation sites published in current literature i.e. brachiocephalic trunk, right common carotid artery, transapical cannulation, although we prefer an innovative method through non dissected aortic wall on lesser curvature at level of Botallo`s ligament using a Seldinger technique.

Our first experience was a 50 year-old man with sudden onset of ripping chest pain, admitted unconscious accompanied by anisochoria. Computed tomography scan revealed an extensive type A aortic dissection. The dissection began exactly over the aortic valve; maximal diameter of ascending aorta measured 60 x 55 mm. On the lesser curvature of arch, particularly at Botallo`s ligament, preservation of the true lumen with an intact wall was observed, although the dissection involved all supraaortic vessels. Visceral arteries originated from the true lumen except the left renal artery. Dissection in both iliac arteries was also present. Rapid deterioration of the patient with cardiovascular instability led us to cannulate at Botallo`s ligament applying a minimal invasive cannulation method with a Seldinger technique [Figure 1, 2]. At Botallo`s ligament the aorta is firmly bound to pulmonary trunk with a mass of connective tissue, which usually protects it from a complete dissection in this area. Position of cannula has to be guided by either transoesophageal or epiaortic ultrasonography. With this rapid and safe cannulation method extracorporeal circulation can be easily established, thus reducing the risk of perioperative shock and increased mortality [13].

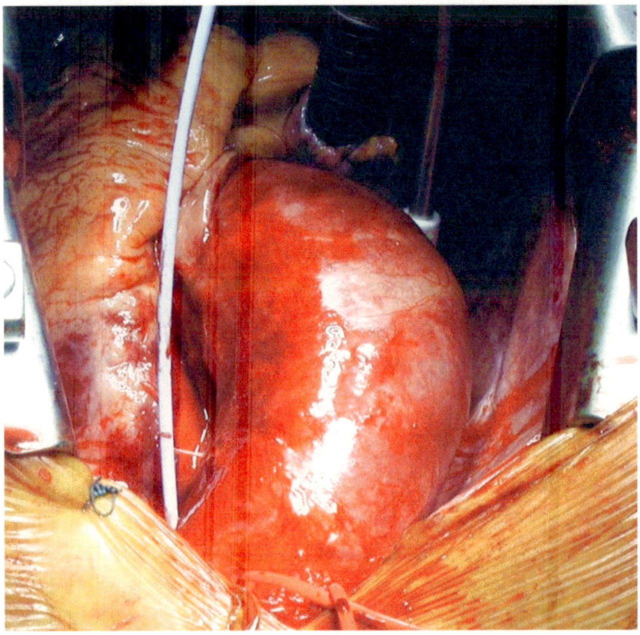

Fig. 1. Seldinger cannulation of a type A aortic dissection (first dialation step)

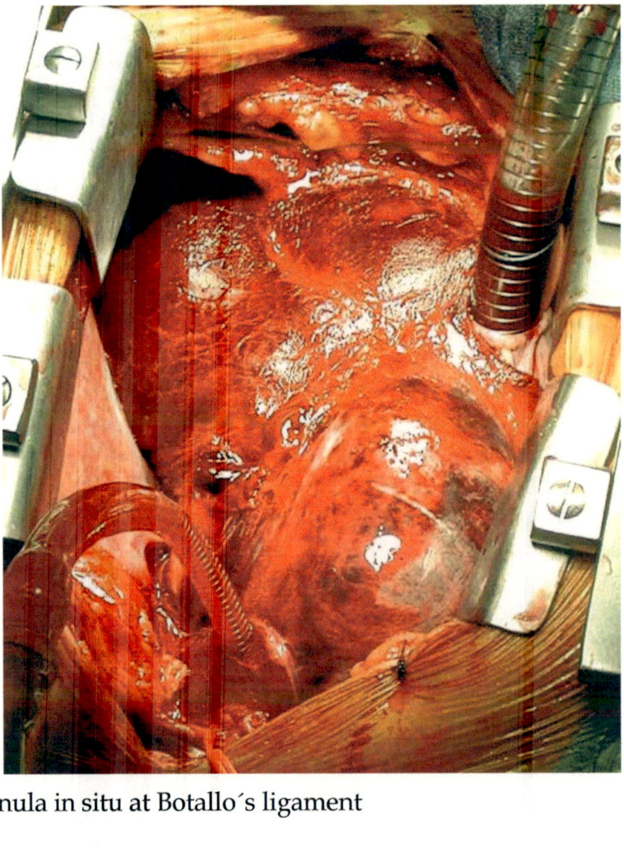

Fig. 2. Arterial cannula in situ at Botallo´s ligament

Cardiopulmonary bypass via axillary/subclavian artery has become an alternative perfusion site in the past decade, predominantly in acute aortic dissections but also for patients with severe aortic atherosclerosis [14-20]. Despite several advantages of axillary/subclavian artery cannulation such as dominantly antegrade perfusion of the aorta, this technique is not without its complications. Establishment of axillary/subclavian artery inflow may not be ideal for providing rapid antegrade perfusion in cases with hemodynamic instability, as dissection and cannulation can take too long. In small patients, a limitation of CPB pump flow due to a narrow axillary artery may be a concern [21, 22]. Applying the standard technique, however, only the right hemisphere is continuously perfused, which can result in malperfusion of the contralateral hemisphere, as Merkkola et al demonstrated, up to 17% of the patients having incomplete circle of Willis [23]. Even with a complete circle of Willis, concern has been raised, if this type of perfusion alone can sufficiently supply the left hemisphere.

Transapical cannulation is another technique for establishing reliable antegrade arterial access, as described by Wada et al [24]. In large cohort of 138 patients, cannula was placed through a 1 cm apical incision into true lumen via aortic valve under transoesophageal echocardiography guidance. Impact of causing an acute aortic insufficiency in this context is not discussed in detail. This technique carries disadvantage of resulting in prolonged cardiopulmonary bypass times, since no additional manipulations can be performed during cooling phase, i.e. inspection and preparation of aortic root.

Right carotid artery cannulation, performed by Urbanski in 100 patients, including 27 with type A dissections, provides another possible alternative, but also carries the risk of left hemisphere malperfusion and potential complications when the vessel is de-cannulated [25]. Experience with innominate artery cannulation by Di Eusanio et al includes 55 patients with only two in acute aortic dissections [26], so it is difficult to evaluate the efficacy of this method due to the small experience.

Fusco at al presented their results in femoral artery cannulation in 2004 [27]. With a conversion rate of 2.5% to ascending aortic cannulation, they conclude that femoral cannulation is appropriate and yields excellent clinical results. They are not aware of having encountered retrograde embolism from the descending aorta, probably since atherosclerosis is less common in dissection patients.

3.2 Cerebral protection in dissection surgery

Avoiding neurological damage is one of the main aims of dissection surgery, as Carrel emphasised a century ago. Deep hypothermia with circulatory arrest (HCA) is the most common technique for cerebral protection in aortic surgery with a well defined safe period for circulatory arrest, of 45-50 minutes at a core temperature of 20°C. Systemic hypothermia to extend the period of safe cerebral ischaemia has been the mainstay of neuroprotection for many decades [28, 29]. Safety of this approach relies on adequate systemic cooling and if this is incomplete, it risks the patient for neurological injury. Introduction of selective antegrade carotid perfusion (ACP) has prolonged this safe period. A combination of cold selective antegrade cerebral perfusion and deep/moderate hypothermic circulatory arrest allows adequate protection for the body and is not associated with higher risk of cerebral microemboli [30, 31]. The efficacy of selective antegrade cerebral perfusion as an adjunctive to hypothermic arrest has been proven by numerous publications [32, 33].

Unilateral brain perfusion, i.e. right subclavian/axillary artery, right carotid artery, brachiocephalic trunk is safe under monitoring with near infrared spectroscopy (NIRS), as nearly 1/5 of the population has an incomplete circle of Willis. Therefore a significant number of patients require bilateral ACP, on the other hand, in the rest population it is still debatable, if in left haemisphere the same temperature can be achieved as the contralateral hemisphere, with unilateral perfusion, after blood has perfused the right side. Further concern is raised with unilateral perfusion, that by aiming for bilateral equal brain saturations, the right haemisphere is may be slightly overperfused, leading to right hemishperal oedema. Near infrared spectroscopy does not provide this type of information, so unilateral perfusion enhances but cannot guarantee cerebral protection. These latter considerations require further research, although applying bilateral ACP may resolve these issues.

In our practice, during HCA, selective antegrade cerebral perfusion is applied through both carotid arteries (DLP Retrograde Coronary Sinus Perfusion Cannula with manual Inflating Cuff®, Medtronic Inc., Minneapolis, USA) at a flow rate adapted to keep a constant cerebral O_2 saturation each side with a perfusion pressure of 35-40 mmHg [Figure 3]. Cerebral monitoring is performed using NIRS, with the aim of maintaining brain tissue oxygen saturation measures at 65-70% continuously during perfusion, which should correspond to the induction values.

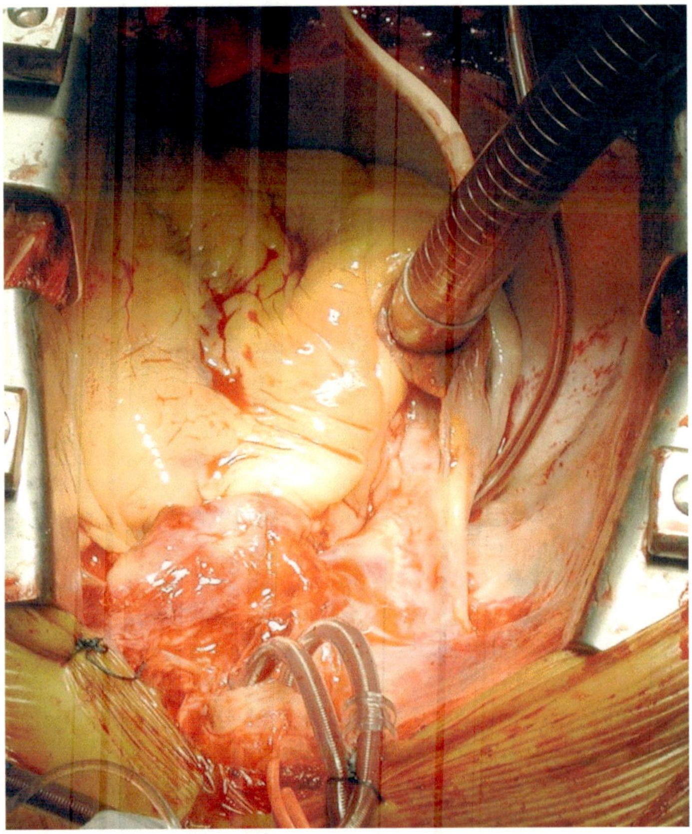

Fig. 3. Selective antegrade carotid perfusion

Retrograde cerebral perfusion via superior vena cava may also be undertaken, although in arch surgery carotids are available for ACP. If the carotids are severely destroyed by dissection, retrograde cerebral perfusion may be considered as an option, so long carotids are replaced by tube grafts. However, retrograde cerebral perfusion is associated with a significantly higher incidence of temporary neurological complications, later extubation, longer ICU-stay, hospitalization, than ACP [34].

In a study of 4670 patients who underwent extensive aortic surgery between 1985 and 2002 at the Heart Centre Leipzig, Germany, superiority of ACP over retrograde cerebral perfusion or stand-alone deep hypothermia was confirmed. ACP was associated with 5-14% mortality and 4-10% permanent neurological deficit, retrograde cerebral perfusion showed 12-22%; 10-20%, stand- alone deep hypothermia 15-30%; 8-24%, respectively.

Rigorous patient temperature monitoring is crucial to a balanced cerebral protection during CPB. As a standard body temperature measurement, rectal monitoring has been widely used for decades in many departments. In the past decade tympanic and urinary bladder temperature monitoring has been studied and suggested as an alternative to gold standard. Tympanic measurements provide a very good estimation of the brain temperature with minimal delay in the changes due to its close proximity to the central nervous system [35, 36]. Tympanic measurements are well established even in everyday body temperature measurement with portable thermometers in general health care. However, to obtain reliable values from the tympanic membrane, debris free status of the ear channel has to be proven by otoscopy prior to placement of probe, followed by a good heat insulation of ears by i.e. using swabs to prevent accidental heat loss due to theatre ventilation system.

Urinary probes are available built into urinary catheters, so their placement is very convenient, although measurement reliability depends slightly on urine flow [37]. Rectal measurements are less reliable, since faecal matter prevents sudden heat exchange [38]. Nasopharyngeal/oesophageal temperature monitoring in HCA as standard measurement site, has limitations as it may significantly over- and underestimate brain temperatures during the cooling and rewarming phases [39-41]. Akata et al have furthermore demonstrated, that pulmonary artery temperatures closely reflect changes in brain temperatures, but nasopharyngeal/oesophageal measurements could not be considered as a reliable index of brain temperature during the rapid induction of moderate/deep hypothermia [42].

4. Follow-up

As aortic dissections often develop on a background of preexisting aortic aneurysms, this mandates regular follow-up in these patients to facilitate elective intervention when required. These elective operations carry less risks as the patient can be thoroughly prepared using the ideal imaging modalities and optimizing the patient's medical condition for major surgery. At the Department of Cardiothoracic Surgery, University Hospital Regensburg, Germany there is a regular aortic day-clinic available on weekly basis for pre- and postoperative follow-ups, that has been running for over a decade, which allows this endangered patient population to be monitored on a 6-monthly basis. Regular postoperative monitoring is essential to provide good long term results with the early discovery of endo-leaks, progression of aortopathy, control of hypertension, etc. As the AAS population is

young, average age of involved is sixty years [3], regular follow up contributes to the restoration of health in this still relatively active age group.
Patients with AAS have a long-term outcome which is less favorable when associated with a past medical history of previous cardiac surgery or generalized atherosclerosis [43]. Surgical repair has been recommended when maximal ascending aortic diameter reaches 50 mm (45 mm at Marfan´s syndrome) or 60 mm when involving the descending aorta, although decision making has to be individualized to patient and other comorbidities [10]. Blood pressure control is essential for these patients, with the aim of maintaining the blood pressure no more than 130/80 mmHg [44]. If there is a well know hereditary component present, the patient´s complete family should be offered the opportunity to be genetically tested and councilled.
Some recent publications have already highlighted the role of angiotensin II in progression of aortic aneurysms, although the relative contribution of its type 1 (AT1) and type 2 (AT2) receptors remain unknown. Habashi et al demonstrated that loss of AT2 expression accelerates the aberrant growth and rupture of aorta in a mouse model of Marfan`s syndrome. Losartan, a selective AT1 blocker reduces aneurysm progression in mice; a full protection required intact AT2 signaling. The angiotensin-converting enzyme inhibitor enalapril, which limits signaling through both receptors, is less effective. Both drugs attenuated transforming growth factor-ß (TGF ß) signaling in the aorta, but losartan uniquely inhibited TGF ß-mediated activation of extracellular signal regulated kinase, by allowing continued signaling through AT2, which shows the protective nature of AT2 signaling and the choice of therapy in aortic aneurysms [45].
International multicentric studies are currently evaluating the possible pharmacological prevention and postoperative medical supportive therapy options in Marfan´s syndrome provided by AT1 blockers, especially losartan in a combination with a ß-blocker, such as nebivolol. The key molecule in aortic aneurysms, TGF ß, normally attached to extracellular matrix, is free and activated. Under experimental circumstances, TGF ß blockade prevents aortic wall damage and dilatation. AT1 blockers exert an anti-TGF ß effect; trials are now ongoing for evaluating the effect of losartan compared with atenolol or nebivolol. The third generation ß-blocker nebivolol retains the ß-adrenergic blocker effects on heart rate and further exerts antistiffness effects, typically increased in aortic aneurysms [46, 47].
After evaluation these ongoing human studies we have more insight to the pharmacological support of AAS and aortic aneurysms, which completes the surgical management possibilities of this severe disease group.

5. References

[1] Hirst AE, Johns Vr, Kime SW. Dissecting aneurysm of the aorta: a review of 505 cases. Medicine (Baltimore) 1958;37:217-279.
[2] Ehrlich MP, Ergin MA, McCullough JN, Lansman SL, Galla JD, Bodian CA, Apaydin A, Griepp RB. Results of immediate surgical treatment of all acute type A dissections. Circulation 2000;102: 248-252.
[3] Hagan PG, Nienaber CA, Isselbacher EM, Bruckman D, Karavite DJ, Russman PL; International Registry of Acute Aortic Dissection (IRAD). New insights into an old disease. JAMA 2000;283:897-903.

[4] Olsson C, Thelin S, Stahle E, Ekbom A, Granath F. Thoracic aortic aneurysm and dissection: increasing prevalence and improved outcomes reported in a nationwide population-based study of more than 14000 cases from 1987 to 2002. Circulation 2006;114:2611-2618.
[5] Mehta RH, Manfredini R, Hassan F, Sechtem U, Bossone E, Oh JK, Cooper JV, Smith DE, Portaluppi F, Penn M, Hutchison S, Nienaber CA, Isselbacher EM, Eagle KA; International Registry of Acute Aortic Dissection (IRAD) Investigators. Chronobiological patterns of acute aortic dissection. Circulation 2002;106:1110-1115.
[6] Millar-Craig MW, Bishop CN, Raftery EB. Circadian variation of blood pressure. Lancet 1978;311:795-797.
[7] Boutouyrie P, Germain DP, Fiessinger JN, Laloux B, Perdu J, Laurent S. Increased carotid wall stress in vascular Ehlers-Danlos syndrome. Circulation 2004;109:1530-1535.
[8] Golledge J, Eagle KA. Acute aortic dissection. Lancet 2008;372:55-66.
[9] Evangelista Masip A. Progress in the acute aortic syndrome. Rev Esp Cardiol 2007;60:428-439.
[10] Erbel R, Alfonso F, Boileau C, Dirsch O, Eber B, Haverich A, Rakowski H, Struyven J, Radegran K, Sechtem U, Taylor J, Zollikofer C, Klein WW, Mulder B, Providencia LA; Task Force on Aortic Dissection, European Society of Cardiology. Diagnosis and management of aortic dissection. Eur Heart J 2001;22:1642-1681.
[11] Kaji S, Akasaka T, Horibata Y, Nishigami K, Shono H, Katayama M, Yamamuro A, Morioka S, Morita I, Tanemoto K, Honda T, Yoshida K. Long-term prognosis of patients with type a aortic intramural hematoma. Circulation 2002;106: 248-252.
[12] Arts CHP, Muhs BE, Moll FL, Verhagen HJM. Endovascular management of type B aortic dissection. In: Davies AH, Mitchell AWM, eds. Vascular and endovascular surgery highlights 2006-2007. Abingdon: Health Press, 2007.
[13] Göbölös L, Philipp A, Foltan M, Wiebe K. Surgical management for Stanford type A aortic dissection: direct cannulation of real lumen at the level of the Botallo's ligament by Seldinger technique. Interact Cardiovasc Thorac Surg. 2008; 6:1107-1109.
[14] Schachner T, Vertacnik K, Laufer G, Bonatti J. Axillary artery cannulation in surgery of the ascending aorta and the aortic arch. Eur J Cardiothorac Surg 2002; 22: 445–447.
[15] Yavuz S, Gönzü MT, Türk T. Axillary artery cannulation for arterial inflow in patients with acute dissection of the ascending aorta. Eur J Cardiothorac Surg 2002; 22: 313–315.
[16] Whitlark JD, Goldman SM, Sutter FP. Axillary artery cannulation in acute ascending aortic dissections. Ann Thorac Surg 2000; 69: 1127–1129.
[17] Neri E, Massetti M, Capannini G, Carone E, Tucci E, Diciolla F. Axillary artery cannulation in type A aortic dissection operations. J Thorac Cardiovasc Surg 1999; 118: 324–329.
[18] Schachner T, Laufer G, Vertacnik K, Bonaros N, Nagiller J, Bonatti J. Is the axillary artery a suitable cannulation site in aortic surgery? J Cardiovasc Surg 2004; 45: 15–19.

[19] Pasic M, Schubel J, Bauer M, Yankah C, Kuppe H, Weng YG, Hetzer R. Cannulation of the right axillary artery for surgery of acute type A aortic dissection. Eur J Cardiothorac Surg 2003; 24: 231-236.

[20] Watanabe K, Fukuda I, Osaka M, Imazuru T. Axillary artery and transapical aortic cannulation as an alternative to femoral artery cannulation. Eur J Cardiothorac Surg 2003; 23: 842–843.

[21] Schachner T, Nagiller J, Zimmer A, Laufer G, Bonatti J. Technical problems and complications of axillary artery cannulation. Eur J Cardiothorac Surg 2005; 27: 634 – 637.

[22] Sinclair MC, Singer RL, Manley NJ, Montesano RM. Cannulation of axillary artery for cardiopulmonary bypass: safeguards and pitfalls. Ann Thorac Surg 2003; 75: 931 – 934.

[23] Merkkola P, Tulla H, Ronkainen A, Soppi V, Oksala A, Koivisto T, Hippelainen M. Incomplete circle of Willis and right axillary artery perfusion. Ann Thorac Surg 2006; 82: 74-79.

[24] Wada S, Yamamoto S, Honda J, Hiramoto A, Wada H, Hosoda Y. Transapical aortic cannulation for cardiopulmonary bypass in type A aortic dissection operations. J Thorac Cardiovasc Surg. 2006; 2: 369-372.

[25] Urbanski PP, Lenos A, Lindemann Y, Weigang E, Zacher M, Diegeler A. Carotid artery cannulation in aortic surgery. J Thorac Cardiovasc Surg 2006; 132: 1398-1403.

[26] Di Eusanio M, Ciano M, Labriola G, Lionetti G, Di Eusanio G. Cannulation of the innominate artery during surgery of the thoracic aorta: our experience in 55 patients. Eur J Cardiothorac Surg 2007; 32: 270-273.

[27] Fusco DS, Shaw RK, Tranquilli M, Kopf GS, Elefteriades JA. Femoral cannulation is safe for type A dissection repair. Ann Thorac Surg 2004; 78: 1285-1289.

[28] Borst HG, Schaudig A, Rudolph W. Arteriovenous fistula of the aortic arch: repair during deep hypothermia and circulatory arrest. J Thorac Cardiovasc Surg 1964;48:443-447.

[29] Hogue CW, Palin CA Jr, Arrowsmith JE. Cardiopulmonary bypass management and neurologic outcomes: an evidence based appraisal of current practices. Anesth Analg 2006;103:1-37.

[30] Kamiya H, Hagl C, Kropivnitskaya I, Bothig D, Kallenbach K, Khaladj N, Martens A, Haverich A, Karck M. The safety of moderate hypothermic lower body circulatory arrest with selective cerebral perfusion: a propensity score analysis. J Thorac Cardiovasc Surg 2007; 133: 501-509.

[31] Kamiya H, Klima U, Hagl C, Logemann F, Winterhalter M, Shrestha ML, Kallenbach K, Khaladj N, Haverich A, Karck M. Cerebral microembolization during antegrade selective cerebral perfusion. Ann Thorac Surg 2006; 81: 519-521.

[32] Hagl C, Khaladj N, Peterss S, Hoeffler K, Winterhalter M, Karck M, Haverich A. Hypothermic circulatory arrest with and without cold selective antegrade cerebral perfusion: impact on neurological recovery and tissue metabolism in an acute porcine model. Eur J Cardiothorac Surg 2004; 26: 73-80.

[33] Khaladj N, Peterss S, Oetjen P, von Wasielewski R, Hauschild G, Karck M, Haverich A, Hagl C. Hypothermic circulatory arrest with moderate, deep or profound

hypothermic selective antegrade cerebral perfusion: which temperature provides best brain protection? Eur J Cardiothorac Surg 2006; 30: 492-498.

[34] Apostolakis E, Koletsis EN, Dedeilias P, Kokotsakis JN, Sakellaropoulos G, Psevdi A, Bolos K, Dougenis D. Antegrade versus retrograde cerebral perfusion in relation to postoperative complications following aortic arch surgery for acute aortic dissection type A. J Card Surg. 2008;23:480-487.

[35] Baker MA, Stocking RA, Meehan JP. Thermal relationship between tympanic membrane and hypothalamus in conscious cat and monkey. J Appl Physiol 1972;32:739-742.

[36] Benzinger M. Tympanic thermometry in surgery and anesthesia. JAMA 1969;209:1207-1211.

[37] Horrow JC, Rosenberg H. Does urinary catheter temperature reflect core temperature during cardiac surgery? Anesthesiology 1988;69:986-989.

[38] Severinghaus JW. Temperature gradients during hypothermia. Ann N Y Acad Sci 1959;80:515-521.

[39] Stone JG, Young WL, Smith CR, Solomon RA, Wald A, Ostapkovich N, Shrebnick DB. Do standard monitoring sites reflect true brain temperature when profound hypothermia is rapidly induced and reversed? Anesthesiology 1995;82:344–351.

[40] Hercus V, Cohen D, Bowring AC. Temperature gradients during hypothermia. BMJ 1959;1:1439–1441.

[41] Stefaniszyn HJ, Novick RJ, Keith FM, Salerno TA. Is the brain adequately cooled during deep hypothermic cardiopulmonary bypass? Current Surgery 1983;40:294–297.

[42] Akata T, Yamaura K, Kandabashi T, Sadamatsu S, Takahashi S. Changes in body temperature during profound hypothermic cardiopulmonary bypass in adult patients undergoing aortic arch reconstruction. J Anesth 2004;18:73–81

[43] Tsai TT, Evangelista A, Nienaber CA, Trimarchi S, Sechtem U, Fattori R, Myrmel T, Pape L, Cooper JV, Smith DE, Fang J, Isselbacher E, Eagle KA; International Registry of Acute Aortic Dissection (IRAD). Long-term survival in patients presenting with type A acute aortic dissection: insights from the International Registry of Acute Aortic Dissection (IRAD). Circulation 2006;114:350-356.

[44] Shores J, Berger KR, Murphy EA, Pyeritz RE. Progression of aortic dilatation and the benefit of long-term beta-adrenergic blockade in Marfan's syndrome. N Engl J Med 1994;330:1335-1341.

[45] Habashi JP, Doyle JJ, Holm TM, Aziz H, Schoenhoff F, Bedja D, Modiri AN, Judge DP, Dietz HC. Angiotensin II type 2 receptor signaling attenuates aortic aneurysm in mice through ERK antagonism. Science 2011;332:361-365.

[46] Gambarin FI, Favalli V, Serio A, Regazzi M, Pasotti M, Klersy C, Dore R, Mannarino S, Vigano M, Odero A, Amato S, Tavazzi L, Arbustini E. Rationale and design of a trial evaluating the effects of losartan vs. nebivolol vs. the association of both on the progression of aortic root dilation in Marfan syndrome with FBN1 gene mutations. J Cardiovasc Med 2009;10:354-362.

[47] Radonic T, de Witte P, Baars MJ, Zwinderman AH, Mulder BJ, Groenink M; COMPARE study group. Losartan therapy in adults with Marfan syndrome: study protocol of the multi-center randomized controlled COMPARE trial. Trials. 2010;12:11:3.

14

Neurologic Injury Following Hypothermic Circulatory Arrest

Elizabeth O. Johnson, Antonia Charchanti, Maria Piagkou, Theodore Xanthos and Theodore Troupis
Department of Anatomy, University of Athens, School of Medicine,
Department of Anatomy, University of Ioannina, School of Medicine,
Greece

1. Introduction

Cardiothoracic surgeons are faced with the challenge of protecting the brain during the sensitive time of interruption of normal cerebral blood flow. The brain is an exceptionally complex organ with a functional anatomy that is difficult both to understand and assess. Experimental and clinical studies have shown that the mechanism of neural injury is multifactorial. As such, discussions regarding the best surgical strategies for neuroprotection during circulatory arrest are formidable, at best. Although we are armed with excellent experimental and clinical studies that demonstrate the deleterious effects of prolonged exposure to cardiopulmonary bypass (CPB) on brain function and structure, the various neuroprotective strategies, particularly that of deep hypothermic circulatory arrest (DHCA) remain an issue of debate. This is related in part to the gap between the basic science understanding of brain injury caused by these events and the clinical application of various neuroprotective strategies and their subsequent clinical outcomes. The goal here is to address the current understanding of the mechanisms underlying brain injury after HCA and relevant strategies of neural protection, supported by primary experimental data from our laboratory.

2. Hypothermic ciruclatory arrest

The use of therapeutic hypothermia dates back to the ancient Egyptians, Greeks, and Romans. In modern times, the use of therapeutic hypothermia progressed from observation case reports to animal studies to clinical use in children and then adults. Initially there were observational reports of therapeutic use of hypothermia in patients with severe cerebral trauma, followed by experimental studies in dogs that suggested a therapeutic role for hypothermia for cerebral protection during cardiac surgery. Later, profound hypothermia (12° C, nasopharyngeal) with circulatory arrest (up to 1 hour) was used in children undergoing surgical repair of the tetralogy of Fallot. (Apostolakis & Shuhaiber, 2007)

The use of deep hypothermic cardiopulmonary arrest (DHCA, 14-18°C) was first applied as a method for cerebral protection during the prosthetic replacement of the aortic arch.(Griepp et al, 1997) Later, the use of a DHCA was extended into other major vascular surgeries such as the repair of thoracoabdominal aortic lesions, clipping of giant and complex cerebral aneurysms, and resection of renal carcinoma with tumor thrombus extending into the inferior vena cava or atrium.

Deep hypothermic circulatory arrest (DHCA or HCA) provides 2 clinical benefits. The circulatory arrest component provides a bloodless surgical field without the need for the use of intrusive clamps and cannulae. The deep hypothermic component significantly decreases brain metabolism and oxygen requirements and thus permits a longer period of interrupted blood perfusion to the brain. The cerebral metabolic rate is related exponentially to brain (core body) temperature, with the cerebral metabolic rate decreasing by about 50% for each 6°C drop in brain temperature. Since the first experimental studies, the use of DHCA has become the standard technique for the surgical repair of certain congenital and acquired cardiovascular lesions. The outcome after these operations improved considerably over the past two decades and surgery requiring HCA can usually be performed with an acceptable risk for the patient. However, it is likely that these improvements are more a consequence of an increasing expertise with this type of surgery, rather than the influence of one particular organ protection method employed. Despite this fact, there is still room for improvement, since prolonged periods of HCA are still associated with significant morbidity and mortality. As the brain is the organ most sensitive to ischemic damage, it is considered to be the limiting factor for the duration of HCA. Nevertheless, despite its protective effects, HCA can be detrimental for other organ systems.

The basic established techniques and perfusion strategies during aortic arch replacement number three: hypothermic circulatory arrest (HCA), antegrade cerebral perfusion (ACP), and retrograde cerebral perfusion (RCP). During the past decade and after several experimental studies, RCP lost its previous place in the armamentarium of brain protection, giving it up to ACP as a major method of brain perfusion during HCA. HCA should be applied at a temperature of ≈20°C with long-lasting cooling and rewarming and should not exceed by itself the time of 20–25 min. RCP does not seem to prolong safe brain-ischemia time beyond 30 min, but it appears to enhance cerebral hypothermia by its massive concentration inside the brain vein sinuses. HCA combined with ACP, however, could prolong safe brain-ischemia time up to 80 min. Cold ACP at 10°–13°C should be initially applied through the right subclavian or axillary artery and continued bihemispherically through the left common carotid artery at first and later the anastomosed graft, with a mean perfusion pressure of 40–70 mm Hg. The safety of temporary perfusion is being confirmed by the meticulous monitoring of brain perfusion through internal jugular bulb O_2 saturation, electroencephalogram, and transcranial comparative Doppler velocity of the middle cerebral arteries (Kouchoukos et al, 2003).

3. Methods of end-organ protection during DHCA

3.1 Hypothermia

Hypothermia acts by reducing the metabolic rate of the brain and improving the balance between energy supply and demand. Hypothermia reduces cerebral blood flow (CBF) in a linear manner, but the decrease in cerebral metabolic rate of oxygen ($CMRO_2$) is not exactly linear. On average, the reduction in $CMRO_2$ is about 7%/1°C. Between 37°C and 22°C, $CMRO_2$ is reduced by about 5%/1°C, and then the reduction accelerates when $CMRO_2$ reaches 20% at 20°C and 17% at 18°C, at which point about 60% of patients achieve electrical silence on electroencephalography (EEG).

3.2 Drug interventions

To increase the tolerance to ischemia, the use of potentially neuroprotective drugs is an appealing concept, especially since the circulatory arrest interval is well defined and allows a preischemic treatment. Therefore, it is evident that the use of these pharmaceuticals is more promising in HCA patients than for the postischemic treatment of patients after embolic strokes. Studies in a chronic porcine model showed that nontoxic drugs are available that have neuroprotective effects, making them potential candidates for clinical use. Additionally, combining drug treatment with selective perfusion techniques, to support adequate delivery of the agent into the target organ, seems to be a promising concept.
Among the various neuroprotective pharmacologic agents are barbiturates, which are believed be protective in focal ischemia by reducing $CMRO_2$, CBF, free fatty acids, free radical and cerebral edema. Steroids decrease proinflammatory responses, while beta-blockers decrease the inflammatory response. Mannitol reduces cerebral edema, scavenges free radicals and protects the kidneys by lowering renal vascular resistance. Furosemide blocks renal reabsorption of sodium, and insulin controls hyperglycemia, which in turn prevents intracellular acidosis. Lidocaine is a selective blocker of Na^+ channels in neuronal membranes and thus, reduces $CMRO_2$. Dexmedetomidine inhibits ischemia-induce norepinephrine release and is protective for both focal and global ischemia. Acadesine appears to mitigate the effects of reperfusion injury.

3.3 Intraoperative neuromonitoring

Neurophysiological monitoring during thoracic aortic surgery using HCA became increasingly popular in the last decade. Besides its value during an ongoing operation, the collection of data in combination with outcome analysis might help to improve or change surgical strategies. Continuous recording of electroencephalograms (EEGs) as well as SSEPs is now routine in most neurosurgical units. The use of neuromonitoring in cardiothoracic surgery is in part hampered by the fact that hypothermia has an impact on the sensitivity of neurophysiological measures, so they cannot be used during deep hypothermia. On the other hand, some surgeons have found this an asset, and use disappearance of the EEG to determine the optimal level of hypothermia before they stop the extracorporeal circulation. Therefore, the value of the EEG as an isolated method for ascertaining whether cerebral protection is adequate is questionable. Furthermore, nonsynaptic metabolic activity may persist even when the EEG is isoelectric. On the other hand, the EEG may provide valuable information for those groups which are using relative high blood temperatures during SCP. Furthermore, EEG seems to be a good tool for detecting electrophysiological recovery in the early postoperative period. Monitoring of SSEPs is generally easier than EEG since electric noise does not play such a substantial role. It is generally less influenced by anesthetic drugs, and it remains detectable as long as cortical activity can be encountered. From clinical experience, SSEPs seem especially valuable during surgery on the descending or thoracoabdominal aorta (which is not subject of the present synopsis) but muscle evoked potentials (MEPs) may be even more sensitive for detection of spinal cord injury.

3.4 Acid-base management during hypothermia

Hypothermia alters the results of analysis of arterial blood gases by increasing the solubility of CO_2 and O_2 in plasma. The increase in CO_2 solubility decreases the concentration of the insoluble portion and, thus, the partial pressure. However, the total content of CO_2 in the blood remains the same. During hypothermia, if a blood sample is taken and warmed to 37°C in the blood gas analyzer, the CO_2 initially dissolved will now contribute to the partial pressure of CO_2 (PCO_2) and the PCO_2 will be within the normal normothermic range. If, on the other hand, the value is estimated at the patient's actual temperature, the PCO_2 will be reduced despite similar arterial CO_2 content. In addition to its effect on gas solubility, hypothermia decreases the metabolic rate and CO_2 production. Maintaining the PCO_2 within the normal range in rewarmed 37°C blood is called "alpha-stat." If the PCO_2 is corrected to the patient's actual temperature and that value is kept within the normal range, the management is called "pH-stat."

4. Duration of DHCA

A number of biochemical and cellular structural changes take place as the duration of circulatory arrest lengthens. After 15 minutes of ischemia at 18°C, the recovery of oxygen consumption is impaired, and after 20 minutes, cerebral lactate is detected in the effluent blood. The safe duration of circulatory arrest at 15°C was predicted to be about 29 minutes and at 10°C about 40 minutes. If ischemic tolerance is considered 5 minutes at normothermia, the calculated safe period of circulatory arrest at 18°C would be 15 minutes. Clinical studies have shown a persistent loss of cognitive function (lasting more than 6 weeks) and deterioration in postoperative cognitive scoring/testing in patients who underwent aortic arch surgery by using DHCA for more than 25 minutes at 10°C.

5. Complications of DHCA

Disadvantages of DHCA include increased cardiopulmonary bypass (CPB) time, edema formation, coagulopathy, and alteration in many organ functions including the kidney, the brain, vascular smooth muscles, intestinal mucosa, alveolar epithelium, the liver, and the pancreas. Based on reports from 8 major cardiac surgery centers in the United States, Europe, and Japan, the risk of permanent neurologic injury after aortic arch surgery using DHCA ranged from 3% to 12%, renal dysfunction from 5% to 14%, pulmonary insufficiency from 5% to 39%, and left ventricular failure or low-cardiac-output syndrome from 7% to 34%. Alternatives to the use of DHCA during aortic arch replacement are the use of normothermic CPB or mild-to-moderate degrees of hypothermia. These alternatives obviously require the use of a perfusion system for the brain, separate from the rest of the body, which might increase the risk of cerebral emobilization.

5.1 Neurologic injury

Neurologic injury is the most troublesome adverse effect of DHCA and CPB, presenting either as transient neurologic deficit (5.9%-28.1%) or irreversible neurologic injury (1.8%-13.6%). Early postoperative mortality markedly is increased (18.2%) in patients with neurologic injury, and long-term cognitive disability is common among survivors. Neurologic deficit after DHCA encompasses a wide scale of disorders ranging from deep coma to subtle, hardly perceptible alterations in cognitive functions or behavior. In the immediate postoperative period, the return of sophisticated neurologic functions is often obscured by the administration of sedative and analgesic agents. Neurologic injury presents at that time mostly as a focal or diffuse deficit. A focal deficit is due to interruption of blood in a terminal vascular territory, usually following embolism of material or gas bubbles. The clinical expression is typically motor-sensory deficit, aphasia, or cortical blindness (Kunihara et al, 2005; Lipton, 1999). Computed tomography and magnetic resonance imaging are usually able to detect a sharply demarcated area of necrosis in the brain.

A focal deficit is usually an embolic phenomenon, whereas a prolonged poor perfusion of the brain may produce necrosis in watershed zones. Age, atherosclerosis, and manipulation of the aorta are risk factors for both. Global cerebral ischemia leads to diffuse neurologic deficit, which may be benign and reversible or more debilitating (seizures, Parkinsonism, and coma). Risk factors include increased duration of circulatory arrest and CPB, diabetes mellitus, and hypertension. Transient neurologic dysfunction appears to be a marker of long-term cerebral injury. Deficits of memory and fine-motor function may persist after hospital discharge. Reductions in $CMRO_2$ and the duration of DHCA reduce the risk of neurologic injury. The length of time on CPB might be a better predictor of postoperative death and stroke than the duration of DHCA time (Hagl et al, 2003).

Aortic procedures requiring hypothermic circulatory arrest have been specifically correlated with increased risk of both stroke and mortality in all patients. This may be accentuated in the elderly, who may have less tolerance for neurological insult. Many physicians think patients >75 years old are too frail and lack the reserve to survive a major cardiothoracic surgery. In particular, there remains some hesitancy in performing procedures with a higher risk of stroke in patients with a higher susceptibility for adverse neurological sequelae. This perceived combination of risk and susceptibility may be a barrier to care for elderly patients requiring hypothermic circulatory arrest to address their aortic pathology. According to Coselli et al. (2008), in a study accessing the safety and efficacy of HCA, there are various major complications associated with HCA. These included death (interoperative, during hospital stay, and within 30 days), stroke, paraplegia, paraparesis, uncontrolled bleeding which required reoperation, renal failure, cardiac complications, and vocal cord paralysis.

6. Strategies for brain protection during DHCA

6.1 Hypothermia – reduction of metabolism

Hypothermia is the most efficient measure to prevent or reduce ischemic damage to the central nervous system when blood circulation is reduced. The central nervous system has a high metabolic rate and limited energy stores, which make it extremely vulnerable to ischemia (Elrich et al, 2002). Hypothermia acts by reducing the metabolic rate of the brain and improving the balance between energy supply and demand, and thus lengthens the period of tolerated ischemia. Hypothermia reduces cerebral blood flow (CBF) in a linear manner, but the decrease in cerebral metabolic rate of oxygen ($CMRO_2$) is not exactly linear. On average, the reduction in $CMRO_2$ is about 7%/1°C. Between 37°C and 22°C, $CMRO_2$ is reduced by about 5%/1°C, and then the reduction accelerates when $CMRO_2$ reaches 20% at 20°C and 17% at 18°C, at which point about 60% of patients achieve electrical silence on electroencephalography (EEG) (McCullough et al, 1999).

6.2 Techniques and perfusion strategies

Although reduction of cerebral metabolism and swift surgery are the two fundamental measures that can prevent or reduce brain damage during circulatory arrest, there are adjunctive protective measures that can be considered. The basic established techniques and perfusion strategies during aortic arch replacement number three: hypothermic circulatory arrest (HCA), antegrade cerebral perfusion (ACP), and retrograde cerebral perfusion (RCP).

7. Experimental investigation of cerebral injury following DHCA

A clearer understanding of the consequences of HCA will be pivotal in clinical decision-making, including when to initiate circulatory arrest and the appropriate interval. Delayed cell death is of special interest because of the potential for intervention. Although apoptosis is believed to play a part in the cerebral injury, its role has generally been identified through histologic techniques. These snapshots do not permit a clear delineation of the time-line of apoptosis. Because its role is not clear, therapies have yet to be designed for the specific purpose of inhibiting apoptosis.

The balance between cell survival and death is under tight genetic control (Almeida et al., 2000). A multiplicity of extracellular signals and intracellular mediators are involved in maintaining this balance. When the cell is exposed to physical, biochemical or biological injury, or deprived of necessary substances, it activates a series of stress-response genes. Although with minimal insults, the cell may recover, with greater insults, single cell death results. The current understanding of the neurons response to insult has been supported by evidence from a series of studies using a porcine model system to investigate the effects hypothermic circulatory arrest and ischemic insult on the integrity of neuronal populations.

7.1 Clinically relevant animal models

Evaluating various strategies and treatments in animal studies in order to determine clinical feasibility remains a challenge. Animal models have contributed immensely to our understanding of cerebral consequences of HCA, with several animal models having been used. To date, the preclinical investigation of cerebral injury mechanisms related to deep hypothermic circulatory arrest has been limited to large-animal models (porcine, canine and ovine). These models are expensive, personnel demanding, cumbersome and are usually performed without validated neuropsychologic assessment. Rodent models have been attempted to overcome some of these disadvantages, although treatment effects cannot always be confirmed in the rat model. Ultimately, however, each experimental model system from cell cultures to rats, to large animals and ultimately to clinical trials, have their advantages and disadvantages, and ultimately their place in these investigations.

Most animal models require an extended period of arrest to produce a reproducible level of neuronal injury that would facilitate elucidating the mechanisms of injury and efficacy of neuroprotective interventions. Many large animal models require DHCA for at least 90-120 minutes to demonstrate neurologic deficits. Although such prolonged DHCA interval might not be considered clinically realistic, they may be more appropriate for demonstrating the molecular pathways behind acute neuronal injury and hence, modes of intervention (Conti et al, 1998).

Study of a neuroprotective strategy includes appropriate selection of an animal model and functional indices. The model is selected with respect to their relevance and feasibility of assessing the parameters of interest. Investigations of promising neuroprotectvie methods require validation (validation study), use in experimental settings to optimize cerebral protection during CPB and DHCA (performance study) and test during routine cardiac surgery (clinical study).

Hypothermia is essential for cerebral protection during HCA. Hypothermia reduces cerebral metabolic activity, oxygen demand, and prevents the release of neurotransmitters and delays the onset of fatal biochemical cascade (Elrich et al., 2002; McCullough et al., 1999). Although reduced, brain metabolism is not suppressed adequately and remains relatively high at 18°C in traditional HCA protocols (McCullough et al., 1999). In light of evidence suggesting that the apoptotic pathway may be reversible in their earlier stages (McCullough et al., 1999), studies from our team were undertaken to assess whether cooling to 10°C can reduce neurological injury during 75 minutes of HCA in an acute porcine model compared to less profoundly cooled (18°C) animals, as assessed by DNA fragmentation, anti-apoptotic protein Bcl-2 expression, and ultrastructural changes in the sensory cortex. Sixteen male juvenile pigs from a commercial farm, 2-3 months of age and weighing 25-35 Kg were used for this study. The animals were divided into three groups: Group A (n=6) underwent hypothermic circulatory arrest at 18°C for 75 min, Group B (n=6) underwent hypothermic circulatory arrest at 10°C for 75 min and Group C (n=4) served as normal controls.

Preparation and surgery were performed as previously described (Ananiadou et al 2005). Briefly, catheters were inserted in an ear vein and the left femoral artery for monitoring purposes and withdrawal of blood samples. Anesthesia was induced with intramuscularly ketamine hydrochloride (15 mg/kg), atropine (0.05 mg/kg), and dormicum (0.1 mg/kg) and was maintained with intravenous fentanyl (50-200 µg/kg), dormicum and 1% to 2% isoflurane. Paralysis was achieved with a bolus intravenous rocuronium (0.6 mg/kg) and was maintained with 20% of the total dose every 30 min.

Animals were ventilated mechanically with 100% oxygen, after endotracheal intubation. Ventilator rate and tidal volume were adjusted to maintain the arterial carbon dioxide tension at 40 mmHg. Hematocrit values during cardiopulmonary bypass (CPB) were maintained between 13%-23%. A temperature probe was placed in the rectum, while brain temperature was determined with bilateral tympanic membrane probes. Urine output was collected through a bladder catheter (Foley 8-10 F). Arterial pressure, end-expired carbon dioxide, electrocardiogram, and blood gases (ABL Radiometer Medical A/S DK-2700, Copenhagen, Denmark) were monitored.

As previously described, the chest was opened via a right thoracotomy in the fourth intercostal space (Ananiadou et al., 2005). After administration of intravenous heparin (300 IU/kg), cannulas were advanced to the ascending aorta (16 F arterial cannula) and to the right atrium (single 26 F cannula). Non-pulsatile CPB, was initiated at a flow rate of 100 ml/kg per min and then adjusted to maintain a minimum arterial pressure of 50 mmHg. To avoid distension of the left ventricle during CPB, a 10 F vent catheter was inserted via the superior pulmonary vein. The lungs were allowed to collapse after CPB was initiated. The CPB circuit was primed with a bloodless solution consisting of 1000cc lactated Ringer's, 50 ml mannitol, and 5000 IU heparin. Sodium bicarbonate was added to adjust the pH to 7.4, as necessary.

CPB was continued for an average 58 or 106 minutes, to reach a deep brain temperature of 18°C or 10°C, respectively. Myocardial protection was afforded by applying iced saline (4°C) topically during the 75-minute interval of hypothermic circulatory arrest. When the tympanic membrane temperature reached 18°C or 10°C, bypass was discontinued, the blood was drained into the oxygenator reservoir, and circulatory arrest was maintained for 75 minutes. Ice bags were positioned around the head to maintain the brain temperature during HCA. At the end of the arrest, bypass was initiated again with gradual rewarming to a rectal temperature of approximately 35°C to 36°C. A temperature gradient exceeding 10°C between the perfusate and the core temperature was avoided. A temperature of 36°C was reached after an average of 83 or 104 minutes of reperfusion for animals treated with 18 °C or 10 °C HCA, respectively. Systemic pressure was maintained above 60 mmHg during reperfusion. Measurements of hemodynamics (heart rate, mean arterial pressure), arterial blood gases, hematocrit, glucose lactate, as well as temperatures were recorded at five time points during the experiment. These were: 1) Baseline at 37°C and prior to CPB; 2) At the initiation of CPB; 3) During CPB, while cooling to a brain temperature of 18°C or 10°C just before HCA; 4) During rewarming; and 5) At the end of CPB.

The mean duration (+SD) of CPB cooling and CPB warming for animals with 18°C HCA was 57.50+17.25 and 82.50+10.37 minutes, and for 10°C was 105.8±21.8 and 104.2±19.8 minutes, respectively. Perioperative physiological variables are shown in Table 1. Although there were some minor variations, no apparent clinically relevant hemodynamic differences were observed between treatment groups. Lactate levels were significantly higher following HCA at 10°C compared to 18°C. PO2 levels were significantly lower in 18°C HCA animals compared to 10°C during cooling, and hematocrit levels dropped to a similar degree in all experimental animals during the procedure.

Variable	Baseline	Init CPB	Cooling	Warming	End CPB
Brain Temperature (°C)					
18 °C	36.5±0.4	34.1±1.8	18.0±0.0	25.8±3.2	36.5±0.8
10 °C	36.5±0.4	33.2±1.6	10.0±0.0	28.2±3.1	36.9±0.2
MAP (mmHg)					
18 °C	114.0±14.9	57.2±16.3	55.2±8.1	67.8±15.7	68.3±25.7
10 °C	118.7±13.0	59.7±10.1	54.0±3.4	69.4±16.5	85.0±8.9
Arterial pH					
18 °C	7.40±0.12	7.26±0.19	7.26±0.12	7.20±0.07	7.35±0.14
10 °C	7.34±0.13	7.32±0.11	7.28±0.11	7.32±0.08	7.38±0.13
pO_2 (mmHg)					
18 °C	409.9±67.8	751.4±202.8	787.1±319.06*	429.0±126.9	424.6±112.1
10 °C	378.4±118.3	689.5±45.5	1066.0±122.8	562.8±123.4	459.4±45.4
pCO_2 (mmHg)					
18 °C	51.32±19.0	73.7±37.8	67.2±31.3	69.3±14.4	38.7±18.7
10 °C	58.1±23.3	60.0±17.7	58.2±12.4	44.0±12.9	31.7±9.0
Hematocrit (%)					
18 °C	26.4±3.8**	16.4±3.4	15.51±3.3	16.6±3.9	15.5±3.1
10 °C	26.0±3.8**	18.5±3.0	18.6±3.7	19.2±3.5	19.2±3.0
Lactate (mmol/L)					
18 °C	2.7±1.8	4.5±2.1	5.6±2.5	6.3±1.7*	11.0±4.3
10 °C	3.1±1.03	4.4±1.6	8.3±3.0	11.6±2.8	11.9±3.5

Table 1. Typical Physiologic Variables During HCA Paradigm in a Porcine Model
All values are expressed as mean + SD. *P<0.05 between animals treated with HCA at 18°C vs 10°C (unpaired, 2-tailed, t-test). **P<0.05 between sample times (ANOVA followed by Fisher PLSD).

8. Neuronal injury and nerve cell death: basic sciences

Neuronal death is normal during development of the nervous system, but it is abnormal in brain and spinal cord disease and injury. The available evidence indicates that the survival of neurons and their death are highly regulated and finely orchestrated dynamic events that depend on a number of internal and external factors. Two types of cell death are recognized: cell necrosis resulting from injury and causes inflammation and apoptosis, observed normally in development and now identified as programmed cell death. Apoptosis and necrosis are types of cell death. They are generally considered to be distinct forms of cell death, but there is mounting evidence supporting an apoptosis-necrosis cell death continuum (Portera-Calliau, et al, 1997). In this continuum, neuronal death can result from varying contributions of coexisting apoptotic and necrotic mechanisms, resulting in some of the distinctions between apoptosis and necrosis becoming blurred. Today it is believed that apoptosis may contribute to the neuronal degeneration in neurological injuries such as cerebral ischemia and trauma (Kerr et al 1972; MacManus and Linnik, 1997; Martin, 2001).

Necrosis can result from acute oxidative stress characterized by passive cell swelling, rapid energy losss, and generalized disruption of internal homeostasis with lysis of the nucleus, intra-nuclear organelles and plasma membranes leading to the release of intracellular components that induce a local inflammatory response that in turn, result in edema and injury to neighboring cells. Morphologically, cell death is characterized by swelling of organelles and rupture. Necrotic cell death is characterized by inflammation and wide-spread damage.

Apoptosis is a process of cell suicide, the mechanisms of which are encoded in the chromosomes of all nucleated cells. Although the capacity to carry out apoptosis appears to be inherent in all cells, the susceptibility to apoptosis varies markedly and is influenced by external and cell-autonomous events. Apoptosis is regulated by complex molecular signaling systems resulting in an orderly, energy-dependent enzymatic breakdown into characteristic molecular fragments, DNA, lipids and other macromolecules. Apoptosis can be induced by cell surface receptor engagement, growth factor withdrawal and DNA damage. In contrast to those observed in cell necrosis, the morphological changes that occur during developmental cell death include cell shrinkage, membrane blebbing, chromatin condensation and DNA fragmentation. Earlier studies showed that one of the biochemical hallmarks of apoptosis is DNA cleavage at internucleosomal linker regions, resulting in ladder formation of DNA of 180-200 bp or multiples thereof. However, this ladder-type DNA fragmentation is also found in some cells dying of necrosis, indicating that DNA fragmentation cannot be the sole criterion, but simultaneous morphological assessment must also be done for identifying apoptosis.

8.1 Mechanisms of apoptotic cell death

Several families of proteins and specific biochemical signal-transduction pathways regulate cell death. Cell death signaling can involve plasma membrane death receptors, mitochondrial death proteins, proteases, kinases and transcription factors. Predominant factors in cell death and cell survival include fas receptor, Bcl-2 and Bax (and their homologues), cytochrome c, caspases, p53 and extra cellular signal-regulated protein kinases. Some forms of cell death require gene activation, RNA synthesis and protein synthesis, whereas other forms are transcriptionally-translationally independent and are driven by posttranslational mechanisms such as protein phosphorylation and protein translocation.

The precise signaling cascade starting from the detection of the signal at the cell surface to the events that occur in the nucleus in apoptosis is not well established, with several grey zones in most suggested pathways. However, many events that occur at the cell surface and intracellularly during apoptosis in the nervous system have been reported. Following an appropriate stimulus, the first stage or "decision phase" of apoptosis is the genetic control point of cell death. This is followed by the second state or "execution phase", which is responsible for the morphological changes of apoptosis. The decision phase or genetic control appears to be mediated by two genes Bcl-2 and p53, while the execution phase appears to result from the activation of caspases. It has become apparent that the Bcl-2 family of proteins constitutes a critical intracellular checkpoint within a distal common pathway of programmed cell death (Almeida et al, 2000).

8.2 Selective vulnerability of neural populations to neural insult after HCA

After assessing acute neuronal injury in various regions of the brain after HCA in a porcine animal model, we found that neurons in the sensory and motor neocortex, as well as those in the hippocampus, were vulnerable to cell injury acutely after 75 min of HCA at 18oC, as determined by a positive TUNEL reaction for DNA fragmentation (Ananiadou et al, 2005). TUNEL positive cells are identified by a red-stained, condensed nucleus with apoptotic bodies, along with a diminutive or absent cytoplasm. (Figure 1) Although nerve cell populations in the cerebellum, thalamus and ventral medulla were also found vulnerable to cell injury, the percentage of TUNEL positive cells in these areas was significantly less than that observed in the primary motor and sensory gray matter, and in the hippocampus. (Table 2)

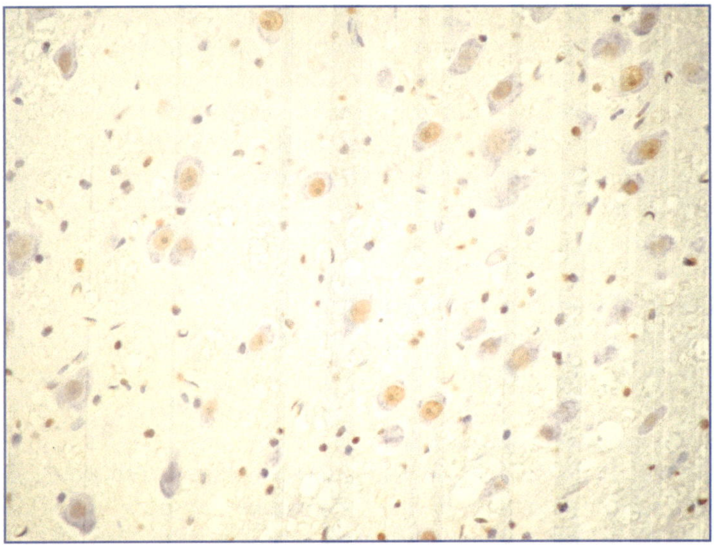

Fig. 1. Typical Presentation of TUNEL Positive Cells.
Photomicrograph showing apoptosis in the brain following HCA in an acute porcine model. Cluster of TUNEL (+) apoptotic neurons (nucleus is red stained) are interspersed among normal neurons in the anteroventral medulla. (magnification x400)

Brain Region	18 °C	10 °C	Control
Motor Cortex	3.28±0.32*	1.79±0.38+	0.50±0.22
Sensory Cortex	3.88±0.13**	1.60±0.31+++	0.14±0.14
Hippocampus	2.67±0.36*	1.39±0.24++	0.17±0.17
Cerebellum	2.13±0.48	1.82±0.23++	0.71±0.18
Medulla	2.00±0.41	2.08±0.23+++	0.57±0.20
Thalamus	2.33±0.67	1.54±0.31+++	0.00±0.00

Table 2. TUNEL Scores in Brain Regions of Animals Treated with HCA
All values are expressed as mean ± SE. *$p \le 0.006$ and **$p \le 0.0001$ compared to values from animals treated with 10°C HCA. +$p \le 0.05$; ++$p \le 0.005$; +++$p \le 0.002$ compared to normal control levels.

Age and temperature appear to influence neuronal injury, by making certain nerve cell populations more vulnerable to injury. In particular, the hippocampus, cerebellum, striatum, thalamus, amygdala and neocortex have been reported vulnerable in adult normothermic ischemia. In contrast, newborns were more vulnerable to injury in the neocortex and striatum. In the present model of hypothermic ischemia in juvenile pigs, the neocortex and hippocampus demonstrated the greatest vulnerability to insult during HCA. The apparent higher level of TUNEL positive cells in the primary sensory cortex (post-central gyrus) is not clear.

Although these previous studies clearly support that some of the cell death observed in HCA is via an apoptotic pathway, the experimental conditions used may underestimate the contribution of apoptosis to the cerebral sequelae after HCA (Kurth et al, 1999; Hagl et al, 2001). In this regard, some authors have expressed concern regarding the temporal pattern of brain damage and apoptosis after HCA. Thus, although recently improved methods of perfusion-fixation and more sophisticated analysis, have clearly shown the HCA initiates a series of events that ultimately leads to cell death via a typical apoptotic pattern, the time course of these events remains unclear. Most of these previous studies use the classic 90-min HCA, 20 °C model, which results in more severe cerebral injury than that usually observed clinically, where HCA is carried out for shorter intervals. The results from earlier studies also demonstrated that serious cell injury exists as early as 6 h after HCA, and that this process continues for at least 72h.

The importance of understanding the time course of events is underscored by an earlier study of long-term survivors of the 90-min, 20 °C protocol. Although treatment with CsA was reported to improve behavioral recovery after 7 days, at the 7 days time point after HCA there was no difference between CsA treated animals and controls for apoptosis measures. The authors concluded that they had missed the peak of apoptosis, and that an effective reduction in nerve cell injury would be found most likely with CsA treatment had they examined brain tissues at an earlier time point.

We found no morphological evidence of apoptosis or necrosis, but significantly greater levels of TUNEL positive cells in the brain regions assessed, compared to normal control animals. We hypothesize, that these findings indicate an early point of activation of the apoptotic

pathway. This is consistent with the rapid cell death observed in normal cell suicide programs that can kill a cell within 2 to 3 h. At an earlier time point, such as that in this study, we would not anticipate completion of the apoptotic mechanism, resulting in cell death with its classic morphological characteristics, but rather the initiation of the cellular response cascade.
Certain cell populations appear to be more vulnerable to injury. In particular, the hippocampus, cerebelleum, striatum, thalamus, amygdala and neocortex are more vulnerable in adult normothermic ischemia. In contrast, newborns are more vulnerable to injury in the neocortex and striatum. Our studies show that hypothermia does not provide equal protection to all regions of the brain. In the juvenile pig model, the neocortex and hippocampus demonstrated the greatest vulnerability to insult during HCA. The apparent higher level of TUNEL positive cells in the primary sensory cortex (post-central gyrus) is not clear, and demands further investigation. (Figure 2)

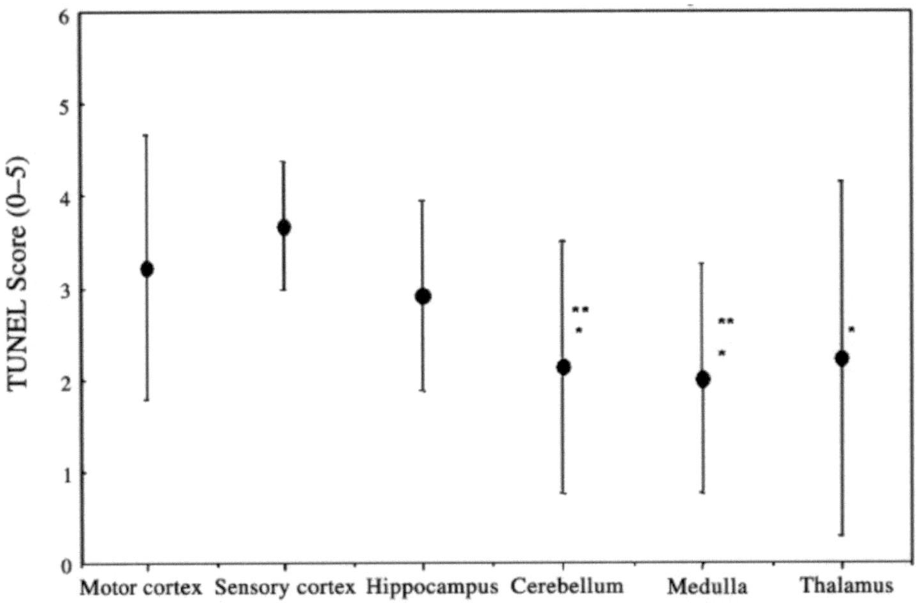

Fig. 2. Positive TUNEL Reaction in Vulnerable Neural Regions
Regional pattern of neuronal death after deep hypothermic circulatory arrest in juvenile pigs. Each point represents the mean score from six experimental animals for each brain region. The brackets indicate the S.D. Among the HCA treated animals, significantly higher concentrations of TUNEL (+) cells were observed in the sensory cortex, motor cortex and hippocampus, compared to the cerebellum, thalamus and medulla ($P < 0.05$ by ANOVA followed by Fisher PSLD). Although not statistically significantly greater than the motor neocortex and hippocampus, the postcentral gyrus had greater TUNEL scores compared to the medulla and thalamus ($P<0.01$). [*$P<0.05$ vs sensory and motor cortex, and hippocampus; ** $P<0.001$ vs sensory cortex}

8.3 Profound hpothermia rduces aoptotic nurologic ijury ater HCA

The use of HCA in aortic repair and congenital heart surgery is based on the idea of reducing the metabolic rate and thus, allowing a more prolonged interval without perfusion that can be safely tolerated by the brain. The brain, in general, is very sensitive to hypoxia-ischemia because it has a high metabolic rate and small reserve of high-energy carbohydrates and phosphates. Several studies have indicated that cerebral metabolism is reduced effectively at profound levels of hypothermia, suggesting that protection of the brain should be greater when HCA is performed at even lower temperatures, such as that used in our studies (Strauch et al, 2005).

We have found that profound hypothermia at 10°C during HCA resulted in a significant reduction in neurological injury in selectively vulnerable brain regions. TUNEL (+) staining was significantly less at 10°C in the motor and sensory cortex and the hippocampus compared to 18°C HCA, indicating that there was increased cerebral protection (Ananiadou et al, 2008). These findings are compatible with previous reports that profound hypothermia results in a superior neurological outcome compared to conventional HCA methods. Although this study does not elucidate the mechanisms, it does affirm that profound hypothermia exerts a neuroprotective effect.

8.4 The decision phase for apoptotic nerve cell death: evidence for Bcl-2

Apoptosis is controlled genetically, and two genes, Bcl-2 and p53 are now believed to be important. It is now established that proteins encoded by the Bcl-2 gene family are major regulatory components of the apoptotic pathway (Kroemer, 1997). Within the apoptotic cascade, several proteins that facilitate neuronal survival compete with molecules that contribute to cell death. Ultimately, the final balance between cell survival-promoting proteins versus cell death-promoting proteins determines the fate of the cell. The Bcl-2 family of proteins plays an important role in this cell survival-cell death decision.

This hypothesis is supported by our findings in Bcl-2 expression. The Bcl-2 family of proteins is important for the regulation of apoptosis during the "decision phase." An increase of Bcl-2 has been suggested as an internal protective mechanism against apoptotic cell death, where Bcl-2 is persistently expressed in neurons that survive in ischemia. In the present study, brain regions that were selectively vulnerable to neurologic injury, particularly the neocortex and hippocampus, showed higher levels of Bcl-2 expression after HCA at 18°C compared with other brain regions (thalamus, cerebellum, and medulla). Moreover, profound hypothermia at 10°C resulted in a significant decrease in TUNEL staining in these brain regions. Although a concomitant increase in Bcl-2 expression was observed in the neocortex, it remains unclear whether profound hypothermia deters from neuronal injury by activation of anti-apoptotic protein Bcl-2 expression (Ananiadou et al, 2007). (Table 3)

Sensory Cortex	18°C	10°C	Control
TUNEL	3.88 ± 0.13**	1.60 ± 0.31***	0.14 ± 0.14
Bcl-2	0.83 ± 0.31	1.8 ± 0.31*	1.8 ± 0.63

Table 3. TUNEL Scores and Bcl-2 Immunoreactivity in the Sensory Neocortex of Animals Treated with HCA at 18°C or 10°C Compared to Controls

All values are expressed as mean $\pm$ SE.

*$p \leq 0.05$ compared to values from animals treated with 18°C HCA.

**$p \leq 0.0001$ compared to values from animals treated with 10°C HCA.

***$p \leq 0.002$ compared to normal control levels

8.5 Morphological and ultrastructural evidence of neural protectin during profound cooling

Necrosis can be characterized by passive cell swelling, rapid energy losss, and generalized disruption of internal homeostasis with lysis of the nucleus, intranuclear organelles and plasma membranes leading to the release of intracellualar components that induce a local inflammatory response that in turn, result in edema and injury to neighboring cells. Morphologically, cell death is characterized by swelling of organelles and rupture. Necrotic cell death is characterised by inflammation and wide-spread damage. In contrast to those observed in cell necrosis, the morphological changes that occur during apoptotic cell death include cell shrinkage, membrane blebbing, chromatin condensation and DNA fragmentaion (Kerr et al., 1972). In continuation of the above studies, we assessed the morphological evidence that profound cooling of the cortex to 10°C can reduce neurological injury during hypothermic circulatory arrest (HCA) in our porcine model. Electron microscopy assessed ultrastructural changes indicative of activation of programmed cell death.

Parafin embedded samples described above were dewaxed in xylene. After rehydration using graded ethanol, slices were washed in cold 0.1 M sodium cacodylate buffer and fixed in 2.5% glutaraldeyde in 0.1 M cacodylate buffer overnight. Samples were washed in cold cacodylate buffer and then post-fixed with 1% osmium tetroxide in the same buffer for 1 hr at room temperature. After osmium tetroxide treatment, the samples were washed with 0.1 M sodium cacodylate buffer. The selected area was identified with a dissecting microscope, and 2x2x2 mm sections were cut out from the coronal slices and dehydrated in a graded series of ethanol, before being embedded in epoxy resin. Blocks were trimmed, and semithin 0.5-µm sections were cut with an ultramicrotome and stained with toluidine blue for light microscopy analysis. Ultrathin (75-90 mm) sections were cut and placed on 200-mesh copper grids for double-staining with uranyl acetate and lead citrate. Samples were examined with a JEOL JEM 100 CX-II electron microscope.

Samples were examined in a blind fashion by one observer using a JEOL 100CX electron microscope who was instructed to find 10 representative neurons (per experimental brain specimen) as identified by a typical nucleus and surrounding perikaryon. Two blinded investigators using an objective grading system analyzed electron micrographs of these neurons. Each investigator was asked to examine each neuron for evidence of nuclear changes (chromatin dispersion or clumping), for the presence of cytoplasmic changes, for the overall shape of the neuron (shrunken, swollen) and the appearance of rough endoplasmic reticulum (RER) compared with matched controls. Similarly, each investigator was instructed to examine the perinuclear neuronal mitochondria for abnormalities in mitochondrial distribution or shape, matrix density, crystal structure, and appearance of any abnormal structures compared with matched controls; each finding was indicated as mild, moderate, or severe depending on its frequency.

Electron microscopic observations in our study provided no appreciable morphological evidence to confirm apoptosis or necrosis of the sensory cortical neurons in this acute paradigm of HCA. In general, neurons showed normal nuclear and cytoplasmic morphology in all three treatment groups, with only minor ultrastructural changes observed ater HCA at 18°C. There was no evidence of cells swelling. The neurons of the sensory cortex in control animals had large round or oval nuclei with an evenly distributed chromatin. No discontinuities were found in cytoplasmic membrane and nucleolemma. Well-developed rough endoplasmic reticulum (RER) that was arranged in parallel stacks was observed in the cytoplasm. Polyribosomes formed characteristic rosettes, and mitochondria appeared normal in all control animals. Blood capillaries were surrounded by thin astrocytic end feet and showed endothelial cells with euchromatic nuclei, tight junctions between the adjacent plasma membranes.

Compared to normal controls, treatment with HCA at 18°C (group A) resulted in minor ultrastructural alterations in the sensory cortex. (Table 4) Most neurons exhibited a pale round or oval nuclei. Nucleoli were intact, although sometimes they were localized in eccentric positions. Plasma and nuclear membranes remained intact, as did the mitochondria, which maintained their normal appearance, with recognizable cristae. While most neurons had slightly dilated RER and Golgi apparatus, some cells displayed more significant edema and morphological modifications of their organelles and dilated mitochondria. (Figure 3). In some cases, polysomes were disassociated, displaying desegregated ribosomes. In addition, some neurons, also exhibited some chromatin clumps. Although some mitochondria were slightly dilated, they showed an otherwise normal morphology.

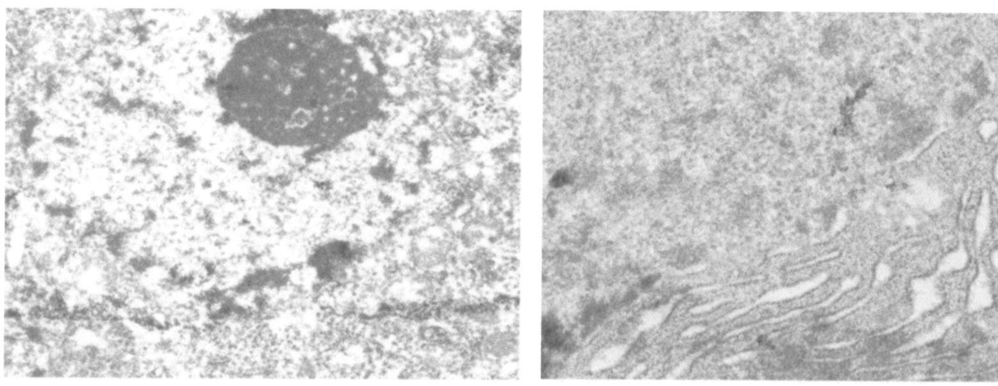

Fig. 3. Ultrastructural Changes in the Sensory Cortex
Sensory cortex from HCA at 18°C. (Left) Electron micrograph following HCA at 18°C with detail of neuron, showing nucleus(x18400). (Right) The same neuron showed dilated rough endoplasmic reticulum (x25200).

Sensory cortex												
Treatment	Overall shape of the neuron				Nuclear changes				Cell organelles			
	Shrunken		*Swollen*		*Chromatin Dispersion*		*Clumping*		*Mitochondrial Swelling*		*RER Swelling*	
	10°C	18°C	10°C	18°C	10°C	18°C	10°C	18°C	10°C	18°C	10°C	18°C
1	-	-	-	-	-	-	-	-	-	+	-	+
2	-	-	-	-	-	-	-	-	-	-	-	-
3	-	-	-	-	-	-	-	-	-	+	-	+
4	-	-	-	-	-	-	-	-	-	+	-	+

Table 4. Ultrastructural Changes in the Sensory Neocortex of Animals Treated with HCA at 18°C or 10°C Compared to Controls
- No changes noted compared to control
+ Positive observation compare to control animals

Deep hypothermia at 10°C resulted in negligent ultrastructural changes in the sensory cortex. Most neurons exhibited pale round or oval nuclei and intact nucleoli. In a few cases, the nucleoli were localized in eccentric positions. Plasma and nuclear membranes remained intact, and the structure of the cytoplasmic organelles was similar to that observed in control animals.

The first stage or the decision phase of apoptosis is initiated after an appropriate stimulus. This is referred to as the genetic control point of cell death and appears to be regulated by the Bcl-2 family of genes. The "execution phase" which follows is responsible for the morphologic changes of apoptosis (Kam and Ferch, 2000). The absence of clear morphologic evidence of apoptosis potentially suggests that these observations may represent an early point of activation of the apoptotic pathway (decision phase), which is supported by the Bcl-2 expression findings. As important regulators of the "decision phase," an increase of Bcl-2 may represent an internal protective mechanism against apoptotic cell death. Bcl-2 is persistently expressed in neurons that survive in ischemia. The sensory cortex is selectively vulnerable to neurologic injury and showed high levels of Bcl-2 expression after HCA at 18°C compared (Ananiadou et al., 2008). Moreover, profound hypothermia at 10°C resulted in a significant decrease in TUNEL(+) staining in this brain region. The concomitant increase in Bcl-2 expression that was observed in the sensory neocortex, suggests that profound hypothermia (at 10°C) may deter from neuronal injury by activation of anti-apoptotic protein Bcl-2 expression (Almeida et al., 2000). Although subtle, electron microscopy showed that at 18°C cells exhibited dilation of the rough endoplasmic reticulum and mitochondria, ribosome detachment and Golgi derived vacuolation, while at 10°C cells exhibited only dilation of the rough endoplasmic reticulum and ribosome detachment, indicating Phase II and Phase I of the apoptotic process, respectively.

The observation that TUNEL labeled cells may eventually, but not necessarily, progress into morphologically distinct apoptotic cells also confirms the idea that different morphologic characteristics may reflect different stages of the same death process. This is supported by our electron microscopy findings. At 18°C HCA, the neurons of the sensory cortex displayed dilation of the rough endoplasmic reticulum and detachment of ribosomes, along with Golgi derived vacuolation. According to Portera-Cailliau and colleagues (Portera-Calliau, et al., 1997), these findings suggest that the sensory cortex was in Phase II of the apoptotic process. At 10°C hypothermia, the ultrastructural findings indicate that the sensory cortex was in Phase I, showing only dilation of the rough endoplasmic reticulum and detachment of ribosomes. Although both groups appear to be in earlier stages of apoptosis, the findings clearly indicate that HCA at 18°C is associated with more morphological characteristics of apoptosis, compared to 10°C.

Although subtle, electron microscopy showed that at 18°C cells exhibited dilation of the rough endoplasmic reticulum and mitochondria, ribosome detachment and Golgi derived vacuolation, while at 10°C cells exhibited only slight changes. Our findings of significantly reduced TUNEL(+) staining, a concomitant increase in Bcl-2 expression and slightly decreased ultrastructural evidence of activation of programmed cell death support that deep hypothermia at 10°C further protects the sensory neocortex.

9. Conclusions

Cardiac surgeons are faced with the challenge of protecting the brain during the sensitive time of interruption of normal cerebral blood flow. The brain is an exceptionally complex organ with a functional anatomy that is difficult both to understand and assess. Experimental and clinical studies have shown that the mechanism of neural injury is multifactorial. As such, discussions regarding the best surgical strategies for neuroprotection during circulatory arrest are formidable, at best. Although we are armed with excellent experimental and clinical studies that demonstrate the deleterious effects of prolonged exposure to cardiopulmonary bypass (CPB) on brain function and structure, the various neuroprotective strategies, particularly that of deep hypothermic circulatory arrest (DHCA) remain an issue of debate. This is related in part to the gap between the basic science understanding of brain injury caused by these events and the clinical application of various neuroprotective strategies and their subsequent clinical outcomes.

Our goal has been to assess a possible mechanism of the neuronal injury (eg apoptosis) following DHCA. As this appears to involve a subtle and complex cascade of events, we decided to apply a paradigm that on the one hand may not be totally clinically relevant, but on the other hand would allow a robust response for assessment. Further study is clearly warranted to unravel relevant mechanisms and sensitive markers, which in turn, would allow us to appreciate the potential clinical relevance of these experimental findings. Evaluating various strategies and treatments in animal studies in order to determine clinical feasibility remains a challenge. Animal models have contributed immensely to our understanding of cerebral consequences of HCA, with several animal models having been used. To date, the preclinical investigation of cerebral injury mechanisms related to deep hypothermic circulatory arrest has been limited to large-animal models (porcine, canine and ovine). These models are expensive, personnel demanding, cumbersome and are usually performed without validated neuropsychologic assessment. Rodent models have been attempted to overcome some of these disadvantages, although treatment effects cannot always be confirmed in the rat model. Ultimately, however, each experimental model system from cell cultures to rats, to large animals and ultimately to clinical trials, have their advantages and disadvantages, and ultimately their place in these investigations.

There is now convincing evidence that there is a general relationship between CNS damage and increasing duration of DHCA. Although one of the goals of experimental studies is to assess the upper safe limit of DHCA, in order to do so we must more clearly understand the mechanism of cerebral injury. In most animal models, an extended period of arrest is necessary to produce a consistent and reproducible level of neuronal injury that would facilitate elucidating the mechanisms of injury, as well as the efficacy of potential neuroprotective interventions. Many large animal models require DHCA for at least 90-120 minutes in order to demonstrate neurologic deficits. Although such prolonged DHCA interval might not be considered clinically realistic, they may be more appropriate for demonstrating the molecular pathways behind acute neuronal injury and hence, modes of intervention.

Profound hypothermia of the brain results in a reduction of cerebral blood flow and steady state cerebral oxygen consumption (considered a true index of brain metabolic activity). Research in laboratory animals and clinical observations have now documented that considerable residual cerebral metabolism remains with cooling to levels of 15-18oC, particularly when cooling interval are short. Both experimental and clinical paradigms are faced with unresolved issues, including cooling gradients, nonuniformity of brain cooling, rewarming, pH management, among others.

Various strategies have been addressed in an effort to reduce neurological complications, including profound hypothermia, antegrade cerebral perfusion, retrograde cerebral perfusion, etc, each with their advantages and disadvantages. Cold reperfusion has shown promising results in animal studies and needs further clinical evaluation, while pharmacological interventions may offer a very promising pathway for preventing cerebral injury.

Experimental study of a neuroprotective strategy includes appropriate selection of an animal model, as well as functional indices. Of the available animal models, selection is made with respect to their relevance and feasibility of assessing the parameters of interest. The later are identified in the context of the available data. Investigations of promising neuroprotectvie methods require validation in an experimental model (validation study), use of the method in experimental settings to optimize cerebral protection during CPB and DHCA (performance study) and test its utility during routine cardiac surgery (clinical study). Despite the plethora of experimental and clinical studies, we still require a clearer understanding of the pathophysiologic consequences of HCA. This information will be pivotal in clinical decision-making, including when to initiate circulatory arrest and the appropriate interval.

Delayed cell death via apoptotic pathways is of special interest because of the potential for intervention. Although apoptosis is believed to play a part in the cerebral injury, its role has generally been identified through histologic techniques in animal models. These snapshots do not permit a clear delineation of the time-line of apoptosis in the course of HCA. Because it clinical role is not clear, therapies have yet to be designed for the specific purpose of inhibiting apoptosis. Both the cascade of events and identification of pharmacologic agents that can act on molecular mediators require active investigation.

Rewarming represents a critical time period, during which any additional harm to cerebral cells might induce permanent injury or even precipitate their death. How rapidly a stable energetic and biochemical homeostasis can be obtained in order to prevent the occurrence of secondary injuries remains unclear.

Optimal perfusion characteristics required to reduce neurologic morbidity remain important issues for experimental study. While there is ample evidence supporting the effectiveness of antegrade perfusion, its optimal delivery and perfusion characteristics remain unclear.

Overall, there are still many gaps in our knowledge about how to best study cerebral outcome following DHCA. The wealth of available evidence suggests that investigations require coordinated efforts by multiple research groups, pursuing systematic, multilevel research - spanning from cell cultures, to various animal model systems ranging from rodents to large animals and ultimately to clinical trials.

10. Acknowledgements

We would like to acknowledge Mr. Alexandros Samolis for his active support in this study.

11. References

Almeida OFX, Conde GL, Crochemore C, et al. (2000) Subtle shifts in the ratio between pro- and antiapoptotic molecules after activationof corticosteroid receptors decide neuronal fate. FASEB journal 14:779-790

Ananiadou GO, Drossos GE, Bibou NK, Palatianos MG, Johnson OE. (2005) Acute regional neuronal injury following hypothermic circulatory arrest in a porcine model. Interact CardioVasc Thorac Surg., 4, 597-601

Ananiadou OG, Bibou K, Drossos GE, Bai M, Haj-Yahia S, Johnson EO. (2008) Hypothermia at 10C reduces neurologic injury after hypothermic circulatory arrest in the pig. J Cardiac Surg., 23, 31-8.

Ananiadou OG, Bibou K, Drossos GE, Charchanti A, Bai M, Haj-Yahia S, Anagnostopoulos CE, Johnson EO. (2007) Effect of profound hypothermia during circulatory arrest on neurologic injury and apoptotic repressor protein BcL-2 expression in an acute porcine model. J Thorac Cardiovas Surg., 133, 919-926

Apostolakis E, Shuhaiber JH. (2007) Antegrade or retrograde cerebral perfusion as an adjunct during hypothermic circulatory arrest for aortic arch surgery. Semin Cardiothoracic Vasc Anesth 11(1):77-85.

Conti AC, Raghupathi R, Trojanowski JQ, McIntosh TK. (1998) Experimental brain injury induces regionally distinct apoptosis during the acute and delayed post-traumatic period. J Neurosci., 18, 5663-72

Coselli JS, Bozinovski J, Cheung C. (2008) Hypothermic Circulatory Arrest: Safety and Efficacy in the Operative Treatment of Descending and Thoracoabdominal Aortic Aneurysms, Ann Thorac Surg 85:956–64.

Elrich MP, McCullough JN, Zhang N, Weisz DJ, Juvonen T, Bodian C, Griepp RB., (2002) Effect of hypothermia on cerebral blood flow and metabolism in the pig. Ann Thorac Surg., 73,191-7

Griep RB, Ergin MA, McCullough JN, Nguyen KH, Juvonen T, Chang N, Griepp EB. (1997) Use of hypothermic circulatory arrest for cerebral protection during aortic surgery. J Card Surg 1997; 12: 312-21.

Hagl C, Khaladj N, Karck M, Kallenbach K, Leyh R, Winterhalter M, Haverich A. (2003) Hypothermic circulatory arrest during ascending and aortic arch surgery: the theoretical impact of different cerebral perfusion techniques and other methods of cerebral protection,Eur J Cardio-thoracic Surg 24: 371–378.

Hagl C, Tatton NA, Khaladj N, Zhang N, Nandor S, Insolia S, Weisz DJ, Spielvogel D, Griepp RB. (2001) Involvement of apoptosis in neurological injury after hypothermic circulatory arrest: a new target for therapeutic interventions? Ann Thorac Surg., 72, 1457–64.

Kerr JFR, Wyllie AH, Currie AR. (1972)Apoptosis: A basic biological phenomenon with wide ranging implication in tissue kinetics Br J Cancer 26:239-257

Kouchoukos NT, Masetti P, Murphy SF. (2003) Hypothermic Cardiopulmonary Bypass and Circulatory Arrest in the Management of Extensive Thoracic and Thoracoabdominal Aortic Aneurysms, Semin Thoracic Cardiovasc Surg 15(4): 333-339.

Kroemer G. (1997) The proto-oncogene Bcl-2 and ist role in regulating apoptosis. Nat Med., 3, 614-20.

Kunihara T, Grün T, Aicher D, Langer F, Adam O, Wendler O, Saijo Y, Schäfers HJ. (2005) Hypothermic circulatory arrest is not a risk factor for neurologic morbidity in aortic surgery: A propensity score analysis, J Thorac Cardiovasc Surg 130:712-718.

Kurth CD, Priestly M, Golden J, McCann J, Raghupathi R. (1999) Regional patterns of neuronal death after deep hypothermic circulatory arrest in newborn pigs. J Thorac Cardiovasc Surg., 118(6), 1068-1077

Lipton P. (1999) Ischemic cell death in brain neurons. Physiol Rev., 79, 1431-1568

MacManus JP, Linnik MD. (1997) Gene expression induced by cerebral ischemia: an apoptotic perspective. J Cereb Blood Flow Metab., 17, 815-32.

Martin LJ. (2001) Neuronal cell death in nervous system development, disease and injury. Int J Mol Med 7(5):455-78

McCullough JN, Zhang N, Reich DL, Juvonen T, Klein J, Spielvogel D, Ergin AM, Griepp RB. (1999) Cerebral metabolic suppression during hypothermic circulatory arrest in humans. Ann Thorac Surg 67, 1895-9

Portera-Calliau C, Price DL, Martin LJ. (1997) Excitotoxic neuronal death in the immature brain is an apoptosis-necrosis morphological continuum. J Comp Neurol 378:70-87

Strauch JT, Spielvogel D, Haldenwang PL, Zhang Ning, Weisz D, Bodian CA, Tatton NA, Griepp RB. (2005) Cooling to 10°C and treatment with cyclosporine A improve cerebral recovery following prolonged hypothermic circulatory arrest in a chronic porcine model. Eur J Cardiothorac Surg., 27, 74-80

15

New Approaches for Treatment and Prevention of Aortic Aneurysms

Stefano Nazari
Foundation Alexis Carrel, Pavia, Italy

1. Introduction

1.1 Background

1.1.1 The beginning

Vascular surgery was quite obviously conditioned by the development and evolution of the techniques for vascular anastomosis, started around the beginning of the past century. Apart in fact from few episodic and lucky clinical cases of lateral laceration repair as well as many experimental endeavours of vascular suture, accurately described and illustrated in a detailed historical italian review (Zannini G 1967), before that point in time vascular surgery clinical practice was substantially confined to vascular ligature.

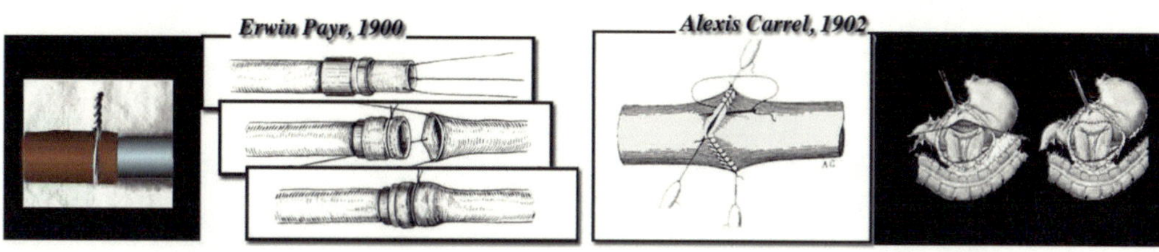

Fig. 1. Payr and Carrel pioneering techniques.
Payr first reported device for vascular anastomosis substantially derived from elaboration of the common method for rubber tubing connection (left square) while Carrel triangulation was apparently derived from refinements of gastrointestinal suture (right square).

In 1900 Erwin Payr reported to the German Surgical Society results on animal experiments of the apparently first device for vascular anastomosis, which is essentially based on external legature of vascular stumps over a rigid and absorbable magnesium ring (Payr E, 1900), thus trying to adapting to surgery a method already universally used for coupling floppy/elastic tubing. In spite of its elegance (intima-to-intima facing, absorbable magnesium ring) one of its implicit mechanical limits was already outlined in the original report: elastic retraction of the vascular wall when clamped significantly reduces its diameter, thus making quite difficult to put in place a rigid ring of appropriate diameter.
In those very years Alexis Carrel, as well as many others in fact (Zannini G 1967), was focusing his attention on suture techniques, already currently adopted in the gastrointestinal tract, and was able to realize blood-tight, low thrombogenic vascular anastomoses by careful refinements of the needles, threads and techniques for their use

(Carrel A, 1902, 1907), thus establishing the standard technique of vascular surgery. Although technically demanding, its versatility allowed to deal with virtually all clinical occurrences, from large aortic to microsurgical anastomosis, so that the many and significant improvements in needles (i.e. curved, atraumatic), threads (i.e. polypropylene) and surgical technique (i.e. parachute, etc) developed throughout more than a century could not break the ideal line linking the Nobel prize acknowledged (1912) Carrel original work with today clinical practice.
Interestingly enough for more than a century vascular anastomosis technique research moved forward, very slowly to say the truth, with occasional brief clinical applications essentially along these two basic principles only, with the possible exception of gluing based methods.

1.2 Vascular staplers

It was in fact substantially a technological evolution of the Carrel coupling principle (full thickness wall stump stitching) that gave origin, around the middle of the past century, to stapling devices with the aim of automating the anastomoses.

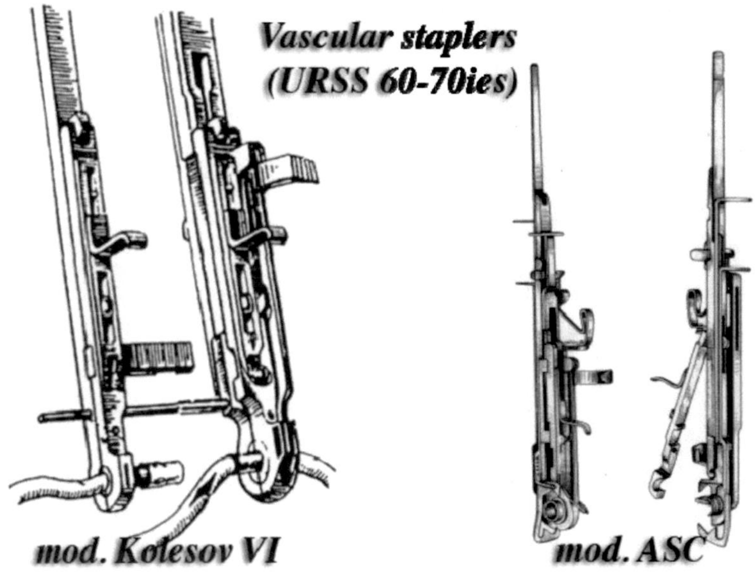

Fig. 2. Models of URSS vascular staplers (1960-70).
Similar bulky and cumbersome devices were also realized at that time in Canada, USA and Japan.

However, while stapling devices have long since allowed standardization and simplification of digestive tract circular anastomosis, despite extensive research (see exhaustive reviews: Tesauro 1967; Tesauro & Persico 1979), including our own (Nazari S et al, 1990), the stapling principle has so far failed to be of significant use for vascular anastomosis, which remains substantially the only basic surgical task still to be automated.
The 60-70ies stapling devices (fig 2) have all quite cumbersome and heavy configuration in particular in relation to the delicate structure of the quite small diameter vessel to which they were intended to be used in those years.

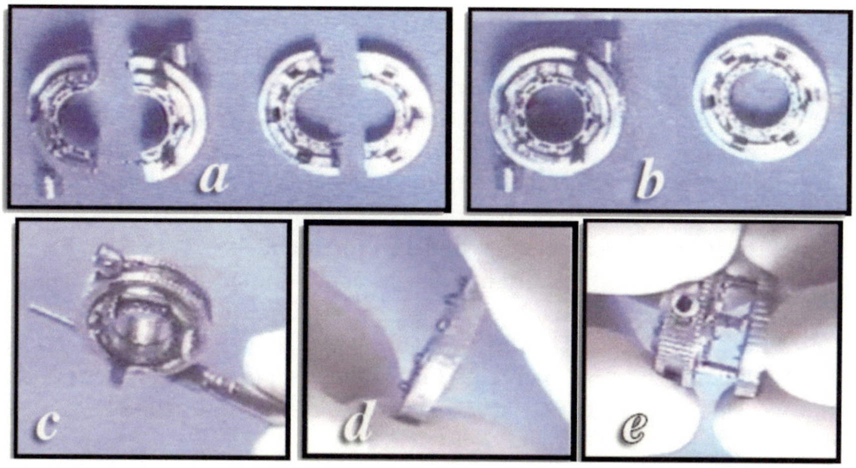

Fig. 3. Vascular stapler for reducing warm ischemia in organ transplantation.
With our model each stapler end can be mounted on donor and recipient by independent surgical teams without care for reciprocal orientation, being the maximal possible vascular axis torsion ≤30°. Activating guide-wire is connected just immediately before firing (Nazari et al 1990). Video at http://www.fondazionecarrel.org/tsb2/tsb2.html

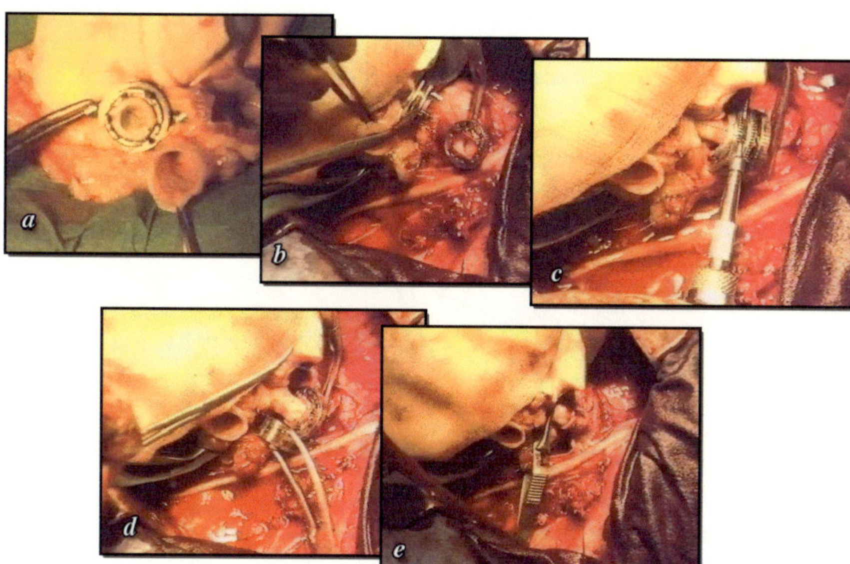

Fig. 4. Vascular stapler for reducing warm ischemia in experimental lung transplantation.
In a canine model of left single lung transplantation one stapler end was applied on donor pulmonary artery at back table (a) and the other by the recipient surgical team; then the two ends are quickly connected together (b), the firing wire connected and activated (c). After having sectioned the two sutures linking the vascular stumps to the device ends, the two stapler parts were divided and removed (d) and anastomosis checked (e) still preventing graft perfusion until atrial connection was established (Nazari et al 1990).
Video at http://www.fondazionecarrel.org/tsb2/tsb2.html

With this in mind first of all we tried to simplify the procedure by severing the stapling device (fig 3) from the activating handle, which in our device consisted in a flexible, camera-type, firing guide-wire that could be connected to the stapler after its coupling with vascular stumps just before firing (fig. 4,c), at the more convenient of the two opposite sides connectors (fig. 3). Moreover the two stapler parts were designed in such a way that each one could be mounted on the vascular stump by independent surgical teams without taking care for their reciprocal orientation; the connectors of the two parts of the stapler in fact allowed to limit the maximal possible vascular axis torsion to 30°.

One of the crucial points mechanically implicit in any vascular stapler model, is related to the requirement of temporary fixation of the vascular stumps to the device ends in preparation for the anastomosis. The vascular stump link to each device end in fact must be, on one side, strong enough to be maintained during device manipulation for ends coupling but, on the other side, should be weak enough to be easily released after stapler firing, to allow the device ends to be divided and removed.

Being our stapler ideated for use in organ transplantation to reduce the warm ischemic phase, we could solve this problem by temporarily suturing vascular stumps to the stapler end by single thread on predisposed little rings (fig 3, d); this can be done independently by the donor surgical team at back table to one stapler end (fig 4, a) and by the recipient team to the other stapler end, without interfering with time critical surgical phases. When the donor organ is at the recipient operative table (fig 4, b) the two stapler ends can be easily and quickly connected and the stapler fired (fig. 4,c). Only when the circulation is resumed the sutures temporarily connecting the vascular stumps to the stapler ends can be sectioned and the device removed (fig 4, d) without impacting on the organ warm ischemia time.

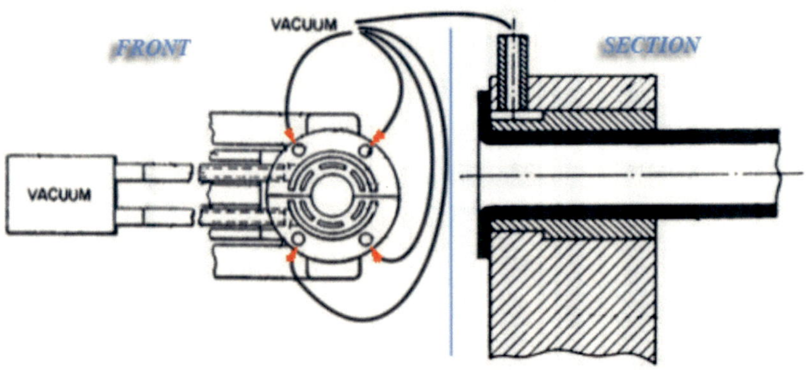

Fig. 5. Kolesov VI vacuum assisted vascular stapler.
To temporarily connect coronary artery stumps to the stapler ends, vacuum is applied to the predisposed device whose surface then sucks and holds the vascular wall (red arrows).

An elegant technical solution to this problem was provided by V. Kolesov (Kolesov VI et al 1970, 1991), credited for the first LIMA-coronary artery by pass (Konstantinov IE, 2004) and the first (and at this point in time the only one) surgeon to have clinically used coronary stapling device. He devised to realize this vascular stump-stapler end temporary link by applying vacuum to each device end whose surface was appropriately predisposed (Fig. 5, red arrows) thus sucking and holding the vascular stump in position. This seems a simple and effective method that can ideally fit with the surgical need and possibly solve this part of the vascular stapler problems.

In synthesis however, even though research restlessly continue to produce new prototypes, the apparently unavoidable critical point is that the intrinsic manual surgical skill required to put in position and operate any stapler on the delicate vascular structure didn't yet (can't?) result in a easier, simpler, quicker and more efficient task than standard hand suture, even when its use is for very large diameter vessel only (Takata et al 2011).

1.3 Intraluminal ringed prosthesis

In the 1970-1980s, a simplified Payr concept was revived with the introduction of intraluminal ringed prostheses, whose use in aortic substitution was quite extensively reported (Lemole et al, 1982; Berger et al, 1983; Crawford ES & JL, 1984).

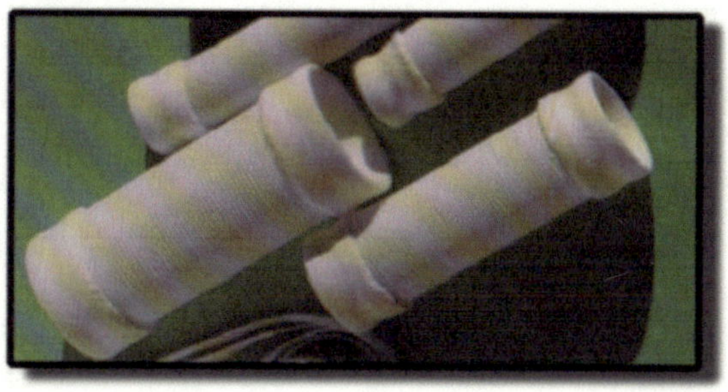

Fig. 6. Intraluminal ringed prosthesis.
Aortic anastomotic device commercially available (FDA) in 70-90ies.

The reasons for their clinical failure have been numerous. Facts mechanically implicit in the method (fig 7) are related both to the elastic retraction of the vessel when is clamped, already outlined in the Payr report (Payr, 1900), and to the floppy consistency of the vascular wall that requires a further significant gap to be left between the clamped internal aortic wall and the external ring diameter to allow the ring to be easily slipped into the vascular stump without friction. Accordingly a ringed prosthesis with a diameter significantly smaller than appropriate must be used to keep the cross-clamping time shorter than that attainable with manual suturing (Nazari, 1996a). Thus when the aorta is re-perfused, the resulting discrepancy between perfused vascular stump and intraluminal ring diameter generates conditions greatly favouring coupling instability (fig. 7, C); moreover possible generation of systolic movements of the aortic wall at ligature hinge may potentially cause mechanical friction/erosion and thus eventually rupture. (fig 7, D).
Many other inappropriate constructive features of those devices were probably responsible for their eventual failure. Thus the rigid ring was too short to be easily identified from outside the aorta, making very difficult the appropriate positioning of the external ligature; moreover the groove shape and dimension were inappropriate to maintain coupling stability.
This latter point offers the occasion for some important consideration. Vascular anastomosis must guarantee two essential mechanical facts: haemostatic sealing and stability of the coupling. This may seem a self-evident, unnecessary distinction since both are obviously provided at once by the standard hand suture; not so however with the "Payr" coupling principle, which is at basis of 70-80ies intraluminal prosthesis as well as of our expandable device.

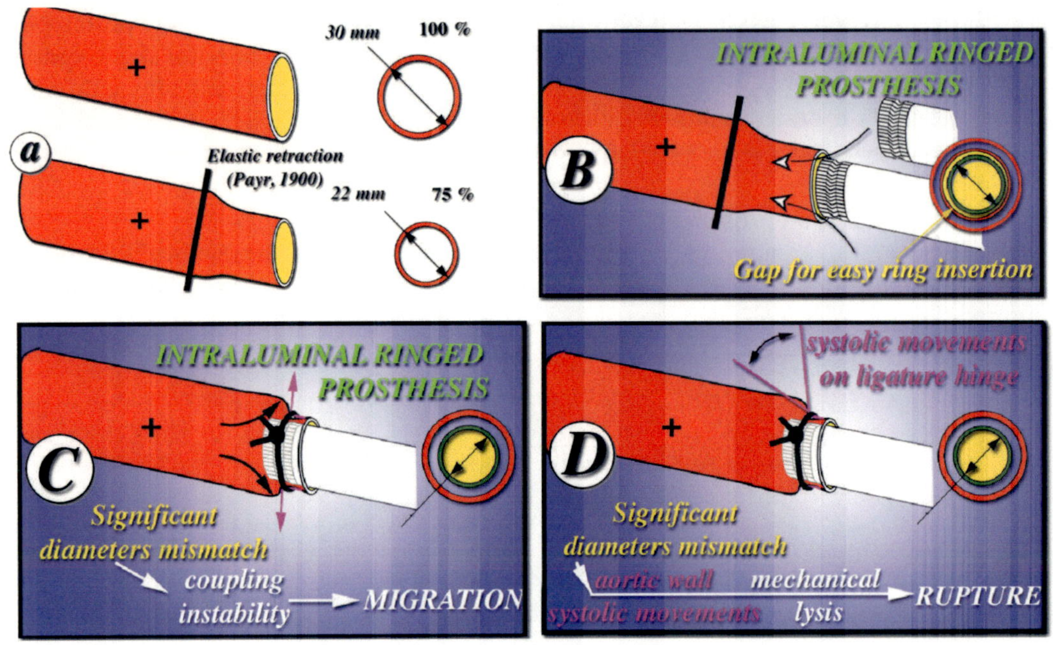

Fig. 7. Facts related to intraluminal ringed prosthesis (Payr type coupling).
When the vessel is clamped there is a significant reduction of the stump diameter due to its elastic retraction (a); moreover because of the floppy consistency of the vascular wall a significant gap (b) must be left between outer ring and inner stump diameter for a rapid positioning. When blood flow is resumed the resulting significant diameter mismatch (c) generates conditions for coupling instability and device dislocation. It may also be hypothesized that systolic movements on ligature hinge (d) may generate mechanical erosion and possibly rupture.

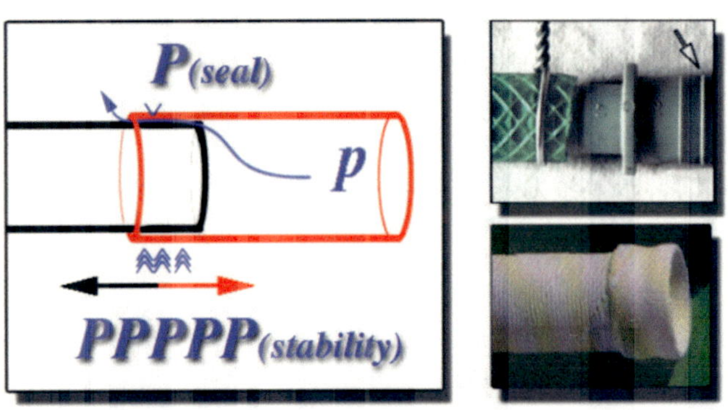

Fig. 8. Haemostasis and stability in Payr coupling type.
While hemostasis can be achieved by applying an external pressure ≥ blood pressure, even much higher pressure may not prevent the stump from slipping over the inner sleeve and split apart (larger square). Grooves on the inner sleeve outer surface can prevent dislocation only if appropriately dimensioned and shaped (right upper square). Intraluminal prosthesis groove appears inappropriate in deepness, length and shape to keep coupling stability (right lower square).

While in fact to achieve haemostatic seal is sufficient to apply on the vascular stump external surface a pressure equal or just exceeding the blood pressure, that pressure or even a much higher pressure may not be enough to prevent the vascular stump from slipping off from the inner sleeve (fig. 8, large square). Then means to increase friction (i.e. groove or hooks, etc) between the opposing surfaces or to permanently link them together (i.e. full thickness stitches) must be put in place to prevent vascular stump from sliding off. Although this was soon appreciated (and solved!) by gardeners since many years (fig. 8, upper right square), the failure of the 70-80ies intraluminal prosthesis may have been caused also by underestimation (fig. 8, lower right square) of this not irrelevant detail.

1.4 Endovascular surgery

In the last decade of the past century, preceded by pioneering work of C. Gianturco (Charnsangavej et al, 1985; Wright et al, 1985; Yoshioka et al, 1988) and popularized by J.C Parodi clinical reports (Parodi 1991, 1994), endovascular techniques burst into clinical vascular surgery, allowing prosthesis positioning into the aneurysm and excluding it from blood stream without open surgery. This provided a less invasive and lower complications rate therapeutic tool that allowed cure for patients previously not amenable to open surgery for age, general conditions or associated risk factors. First successfully popularized in infrarenal aortic aneurysm, techniques and materials continuing improvements allowed endovascular prosthetic substitution of virtually all segments of aorta, including arch, even though sometime with hybrid procedures (Canaud et al, 2010;Antoniou et al, 2010; Tsagakis et al, 2010, Di Eusanio, 2011).

It is not the aim of this chapter to describe, even summarily, the historical evolution of these techniques, but rather to try to outline the proved facts of these new therapeutic tools at this point in time.

While obviously technological evolution will further extend indications and improvements in clinical results, superiority of endovascular method vs open surgery at this point in time was conclusively proved in infrarenal aortic aneurysms and in uncomplicated, non genetic, isolated descending aorta aneurysms (Gopaldas et al, 2010). An interesting result of several recent studies (The UK EVAR Trial Investigators, 2010; De Bruin, 2010; Schermerhorn, 2008) showed that, despite a two-thirds decrease in 30-day operative mortality rate after endovascular abdominal aortic aneurism repair (EVAR) compared with open repair, the all-cause mortality curves converge during the first 2-3 years thereafter, with no significant difference in all-cause mortality beyond this time. A recent study (Brown et al, 2011) seems to indicate that more cardiovascular deaths in the EVAR patients group contribute to the convergence in all-cause mortality during the first 2 years.

Quite wide clinical experience however already showed that endovascular procedures cannot protect from spinal chord ischemia and consequent paraplegia in extended descending aorta prosthetic substitution. It has been hypothesized that this could be due, at least in some case, to the fact that while endoprosthesis immediately prevents intercostal branches to be physiologically perfused, cannot prevent, at least for a certain time in the initial phase, backwards blood flow into the space between endoprosthesis and aortic wall, thus generating conditions for a blood flow "steal" from perfusion of the spinal chord (Kawaharada et al, 2010).

Last but not least overall recent USA Nationwide Inpatient Sample data 2006-2007 review (Gopaldas et al, 2010) showed that only 23% (2,563/11,669) of ideal candidate to endovascular treatment (uncomplicated, elective descending aortic aneurysms) underwent endovascular procedure (TEVAR), while the remaining 77% (9,106/11,669) still underwent open surgical repair.

These facts prompted us to consider new strategies against aortic aneurysm based on new tools we developed for its treatment and prevention.

2. New expandable devices for easier, safer and more efficient open surgery for large thoracic or thoracoabdominal aneurysms

Even though endovascular techniques will continuously gain wider indications for prosthetic substitution of the aorta, more complex cases will always remain in which open surgery is the only or the best option. Moreover while acute aortic syndrome is obviously spread throughout the territory only highly specialized centers can offer endovascular techniques as an emergency measure; current data show that vast majority (77%) of uncomplicated, non genetic elective descending aorta aneurisms still underwent standard open surgery in US (Gopaldas et al, 2010). On the other hand open thoracic aorta prosthetic substitution still carries significant risk of serious complications that cannot be prevented even in very highly specialized centers, in particular to CNS and spinal cord.

Although the pathogenesis of these complications is multifactorial, there is general agreement that the length of clamping/circulatory arrest time is an extremely important factor. Since nearly all the clamping/arrest time is spent for vascular anastomosis construction, a device able to quicken and simplify the vascular anastomosis can be expected to have a significant impact on the incidence of these complications.

Suture line haemostasis is another important source of intra- and postoperative complications with standard open technique. In fact due to the altered aortic wall mechanical features, impaired by the underlying aortic pathology (arteriosclerosis, medial cystic degeneration, Marfan disease etc.), the suture line haemostasis may be difficult to achieve in spite of appropriate surgical technique or may require additional surgical maneuvers (buttressing, gluing etc.) that imply prolongation of the ischemia time.

Moreover in cases of dissection, it may be difficult to achieve firm layers approximation and to prevent re-dissection and false lumen persistent perfusion, in particular at suture lines.

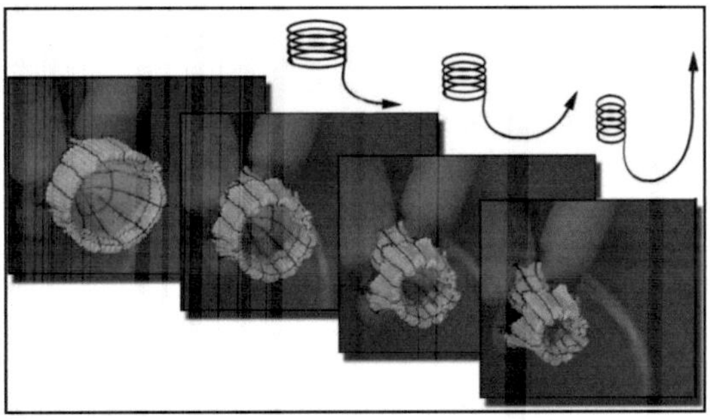

Fig. 9. Expandable device working principle.
Loops of nitinol wire wrapped by Dacron fabric form a rigid sleeve whose diameter can be modified by varying the diameter of the nitinol loops, while the regular cylindrical shape is maintained.

For these reasons several years ago we started research (Nazari et al, 1994) to develop a new expandable device aimed: **1**-to simplify the surgical technique; **2**-to significantly reduce the ischemic time and thus the ischemic complications rate; **3**-to enhance suture line anastomosis; **4**-to achieve firm and reliable dissected layers approximation, thus preventing

re-dissection and/or false lumen persistent perfusion at suture lines, particularly in acute dissection repairs.
The device consists of loops of nitinol wires, wrapped within a Dacron fabric and connected to a prosthesis end (Type I). The nitinol wire loops can be expanded and tightened by activating a removable guide in such a way that device end varies its diameter, while maintaining a regular cylindrical shape. This allows the easy and quick insertion of the retracted device into the vascular stump and then its expansion to perfectly fit with the vessel diameter; haemostasis and permanent device fixation is provided by external ligature/suture.

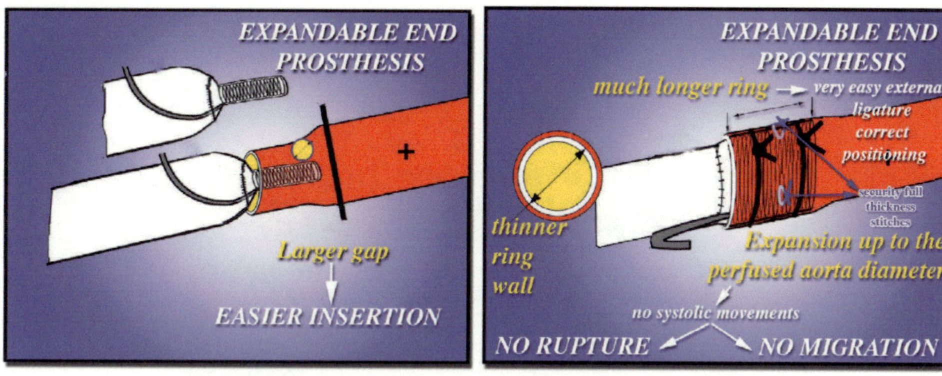

Fig. 10. Expandable device vs intraluminal ringed prosthesis.
The expandable configuration of the ring allows to solve all the insertion, positioning and diameter mismatch problems of the 70ies intraluminal prosthesis.

Its quite evident that the expandable configuration of the ring allows to solve all the insertion, positioning and stability problems of the 70ies intraluminal prosthesis (fig. 10). That makes performing an anastomosis a very simple task, which can be carried out in seconds vs the 10-15 min per anastomosis at best required with standard hand suture.
The aortic wall being not perforated by the suture, the coupling is immediately blood-thigh ("air-tight" in fact!) and independent by the integrity of the physiological coagulation mechanisms.
The device underwent many modifications and refinements, finally resulting in three main models (Type I, II and III) applying the same working mechanism, but with different shape to fit with all aorta segments as well as special conditions of use.
Extensive "ex vivo" and "in vivo" animal experiments (Nazari et al 1994, 1996a, 1996d, 1997, 2006, 2009; Rossella et al 2008) were carried out and few clinical cases were also successfully treated with this device (Nazari et al.1999; Aluffi et al, 2002, Buniva et al 2002).

2.1 Device description and operational details

2.1.1 Device type I and II

Device type I and II differ because of the orientation of the activating guide in respect to the main axis of the device wireframe expandable sleeve (fig 11, upper right and lower left squares); that allows the devices to be ideally used for the first and second anastomosis respectively. Thus the type I device, activated by guide-wire coaxial to the lumen, is sutured at one end of the tube graft of appropriate size before clamping, can be quickly and easily positioned either in the proximal or distal end of the aortic tract to be replaced (fig. 11, top

strip). Any further manipulation of the tube graft is then easily possible, including accessory side anastomosis with aortic branches, without any hindrance. The tube graft can then be sectioned at its exact required length and fixed with a single stitch at the rear anastomosis side (fig 11, middle strip); type II device, activated by guide-wire orthogonal to the vascular axis allowing stump connection at both sides, is then inserted, expanded and fixed by external ligature (fig 11, lower strip) ending the ischemia phase.
When the perfusion is resumed, permanent fixation is carried out by tying ligature and applying few full thickness polypropilen 4-0 equidistant stitches, to further stabilize the device thus virtually preventing any possible late dislocation. Activating guide can then be removed by predisposed tools.

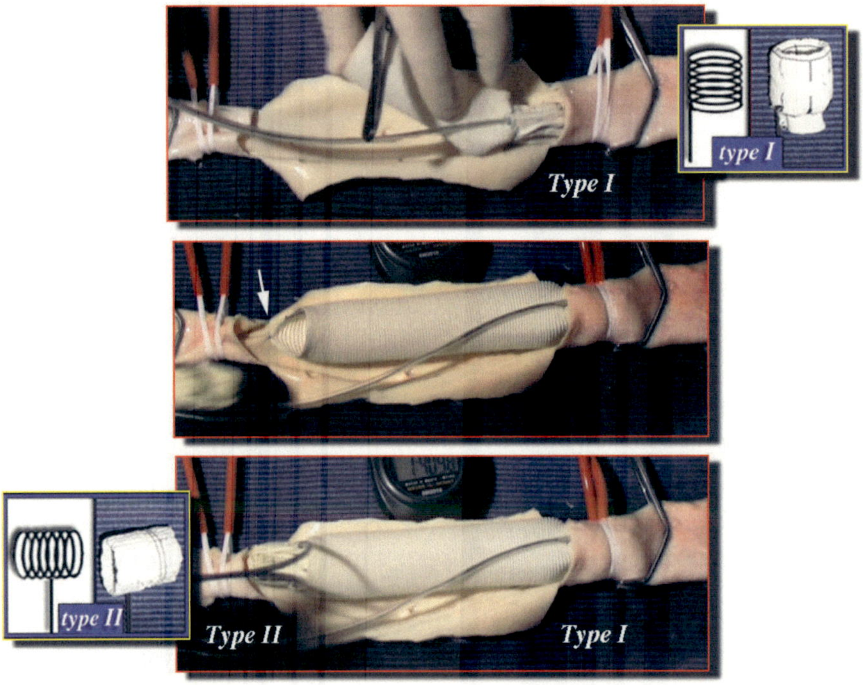

Fig. 11. Device Type I and II.
Device type I, previously sutured to the appropriate diameter tube graft end, is used for the first anastomosis; then after having carried out any other collateral branch anastomosis possibly required, the tube graft is cut at its final measure, fixed with a single stitch at rear anastomosis side (arrow) and device Type II is applied for the anastomosis. Circulation can be immediately resumed after tourniquets tightening. Thus final ligature, full thickness stabilizing stitches (3 at each anastomosis) and activating guide removal can be carried out without prolonging the ischemic phase.

Use of the external ligature (umbilical tape or polipropilene) allows to minimize ischemic time, since the blood flow can be resumed after the simple tourniquet tension, the final stabilization being carried out afterward. With a very little prolongation of ischemia time however a polypropilene suture can be passed in a purse-string fashion also in the vascular intimal surface, totally or partially, with the same functional results (fig. 12). Even in this case it is important to pass the suture full thickness through the device at least in 3 roughly equidistant points in order to prevent any possible late dislocation.

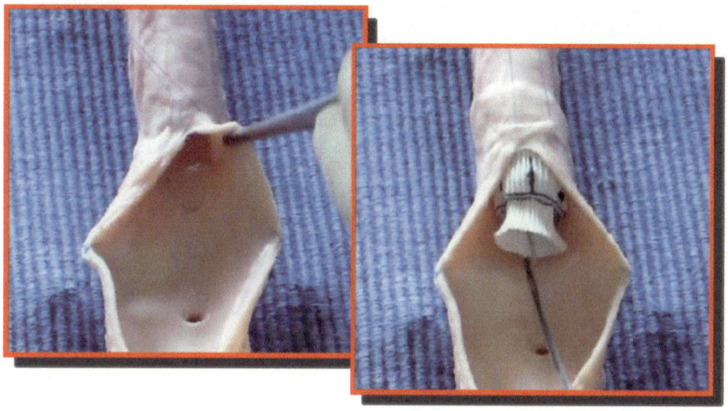

Fig. 12. Purse-string device fixation.
With type I and II devices, the vascular stump encirclement can be avoided and substituted by endovascular (full or partial) purse-string polipropilene suture prepared at the site of expandable device positioning. The required full thickness security stitches can be passed after the circulation has been re-estableshed (from Nazari, 2010).

The solution of positioning and stability problems of the 70ies intraluminal prosthesis (fig. 10) allows for the first time the clinical appreciation of the most important feature of the "Payr principle" of anastomosis (vascular stumps compression against/between rigid structures i.e. an inner rigid ring and external ligature/outer rigid ring) *which is to achieve an immediate hermetic seal* ("air-tight" in fact) ensuring reliable haemostasis at the anastomosis line, not dependent from coagulation. Interestingly enough were just the positioning problems of Payr model as well as of its more recent modification (Intraluminal ringed prosthesis), that prevented in fact the clinical implementation of this coupling method, which is the most intuitive (and in fact was the first to be attempted in vascular surgery) and whose application failed only in the surgical field, while was in use (and still is) in all other technological fields where connectors between elastic/floppy tubing are required.

Of course clinical experience over more than a century has shown that the standard suturing technique does not need to provide an "air-tight" anastomosis to ensure perfect hemostasis in virtually all clinical circumstances. In particular cases however (acute dissection, cystic medial necrosis, etc.), structural impairments of the aortic wall may necessitate additional maneuvers including graft strips buttressing, gluing and a variety of accessory techniques, whose efficacy at achieving hemostasis are not always fully predictable and that obviously further significantly prolong the period of ischemia in this most critical area. A coupling method that provides haemostasis by compression of the stumps' vascular wall between two rigid structures (i.e. inner and outer expandable rigid sleeves) without perforation may be then particularly useful in these cases, not only because of its ease and quickness, but also because it offers the best mechanical chance of immediate blood-tightness. The expected advantages with regards to approximation of dissecting layers and false lumen permanent sealing rely on the same concept.

An other important difference with 70-80ies intraluminal ringed devices is that the expandable sleeve is much more thin and porous, being formed substantially by a double layer of standard vascular dacron fabric, and can, therefore, be wholly and quickly colonized by fibroblasts and integrated with the aortic wall.

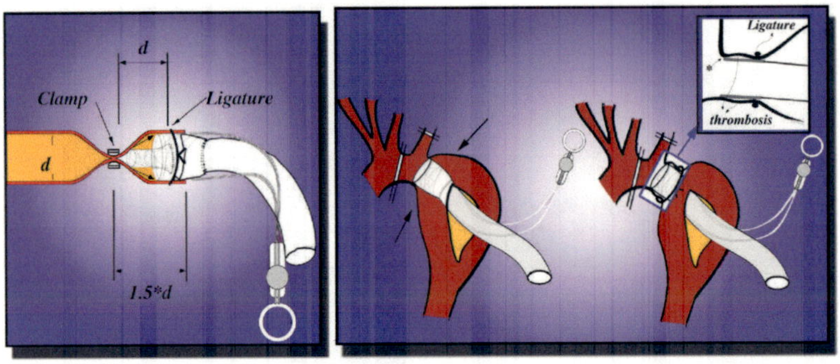

Fig. 13. Expandable device operational details.
Left square. When a clamp is applied the linearization of the stump requires to keep its length significantly longer than usual in order to leave the space necessary for full expansion of the expandable end. It is also important to avoid full longitudinal vascular opening as carried out with current technique and thus keeping intact the entire circumference of the vascular stump for a tract long enough to host the whole device expandable end.
Right square. The expandable end also can be positioned against aneurysmal wall, provided that its distal end would reach the healthy vascular wall. Thrombosis of the tract between the ligature and the prosthesis end will soon move the effective anastomosis line (upper right square*) where it would be with standard suture (mod from Nazari et al, 1997).

The nitinol wire-frame in fact forms a very thin and wide mesh net that accounts for a very small proportion of the device's volume and that offers no significant barrier to fibroblastic invasion of the dacron fabric and thus to stable biological integration of the device.
Few technical details must be considered with the expandable devices.
First of all care must be taken when entering the aneurysm not to extend the incision up to both the distal and proximal ends as usually carried out with standard suture; it is in fact very important to keep intact the entire circumference of the vascular stump for a tract long enough to host the device expandable end.
Due to the linearization of the vessel diameter induced by the clamp, the length of the vascular stump distal to it must be significantly longer than imagined before clamping; in practice it is advisable to isolate the vessel for a length exceeding its diameter (Fig. 13, left square).
It may be argued that the use of the device may require a distinct healthy vascular neck, as with endovascular techniques. This is not necessary; the device in fact can be expanded even within the aneurysmal wall and fixed there by the external ligature, provided that its end reaches the healthy vascular wall limit, where ideally the standard suture would be placed (Fig 13, right square). The thrombosis developing in the tract between the ligature and the prosthesis end will soon exclude the brief tract of aneurysmal wall from the bloodstream, thus moving the effective anastomosis line (fig 13,* at upper right square) where it would be with standard suture.
Thus devices type I and II can be ideally used anywhere in descending and abdominal aorta and allow to carry out any required additional surgical maneuver on the tube graft, i.e. collateral branch anastomosis, as well as its appropriate tailoring at the required length measured directly on the operative field as in standard technique without obstacle or hampering condition. Its great simplicity of use allows the devices to be used also in condition of suboptimal operative field exposure. Thus for example both proximal and distal

anastomosis in extended descending thoracic aorta substitution be easily and safely carried out though a single space thoracotomy; moreover aortic prosthetic substitution via mini-access thoracotomy or laparotomy video-assisted setting may be also predictably considered.

2.1.2 Device type III

In this version of the device the external ligature is substituted by an expandable sleeve, which is based essentially on the same working principle as the inner sleeve, but activated contrariwise. Thus, the vascular stump is compressed between two sleeves (Fig. 14, upper left little squares), with variable and controllable diameters, allowing full control of the pressure (amount and surface of its application) applied to the vascular stump.

Operative technique for device type III is illustrated in fig 14 in ascending aorta "ex vivo" model and it is really very simple. First of all both sleeves diameter is set at the predicted value of the aortic tract where the device will be applied. Then the inner sleeve diameter only is reduced as much as possible by acting on its guide-wire; this causes also the backwards eversion and partial rotation of the outer sleeve thus greatly enhancing inner sleeve visibility and then its easy positioning into the vascular stump. The inner sleeve is then re-expanded against the vascular stump inner surface; at this point the outer sleeve is gently retracted acting on its own activating guide to compress the vascular stump.

The primary aim of this new version of the device is to make possible and convenient to apply this coupling principle also to acute ascending aorta and arch dissection, in order to simplify the technique, to reduce the ischemic time, to improve hemostasis of the anastomosis line and to achieve reliable, stable sealing of the dissection layers in this very complex surgical setting. The device in fact allows to actually automate substantially the same aortic wall sandwiching between two graft strips procedure usually carried out in the dissection cases and realizing at once the prosthesis anastomosis, being the tube graft (not shown in the figure) obviously previously sutured to the inner sleeve proximal end. Interestingly enough the particular configuration of the device allows full and easy compliance with aortic anatomy, perfectly adapting also to the elliptic, asymmetric "oblique"stump resulting from inclusion of the arch concavity in the anastomosis line (Fig. 15, B). Full and persistent air-tight sealing of the device-aortic wall coupling was verified at endovascular pressures of up to 150 mmHg in "ex vivo" swine aortic models, including those involving an elliptic, 'oblique' anastomosis (Fig. 15, b) (Nazari, 2010). As expected, standard vascular sutures were not air-tight even at pressures below 10 mmHg (Fig. 15, c).

Type III device use is then ideally indicated in dissection cases for distal anastomosis sited at distal ascending aorta, including as much as required of the concavity of the arch during a very brief circulatory arrest phase; proximal anastomosis will be then carried out either by hand suture or with the expandable device version most appropriated for the particular anatomical condition, in normal CEC in no rush and after having performed any additional procedure possibly required, for example on the valve.

Anastomosis at the distal arch/proximal descending aorta in case of full arch substitution is also an ideal indication for type III device use in case of dissection or whenever, for particular aortic wall fragility, graft strips sandwiching buttressing may be advisable. Supra-aortic trunks in these cases can be ideally re-vascularized by devices type I previously appropriately connected to the main tube graft so that they can be plugged in and there fixed by purse-string partially or entirely passed from inside the vascular lumen (fig. 11).

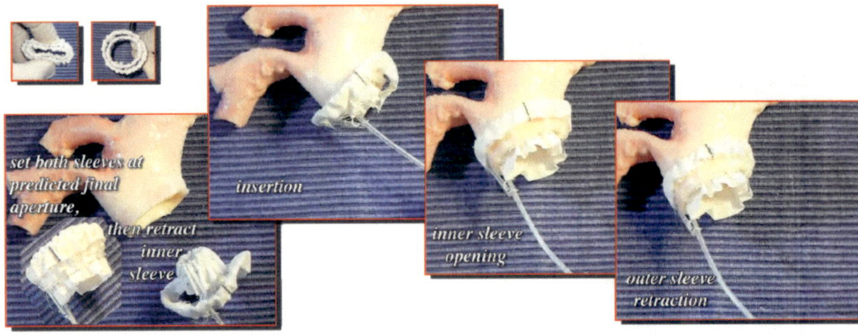

Fig. 14. Device type III.
The type III device incorporates an external sleeve that substitutes the external ligature, thus allowing standardization of the pressure applied to the vascular stump wall. The wire-frame of the device is quite soft and compliant, and can be easily compressed and widely deformed while maintaining perfect reciprocal alignment of the internal and external sleeves (top left squares). Lower squares: First of all both sleeves are set at predicted final aperture. Acting only on the activating guide of the inner sleeve results in outer sleeve backwards rotation and eversion, bringing the retracted inner sleeve in full visibility, so that can be easily inserted into the vascular stump. Then inner ring is expanded as much as the vascular wall can be distended by acting contrariwise on the same guide. At this point, the outer sleeve is only slightly retracted towards the aortic wall using its own guide. (Nazari, 2010) Video at http://www.fondazionecarrel.org/tsb2/tsb2.html

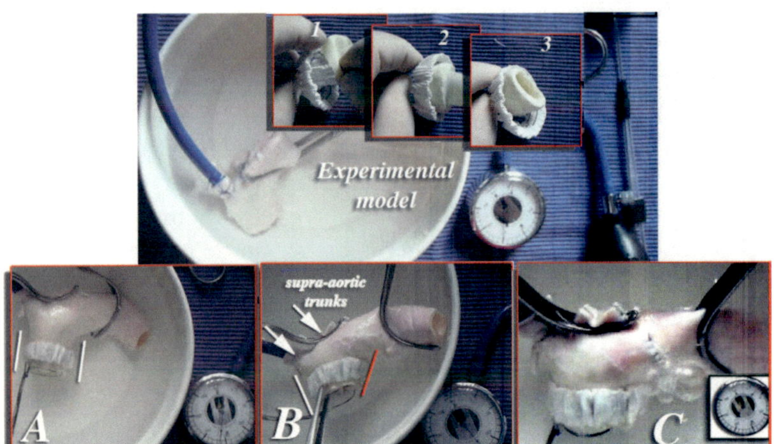

Fig. 15. Device type III seal test.
The outer surface of the inner sleeve was wrapped by a latex cuff (top squares) in order to overcome the problem of the porosity of the dacron graft and the requirement for the connection of the tube graft to the proximal end of the inner sleeve as in its final clinical use. A) The air-tightness of the connection was verified at endovascular pressures of up to 150 mmHg in a regular cylindrical anastomosis of ascending aorta (white bars). (B) The same was verified when the anastomosis is irregularly oriented, such as when involves the arch concavity. (C) As easily predictable, a standard suture (4–0 prolene) of an approximately 3 cm incision of the aortic wall cannot be proved airtight even at minor endovascular pressure. (Nazari, 2010). Video at http://www.fondazionecarrel.org/tsb2/tsb2.html

Thus in all cases where sandwiching buttressing is planned the use of the device type III requires exactly the same aortic stump external wall preparation required for hand suture double graft strips application. When anatomical conditions do not require sandwiching buttressing, device type I or type II may be also used even without external vascular stump encircling, being possible to fix the expanded device end by purse-string passed entirely or partially from inside the aortic lumen (fig. 11).
The great simplification and the very significant quickening of this complex surgical part together with the higher accuracy and "mechanical" reliability of this coupling method in comparison with manual suture could potentially have impact that may exceed that strictly related to the anastomosis. For example being possible to carry out even the entire arch re-vascularization in few minutes of circulatory arrest, the level of hypothermia may be very significantly reduced and even the type of cerebral protection may be tailored to these very restricted time lapses, just to say the firsts coming in mind.

2.1.3 Other expandable device models

We also realized a variety of modified versions of the device to better fit with the anatomical configurations occurring in particular clinical circumstances.

2.1.3.1 Type I - SOLD (Single Outer Layer for small Diameters)

In small vessel diameters obviously device dimensions can interfere more significantly with physiological lumen amplitude in their range of use. More in particular the unpredictable way of folding of the inner fabric layer when the device is incompletely opened may significantly reduce the lumen available for the blood flow. Accordingly for diameters ≤ 12 and ≥6 mm we decided to use devices wrapped by fabric only at external layer (fig. 16). Two sizes were prepared respectively for diameter from 6 to 9 (SS) and from 10 to 12 mm (S). This may fit for renal artery, celiac axis and supraortic trunks. The device is previously prepared at the end of collateral branch of the main tube graft tailored at the expected appropriated length or directly on the main tube graft. The particular fabric disposition implies a mandatory blood flow direction, which however allows the use as main tube graft lateral branches for the major aortic branches.

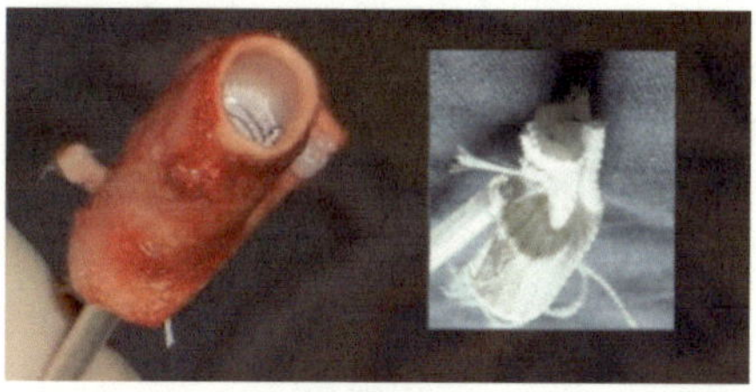

Fig. 16. Device type I - SOLD.
For small diameters vessels (≥6mm ≤12mm) device type I was prepared with single outer fabric graft in order to prevent the possible significant interference with vascular lumen of unpredictable way of folding of the inner layer when the device cannot be fully expanded. These devices allow one way flow direction only.
Video at http://www.fondazionecarrel.org/tsb2/tsb2.html

2.1.3.2 Type II - BIO (Bending and Independent Opening)

This type II device modified version is intended for use in ascending aorta substitution in absence of dissection. The two ends of the device can vary their reciprocal axis up to 90° to better fit with the curvature of the ascending aorta; their aperture can be independently controlled in order to comply with possible differences in diameter of the proximal and distal stumps. In this way the ascending aorta substitution can be carried out very quickly by one single device.

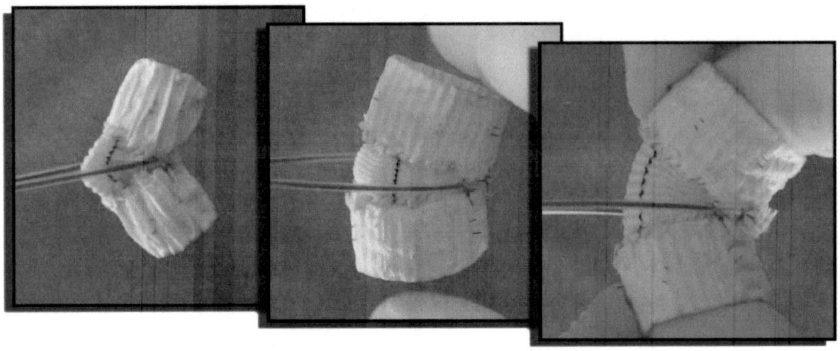

Fig. 17. Device Type II - BIO.
This type II device version allows the bending up to a 90° degree angle of the axis of their ends, whose aperture can be independently controlled. This allows to fit curved anatomy of ascending aorta and possible variations in diameter of the vascular stumps.
Video at: http://www.fondazionecarrel.org/tsb2/tsb2.html

In case of dissection however type III device previously connected with graft tube should be better used for distal anastomosis. Proximal anastomosis can be carried out with standard suture, time being not here a critical factor, or by a second type III device if dissection involves also the proximal anastomosis line.
This device version can also be used in isthmus rupture repair, having care of entering the aorta through or close to the laceration in order to preserve integrity of the vascular wall at site of device ends deployment.

2.1.3.3 Recent refinements

The extensive past experience provided full mechanical reliability of devices in all their versions and proved their easy applicability to aortic stump in all conditions. While the expandable device allows a much easier, quicker and more efficient ("airtight" seal) graft-aortic stump coupling than standard suture (Nazari 2010), it implies however the permanence of endovascular tubular wireframe and external ligature that could, at least theoretically, mechanically conflict with aortic wall, particularly at device ends, and with confining tissues/organs.
Aorto-digestive fistula is an infrequent but well documented occurrence after aortic open (Geraci et al 2008; Luo et al, 2010) as well as after endovascular (Ruby & Cogbill, 2007; Marone et al, 2007; Chiesa et al, 2010) repair. While graft or/and suture line contamination/infection may occasionally be suspected as the primary etiological factor, pure mechanical erosion from systolic movements of graft and even from the suture line only (Tanaka et al, 2009) may probably represent the first triggering factor in a portion of cases difficult to quantify.
The pure mechanical effect of these movements on the confining tissue/organ is predictably higher the harder/less compliant is the prosthetic material as well as the more conflicting is its orientation in relation to the confining tissue/organ.
We then recently focused on optimal consistency of the expandable wireframe and on means to provide external fixation with the final aim of achieving mechanical forces of coupling as much as possible similar to those taking place in standard hand suture anastomosis.

For this purpose, on one side, the wireframe consistency was decreased by variably reducing the gauge of nitinol wires and their respective position within wireframe and, on the other side, the external ligature was carried out with the thinnest possible prolene (5-0) encircling suture, transfixing full thickness the device and aortic wall at three equidistant points. The limit of the former was the ability to sustain the external ligature without wireframe deformation/collapse at pressure providing "airtight" seal; the limit of the later was the ability to provide stability of the aortic stump-expandable device coupling at stretch test.
The present versions of the devices with minimal consistence and great compliance minimize the risk of mechanical conflict and erosion with the confining tissue/organs; moreover wireframe consistency was settled in such a way that is minimal at the device end where the possible conflict with aortic wall could be higher.
Concerning the external ligature and its many possible ways of application, it may be useful to recall that vascular anastomosis must guarantee haemostatic sealing and stability of the coupling which, contrariwise to standard suture, rely on different mechanisms with this type of coupling (Fig. 8).
Thus even though external devices surface is provided with short needles perpendicularly positioned around its circumference at 4-6 equidistant points, reduction of the wireframe consistency may probably decrease their reliability in keeping coupling stability.
To optimize coupling stability in this lighter expandable wireframe we successfully tested 5-0 prolene encircling suture, transfixing full thickness the device and aortic wall at three equidistant points (fig. 18). In this way in fact the minimal expandable wireframe consistence to sustain the external ligature can be further significantly reduced and stability increased, by splitting the external ligature circumference in three separate and equivalent segments. In this embodiment the expandable ring will be then really only a bit more consistent of a common graft tube.

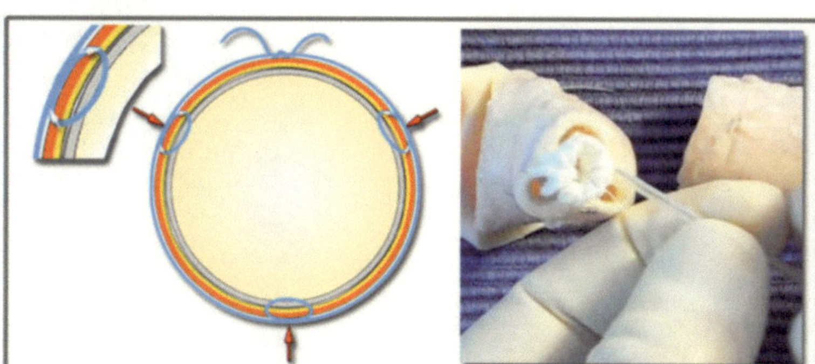

Fig. 18. Carrel's triangulation - back to the future.
To provide reliable coupling stability, instead of simple external ligature, 5-0 prolene encircling suture, transfixing full thickness the device and aortic wall at three equidistant points, was passed and tied as shown, in a sort of revival of the Carrel triangulation historical technique. Video at http://www.fondazionecarrel.org/tsb2/tsb2.html

This coupling stability was proved by a stretch test consisting in a sequence of manoeuvres carried out on the anastomosis that includes: **1)** complete compression of the anastomosis in orthogonal directions and then **2)** vigorous manual stretching of the anastomosis in the coaxial plane separately at four points of its circumference. The sequence was repeated three times and the anastomosis checked for any significant vascular stump backwards dislocation on the expandable wireframe throughout the entire circumference.

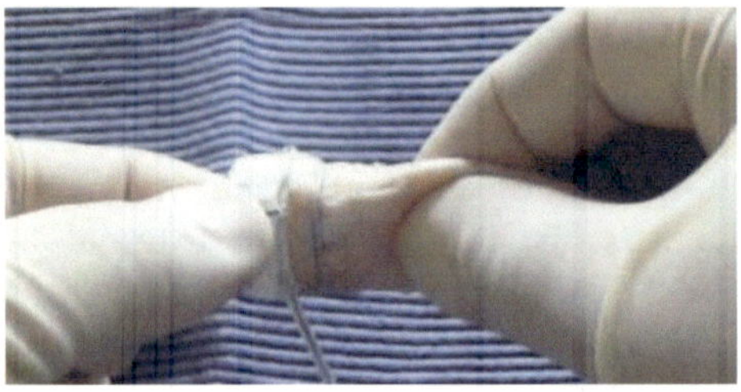

Fig. 19. Stretch test.
Stability coupling was validate by stretching test consisting in vigorous manual stretching of the anastomosis in the coaxial plane separately at four points of its circumference; the anastomosis was than checked for any significant vascular stump backwards dislocation on the expandable wireframe throughout the entire circumference.
Video at: http://www.fondazionecarrel.org/tsb2/tsb2.html

Device type III stability was also increased by further buttressing the inner and outer Dacron wrapping by 4-0 prolene suture transfixing the circumference in 3-6 points (fig. 20), a manoeuvre that however can be predictably carried out after perfusion is resumed.
While it's certainly easier and also a bit quicker to use expandable device wireframe strong enough to block the aortic stump between simple external ligature and outer surface of the device fixing needles, I think that it's much more technically appropriate and probably safer to realize a vascular/graft coupling where the forces applied are as much as possible similar to those involved in standard vascular suture, even though this can mean a minimal increase of ischemic time, required for placing the 3 full thickness stitches around the positioned device.

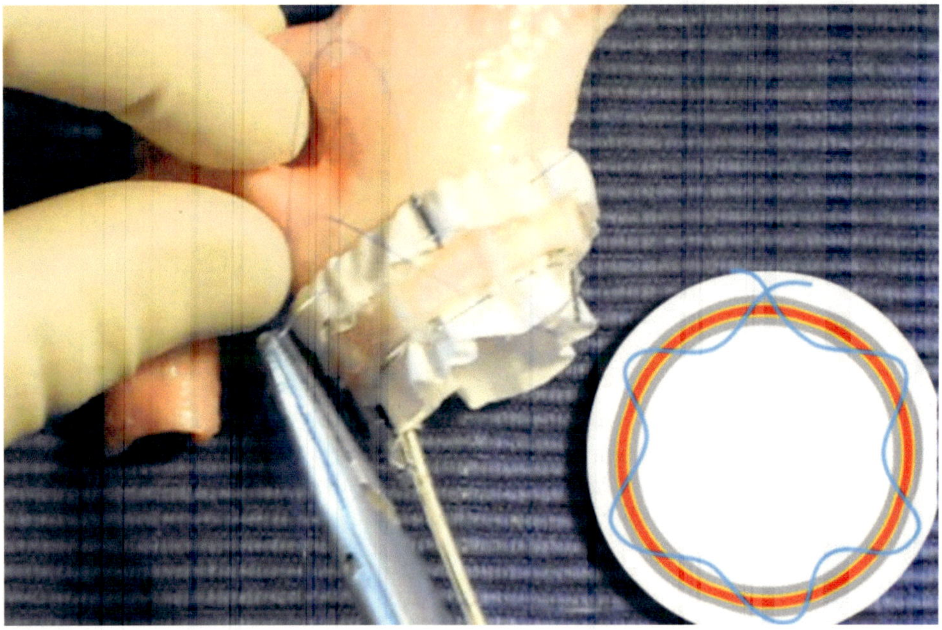

Fig. 20. Type III security fixation.
A simpler in and out 4-0 prolene buttressing in 4-6 points of the inner and outer device wireframe will greatly increase coupling stability.
Video at http://www.fondazionecarrel.org/tsb2/tsb2.html

In synthesis this method ideally allows to change any vascular-graft anastomosis ≥ 6 mm in diameter from the current facing ends Carrel suture into a simpler, quicker and more efficient ("airtight" seal) telescoping anastomosis, sealed and fixed by single thread external ligature passed full thickness at three points (or more when appropriate), in a sort of ideal re-elaboration of the historical Carrel triangulation technique.
The hypothesizable potential impact (table 1) may exceed that expected on complication rate of open prosthetic substitution of all aortic tracts and in particular in those higher risk conditions as acute dissection. In fact the technical simplification with increased reliability of anastomosis haemostasis and dissection layer approximation with false lumen permanent seal has the logical direct consequence, for example, of enabling also lesser expert cardiovascular surgeons to deal with these clinical cases very often requiring immediate surgical attention, thus increasing surgical team efficiency and hospital unit productivity.

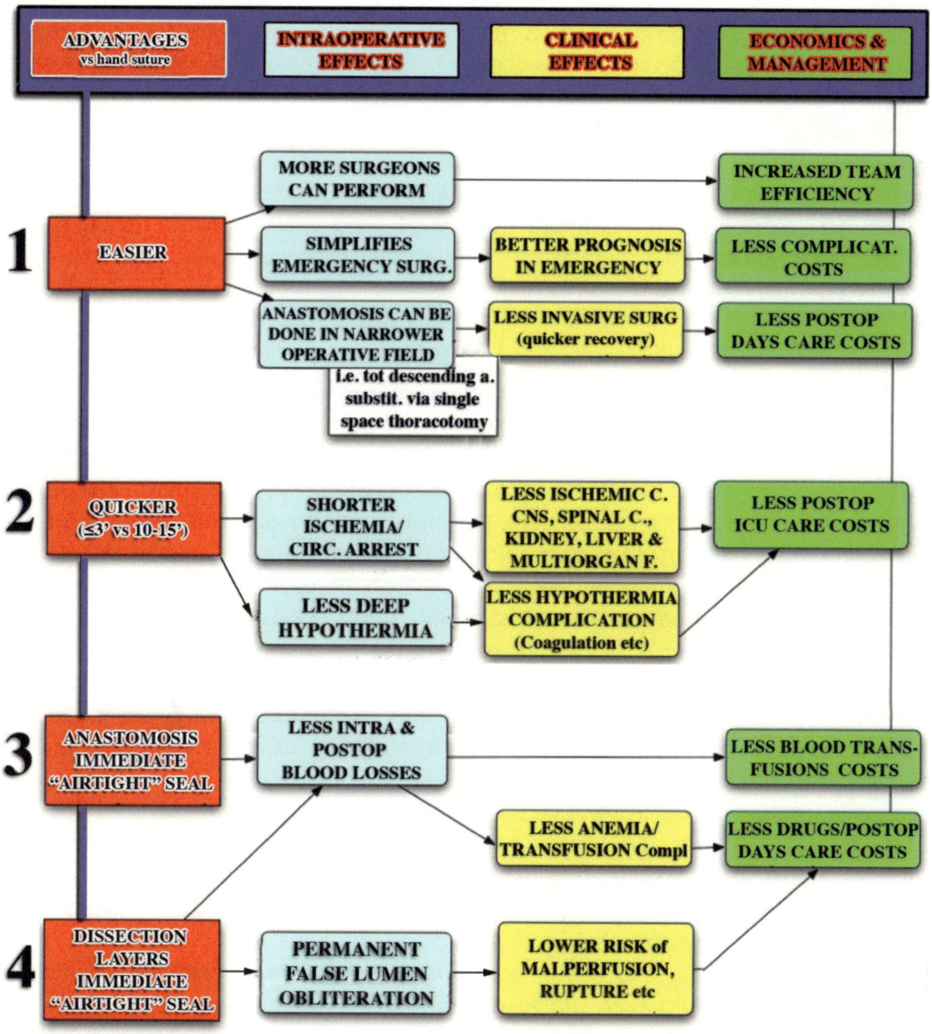

Table 1. Potential impact of expandable device aortic anastomosis compared with current hand suture technique

3. New endovascular "net" prosthesis for aortic wall strengthening without blocking aortic branches perfusion to early stop aneurysm progression or to prevent its formation in high risk patients

3.1 Background

While endovascular procedures already proved lower mortality and complications rate than open surgery and as good long term results in infrarenal and upper descending aorta, in all other aortic tracts endovascular techniques are much more complex and long term results less predictable mainly due to the presence of significant collateral branches, that require additional maneuvers to avoid their obstruction by the endoprosthesis (i.e. hybrid procedure with open surgery for supraortic trunks de-branching).
Moreover endovascular procedures failed to protect from spinal chord ischemia and consequent paraplegia in extended descending aorta prosthetic substitution; it has been hypothesized that this could be due, at least in some case, to the fact that while endoprosthesis prevents intercostal branches to be physiologically perfused, cannot prevent, at least for a certain time in the initial phase, backwards blood flow into the space between endoprosthesis and aortic wall, thus generating conditions for a blood flow "steal" from perfusion of the spinal chord (Kawaharada et al, 2010).
On the other hand current data (Gopaldas et al, 2010) show that only less than 1/4 of ideal candidates to endovascular treatment (uncomplicated, non genetic, isolated, elective descending aortic aneurysms) underwent endovascular procedure, while the remaining 3/4 still underwent open surgical repair in US.

3.2 The rational

The relative slowness of aneurysm formation and progression to rupture indicates that the decrease in the strength of the arterial wall under the aneurysm formation threshold may be very gradual and limited. Consequently one can imagine that measures to increase, even moderately, the mechanical strength of the arterial wall, for example by means of a dacron fabric network, should be successful in preventing aneurysm formations and thus its complications (dissection and rupture), without requiring complete prosthetic substitution. Moreover the conclusive understanding that a destruction of the elastin fibrils network is at the basis of aneurysm formation [Gott et al, 1996], might acknowledge the re-establishment of a uniform and regular network strengthening of the vascular wall with a net prosthesis as a logic, direct correction of the primary defect. On the other hand this mechanical approach since long time is already in use in many other technology fields for prevention of deformation of elastic/floppy tubes or structures subject to inner high pressure, as for example gardening tubes, tires, rubber boat etc.
In previous animal experiments we showed that the endovascular positioning of polypropilen "net" prosthesis, if kept in contact with the inner vascular surface, is spontaneously covered by new intima and included in the aortic wall in few weeks (fig 21 and fig 22), still keeping perfusion of some intercostals vessels, even though the net meshes used in those experiments were certainly too tight to assure their long term patency.
The experimental hypothesis is based on the fact that the net prosthesis positioned and maintained in stable contact with the aortic walls (A) is spontaneously, gradually covered by the neo-intima (B), invaded by fibroblasts and thus stably associated to the aortic wall. If the net mesh is appropriately dimensioned, it may be expected that the blood flow through the collateral branches is not affected (arrows) (from Nazari et al, 1996c)

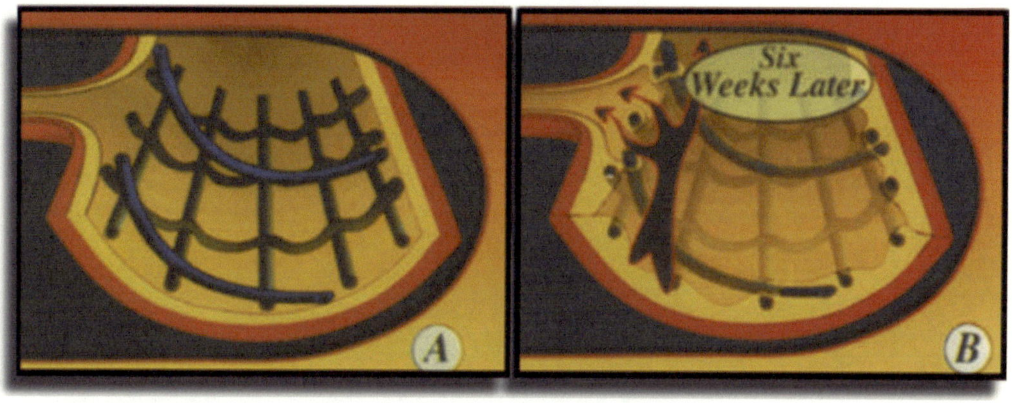

Fig. 21. The Rational. The experimental hypothesis is based on the fact that the net prosthesis positioned and maintained in stable contact with the aortic walls (A) is spontaneously, gradually covered by the neo-intima (B), invaded by fibroblasts and thus stably associated to the aortic wall. If the net mesh is appropriately dimensioned, it may be expected that the blood flow through the collateral branches is not affected (arrows) (from Nazari et al, 1996c)

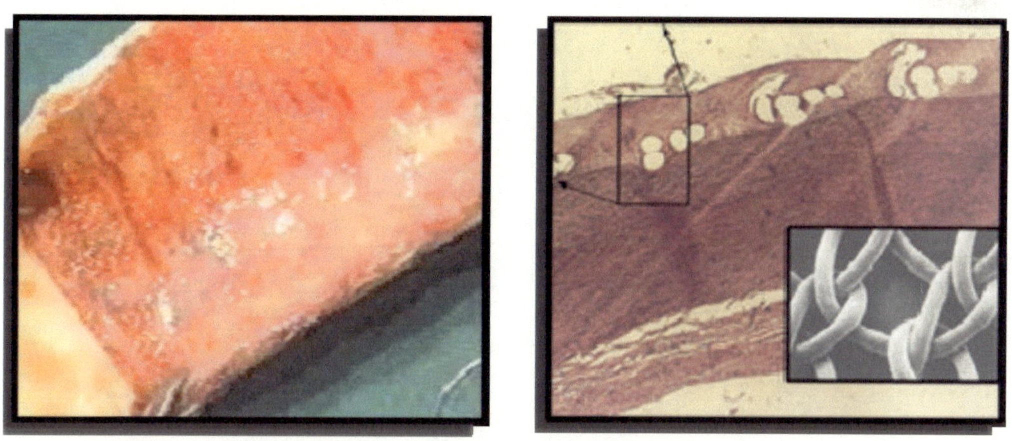

Fig. 22. Swine experimental model.
Left square. After 6 weeks the net prosthesis, a braided polipropilene fitted with a co-axial thin stainless steel coil surgically positioned in swine upper descending aorta, was found to be covered by the new intima and well attached to the aortic wall. In the lower right side of the prosthesis segment the net is no longer visible and presumably, with little more time, this smooth, normal intimal surface would extend to completely cover the whole net prosthesis (metallic coil was removed). *Right square.* Histology shows the net prosthesis completely included into the intima layer and lying in contact with the media. The square area shows the magnified polypropylene mesh net pattern. (mod from Nazari et al 1996 c) Video http://www.fondazionecarrel.org/tsb2/tsb2.html

The fabric framework linked to the aortic wall would then condition its significant, regular and uniform mechanical strengthening that fractionates and absorbs the centrifuge systolic stress of the bloodstream. The significant mechanical strengthening achieved in this way was measurable by comparison of compliance ($\Delta V/\Delta P$) of the treated aortic tract with that of the immediately confining segment (fig 23)

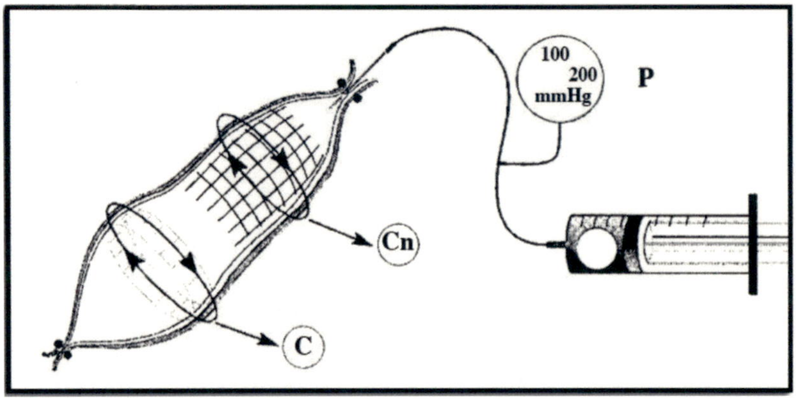

Fig. 23. Aortic wall compliance ($\Delta V/\Delta P$).
To quantify aortic wall strengthening induced by the net prosthesis its compliance ($\Delta V/\Delta P$). was compared with that of the confining segments that was found significantly higher. (from Nazari et al 1996b) Video at http://www.fondazionecarrel.org/tsb2/tsb2.html

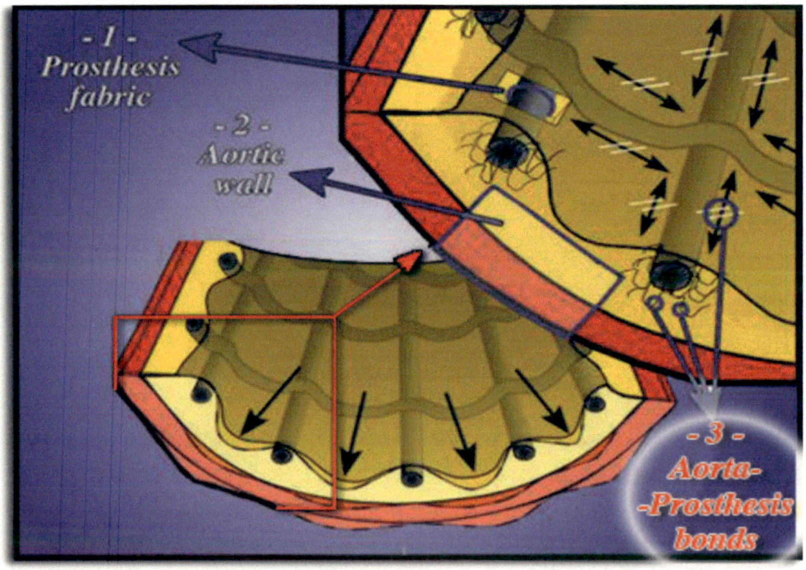

Fig. 24. Aortic wall strengthening factors.
The structural properties of the aortic wall associated to the intraluminal net prosthesis rely on three factors: **1)** the structural properties of the net prosthesis, **2)** the structural properties of the aortic wall, **3)** the strength of the bonds between the aortic wall and the net prosthesis, based substantially on fibroblastic invasion of the net fabric and its permanent integration with aortic wall. The latter is the crucial point and can be viewed as the true "functional unit" of this model. In fact if this link is sufficiently strong and stable in the time it can be hypothesized to be able to stabilize aortic wall and prevent dilatation even independently from the "net" prosthesis own diameter, which could not be further distended after that their fabric threads have been integrated into the aortic wall. (mod. from Nazari et al 1996b)

The structural properties of the aortic wall associated to the intraluminal net prosthesis rely on three factors (fig 24): 1) the structural properties of the net prosthesis, 2) the structural properties of the aortic wall, 3) the strength of the bonds between the aortic wall and the net prosthesis, based substantially on fibroblastic invasion of the net fabric and its permanent integration with aortic wall. Given the structural adequacy of the net prosthesis (polypropylene net prosthesis squared mesh 5x5 mm with a thread diameter of 0.5 mm sustaining a pressure of 300 mmHg (0.04 Nmm^2) is charged at 50% of its failure tension (Nazari at al, 1996b, 1996c) and the mechanical effect of fractioning the aortic wall in the small area of the net meshes (fig 24, lower part), the important point of this model is the strength of the links biologically established between the threads of the mesh and the aortic wall tissues (point 3 in fig. 24) during the 4-6 weeks integration process.
It may be hypothesized that its strength relies mainly in the degree of integration of the net thread with the intimal layer mainly due to fibroblastic invasion and is then predictably stronger with porous material (PTFE) or multifilament braided polyester (Dacron).

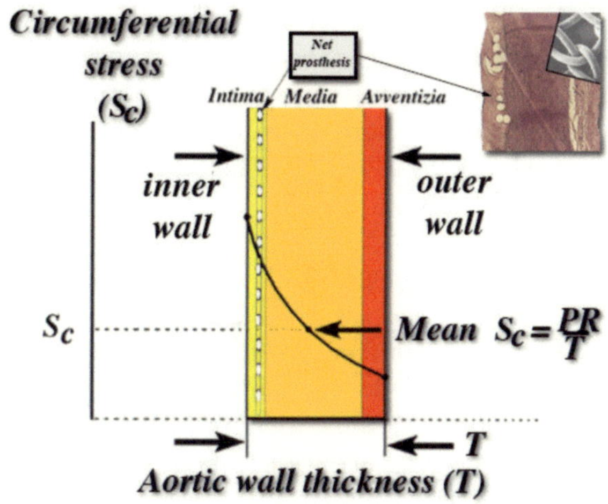

Modified from Robicsek and Thubrikar, Ann Thorac Surg 1994;58:1247

Fig. 25. Variation of the circumferential stress through the aortic wall thickness.
For a thick cylinder (thickness > 8% of the radius (R)) such as the aorta, the stress is not uniform throughout the wall; it is maximal on the inner wall, it decreases through the thickness of the wall and is minimal on the outer wall. This explains the pathogenic mechanism of dissection, where only stress to the inner part of the wall is strong enough to cause tear; moreover it adds arguments to the rationale of intraluminal positioning of the net prosthesis in order to achieve the structural strengthening just where this is most needed, i.e. where the circumferential stress is maximal. This allows for the required strengthening with optimization of the amount of prosthetic material (thinner threads) (Mod from Robicsek and Thubrikar 1994)

The latter is the crucial point of this model. In fact if this link is sufficiently strong and stable in the time, it can be hypothesized to be able to stabilize aortic wall and prevent dilatation even independently from the "net" prosthesis own diameter, which could not be further distended after that their meshes have been firmly integrated into the aortic wall (Redaelli & Fiore, 2011). The practical consequence is that the precise equivalence between diameter of the net prosthesis and aortic diameter is not necessary; the prosthesis in fact can be

significantly redundant in respect to the effective aortic diameter, thus allowing for its easier adaptability to geometrical irregularity of aneurysm wall without consequences on its efficiency in keeping stable aortic diameter. The final "functional unit" of this model for aortic wall strengthening is then the single mesh of the net integrated into the aortic wall, whose efficiency relies then on the bonds between net threads and aortic tissue.
Interestingly enough in this model the endovascular net prosthesis provides aortic wall mechanical support just where the mechanical stress is higher (Robicsek & Thubrikar, 1994) (fig. 25), and thus just where it's most needed both to prevent further dilatation, theoretically preventable also by external aortic wall wrapping (Pepper et al 2010), and to avoid partial (dissection) or total rupture, with optimization of the amount of prosthetic material. The reduced volume of the net prosthesis in comparison with current endoprosthesis (≤1/6th approximately) further greatly enhances its introduction through peripheral vessel often tortuous and restricted by atherosclerosis.

3.3 Methodology

The previous experimental work as well as structural mechanical theoretical considerations allow to predict applicability and reliability of the method in the clinical setting of preventing aneurysm formation or arresting its progression at an early stage.
The organizative plan for achieving this final goal however includes several further distinct steps.

3.3.1 Ideal "net" prosthesis prototypes setup

This part of the project includes

- the selection of the best fabric material (PTFE, multifilament polypropylene, etc) with the best chances of the strongest links with aortic wall
- identification of its appropriated dimensioning and mechanical features, including elasticity, to provide the best support to the stream pressure stress up to its extreme pathological limit (300 mm hg)
- identification of the most appropriate net prosthesis embodiment able to maintain it in permanent contact with intimal surface, which is essential to its quick and spontaneous incorporation into the aortic wall. This may include a thin nitinol wireframe associated to the main net prosthesis; a prototype for descending aorta currently in study is illustrated at fig. 26. However fluid-dynamic shapes of the net threads will be also evaluated in mechanical models with the aim to verify if it is possible to achieve conduit inner wall contact by means of pure fluid stream
- Ascending aorta and Arch require variably curved net prosthesis (fig 26, right); for these tracts however bespoke prosthesis on the individual TC scan, maybe with wider meshes for the supraortic trunks area, is an option to be considered for clinical use; bespoke prosthesis however have being already realized in a external ascending aorta wrapping protocol (Pepper et al, 2010)).
- Endovascular delivery system is also to be realized

The nitinol wireframe adds to the net further structural strengthening then greatly exceeding that required; an accurate structural mechanics computation would theoretically allow the achievement of the necessary aortic wall structural strengthening to permanently fix aortic diameter with really a very thin and wide meshes net prosthesis.

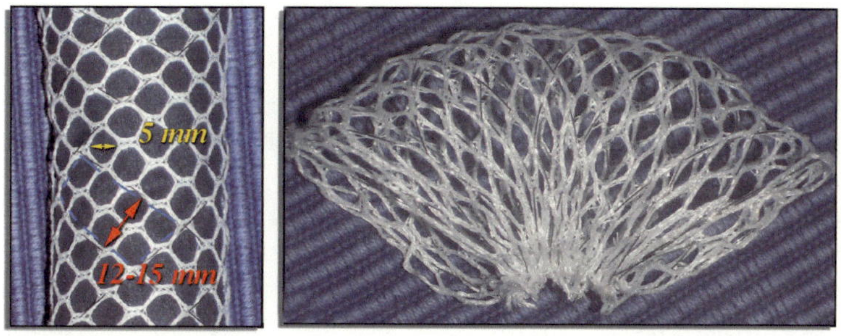

Fig. 26. "Net" prosthesis prototypes.
Possible prototypes versions were realized by 5x5mm meshes of braided fabric embodied with very thin nitinol wider helicoidal wireframe (*left*:blu lines, red arrows, 12-15 mm). Ascending aorta and arch would require curved prosthesis (*right*), maybe bespoke to the patient aortic anatomy on CT scans.

A more straight, ready, maybe oversimplified method, but still mechanically efficient, could consist in the simple substitution of the Dacron tube with a fabric net prosthesis in any of the current endovascular devices.

3.3.2 Experimental protocol

The prototypes resulting from the above project phase will undergo "in vivo" animal experiments. Ideally these experiments should include long term (≥12 months) evaluation in an appropriate animal (sheep) models. These may consist in prototypes positioning in the thoraco-abdominal aorta (model 1) and in the aortic arch (model 2) surgically or, possibly, as endovascular procedure if the endovascular delivery system is realized and suitable with the animal model peripheral vascular diameter. Half surviving animals could be sacrificed at 12 months and examined to verify:

- regular integration of the net prosthesis into the intimal layer, looking for site and extension of possible areas on lacking integration with aortic wall
- preserved perfusion of all collateral branches for the extent of the net prosthesis
- the real structural strengthening achieved by measuring the aortic wall compliance ($\Delta V/\Delta P$) compared to that of the confining aortic segment (Fig. 5)
- absence of complications such as migration, ulceration, perforation etc

The remaining animals could be followed indefinitely and examined in case late complication or death.

3.3.3 Preparation of clinical trial

Ideally during the experimental phase will be identified and monitored Marfan patients with still normal or initial dilatation of any tract of the aorta in order to select those to be offered/accepting the prophylactic endovascular aortic strengthening. Obviously associated risk factors, in particular familiar history of aneurism and rupture, as well as other inclusion and exclusion criteria indicated by the Marfan Associations and clinical Institution Marfan Centers, will form the basis for planning the possible future clinical trial.
Marfan diseases is a condition where pure prophylaxis of aortic aneurism would be in most cases "per se" appropriate, due to its very high incidence and rather early in the patient life; on the other hand prophylactic surgical aortic substitution is an already considered option

in occasional patients. Prophylaxis is then particularly suitable for these patients with this new method when its long term safety, efficacy, simplicity and predictably low cost are proved; the re-establishment of an artificial elastic network in fact will represent a logic, direct correction of the primary defect, i.e. fragmentation and destruction of vascular wall physiological elastin fibrils network (Gott et al 1996).

This will otherwise open interesting new perspectives in the "very early treatment" of any type of aortic aneurisms as soon as they appear, well in advance the current endovascular or surgical treatments are indicated, when the still limited aortic geometry distortion both simplifies net prosthesis positioning and integration into the aortic wall and increase its efficiency.

The final goal is then the mininvasive, low cost, full prevention of the costly and still risky endovascular or surgical treatments of overt aortic aneurysm of any nature, ideally in all aortic tracts.

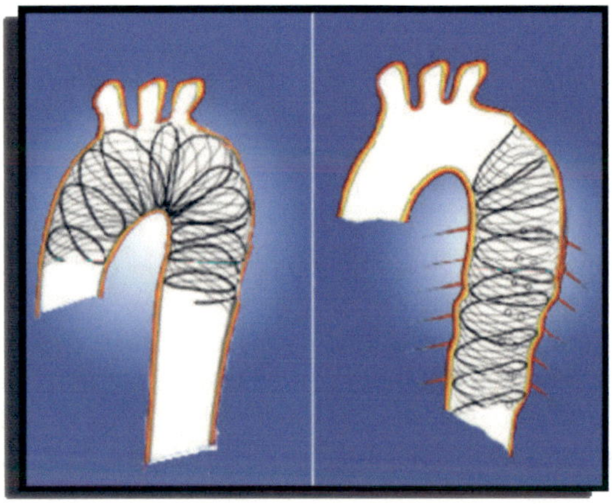

Fig. 27. Prophylactic or very early strengthening of Aortic Arch and Descending Aorta. Sketches illustrate an hypothetical application of the method in high risk aortic area as a pure prophylactic measure for example in Marfan patient. In extended descending aorta this method is the only one that may theoretically provide full prevention of spinal chord complications, not yet fully achieved neither by surgery nor by endovascular techniques. (From Nazari et al 1996b)

Last but not least this method could be the only one theoretically able to totally annul complications related to spinal chord ischemia due to critical intercostal collaterals, still a major problem not yet solved by any surgical nor endovascular technique.

4. References

Aluffi A, Buniva P, Rescigno G & Nazari S. (2002) Improved device for sutureless aortic anastomosis applied in a case of cancer. Tex Heart Inst J. 29: 56–59.

Antoniou GA, El Sakka K, Hamady M & Wolfe JH. (2010) Hybrid treatment of complex aortic arch disease with supraaortic debranching and endovascular stent graft repair. Eur J Vasc Endovasc Surg. 39:683-90.

Berger RL, Romero L, Chaudhry AG & Dobnik DB.(1983) Graft replacement of the thoracic aorta with a sutureless technique. Ann Thorac Surg. 35:231–239.

Brown LC, Thompson SG, Greenhalgh RM & Powell JT (2011): Incidence of cardiovascular events and death after open or endovascular repair of abdominal aortic aneurysm in the randomized EVAR trial 1. British Journal of Surgery 98: 935–942

Buniva P, Rescigno G, Salvi S, Aluffi A, Berti A. Salsi F, Nazari S (2002) Sutureless expandable end prosthesis for descending aorta substitution invaded by bronchogenic cancer. Video, Proceedings Aortic Surgery Symposium VIII, New York, May 2-3, 2002

Canaud L, Hireche K, Berthet JP et al.(2010): Endovascular repair of aortic arch lesions in high-risk patients or after previous aortic surgery: midterm results. J Thorac Cardiovasc Surg. 140:52-8.

Carrel A. (1902) La technique operatoire des anastomoses vasculaires et la transplantation des visceres. Lyon Med. 98:859–864.

CarrelA. (1907) The surgery of blood vessels. Bull Johns Hopkins Hosp;18: 18–27.

Charnsangavej C, Wallace S, Wright KC, Carrasco CH & Gianturco C. (1985) Endovascular stent for use in aortic dissection: an in vitro experiment. Radiology.157:323-4.

Chiesa R, Melissano G, Marone EM, Marrocco-Trischitta MM & Kahlberg A (2010)Aorto-oesophageal and aortobronchial fistulae following thoracic endovascular aortic repair: a national survey. Eur J Vasc Endovasc Surg. 39:273-9.

Crawford ES & Crawford JL, editors (1984). Diseases of the aorta. Baltimore: Williams and Wilkins, 61–77.

De Bruin JL, Baas AF, Buth J, Prinssen M, Verhoeven EL, Cuypers PW et al.; DREAM Study Group.(2010) Long-term outcome of open or endovascular repair of abdominal aortic aneurysm. N Engl J Med 362:1881–1889.

Di Eusanio M, Armaro A, Di Marco L, Pacini D, Savini C, Martin Suarez S, Pilato E & Di Bartolomeo R (2011) Short- and midterm results after hybrid treatment of chronic aortic dissection with the frozen elephant trunk technique. Eur J Cardiothorac Surg 2011 Mar 5. (Epub ahead of print)

Geraci G, Pisello F, Li Volsi F, Facella T, Platia L, Modica G & Sciume C (2008) Secondary aortoduodenal fistula. World J Gastroenterol. 14:484-6.

Gopaldas RR., Huh J, Dao TK, LeMaire SA, Chu D, Bakaeen FG & Coselli JS (2010) Superior nationwide outcomes of endovascular versus open repair for isolated descending thoracic aortic aneurysm in 11,669 patients. J Thorac Cardiovasc Surg. 140:1001-10

Gott VL, Laschinger JC, Cameron DE, Dietz HC, Greene PS, Gillinov AM, Pyeritz RE, Alejo DE, Fleischer KJ, Anhalt GJ, Stone CD & McKusick VA:(1996) The Marfan syndrome and the cardiovascular surgeon. Eur J Cardiothorac Surg. 10:149-158

Kawaharada N, Ito T, Koyanagi T, Harada R, et al (2010) Spinal cord protection with selective spinal perfusion during descending thoracic and thoracoabdominal aortic surgery. Interact CardioVasc Thorac Surg. 10:986-991

Kolesov VI, Kolesov EV, Gurevich IY & Leosko VA.(1970) Vasosuturing apparatuses in surgery of coronary arteries. Med Tekhnika 6:24–8

Kolesov VI & Kolesov EV. (1991) Twenty years' results with internal thoracic artery-coronary artery anastomosis [letter]. J Thorac Cardiovasc Surg. 101:360–1

Konstantinov I E. (2004): Vasilii I. Kolesov A Surgeon to Remember. Tex Heart Inst J. 31: 349–358.

Lemole GM, Strong MD, Spagna PM & Karilomicz MD(1982). Improved results for dissecting aneurysms: intraluminal sutureless prosthesis. J Thorac Cardiovasc Surg. 83:249–255.

Luo CY, Lai CH, Wen JS & Lin BW (2010) Secondary aortocolic fistula: case report and review of the literature. Ann Vasc Surg.24:256.e5-12.

Marone EM, Esposito G, Kahlberg A, Tshomba Y, Brioschi C, Zannini P & Chiesa R. (2007) Surgical treatment of tracheoinnominate fistula after stent- graft implantation. J Thorac CardioVasc Surg. 133:1641–1643.

Nazari S, Manelli A, Gastaldo A, Rinaldo A, Barana L & Zonta A. (1990) A new vascular stapler for pulmonary artery anastomosis in experimental single lung transplantation. Video, Proceedings of the 4th Annual Meeting of the Association for Cardio-Thoracic Surgery, Naples, September 16–19, 1990

Nazari S., Mourad Z, Luzzana F. (1994) Prosthetic substitution of the descending aorta without blood flow interruption. Proceedings of the IV Aortic Surgery Symposium, New York, April 20-22, 1994

Nazari S, Luzzana F, Banfi C, Mourad Z, Salvi S, Gaspari A & Nazari-Coerezza F.(1996a) Expandable prosthesis for sutureless anastomosis in thoracic aorta prosthetic substitution. Eur J Cardiothorac Surg. 10:1003– 1009.

Nazari S, Luzzana F, Carli F et al:(1996b) Rinforzo strutturale della parete aortica con una protesi a rete per arrestare la progressione dell'aneurisma e prevenirne la dissezione e la rottura. Sperimentazione sull'animale di una nuova modalità terapeutica. CHIRURGIA. 9:412-23

Nazari S, Luzzana F, Carli F et al (1996c) Aortic wall structural strenghtening by intraluminal net prosthesis to arrest aneurysm prograssion and to prevent dissection and rupture. Experimental assessment of a new therapeutic approach. Eur J Cardiothor Surg, 10:264-272

Nazari S, Mourad Z, Banfi C, Salvi S, Visconti E, Aluffi A. (1996d) Composite graft with expandable ends for total arch replacement. Video & Poster, Proceedings Aortic Surgery Symposium V, New York, April 23-26, 1996

Nazari S, Salvi S, Aluffi A, Visconti E, Rescigno G & Buniva P (1997) A new prosthesis for aortic arch substitution. Ann Thorac Surg. 64:1339–1344.

Nazari S, Salvi S, Visconti E, Caramella F, Rossi C, Rescigno G, Banfi C & Buniva P. (1999) Descending aorta substitution using a prosthesis with expandable ends. Case report. J Cardiovasc Surg (Torino) 40:417–420.

Nazari S, Thoracic Aorta Substitution in less than 2 minutes. (2006)Video, Proceedings 16th World Congress of World Society of Cardio- Thoracic Surgeons, Ottawa, August 17-20, 2006

Nazari S. (2009) Modified Expandable Device for Easy and Realiable Dissection Layers Approximation in Sutureless Aortic Anastomosis. Video, proceedings of The Houston Aortic Symposium, Houston, March 26-28, 2009

Nazari S (2010) Expandable device type III for easy and reliable approximation of dissection layers in sutureless aortic anastomosis. Ex vivo experimental study. Interact CardioVasc Thorac Surg. 10:161-164; originally published online Nov 20, 2009; DOI: 10.1510/icvts.2009.216291

Parodi JC, Palmaz JC & Barone HD (1991) Transfemoral intraluminal graft implantation for abdominal aortic aneurysms. Ann Vasc Surg. 5:491-9.

Parodi JC. (1994) Endovascular repair of abdominal aortic aneurysms and other arterial lesions. Surg Technol Int. 3:431-6.

Payr E. (1900) Beitrage zur Technik der Blutgefass und Nervennaht nebst Mittheilungentiber die Verwendung eines resorbierbaren Metalles in der Chirurgie. Arch Klin Chir; 62:67–93

Pepper J, Golesworthy T, Utley M, Chan J, Ganeshalingam S, Lamperth M, Mohiaddin R & Treasure T.(2010) Manufacturing and placing a bespoke support for the Marfan aortic root: description of the method and technical results and status at one year for the first ten patients. Interact Cardiovasc Thorac Surg. 10:360-5. Epub 2009 Dec 11.

Robicsek F & Thubrikar MJ (1994) Hemodynamic considerations regarding the mechanism and prevention of aortic dissection. Ann Thorac Surg 58:1247-1253

Redaelli A & Fiore GB. Personal communication. Politecnico di Milano, 18 Gennaio 2011

Rossella C, Rescigno G, Nazari S. (2008) Modified expandable device for easy, quick and blood-tight sutureless anastomosis in ascending aorta. Proceedings of The Houston Aortic Symposium, April 2008

Ruby BJ & Cogbill TH (2007) Aortoduodenal fistula 5 years after endovascular abdominal aortic aneurysm repair with the Ancure stent graft. J Vasc Surg. 45:834-6.

Schermerhorn ML, O'Malley AJ, Jhaveri A, Cotterill P, Pomposelli F, Landon BE. (2008) Endovascular vs. open repair of abdominal aortic aneurysms in the Medicare population. N Engl J Med 2008; 358: 464–474.

Takata M, Watanabe G, Ohtake H, Ushijima T, Yamaguchi S, Kikuchi Y & Yamamoto Y (2011): Automatic aortic anastomosis with an innovative computer-controlled circular stapler for surgical treatment of aortic aneurysm. J Thorac Cardiovasc Surg. 141:1265-9

Tanaka S, Kameda N, Kubo Y, Obatake N, Wakasa T, Ohsawa M & Wakasa K. (2009) Secondary aortoduodenal fistula caused on the suture line of the wrapping. Pathology International 59: 598–600 doi:10.1111/j.1440-1827.2009.02414.x

Tsagakis K, Pacini, D, Di Bartolomeo R et al (2011).: Arch replacement and downstream stent grafting in complex aortic dissection: first results of an international registry. Eur J CardioThor Surg. 39:87-94

Tesauro B. (1967) Impiego degli adesivi plastici e delle cucitrici meccaniche in chirurgia vascolare. Atti del 698 Congresso della Societa` Italiana di Chirurgia, Firenze 18–20 Ottobre 1967. In: Fegiz G, editor. Archivio ed atti della Societ`a Italiana di Chirurgia. Roma: EMES, 1:663–790.

Tesauro B & Persico G. (1979) Valutazione critica delle suture meccaniche in chirurgia vascolare. Atti dell'818 Congresso della Societa` Italiana di Chirurgia, Catania 8–11 Ottobre 1979. In: Fegiz G, editor. Archivio ed atti della Società Italiana di Chirurgia, Bologna: CLUEB, 1:633– 652.

The UK EVAR Trial Investigators, Greenhalgh RM, Brown LC, Powell JT, Thompson SG, Epstein D, Sculpher MJ.(2010) Endovascular versus open repair of abdominal aortic aneurysm. N Engl J Med 2010; 362: 1863–1871.

Wright KC, Wallace S, Charnsangavej C, Carrasco CH & Gianturco C (1985) Percutaneous endovascular stents: an experimental evaluation. Radiology. 156:69-72.

Yoshioka T, Wright KC, Wallace S, Lawrence DD Jr & Gianturco C.(1988) Self-expanding endovascular graft: an experimental study in dogs. AJR Am J Roentgenol. 151:673-6.

Zannini G (1967) Introduzione storica. In Atti del 69° Congresso della Societa` Italiana di Chirurgia, Firenze 18–20 Ottobre 1967. In: Fegiz G, editor. Archivio ed atti della Società Italiana di Chirurgia. Roma: EMES, 1:7-32

Part 4

General Thoracic Surgery

16

Lung Transplantation

Wickii T. Vigneswaran
Lung and Heart-Lung Transplantation, University of Chicago, USA

1. Introduction

1.1 History

The foundation for lung transplantation was laid in the early 1900 by Guthrie and Carrel. In recognition of his work in vascular anastomosis, Dr. Carrel received the first Nobel Prize in Medicine. Following this early work, in 1946 Demikov in Russia performed a canine lung transplant as a unit. The dog subsequently died of bronchial dehiscence. The first human lung transplant was performed by Hardy at the University of Mississippi in 1963. Patient survived a few days and succumbed to complications. Derom in Belgium was credited with the first successful human lung transplantation when he reported 10 month survival of a patient who had undergone lung transplant for end-stage pulmonary fibrosis in 1971. By 1978, 38 lung transplants had been performed worldwide but Derom's patient was the only one that had approached a beneficial outcome. Consistently noted poor outcome in the 60s and 70s led to a moratorium on clinical lung transplantation in the late 70s. Rejection and infection were the common causes of death in this early group and bronchial anastomotic healing was the barrier for transplant survival beyond 2 weeks (1).

Cyclosporine based immune suppression in kidney and liver transplantation in the early 1980s resulted in dramatic improvements in organ function and patient survival. With this experience Shumway and Reitz successfully transplanted heart-lung blocks using a cyclosporine based immune suppression on primates. Airway complications were rare in heart-lung transplantation due to the non coronary collaterals, where as this was a major drawback of isolated lung transplantation. The success of the Stanford group led to the reinstitution of clinical heart-lung transplantation in the 80s (2).

Meanwhile in Toronto, significant experimental work were done by Pearson and Cooper to solve the bronchial healing problem in animal models. The technique of omental wrap around the bronchial anastomosis was developed by Cooper et al. In 1986 the Toronto Lung Transplant Group reported successful single lung transplantation for pulmonary fibrosis in two patients (3). Technique of en-bloc double lung transplant failed due to the tracheal anastomotic complication related to ischemia. Finally bilateral sequential transplantation was developed as a method of transplanting both lungs without the heart. Currently around 147 centers perform over 2000 isolated lung transplants a year. The bronchial anastomotic technique has evolved since and bronchial wrapping is no longer considered necessary.

2. Patient selection for lung transplantation

2.1 Indications

Lung transplant is indicated for patients with chronic, end-stage lung disease for whom no effective medical therapy is available (4,5). The primary goal of lung transplantation is to provide a survival benefit. Such benefit can be conferred to patients with advanced pulmonary fibrosis, cystic fibrosis and primary pulmonary hypertension. Reports for emphysema are conflicting and for Eisenmenger's syndrome transplant did not find a survival benefit. However, as lung transplantation is a palliative treatment, improvements in quality of life in addition to survival benefit should be used to assess effectiveness of this therapy.

2.2 Contraindications

2.2.1 Major contraindications

A history of malignancy during the past two years, except for skin cancers. In general 5 year disease free survival is expected (4).

Untreatable advanced disease of another organ system, except the heart, where a heart-lung transplantation could be considered.

Untreatable extra-pulmonary infections, including chronic, active viral hepatitis and HIV infection.

Significant chest deformity.

Unreliable social support, medical non-compliance or major psychiatric or psychological disorder.

Active substance abuse or use within the past 6 months.

2.2.2 Relative contraindications

Older age; older patients have less optimal survival following lung transplantation.

Critical or unstable conditions, such as Extra Corporeal Membrane Oxygenation or mechanical ventilation.

Severely limited functional class with poor rehabilitation potential.

Colonization with highly virulent or antibiotic resistant organism.

Obesity or malnutrition (BMI>30 or BMI<17).

Mechanical Ventilation except in carefully selected patients

Severe or untreated gastroesophageal reflux disease.

2.3 Timing of referral

In general referral for transplantation evaluation is recommended when the patient's median survival (50%) is about 2 years or less or New York Heart Association class 3 or 4. Due to the natural history of underlying disease, the referral time will depend on the underlying disease. The waiting period for transplant depends on underlying disease, waiting time, blood group, height of patient and presence of pre-formed antibodies in the recipient.

3. Lung transplantation procedure

3.1 Donor selection and operation

The donor is evaluated for ABO compatibility, size, medical and social history, function, associated pathological findings on CXR or CT scan and bronchoscopic findings. Given the improvements in clinical results and shortage of donor organs the generally accepted donor criteria are continually being challenged and expanded. Donor lung selection also depends on subjective assessment at the time of exploration in the operating room and judgment of the donor surgical team (6).

The donor pneumonectomy is approached via a midline sternotomy. The lung is inspected to evaluate its suitability for transplantation by the donor surgical team. Heparin is administered and a pulmonary plegia cannula is inserted into the main pulmonary artery ensuring both main pulmonary arteries are perfused by the cannula. A clamp is placed on the left atrial appendage and the tip of the appendage is excised for free drainage of the pulmonary effluent during the pulmonary plegic infusion. Prostaglandins and pulmonary vasodilators are administered into the main pulmonary artery followed by cold pulmonary plegia that also contains vasodilator medications. The lung is inflated to moderate amount and the trachea is stapled with lung inflated. The lung block is dissected away from the mediastinal structure with the heart or separately after the heart is excised by the 'cardiac' team. Left atrium is divided midway between the confluence of the pulmonary veins and the atrial groove ensuring that an adequate "atrial cuff" will be available with the lungs for implantation. The ligamentum arteriosum is divided toward the descending aorta avoiding injury to the left main pulmonary artery and the entire lung block is dissected away from the descending aorta and esophagus. The lungs are separated from each other at the back table by dividing the left main bronchus with the staples, pulmonary artery at the bifurcation, and left atrium between the right and left pulmonary veins. Retrograde cold flush of the preservation solution is performed through the pulmonary veins before packaging the organs in sterile fashion for transportation to the recipient operating room (8,9).

Satisfactory early and midterm outcomes had been reported with using lung donation after cardiac death expanding potential lung donors (10). Recent exciting developments on normothermic ex-vivo perfusion allowing repair of injured lung and the ability to evaluate function of the lung prior to transplantation has potential benefit of increasing the donor pool even further (11).

Age < 60
ABO Compatibility
Clear Chest Radiograph
$PaO_2 > 300$ on $FIO_2 = 1.0$ and PEEP of 5 cm H_2O
Tobacco history < 20 pack years
Absence of significant chest trauma
No evidence of sepsis or blood borne infections (Hepatitis B, C or HIV)
Prior cardiopulmonary surgery
Presence of lung pathology on CT scan
Purulent secretion on bronchoscopy or evidence of aspiration

Table 1. Established Criteria for Donor Selection

3.2 Recipient operation

3.2.1 Single lung transplant

Once a donor is verified and deemed suitable for transplant, the recipient is brought into the operating room for transplantation (12). Generally the contra-lateral lung is used to support the recipient during the transplantation procedure. Some patient will require cardiopulmonary bypass to perform the lung transplantation safely. General anesthesia is provided via a double lumen endo-tracheal tube, a left sided tube is preferred thus avoiding the potential complication of obstructing the right upper lobe orifice. Following placement of arterial and venous access lines as well as a Trans-esophageal Echo (TEE) probe, the patient is placed in a lateral decubitus position, with groin exposed on the same side to allow canulation of femoral vessels, if needed. A variety of incisions may be used to enter the thorax including a posterolateral incision, anterior submammary incision, or a lateral incision that either spares or partially divides the muscle.

Hilar dissection is performed exposing the pulmonary vessels while preserving the phrenic nerve. Vagus neurovascular bundles are carefully preserved particularly on the left side where the recurrent laryngeal nerve emerges and encircles the ligamentum arteriosus. The recurrent laryngeal nerve may be injured during the dissection of the left main pulmonary artery and a heightened awareness of this will help to avoid injury. Dissection around main bronchus is kept to minimum to preserve its blood supply. The pericardium is opened around the pulmonary veins to release the left atrium for placement of vascular clamp. When the donor lung is in the room the recipient is given heparin intravenously and the pulmonary veins and artery are divided as distal as possible. We use a linear cutting vascular stapler. The main bronchus is divided at the lobar branch level initially and then divided with a sharp knife about 2-3 cartilage rings from the carina.

At the back table, final dissections are made to the donor lung. This includes removal of excess mediastinal tissue, mobilization of the main pulmonary artery and the left atrial and venous structures from pericardial attachments. We perform a repeat cold retrograde flushing of the pulmonary vascular bed with the preservation solution prior to implantation to evacuate any residual debris from the pulmonary vascular bed and improve preservation (9). The main bronchus of the donor is opened and microbiological specimens are collected. The bronchus is then divided with a knife leaving two rings of cartilage from the origin of the upper lobe bronchus. The donor lung is then brought to the operative field. We perform the bronchial anastomosis as to "frame" the lung in position first. The membranous portion of the bronchus is anastamosed using a running 4-0 absorbable monofilament suture while the cartilaginous portion is secured with interrupted figure-of-eight suture of the same type. Single-running suture techniques have also been described in the literature and appear to be equally effective. Next, attention is turned to the venous anastomosis. A vascular clamp is placed along a portion of the left atrium and the recipient left pulmonary vein orifices are connected by dividing the bridge of atrial tissue in-between to create a single oval "atrial cuff". The donor atrial cuff is then anastamosed to the recipient atrial cuff in an end-to-end fashion using a single, double-armed running 4-0 polypropylene suture. Finally the pulmonary artery is prepared for the final anastomosis. Excess length of pulmonary artery is removed after appropriately sizing the vessel. This is particularly important on the right side, as there is a long length available on the donor. The donor pulmonary artery is anastomosed to the recipient in an end-to-end fashion with a single, double-armed running 5-0 polypropylene suture. Occasionally, a size mismatch exists where the recipient pulmonary artery is larger than the donor pulmonary artery. In this case, the larger inferior pulmonary trunk arising from the main pulmonary artery is anastomosed end-to-end with the donor main pulmonary artery. In this situation the upper branch is divided flush with the main artery to prevent any clots forming in the 'blind-end'. Attention is paid to keep the donor lung cold during the entire period using ice slush and cold sponges, until reperfusion. Bolus of solumedrol is given intravenously (we give 500 mg) prior to reperfusion of the graft. In preparation for reperfusion, the patient is placed in the Trendelenberg position, air and debris are vented through the pulmonary artery anastomosis first. Then pulmonary plegia solution is allowed to vent from the left atrial cuff anastomosis by releasing the arterial clamp to allow a slow flush. While the left atrium is observed by TEE for air bubbles the left atrial clamp is removed and the anastomosis is secured. The reperfusion is controlled by slow release of the arterial clamp and any hypotension is treated promptly by alpha-agonists. The lung is inflated while monitoring the left atrium on TEE. A leak test may be performed at this time by carefully ventilating the new lung with the bronchus submerged in warm normal saline and inspecting for air bubbles. After placement of chest tube, with satisfactory hemostasis, hemodynamics and oxygenation the chest is closed in layers with absorbable sutures. With the patient in the supine position the double-lumen endotracheal tube is changed to a single lumen tube and a fiber-optic bronchoscopy is performed to inspect the bronchial anastomosis and remove any clots or secretions present in the bronchial tree.

3.2.2 Bilateral sequential lung transplant

A bilateral anterolateral thoracotomy is a preferable incision for bilateral sequential lung transplant as it preserves the structural integrity of the sternum and prevents significant incision-related morbidity (13). In a patient with small chest cavity or when there is potential need for cardiopulmonary bypass, a clamp-shell incision is made dividing the sternum across for the transplantation. The dissection of the lung and the donor lung preparation is performed as described above. The lung with the lesser physiologic contribution is transplanted first as the other lung support single-lung ventilation.

The single lung transplants are performed sequentially while the patient is supported by the contra-lateral lung. If the operation is being performed without cardiopulmonary bypass (CPB), it is important to stabilize the patient after the first lung implantation before proceeding with the next. Following implantation of the second lung and patient stable, chest tubes are placed and sternum approximate using metal plates or sternal wires. Then the wound is closed in layers with absorbable sutures.

4. Post-operative management

Patient undergoing lung transplantation requires a team of caregivers who are committed, familiar with the protocols and able to ensure ongoing communication between members of the team. The team members include, transplant coordinators, transplant pulmonologist, transplant surgeon, anesthesiologist, pain management team, critical care specialist, ICU nurses, Infectious disease specialist, pharmacologist, physical and occupational therapist, nutritionist and social worker. Clinical pathways are developed addressing complete patient care with incorporation of immunosuppressive and infection prophylaxis protocols (14). Despite clinical pathways, regular team meeting discussing daily care of patient facilitate efficient and timely interventions and improve post-operative care.

5. Respiratory management

Despite advances in the donor management and preservation of lung, primary graft dysfunction is not uncommon following lung transplantation (15). In the majority however the degree of dysfunction is minor to moderate and reversible, therefore does not progress to graft failure. The incidence of primary graft dysfunction has been reported between 11-57

% (16). When there is primary graft failure, extra corporeal membrane oxygenation (ECMO) may be required. Early institution of ECMO had been shown to be more successful than late (17-19). When the graft dysfunction is mild to moderate, management strategies are employed as used in patients with significant lung injury.

The ventilatory management would be influenced, if the patient received a single or bilateral lung transplant. In patients with bilateral lung transplant it would be aimed at minimizing barotraumas by using low inflation volumes and moderate levels of positive end expiratory pressure (PEEP, less than 10 cm water). In patients with single lung transplant the patho-physiology of the remaining native lung will influence ventilatory strategy. Significant air trapping and auto PEEP is not uncommon in patients with emphysema. Low ventilatory volumes, adequate expiratory time and avoidance of excessive PEEP will help to prevent air trapping and significant hemodynamic instability in these patients. Positioning patients with the allograft side up and bronchodilator therapy are useful strategies in patients with single lung transplant. Very rarely isolated lung ventilation with double lumen tube is necessary to effectively ventilate when there is significant graft dysfunction.

Inhaled Nitric Oxide (NO) through the ventilator has been shown to reduce reperfusion injury in experimental models and clinical transplantation, when used as prophylaxis. It's usefulness in established graft dysfunction is controversial. Selective use of inhaled NO in peri-operative period in patients with pre-existing pulmonary hypertension is not an uncommon practice. The aim of the inhaled NO use is to reduce pulmonary artery pressures during the operation and immediately afterwards thereby assisting the right ventricular function.

As a rule aggressive weaning off the ventilator is practiced following lung transplantation to prevent nosocomial infection and promote early rehabilitation. Sedation should be carefully monitored and sparingly used. It is advisable to use short acting agents while patient is intubated. Majority of the patients are extubated within the first 24 hours after transplantation. After extubation we advocate use of epidural analgesia and avoidance of narcotics and benzodiazepines. Aggressive bronchial hygiene is mandatory to prevent collapse and development of pneumonia. While patients are intubated using soft suction catheters to clear secretion should be performed routinely. Once the patient is extubated incentive spirometry, chest physiotherapy and ambulation are necessary to promote clearance of bronchial secretions. In patients who are debilitated and have retention of secretion we have employed 'mini-tracheostomy' to facilitate removal of the secretion with a soft tip 10 french catheter. Alternatively patients will require repeat bronchoscopic suction of secretions. When a patient fails trial extubation, early tracheostomy facilitates rapid weaning of ventilation, assist in effective management of secretions and promote early physical rehabilitation.

6. Hemodynamic management

Patients selected for lung transplant undergo a detailed cardiac evaluation. Isolated single vessel coronary artery disease alone is not a contra-indication for lung transplantation. These patients would be candidates for pre-transplantation, percutaneous revascularization or would be candidates for simultaneous surgical re-vascularization (19,20). Correctable cardiac lesions such as ASD or simple VSD they are repaired during lung transplantation. Patients with primary or secondary pulmonary hypertension will have varying degrees of right ventricular dysfunction but this improves with successful lung transplantation. Perioperative use of inhaled NO or other pulmonary vasodilator pharmacotherapy is not uncommon and certainly useful to reduce post-operative pulmonary hypertension and the fluctuations in pressures and reduce the hemodynamic instability.

The most common hemodynamic disturbance following lung transplantation is hypotension and supra-ventricular tachyarrhythmia. The principle of keeping these patients in a relative hypovolemic status, make them susceptible to hypotension, if there is any degree of vasodilation. It is important to maintain adequate intravascular volume to maintain adequate cardiac output as well as urine output. The fluid therapy is aimed at maintaining low or low normal cardiac filling pressures. It is however not necessary to monitor pulmonary artery wedge pressures in all patients and monitoring of right atrial filling pressures are most often adequate. The fact that the lymphatic drainage is interrupted from the lung allograft following transplantation, any capillary leak in to the lung parenchyma will be cleared less efficiently. It had been shown that fluid restriction in patients with lung injury promotes early recovery (21). This may be an important factor to consider during the post operative period, due to the fact that majority of the lung grafts suffer some degree of reperfusion injury. Systemic vasodilation whether it is produced by medications or sympathetic blockade due to epidural or release of cytokines, best treated with vasoconstriction using intravenous short acting alpha-blockers than by volume. Neosynephrine is the drug of choice in the treatment of systemic vasodilation in these patients. Vasopressin is an effective systemic vasoconstricor but also appears to cause profound bronchial vasoconstriction and may cause bronchial ischemia in these patients and may affect bronchial anastomotic healing, therefore its use is avoided.

The incidence of supraventricular arrhythmias are not uncommon following lung transplantation (22). The commonest arrhythmias are supraventricular tachycardia and atrial fibrillation. Many programs take preventive measures for atrial fibrillation in the post-operative period which can reduce the incidence of this complication but unlikely to prevent it completely. The effects and complication due to atrial fibrillation are systemic hypotension and systemic embolization, perhaps made worse by fresh suture line on the left atrium. Although amiodarone is generally avoided due to its effects on the lung, we have used amidarone in patients who are resistant or unsuitable for treatment with calcium channel blockers or beta blockers. Anticoagulation will be necessary as in other patients with atrial fibrillation and the biopsy schedules needed to be considered and preferentially treated with short acting agents in the post operative period. It will be prudent to check clotting studies prior to transbronchial biopsy or endobronchial intervention as uncontrollable bronchial hemorrhage is invariably fatal.

7. Diagnosis and management of early surgical complication

The major surgical complications are bleeding, anastomotic complications and mal-rotation of the graft (24). The latter two are rare with current understanding and experience. Bleeding is less common and is due to refinement in surgical techniques, judicious use of pharmacological agents and blood products. The patients at high risk are the ones with extensive pleural adhesions, large and extensive mediastinal collateral vessels and patients with connective tissue disorders with secondary pulmonary hypertension. Patients with right heart failure and congested liver or patients on chronic anticoagulation or anti-platelet therapy are particularly susceptible and correction of coagulation defect is mandatory in these patients. If a patient persists with significant blood loss (>100 cc/hr), for 4-6 hours, the patient needs to return to the operating room unless there is evidence of significant coagulation abnormalities.

The dreaded complication of complete bronchial anastomotic dehiscence is rarely seen now but stenosis at the anastomotic site is not that uncommon, being reported between 5-25% of the anastomoses. This complication is usually delayed for several weeks following transplantation (25). In the presence of anatamotic site infection or significant donor bronchial ischemia minor bronchial dehiscence may present as early as 1-2 weeks.

Vascular anastomotic complications are infrequently reported, and their real incidence may be higher than that reported in the literature. The venous complication if severe enough can present few hours following transplantation as acute graft dysfunction. This presents as rapidly progressing pulmonary edema, with diffuse, dense infiltrate of the affected lung or lobe. This is a potentially lethal condition and diagnosis require high index of suspicion. TEE is helpful to confirm diagnosis. Surgical correction is required if this is due to anatomotic narrowing due to surgical technique. Thrombus formation at the anastomotic site can also cause venous obstruction and this is insidious in origin and progressive. Thrombolytic agents had been successfully used in these circumstances. Arterial anastomotic stenosis presents as hypoxemia, usually associated with exercise. This should be suspected if there is no other reason for hypoxemia. Pulmonary angiogram is diagnostic and catheter based intervention including stent placement has been successfully employed.

Mal-rotation of Lobar or lung on its axis is a rare complication and if not corrected immediately will result in necrosis of the lobe or lung. Complete opacification of the lobe or lung is noted in chest radiograph. Bronchoscopic examination is confirmatory of the bronchial torsion.

8. Pain management

Patients undergoing thoracic surgery require effective pain relief to allow deep breathing, coughing and facilitate early ambulation. In lung transplant patients this becomes crucial as they are chronically debilitated and have difficulty clearing secretions. While providing effective pain relief it is necessary to prevent sedation to promote early ambulation and therefore avoidance of narcotics is preferred. Thoracic epidural analgesia is effective in providing pain relief without causing sedation. We advocate placement of the thoracic epidural pre-operatively or place it soon after patient is extubated. NSAID are avoided because of the potential interactions with other nephrotoxic agents particularly the calcineurin inhibitors. Transitioning to oral pain medication is monitored carefully prior to discharge from the hospital.

9. Immunosuppression

Immunosuppression after lung transplantation includes three major categories of immunosuppressive agents; calcineurin inhibitors (tacrolimus, cyclosporine A), antimetabolites (azathioprine, mycophenolate mofetil) and corticosteroids. In addition, approximately 45% of lung transplant patients receive induction therapy after lung transplantation. The calcineurin inhibitors are administered within hours after transplantation and may be given either intravenously or sublingually. In general, tacrolimus is dosed at 0.05-0.1 mg/ kg over 24 hours by continuous infusion and may also be given sublingually at a dose of 0.03 mg/kg twice daily. Target tacrolimus trough levels range between 10-20 ng/ml in the first six months after transplantation, followed by levels around 10ng/ml thereafter. Cyclosporine is administered at a rate of 3 mg/kg over 24 hours with target trough levels between 350-450 ng/ ml in the first month, between 300-350 ng/ml during the first year and between 200-300 ng/ml thereafter. Both of these medications are available in oral formulation and should be given orally after extubation. Although current data have not shown a superiority of one of the calcineurin inhibitors, there has been an increasing use of tacrolimus in the lung transplant population due to reports of improved pulmonary function and possibly a reduction in the incidence of bronchiolitis obliterans syndrome (26,27).

Antimetabolites (either azathioprine or mycophenolate mofetil) are the second immunosuppressive medication that are used in the treatment of lung transplant recipients. The first dose may be initially administered prior to implantation of the lung allograft. Azathioprine is dosed at 2mg/kg daily and can be administered either intravenously or orally. Mycophenolate mofetil is dosed orally at 2-3 gram in daily divided doses. In general, antimetabolites may be associated with myelosuppression and gastrointestinal distress and doses may be adjusted based on these side effects. Two randomized multicenter studies that have not shown any difference in acute rejection, or survival between these two agents (28,29).

Corticosteroids have been the mainstay of immunosuppression since the advent of successful lung transplantation in the 1980s. First dose of methylprednisolone (between 500 to 1000 mg intravenously) is usually given prior to reperfusion of the graft in the operating room. Subsequent doses of corticosteroids range between 0.5-1 mg/kg during the first few weeks after transplantation. In general, corticosteroids are tapered to the equivalent of 5-10 mg of prednisone daily by three to six months after transplantation.

The role of induction therapy in lung transplantation has yet to be defined. There are several different types of induction therapy that are currently being used in lung transplantation including the interleukin- 2 receptor antagonists (daclizumab, basiliximab), the polyclonal agents(ATGAM, thymoglobulin) and the monoclonal antibody (OKT3). Several reports have suggested that induction therapies may reduce the incidence of acute rejection during the first six months after lung transplantation. However, longer term outcomes including prevention of chronic rejection or improving survival have not been associated with the use of induction therapy after lung transplantation (30-32).

10. Infection prophylaxis

Infections remain a major source of morbidity and mortality after lung transplantation. Prophylaxis against bacterial, viral and fungal organisms usually starts immediately postoperatively in the recipients. Initial antibiotic prophylaxis should be directed towards adequate anaerobic coverage and tailored towards any positive donor or recipient culture detected prior to transplantation. These antibiotics are usually continued between three to fourteen days post transplant depending upon the individual transplant center's protocol. Lung transplant recipients with septic lung disease (cystic fibrosis, bronchiectasis) who may be colonized with resistant organisms often receive two synergistic antibiotics based on prior sensitivities during this time period.

Viral prophylaxis is most commonly targeted against cytomegalovirus (CMV). Aggressive prophylactic therapy is directed towards this organism because of its high virulence and association with mortality in the lung transplant population. Lung transplant recipients with either donor or recipient serology that is positive for CMV usually receive prophylactic therapy with valganciclovir anywhere between three months to lifelong therapy. CMV negative lung transplant recipients who received a CMV positive donor lung may also receive CMV immunoglobulin in addition to their current valganciclovir therapy. Unfortunately, while valganciclovir prophylaxis decreases the incidence of CMV infection during the time of administration, prophylaxis does not completely prevent the development of CMV infection especially after prophylaxis therapy is discontinued. The optimal duration and type of therapy are still a matter of debate. Acyclovir and its derivatives are given to CMV negative lung transplant recipients who receive CMV negative donors in order to prevent the development of Herpes infections.

Fungal prophylaxis varies among the different transplant centers depending upon prior colonization, mechanical airway complications and environmental factors. In general some centers provide general fungal prophylaxis while others consider preemptive therapy depending upon surveillance bronchoscopy findings. Lung transplant recipients are at increased risk for developing *Aspergillus spp.* colonization of the airways leading to anastomotic infections and ulcerative tracheobronchitis. Itraconazole (or other azole substitutes) and inhaled amphotericin are the most common fungal prophylactic agents that are currently used. The azoles will increase the levels of the calcineurin inhibitors (cyclosporine and tacrolimus) so that the doses of these immunosuppressive medications should be decreased by at least 1/3 of their original dose. Calcineurin levels should be checked approximately one week after starting an azole. Of note, voriconazole and sirolimus should not be used together due to the significant rise in sirolimus levels.

11. Transplant outcomes

Significant improvements have been achieved in the past two decades with organ preservation, surgical techniques, critical care and immunosuppression. At present over 80% of patients receiving a lung transplant for end-stage lung disease are alive at 1 year and half of them are at 5 years (33). There are differences in the survival for different etiology for the underlying end-stage lung disease (Figure 1). Primary graft dysfunction is an important cause of post-operative mortality (33). The major cause of early and late mortality is infectious complications and bronchiolitis obliterans, a condition of progressive airflow obstruction associated with chronic airway fibrosis a pathologic finding known as bronchiolitis obliterans (BO). Majority of the late mortality is directly or indirectly due to the development of bronchiolitis obliterans syndrome or OB (Table 2) (34,35). Although the pathological mechanism that lead to BO is not well understood there have been many associations reported. A significant predictor of OB is prior acute rejection. Other conditions are primary graft dysfunction, gastroesophageal reflux or infections (36). Currently there are few well established therapies available for prevention or treatment of OB. Ongoing research continues to advance our understanding of the pathogenesis which may lead to effective treatment strategies in the future.

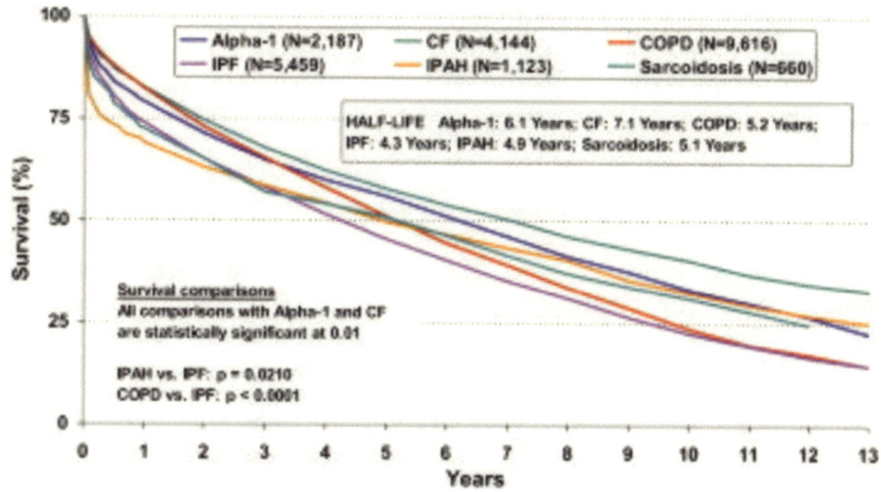

Fig. 1. Kaplan-Meier survival by diagnosis for adult lung transplants performed between January 1990 and June 2008. AT Def, α1-antitrypsin deficiency emphysema; CF, cystic fibrosis; COPD, chronic obstructive pulmonary disease; IPAH, idiopathic pulmonary arterial hypertension; IPF, idiopathic pulmonary fibrosis.
J Heart Lung Transplant. 10: 1083-1141, 2010

	0–30 days	**31 days–1 year**	**>1–3 years**	**>3–5 years**	**>5–10 years**	**>10 years**
	(*n* = 1,966)	**(*n* = 3,387)**	**(*n* = 3,073)**	**(*n* = 1,737)**	**(*n* = 2,014)**	**(*n* = 483)**
Cause of death	**No. (%)**	**No. (%)**	**No. (%)**	**No. (%)**	**No. (%)**	**No. (%)**
Bronchiolitis	6 (0.3)	159 (4.7)	781 (25.4)	508 (29.2)	507 (25.2)	95 (19.7)
Acute rejection	74 (3.8)	61 (1.8)	48 (1.6)	10 (0.6)	15 (0.7)	1 (0.2)
Lymphoma	1 (0.1)	86 (2.5)	63 (2.1)	28 (1.6)	46 (2.3)	23 (4.8)
Other malignancy	4 (0.2)	100 (3.0)	202 (6.6)	151 (8.7)	219 (10.9)	47 (9.7)
Infection						
CMV	0	96 (2.8)	29 (0.9)	5 (0.3)	4 (0.2)	0
Non-CMV	396 (20.1)	1,205 (35.6)	710 (23.1)	329 (18.9)	363 (18.0)	81 (16.8)
Graft failure	557 (28.3)	589 (17.4)	591 (19.2)	327 (18.8)	379 (18.8)	87 (18.0)
Cardiovascular	213 (10.8)	144 (4.3)	118 (3.8)	82 (4.7)	99 (4.9)	36 (7.5)
Technical	162 (8.2)	76 (2.2)	18 (0.6)	8 (0.5)	12 (0.6)	6 (1.2)
Other	553 (28.1)	871 (25.7)	513 (16.7)	289 (16.6)	370 (18.4)	107 (22.2)

Table 2. Causes of Death Following Lung Transplantation in Adult Recipients.
J Heart Lung Transplant. 10: 1083-1141, 2010

12. Conclusion

Lung transplant remains an effective treatment for selected patients with end-stage lung disease. The major rate limiting step for lung transplantation at present is the available donor organs. Chronic allograft dysfunction remains a major source of morbidity and mortality after lung transplantation. Investigations into improving donor lung availability, preventive and therapeutic approaches for OB and alternative for transplantation for end-stage lung disease are subjects currently under intense investigation aimed at improving short and long term result of therapy for end-stage lung disease.

13. References

[16] Barr ML, Kawut SM, Whelan TP, Et al. Report of the ISHLT working group on Primary Graft Dysfunction part IV: recipient related risk factors and markers. J Heart Lung Transplant. 24:1468-82, 2005.

[30] Beniaminovitz A, Itescu S, Lietz K, et al. Prevention of rejection in cardiac transplantation by blockade of the interleukin-2 receptor with a monoclonal antibody. *N Engl J Med* 342:613-9, 2000.

[10] Bernat JL, D'Alessandro AM, Port FK et al. Report of a National Conference on Donation after cardiac death. Am J Transplant 6: 281-291, 2002.

[7] Bhorade SM, Vigneswaran WT, Mc Cabe MA et al. Liberalization of donor criteria may expand donor pool without adverse consequence of lung transplantation. J Heart lung Transplant 19: 1199-1204, 2000.

[32] Brock MV, Borja MC, Ferber L, et al. Induction therapy in lung transplantation: a prospective, controlled clinical trial comparing OKT3, anti-thymocyte globulin, and daclizumab. *J Heart Lung Transplant* 20: 1282-90, 2001.

[35] Chatila WM, Furukawa S, Gaughan JP Criner GJ. Respiratory failure after lung transplantation. Chest 123: 165-173, 2003.

[21] Choong CK, Meyers BF, Guthrie TJ, Trulock EP, Patterson GA, Moazami N. Does the presence of preoperative mild or moderate coronary artery disease affect the outcome of lung transplantation? Ann Thorac Surg 82: 1038-42, 2006.

[34] Christie JD, Edwards LB, Kucheryavaya AY, Aurora P, Dobbels F, Kirk R, Rahmel AO, Stehlik J, Hertz MI. The registry of the International Society of Heart Lung Transplantation: Twenty seventh official adult lung and heart lung transplant report-2010. 29: 1104-1118, 2010.

[33] Christie JD, Kotloff RM, Pochettino A, et al. Clinical risk factors for primary graft failure following lung transplantation. Chest 124: 1232-1241, 2003.

[11] Cypel M, Yeung JC, Liu M et al. Normothermic ex vivo lung perfusion in clinical lung transplantation. N Engl J Med 364: 1431-1440, 2011.

[36] Davis RD Jr., Lau CL, Eubank S, et al. Improved lung allograft function after fundoplication in patients with gastroesophageal reflux disease undergoing lung transplantation. J Thorac Cardiovasc Surg 125: 533-542, 2003.

[31] Garrity, ER Jr., Villanueva J, Bhorade SM, Husain AN, and Vigneswaran WT. Low rate of acute lung allograft rejection after the use of daclizumab, an interleukin 2 receptor antibody. Transplantation 71:773-7, 2001.

[15] JD, Carby M, Bag R, Corris P, Hertz M, Weill D. Report of the ISHLT working group on Primary Graft Dysfunction Part II. Definition. A consensus statement of the International Society for Heart and Lung Transplantation. J Heart Lung Transplant 24:1454-1467, 2005.

[26] Keenan R.J, Konishi H, Kawai, et al. Clinical trial of tacrolimus versus cyclosporine in lung transplantation. Ann Thorac Surg 60: 580-5, 1995.

[12] Loor G, Vigneswaran WT. Single lung transplant.ation. in Lung Transplantation (Eds.) Wickii T. Vigneswaran and Edward Garrity Jr Informa Healthcare, Essex, UK, pp 190-197, 2010.

[1] Mahidhara R, Benfield JR, The History of Lung Transplantation. Lung Transplantation (Eds.) Wickii T. Vigneswaran and Edward Garrity Jr Informa Healthcare, Essex, UK, pp 1-7, 2010.

[29] McNeil K., Glanville AR, Wahlers T, et al. Comparison of Mycophenolate Mofetil and Azathioprine for Prevention of Bronchiolitis Obliterans Syndrome in De Novo Lung Transplant Recipients. *Transplantation* 81:998-1003, 2006.

[18] Myers BF, Sundt TM III, Henry S, et al. Selective use of extracorporeal membrane oxygenation is warrranted after lung transplantation. J Thorac Cardiovasc Surg 120: 631-636, 2000.

[24] Nielsen TD, Bahnson T, Davis RD, Palmer SM. Atrial Fibrilation after pulmonary transplant. Chest 126: 496-500, 2004.

[4] Orens JB, Estenne M, Arcosoy S etal. International guidelines for selection of lung transplant candidates: 2006 update - a consensus report from pulmonary scientific council of the International Society of Heart and Lung Transplantation. J Heart Lung Transplantation. 25: 745-755, 2006.

[6] Pak SW, Sonett J. Lung Donor Selection Criteria. in Lung Transplantation (Eds.) Wickii T. Vigneswaran and Edward Garrity Jr Informa Healthcare, Essex, UK, pp 125-134, 2010.

[28] Palmer SM., Baz MA, Sanders L, et al. Results of a randomized, prospective, multicenter trial of mycophenolate mofetil versus azathioprine in the prevention of acute lung allograft rejection. *Transplantation* 71:1772-6, 2001.

[20] Patel VS, Palmer SM, Messier RH, Davis RD. Clinical outcomes after coronary artery revascularization and lung transplantation. Ann Thorac Surg 75:372-377, 2003.

[8] Puri V, Patterson GA. Adult lung transplantation: technical consideration. Semin Thorac Cardiovasc Surg 20: 152-164, 2008.

[13] Puri V, Patterson GA. Bilateral sequential lung t transplantation: Technical aspects. In Lung Transplantation (Eds.) Wickii T. Vigneswaran and Edward Garrity Jr Informa Healthcare, Essex, UK, pp 198-207, 2010.

[2] Reitz BA, Wallwork JL, Hunt SA, et al. Heart-lung transplantation: successful therapy for patients with pulmonary vascular disease. N Eng J Med 306: 557-564, 1982.

[17] Shargall Y, Guenther G, Ahya VN, Ardehali A, Singhal A, Keshavjee S. Report of the ISHLT working group on Primary Graft Dysfunction Part VI: Treatment. J Heart Lung Transplant 24:1489-1500, 2005.

[5] Stern E, Garrity ER. Patient Selection. in Lung Transplantation (Eds.) Wickii T. Vigneswaran and Edward Garrity Jr Informa Healthcare, Essex, UK, pp 83-98, 2010.

[3] Toronto Lung Transplant Group. Unilateral lung transplantation for pulmonary fibrosis. N Engl J Med 314: 1140-1145, 1986.

[9] Van De Wauwer C, Neyrinch AP, Geudens N et al. Retrograde flush following topical cooling is superior to preserve the non heart-beating donor lung. Eur J Cardiothorac Surg 31: 1125-33, 2007.

[14] Vigneswaran WT, Bhorade SM Wolfe M et al. Clinical pathway following lung transplantation shortens hospital length of stay without affecting outcome. Int Surg 92: 93-99, 2007.

[32] Vigneswaran WT, Bhorade SM. Postoperative care of lung transplant patient in Surgical Intensive Care Medicine (Eds) John M O'Donnel and Flavio E Nacul. Springer Science + Business Media, New York, NY (USA) 2nd Ed, pp 621-628, 2010.

[25] Vigneswaran, WT, Sakiyalak P, Bhorade SM, Bakhos M. Airway complications after isolated lung transplantation, Transplantation Reviews (Eds) Peter J Morris and Nicholas L. Tilney. Elsiver Science (USA). 16(2) pp 87-94, 2002.
[22] Wiedemann HP, Wheeler AP, Bernard GR, et al. Comparison of two fluid management strategies in acute lung injury. N Engl J Med 15:2564-75, 2006.
[19] Zenati M, Pham SM, Keenan RJ, Griffith BP. Extracorporeal membrane oxygenation for lung transplant recipients with primary severe donor lung dysfunction. Transplant Int 1996;9:227-30.
[27] Zuckermann, AH, Reichenspurner T, Birsan H, et al. Cyclosporine A versus tacrolimus in combination with mycophenolate mofetil and steroids as primary immunosuppression after lung transplantation: one-year results of a 2-center prospective randomized trial. J Thorac Cardiovasc Surg 125: 891-900, 2003.

17

Systematic Review of the Literature: Comparison of Open and Minimal Access Surgery (Thoracoscopic Repair) of Esophageal Atresia with Tracheo-Esophageal Fistula (EA-TEF)

M. W. N. Oomen
*Pediatric Surgical Centre of Amsterdam,
VU Medical Centre & Emma's children hospital of the AMC,
The Netherlands*

1. Introduction

Surgical correction of esophageal atresia with tracheo-esophageal fistula (EA-TEF) has been performed since 1943 (Cameron Haight) via postero-lateral thoracotomy using an extra-pleural approach in most cases. This procedure can be considered as the standard treatment of EA. The pitfalls of the operation, the incidence of complications and the outcomes, both short term and long term, have been analysed and reported by many pediatric surgeons around the world.

Since 1999, minimal access surgery (MAS) has been practised for the correction of EA [1]. The risk of complications and short term outcomes have been reported as equal to the open approach. MAS has been advocated because of a possibly reduced risk of impairment of shoulder function, and a possible reduction in occurrence of postoperative scoliosis. Next to that, it has been postulated the MAS repair might lead to a better cosmesis.

Several advantages and disadvantages of both procedures have been described. The open approach is well standardized and is resorted to in difficult cases. Disadvantages of the open approach are the presence of a scar, possible chest wall deformities and rib fusion. The occurrence of scoliosis and possible shoulder function impairment has been related to the open approach as well.

The thoracoscopic approach has the advantage of magnification of view. Next to that the chance on a postoperative scoliosis and impaired shoulder function may be reduced due to the small incisions which also might lead to better cosmesis. Technically, the thoracoscopic approach is more demanding than the open approach which has consequences for training and education.

So far, it seems that there is no difference between open and MAS approach in the frequency of anastomotic leakages, strictures, recurrent fistulas, tracheomalacie or GERD.

In 2005, Holcomb et al presented their results of MAS (thoracoscopic) EA-TEF repair in 104 patients in multiple centres. This landmark paper has been extensively discussed by leaders in the field and highlights the need for a randomized clinical trial. Since that discussion, several more articles have been published on MAS repair of EA-TEF, but no prospective comparative studies, let alone RCT's. The Clinical Trials Register (www.clinicaltrials.gov) does not list a study on this subject.

	Al Thokais,2008 MAS	Al Thokais,2008 open	Szavay 2011MAS	Szavay 2011 open	Kawahara MAS	Kawahara open	Lugo MAS	Lugo open
no of patients	21	22	25	43	7	10	8	25
type EA	C (dist fist)	C (dist fist)	C (dist fist)	C (dist fist)	C (dist fist)	C (dist fist)	C (dist fist)	C (dist fist)
ass malform	9(39.1%)	13(59.1%)	47%	47% (all only)			87,50%	72%
weight at op	2735±744	2427±726	2720	2090	2.814(2.46-3.71)	2.45(1.46-2.9)	2,7	2,4
age at op			1 (median)	1 (median) (all only)	2(0-12)		36,9	36,7
gestat age	36,3	36,3	35	35 (all only)	38(33-41)	34.5-41.6		
anastom leak	4 (18%)	3(14%)			3(30%)	2(25%)	14%	20%
dilat >1	2 (9%)	4 (18%)			1	2	14%	52%
recurr fist	NR	NR						
mortality related	0	2(9%)					0	0
duration op	149±47	179±65	141(median)	106(median)			156(75-240)	123(82-205)
post ventil	no difference						4.6(1-12)	19(3-150)
l.o.s	NR	NR					21.8(11-38)	66(8-280)
conversion rate	3(14%)	NR					1	
antireflux	NR	NR			2	2		
aortopexy	NR	NR						
follow-up	14.4(6-46)mo	29.8(6-119)mo						
other	incl 2 A				antirefluxstudy	antirefluxstudy		
pCO2 max intraop.			62	48				
pCO2 max postop.			53	47				
Base excess postop.			-1	-3				
PH postop.			7.16	7.20				

Table 1.

2. Methods

Search strategy:

EmBase and PubMed (Medline) search using keywords (MESH terms): <Minimal access surgery> OR <thoracoscopic surgery> OR <thoracoscopy> AND <esophageal atresia>

Only full text papers in English were included. If more than one paper had been published by the same author or group of authors [2], only the most recent paper was included in order to avoid duplications.

Two authors reviewed all papers and selected those that contained sufficient data on patients characteristics and outcome parameters to enable comparison with reports on open repair of EA-TEF of patients operated after 1995.

Parameters recorded are represented in table 1.

Three categories can be discerned

1. patients' characteristics
2. intra-operative and post-operative data, including complications
3. follow-up data

3. Results

The initial search resulted in 55 articles. After critical review by two independent reviewers twenty-one articles were included, based on the criteria stated above.

There were no RCT's or prospective studies. All papers were based on retrospective analysis, mostly single center cohort or case studies. The largest population was reported in a multicenter review by experts in minimally invasive pediatric surgery combining the experience in 104 patients.

Together the 22 articles contained 332 patients who had (type C) EA-TEF repair via the thoracoscopic approach, 11 patients with isolated (type A) [3,4,5,6] and one case report of type D (proximal and distal fistula) [7].

At a closer look there are different study-designs in those 22 articles in which only four papers [4,8,9,10] did a retrospective analysis with historic [4] or contemporary [8,9,10] open approaches as controls. (Table 1) Seven papers reported the results of thoracoscopic EA-TEF repair containing at least 20 patients per report for a total of 312 patients [4,11,5,12,13,2,10]. (Table 2)

Several papers, particularly in the early period, concentrated on technical and feasibility aspects dealing with the initial diagnosis of esophageal atresie. Other studies highlighted special characteristics of the patients, like cardiac malformations [14]. Also on anesthesiological subjects, including the effects of CO2 inflation [15,16] and pain after thoracoscopic repair was studied [17].

	Author,year Holcomb,2005	Al Thokais,2008 MAS	Rothenberg	MacKinlay,2009	Patkowski,2009	vanderZee, 2007	Szavay 2011MAS
no of patients	104	21	26	20	23	50	25
type EA	C (dist fist)	C (dist fist)	C	C (dist fist)	C (dist fist)	C (dist fist)	C (dist fist)
ass malform		9(39.1%)	50%	13(65%)	9(38%)	31(61%)	47%
weight at op	2.6±0.5	2735±744	1.8-3.8	1,4-3.9	1070-3390	2620(1025-4030)	2720
age at op	1.2±1.1					1-7 d	1 (median)
gestat age		36,3		31-41		37.2(31.3-42.2)	35
anastom leak	8 (8%)	4 (18%)	3.6%	7(35%)	3 (13%)	9 (18%)	
dilat >1	21 (21%)	2 (9%)	30%	3(15%)	4 (18%)	22 (45%)	
recurr fist	2 (1.9)	NR	0	1(5%)	NR	2 (4%)	
mortality related	1(1%)	0		1(5%)		1(2%)	
duration op	129.9±55.5	149±47	95(55-120)	NR	131(55-245)	178(90-390)	141(median)
post ventil	3.6±5.8	no difference	1-4dd	NR	NR	4(1-95) med	
l.o.s	18.1±18.6	NR		NR	NR	16.5(7-150) med	
conversion rate	5 (5%)	3(14%)	1	1 (5%)		2(4%)	
antireflux	26 (25%)	NR		NR		11(22%)	
aortopexy	7 (6.8%)	NR		NR	1(4%)	6(12%)	
follow-up		14.4(6-46)mo		NR	14 (1.5-33)mo	27(10-145)	
other	Rt arch 6	incl 2 A			2 trach perf		
pCO2 max intraop.							62
pCO2 max postop.							53
Base excess postop.							-1
PH postop.							7.16

Table 2.

To compare the results of the minimal invasive operations with open operations, data were distilled from the literature (Table 3). This represents the results from textbooks and standard papers on open repair of EA-TEF. Also these results on open approach are based on retrospective studies and did not comprise RCT's or prospective studies.

	Ashcraft	Prem Puri	Engum	Spitz	Randolph	Manning	Yanchar
no of patients			174	148	39	63	90
type EA							
ass malform							
weight at op							
age at op							
gestat age							
anastom leak	17%	11-21%		21%	10.2%	17%	16.6%
stricture	17-59%	37-55%	32.7%	17.7 %	33.3%	4.3%	17%
recurr fist	3-15%	5-15%	2.2%	12%	5.1%	6.4%	3.3%
mortality EA/TEF related			4.5%	14.8 %	0%	3.1%	1.1%
duration op							
post ventil							
l.o.s						24(9-174)	
GER	40%	40-50%					
antireflux-operatie	20%	6-45%	25.2%	18%	15.3%	16.9%	32.2%
aortopexy				16%		4.8%	

Table 3.

4. Patiens' characteristics

The *gestational age and the birth weight* of MAS patients were not different from open repairs in the comparative studies (2.7-2.8 kg MAS vs 2.0-2.4 open Table 1). In the minimal invasive group the thoracoscopic approach was succesfully performed even in premature babies with weights below 1500 g [18,5,2] but these are not different from data in the literature for open repair ([19], mean 2557 with range 1100-4460 g).

Concerning the *associated malformations and risk classification* only Holcomb [11] et al present data on Waterston classification(A 62, B 30 and C12) respectively. The reported associated malformations were seen in up to 87.5% [9] of the thoracoscopically repaired babies, but in the comparative studies no difference is seen between MAS (39-87%) and open (47-72%) concerning these associated malformations

5. Perioperative data

Mean *duration of operation* was recorded in 12 articles and ranged between 95 and 260 minutes. In the comparative studies the paper of Szavay [10] reveals a significantly longer operation time (open 106 min versus MAS 141). But Al Tokhais [4] and Lugo [9] did not find a significant difference in operation time between them with 179 and 123 min open and 149 and 156 min.for MAS.

The conversion rate was reported in 15 papers, in which no conversion was done in 9 papers and in the remaining 6 papers the rates varied between 5 and 16%.

The *duration of postoperative ventilation* was mentioned in 10 papers. One reported no difference between open and MAS patients [4], others reported mean duration of 4 days post-

operative ventilation [11,3,20,9,13] (range 1-4.6). Of interest is the paper of Krosnar [16] where, although in a small number, a comparison between open and MAS approach is done concerning extubation time (extt) and discharge to PICU(DPICU) .
These results were for an open approach with an extt of 54 hrs and DPICU discharge of 3.4 days and for the MAS approch extt 37.6 hrs and DPICU of 2.75 days. This numbers suggest a better postoperative recovery of the MAS approach.
Length of hospital stay was reported in 7 articles, some giving mean, others median values so a good comparison of these numbers is not justified. The mean length of stay in Hollcombs' paper compares favorably with open repairs as reported by Manning [21] 18.1 days for MAS and 24 for the open method. This historic group however might not be representative for present l.o.s so the evidence is not clear. Also Lugo [9] found a difference in l.o.s as it is 21 days in MAS (n=8) and 66 days in the open approach (n=25) but in here hard evidence seems to be scarce as the numbers are small. *Mortality* related to the procedure was recorded in 14 articles and 11 reported no mortality; in the other three it varied between 1 and 16%. But these were small numbers also [18]. In the series reported by Holcomb the mortality rate was 0.9 %. Yanchar [22], reported 1.1 % mortality after open repair in 90 patients. For this parameter no difference could be demonstrated.

6. Complications

The main short term complications are leakage of the anastomosis, anastomotic strictures and recurrent TEF. (Table 1, 2, 3)
Anastomotic leakage was reported in 18 papers. Important is that the definition may differ between the papers depending on whether routine esophagograms were performed or not. Most leaks were described as minor and healed spontaneously. The incidence varies between 0 and 30% with a median 15%. There is no difference with the reported leak rates in the open thoracotomies in the papers [8,9,23,24,22] and in the literature.(Table 3)
A clear definition of *anastomotic stricture* is an important factor. Most authors define stricture by the need for (repeated) dilatations however others state that narrowing of more than 50% of the lumen or every narrowing detected on an esophagram with a symptomatic patient can be seen as an anastomic stricture [25,26]. Sixteen papers reported an incidence between 9 and 45%, with a median of 22%. This incidence is comparable to the rates reported after open repair (6-52%) by Holland [24] and in the literature (Table 3).
The incidence of the serious complication of a *recurrent tracheo-oesophageal fistula* was noted in 8 articles. The incidence varied between 0 (in 5 papers) and 4%. In the open repair series and in the literature, similar incidences have been reported (Table 3).

7. Other complications

Allthough *gastro-oesophageal reflux* is often seen after repair of esophageal atresia with TEF, the need for anti-reflux surgery was mentioned in 4 articles. The incidence of anti-reflux surgery varied from 22 to 50% (1,3,4,19). Procedures performed, if reported, were Thal or Nissen-fundoplication. Antireflux surgery numbers after open approach was performed in 18 to 32.2% of cases [19,27,28,21,22].
The need for aortopexy in case of a severe *tracheomalacia* is mentioned in only one paper [11] were it was performed in 6.8% of the cases. This is compatible with the rate of 4.7% and 16% after open repair [21,27].

There were no reports on any cosmetic benefit in any of the papers on MAS. And although there is more awareness of the effect of thoracotomy on shoulder-function and *scoliosis* this was not reported in any of these papers.
The duration of follow-up after discharge from the hospital was reported in 7 papers with means varying between 6 and 30 months. No further *long-term complications* as dysphagia, late pulmonary disease both restrictive and obstructive and late sequelae from GER are reported.

8. Discussion

In summary a total of 22 papers reporting on 332 EA-TEF repairs performed via MAS revealed no prospective studies and only four comparative studies with historic and contemporary open repairs as controls.
The focus of this chapter is on the type C, or esophageal atresia with fistula (TEF) as this is the most common form in esophageal atresia. Even with these numbers data are sometimes scarce and difficult to compare.
Allthough it is not the aim of this chapter a special mention has to be made of the role of MAS in correction of type A (long gap) EA. In some of the reviewed papers, these patients have been included because a esophago-esophagostomy was performed 3,5,6. And there are a number of other reports on the role of MAS in esophageal replacement. For example Stanwell 29 describes 7 patients in whom gastric transposition was performed and were laparoscopically assisted. In this study five of these had a long gap EA. Esteves 30 reported on laparoscopically assisted colon interposition in 5 children with long gap EA. Nevertheless because of the small numbers in these studies, the different nature and the conflicting views on the various procedures (primary anastomosis vs replacement by stomach, colon or jejunum), these papers have not been included in this review.

9. Clinical outcomes

When analyzing the results on *patients characteristics* it does not appear that there is a difference in the selection of patients in favour of any of the procedures. The gestational age, birth weight and associated malformations were similar to data recorded in open repair.
There is a wide variety between reports when focusing on post-operative results and complications. Consistent differences are lacking when compared with results reported for open thoracotomies as is seen in Table 1 and 2. The biggest problem however is the definition of a complication in these cases like anastomotic leakage and anastomotic stricture. For example esophagrams are not made routinely everywhere. Therefore, a difference in the incidence of esophageal strictures is likely to be present due to the difference in classification and not due to an incidence of occurrence of anastomotic strictures.
Also the follow-up data on MAS repair of EA-TEF is scarce, but again, they do not indicate that the incidence of *gastro-oesophageal reflux (GER)* and GER requiring anti-reflux surgery is different from that in patients who had open repairs of the esophageal atresia with TEF. Kawahara [8]et al studied the influence of MAS on esophageal motor function and gastro-esophageal reflux in 7 patients in comparison to 10 patients who had an open repair.

Manometry and 24-hours pH monitoring did not demonstrate any differences between MAS and open repair.
There is only one paper [11] mentioning the consequences of *tracheomalacia* requiring aortopexy. There seem to be no differences between MAS and studies after open repair.

10. Studies on systemic effects of MAS

In several papers the systemic effects of thoracoscopy in neonates are emphasized. In the findings of Bishay [15] (6 Congenital Diafragmatic Hernias and 2 EA-TEF) on decreased cerebral oxygen saturation measured by Near Infra Red Spectrometry (NIRS) might cause concern. These changes and also the decreased arterial pH values had not recovered after 24 hours. However the real value of NIRS is still not clear and is extensively discussed in a study by Pennekamp [31]. So far, the long term effect on brain development remains unknown but will have to be followed very carefully.
In the study by Kalfa et al [32] a cohort of 49 neonates who underwent MAS was investigated, among them five with esophageal atresia. They also found decreased values of saturation due to thoracic insufflation of CO_2. Some other data are reported, such as thermic loss, which is proportional to duration of operation, and a decreased systolic arterial pressure, responding to vascular expansion. But these data are not comparative to open surgery.
Krosnar [16] also noted a decrease of oxygen saturation, and their patients required 100% inspired oxygen in order to maintain the saturation above 85%. They also experienced difficulties in end-tidal CO_2 monitoring. But on the other hand Szavay [10] in his retrospective comparative analysis in 68 patients of which 25 were operated via MAS showed no differences in postoperative pCO_2 max levels as in postoperative PH and base excess.
What do these findings mean?
To begin with, all papers are retrospective studies with inconsistent reporting of results. Obviously, the multi-center study by Holcomb [11] et al should be seen as the standard at this moment with only few institutions reporting on datasets of more than 20 MAS procedures [5,13,2,10,12,4] of which one comparative multicenter study [4]. Even if these papers are compiled no consistent pattern arises to show superiority or inferiority of MAS versus open repair in terms of early post-operative results.
Secondly, almost all reports come from pioneers in this field who have endeavoured with great zeal to advance the skills in pediatric MAS. On one hand, this implies that these studies represent early experiences and learning curves. On the other hand, these results were obtained by the experts and therefore may be difficult to attain by less experienced surgeons. There is still a world to win in MAS as spreading of MAS is possible in centres without pioneers. After passing their learning curves their results would become better and the patients could benefit from it. Already from adult literature we know that there are benefits of minimal invasive surgery when compared with open surgery by means of better cosmesis, body-image, lenght of stay and reduced postoperative complications [33 34 35].
One of the reasons to advocate MAS for EA-TEF repair is the cosmesis and elimination of shoulder function disturbances and scoliosis, that in the past has been reported after open thoracotomies. But until now hard evidence is not available for either for the contention that MAS gives better cosmetic and functional results, or for the better results of muscle-sparing thoracotomies in children. It is interesting that also breast-development, chronic pain (in 50%) and even paraplegia is reported after thoracotomy [36,37,38].

Another argument for MAS could be the reduced need for opioid administration postoperatively.The effects of MAS on *post-operative pain* as measured by opioid requirements were studied by Ceelie [17] et al in 10 CDH and 14 EA patients. No differences were found compared to matched controls (20 CDH and 28 EA) concerning cumulative opioid doses at different time points postoperatively.
An improved esophageal function after thoracoscopic repair, represented by more effective motility and less gastro-esophageal reflux have not been demonstrated in the patients series of Kawahara [8].
Could MAS have negative influences in comparison to open repair?
The insufflation of the pleural cavity appears to have greater impact on arterial oxygen saturation particularly in cerebro than open repair, as demonstrated by Bishay [15] using NIRS. But as mentioned earlier no comparative study has been done and the validation in open surgery for EA with TEF has not been done.
In summary, making up the balance between MAS and open repair, there appear to be no differences in short term results, both in terms of complications and postoperative pain or ICU-stay. Little is known about the long term outcomes, but again, no differences have been recorded. So far there is no data available on the cosmetic or shoulder/spine/chestwall outcomes after MAS. However Holcomb is mentioning that ample literature is now available about long term sequelae from thoracotomies such as, besides scoliosis, mammary maldevelopment and chronic postoperative pain, even after muscle-sparing thoracotomy [39]. Some concern has been raised about the harmful effects of MAS in newborns on cerebral perfusion and subsequent development.
This emphasises the need for a prospective, randomised trial as has already been stated by Holcomb [11] in 2005.

11. References

[1] Lobe TE. Thoracoscopic Repair of Esophageal Atresia in an Infant: A Surgical First. *Pediatric Endosurgery & Innovative Techniques* 1999; 3(3):141-148.

[2] van der Zee DC, Bax KN. Thoracoscopic treatment of esophageal atresia with distal fistula and of tracheomalacia. *Semin Pediatr Surg* 2007; 16(4):224-230.

[3] Allal H, Perez-Bertolez S, Maillet O, Forgues D, Doan Q, Chiapinelli A et al. [Comparative study of thoracoscopy versus thoracotomy in esophageal atresia]. *Cir Pediatr* 2009; 22(4):177-180.

[4] Al TT, Zamakhshary M, Aldekhayel S, Mandora H, Sayed S, AlHarbi K et al. Thoracoscopic repair of tracheoesophageal fistulas: a case-control matched study. *J Pediatr Surg* 2008; 43(5):805-809.

[5] MacKinlay GA. Esophageal atresia surgery in the 21st century. *Semin Pediatr Surg* 2009; 18(1):20-22.

[6] Shimotakahara A, Sueyoshi R, Lane GJ, Okazaki T, Nishimura K, Inada E et al. The benefit of stay sutures during thoracoscopic esophagoesophagostomy in patients with esophageal atresia: a technical report. *Pediatr Surg Int* 2010; 26(4):443-446.

[7] Rice-Townsend S, Ramamoorthy C, Dutta S. Thoracoscopic repair of a type D esophageal atresia in a newborn with complex congenital heart disease. *J Pediatr Surg* 2007; 42(9):1616-1619.

[8] Kawahara H, Okuyama H, Mitani Y, Nomura M, Nose K, Yoneda A et al. Influence of thoracoscopic esophageal atresia repair on esophageal motor function and gastroesophageal reflux. *J Pediatr Surg* 2009; 44(12):2282-2286.

[9] Lugo B, Malhotra A, Guner Y, Nguyen T, Ford H, Nguyen NX. Thoracoscopic versus open repair of tracheoesophageal fistula and esophageal atresia. *J Laparoendosc Adv Surg Tech A* 2008; 18(5):753-756.

[10] Szavay PO, Zundel S, Blumenstock G, Kirschner HJ, Luithle T, Girisch M et al. Perioperative Outcome of Patients with Esophageal Atresia and Tracheo-esophageal Fistula Undergoing Open Versus Thoracoscopic Surgery. *J Laparoendosc Adv Surg Tech A* 2011; 21(5):439-443.

[11] Holcomb GW, III, Rothenberg SS, Bax KM, Martinez-Ferro M, Albanese CT, Ostlie DJ et al. Thoracoscopic repair of esophageal atresia and tracheoesophageal fistula: a multi-institutional analysis. *Ann Surg* 2005; 242(3):422-428.

[12] Patkowsk D, Rysiakiewicz K, Jaworski W, Zielinska M, Siejka G, Konsur K et al. Thoracoscopic repair of tracheoesophageal fistula and esophageal atresia. *J Laparoendosc Adv Surg Tech A* 2009; 19 Suppl 1:S19-S22.

[13] Rothenberg SS. Thoracoscopic repair of esophageal atresia and tracheo-esophageal fistula. *Semin Pediatr Surg* 2005; 14(1):2-7.

[14] Mariano ER, Chu LF, Albanese CT, Ramamoorthy C. Successful thoracoscopic repair of esophageal atresia with tracheoesophageal fistula in a newborn with single ventricle physiology. *Anesth Analg* 2005; 101(4):1000-2, table.

[15] Bishay M, Giacomello L, Retrosi G, Thyoka M, Nah SA, McHoney M et al. Decreased cerebral oxygen saturation during thoracoscopic repair of congenital diaphragmatic hernia and esophageal atresia in infants. *J Pediatr Surg* 2011; 46(1):47-51.

[16] Krosnar S, Baxter A. Thoracoscopic repair of esophageal atresia with tracheoesophageal fistula: anesthetic and intensive care management of a series of eight neonates. *Paediatr Anaesth* 2005; 15(7):541-546.

[17] Ceelie I, van DM, Bax NM, de Wildt SN, Tibboel D. Does minimal access major surgery in the newborn hurt less? An evaluation of cumulative opioid doses. *Eur J Pain* 2011; 15(6):615-620.

[18] Nguyen T, Zainabadi K, Bui T, Emil S, Gelfand D, Nguyen N. Thoracoscopic repair of esophageal atresia and tracheoesophageal fistula: lessons learned. *J Laparoendosc Adv Surg Tech A* 2006; 16(2):174-178.

[19] Engum SA, Grosfeld JL, West KW, Rescorla FJ, Scherer LR, III. Analysis of morbidity and mortality in 227 cases of esophageal atresia and/or tracheoesophageal fistula over two decades. *Arch Surg* 1995; 130(5):502-508.

[20] Bax KM, van der Zee DC. Feasibility of thoracoscopic repair of esophageal atresia with distal fistula. *J Pediatr Surg* 2002; 37(2):192-196.

[21] Manning PB, Morgan RA, Coran AG, Wesley JR, Polley TZ, Jr., Behrendt DM et al. Fifty years' experience with esophageal atresia and tracheoesophageal fistula. Beginning with Cameron Haight's first operation in 1935. *Ann Surg* 1986; 204(4):446-453.

[22] Yanchar NL, Gordon R, Cooper M, Dunlap H, Soucy P. Significance of the clinical course and early upper gastrointestinal studies in predicting complications associated with repair of esophageal atresia. *J Pediatr Surg* 2001; 36(5):815-822.

[23] Castilloux J, Noble AJ, Faure C. Risk factors for short- and long-term morbidity in children with esophageal atresia. *J Pediatr* 2010; 156(5):755-760.

[24] Holland AJ, Fitzgerald DA. Oesophageal atresia and tracheo-oesophageal fistula: current management strategies and complications. *Paediatr Respir Rev* 2010; 11(2):100-106.
[25] Ashcraft. Ashcraft's Pediatric Surgery. Fifth edition ed. Elsevier; 2010.
[26] Prem Puri. Newborn Surgery. Second ed. Arnold Publisher; 2003.
[27] Spitz L, Kiely E, Brereton RJ. Esophageal atresia: five year experience with 148 cases. *J Pediatr Surg* 1987; 22(2):103-108.
[28] Randolph JG, Newman KD, Anderson KD. Current results in repair of esophageal atresia with tracheoesophageal fistula using physiologic status as a guide to therapy. *Ann Surg* 1989; 209(5):526-530.
[29] Stanwell J, Drake D, Pierro A, Kiely E, Curry J. Pediatric laparoscopic-assisted gastric transposition: early experience and outcomes. *J Laparoendosc Adv Surg Tech A* 2010; 20(2):177-181.
[30] Esteves E, Sousa-Filho HB, Watanabe S, Silva JF, Neto EC, da Costa AL. Laparoscopically assisted esophagectomy and colon interposition for esophageal replacement in children: preliminary results of a novel technique. *J Pediatr Surg* 2010; 45(5):1053-1060.
[31] Pennekamp CW, Bots ML, Kappelle LJ, Moll FL, de Borst GJ. The value of near-infrared spectroscopy measured cerebral oximetry during carotid endarterectomy in perioperative stroke prevention. A review. *Eur J Vasc Endovasc Surg* 2009; 38(5):539-545.
[32] Kalfa N, Allal H, Raux O, Lopez M, Forgues D, Guibal MP et al. Tolerance of laparoscopy and thoracoscopy in neonates. *Pediatrics* 2005; 116(6):e785-e791.
[33] Klarenbeek BR, Bergamaschi R, Veenhof AA, van der Peet DL, van den Broek WT, de Lange ES et al. Laparoscopic versus open sigmoid resection for diverticular disease: follow-up assessment of the randomized control Sigma trial. *Surg Endosc* 2011; 25(4):1121-1126.
[34] Eshuis EJ, Slors JF, Stokkers PC, Sprangers MA, Ubbink DT, Cuesta MA et al. Long-term outcomes following laparoscopically assisted versus open ileocolic resection for Crohn's disease. *Br J Surg* 2010; 97(4):563-568.
[35] Bertleff MJ, Halm JA, Bemelman WA, van der Ham AC, van der Harst E, Oei HI et al. Randomized clinical trial of laparoscopic versus open repair of the perforated peptic ulcer: the LAMA Trial. *World J Surg* 2009; 33(7):1368-1373.
[36] Khan IH, McManus KG, McCraith A, McGuigan JA. Muscle sparing thoracotomy: a biomechanical analysis confirms preservation of muscle strength but no improvement in wound discomfort. *Eur J Cardiothorac Surg* 2000; 18(6):656-661.
[37] Shapira OM, Shahian DM. Postpneumonectomy pulmonary edema. *Ann Thorac Surg* 1993; 56(1):190-195.
[38] Bal S, Elshershari H, Celiker R, Celiker A. Thoracic sequels after thoracotomies in children with congenital cardiac disease. *Cardiol Young* 2003; 13(3):264-267.
[39] Jaureguizar E, Vazquez J, Murcia J, Diez Pardo JA. Morbid musculoskeletal sequelae of thoracotomy for tracheoesophageal fistula. *J Pediatr Surg* 1985; 20(5):511-514.

Part 5

Cardiothoracic Anaesthesia

18

Ventilator-Induced Lung Injury: Mechanisms and Future Therapeutic Interventions

Maria A. Hegeman[1,2], Marcus J. Schultz[1,2],
Adrianus J. van Vught[3] and Cobi J. Heijnen[4]
[1]*Laboratory of Experimental Intensive Care and Anesthesiology (LEICA),*
[2]*Department of Intensive Care Medicine, Academic Medical Center, Amsterdam,*
[3]*Department of Pediatric Intensive Care,*
[4]*Laboratory of Neuroimmunology and Developmental Origins of Disease (NIDOD),*
University Medical Center Utrecht, Utrecht,
The Netherlands

1. Introduction

Mechanical ventilation has become a standard technique to support the life of the critically ill patient in the intensive care unit (ICU) (Tobin, 2001). In general, mechanical ventilation is applied when the patient's spontaneous ventilation is inadequate to maintain life. Especially patients who have developed acute respiratory failure require mechanical ventilation (Slutsky, 1993). Patients diagnosed with acute lung injury (ALI) suffer from severe pulmonary dysfunction which may persist for a long period of time. The extent and severity of ALI differs among patients, with the acute respiratory distress syndrome (ARDS) being the most severe manifestation of this lung disease (Schwarz, 2001). ALI and ARDS are characterized by the acute onset of diffuse neutrophilic alveolar infiltrates, protein-rich edema due to enhanced alveolar-capillary permeability and hypoxemic respiratory failure (ratio of arterial oxygen partial pressure to fractional inspired oxygen concentration, $PaO_2/FiO_2 < 300$ for ALI or < 200 for ARDS) (Ashbaugh et al, 1967; Petty & Ashbaugh, 1971). These pulmonary disorders may result from local injuries like pneumonia, gastric aspiration, near-drowning and lung contusion, but also from systemic events like severe sepsis, shock and blood transfusions (Hudson et al, 1995; Ware & Matthay, 2000).
Although mechanical ventilation is a life-saving procedure, it has the potential to cause damage in healthy lung tissue or aggravate damage in diseased lung tissue (Dreyfuss & Saumon, 1998; Slutsky, 1999). The pulmonary complications secondary to mechanical ventilation are frequently referred to as ventilator-associated lung injury (VALI) in the clinical setting and ventilator-induced lung injury (VILI) in the experimental setting. As this chapter will primarily focus on experimental findings, the term VILI will be used.

2. Pathogenesis of ventilator-induced lung injury

VILI is characterized by enhanced alveolar-capillary permeability, accumulation of protein-rich lung edema, disturbed alveolar fibrin turnover, production of inflammatory mediators, and - ultimately - impaired gas exchange. Interestingly, these patterns of injury are very similar to those seen in ALI and ARDS (Tsuno et al, 1991).

Over the years, various experimental models have been used to gather further insights into the mechanism(s) that may underlie the pathogenesis of VILI. These *in vitro* and *in vivo* studies support the clinical observations that mechanical ventilation evokes stretch trauma due to cyclic opening and collapse and/or overdistention of alveoli (Dreyfuss et al, 1985; Webb & Tierney, 1974). Ventilator-induced cyclic opening and closing of alveoli results in depletion of surfactant and renders the lung more prone to collapse (Dreyfuss et al, 1988; Mead et al, 1970). Extensive research demonstrated that surfactant depletion initiates loss of alveolar-capillary barrier function (Lachmann et al, 1987; Seeger et al, 1993; Verbrugge et al, 1997). In turn, serum proteins will leak from the circulation into pulmonary tissue. Protein accumulation in the lung will lead to surfactant inactivation, causing even more protein leakage and edema formation and eliciting a vicious circle of progressive lung injury (Ikegami et al, 1984; Lachmann et al, 1994). Besides surfactant dysfunction, other mechanisms have been proposed to be crucially involved in the development of VILI as well. It is reasonable to assume that these underlying mechanisms are interconnected.

2.1 Inflammatory response

Leukocyte-endothelial interactions have been described to be important in the pathogenesis of severe inflammatory diseases related to VILI, like ALI/ARDS (Abraham, 2003; Moraes et al, 2003). In inflammation, pulmonary endothelial cells undergo a phenotypic shift (Orfanos et al, 2004). Activated endothelial cells secrete chemotactic cytokines (chemokines) which are essential for the recruitment of leukocytes to the site of inflammation (Luscinskas & Gimbrone, Jr., 1996). The main pulmonary chemoattractant is interleukin (IL)-8 or its rodent equivalents macrophage inflammatory protein (MIP)-2 and keratinocyte-derived chemokine (KC) (Donnelly et al, 1993). Besides release of chemokines and other inflammatory mediators, activated endothelial cells express various adhesion molecules on their cell surface thereby directing the multi-step cascade of leukocyte transmigration from blood vessels into affected tissue (Luscinskas & Gimbrone, Jr., 1996). The initial step of transmigration involves members from the selectin family (P- and E-selectin) which tether circulating leukocytes to vascular endothelium and facilitate rolling of leukocytes along the blood vessel wall (Carlos & Harlan, 1994). Subsequent leukocyte adhesion and extravasation are mediated by the immunoglobulin (Ig) superfamily comprising vascular cell adhesion molecule (VCAM)-1, intercellular adhesion molecule (ICAM)-1 and platelet-endothelial cell adhesion molecule (PECAM)-1. In ALI and ARDS patients, Gando et al. observed that soluble P-selectin, E-selectin, ICAM-1 and VCAM-1 levels were elevated within 24 hours after diagnosis (Gando et al, 2004). In addition, these authors showed a marked increase in these soluble adhesion molecules when subdividing patients into survivors and non-survivors. Together, these findings imply that adhesion molecules may have a prognostic value for development and clinical outcome of inflammatory lung diseases (Gando et al, 2004).

Activated leukocytes release oxygen-based free radicals and proteolytic enzymes to restore physiological conditions of inflamed tissue. However, activated leukocytes may obstruct micro-capillaries in the lung due to an increased cellular size leading to ischemia and augmented oxygen-based free radical production. Accumulation of these inflammatory cells in the alveoli may therefore cause severe disruption of pulmonary epithelial-endothelial barriers leading to impaired gas exchange (Abraham, 2003; Lee & Downey, 2001).

Kawano et al. were the first to describe that granulocyte depletion prior to injurious mechanical ventilation ameliorates pulmonary dysfunction in a rodent model of surfactant deficiency, stressing the importance of inflammatory mediators in the pathogenesis of VILI (Kawano et al, 1987). Later, Tremblay et al. revealed that alveolar stretch imposed by *ex vivo* mechanical ventilation caused IL-1β, tumor necrosis factor (TNF)-α, IL-6, MIP-2, interferon

(IFN)-γ and IL-10 expression and introduced the term "biotrauma" to describe the ventilator-induced secretion of inflammatory mediators (Tremblay et al, 1997; Tremblay & Slutsky, 1998). In line with this concept, it has been shown that alveolar macrophages secrete cytokines and chemokines upon *in vitro* applied mechanical stretch (Pugin et al, 1998). Although alveolar macrophages are considered to be the most important source of pulmonary cytokines and chemokines, other cell types like fibroblasts, leukocytes, epithelial and endothelial cells are also capable of producing inflammatory mediators (Kelley, 1990). In this respect, *in vitro* studies clearly showed that alveolar epithelial and capillary endothelial cells indeed release cytokines and chemokines upon mechanical stretch (Iwaki et al, 2009; Vlahakis et al, 1999). Ranieri et al. were the first to provide clinical evidence for the biotrauma-hypothesis (Ranieri et al, 1999). In a randomized controlled trial, these authors observed elevated concentrations of IL-1β, TNF-α, IL-6 and IL-1 receptor antagonist in the bronchoalveolar lavage fluid (BALf) of ALI/ARDS patients when excessive tidal volumes were used for 36 hours (Ranieri et al, 1999).
Based on experimental and clinical observations, it has been hypothesized that the ventilator-induced inflammatory response in the lung may lead to pulmonary injury (Haitsma et al, 2003; Wilson et al, 2003; Wilson et al, 2005). Most experimental models of VILI, however, applied excessively high tidal volumes and/or inspiratory pressures compared to those applied in the clinical setting (Copland et al, 2004; Haitsma et al, 2003; Wilson et al, 2003). In an attempt to better reflect the human situation, we used clinically more relevant ventilator settings in our animal studies (Hegeman et al, 2010). In this way, we were able to prevent shock, metabolic acidosis and substantial damage to lung architecture commonly associated with high tidal volumes and/or inspiratory pressures (Wolthuis et al, 2009b). However, even in our relatively mild model of VILI, mechanical ventilation with either low (LV_T) or high tidal volumes (HV_T) caused increased cytokine, chemokine and adhesion molecule expression compared to non-ventilated control (NVC) animals, which was accompanied by marked granulocyte infiltration (Hegeman et al, 2011b). BALf neutrophil numbers and inflammatory mediator levels were even higher when comparing lungs of HV_T-ventilated mice to lungs of LV_T-ventilated mice (Hegeman et al, 2011b). Since lower PaO_2/FiO_2 ratios were only observed after HV_T-ventilation, it seems plausible that ventilator-induced lung inflammation ultimately impairs gas exchange. In this respect, investigators suggested that enhanced pro-inflammation due to mechanical ventilation makes the patient more susceptible to a "second hit" (Bregeon et al, 2002). Mechanical ventilation itself may be the "second hit" when ventilating critically ill patients suffering from pulmonary injuries like ALI/ARDS or systemic events like sepsis (Headley et al, 1997; Meduri et al, 1995; Slutsky & Tremblay, 1998).

2.1.1 Local versus systemic inflammation

An important clinical observation is that most ventilated critically ill patients do not succumb to acute respiratory failure but rather to progressive multiple organ failure (MOF) (Ferring & Vincent, 1997; Montgomery et al, 1985; Valta et al, 1999). A definition of MOF has been provided by John Marshall, who defined it as "the development of potentially reversible physiologic derangement involving two or more organ systems not involved in the disorder that resulted in ICU admission, and arising in the wake of a potentially life-threatening physiologic insult" (Marshall, 2001). In a clinical study, comprising 3147 patients from 198 ICUs in 24 European countries, Vincent et al. observed significant organ dysfunction in 71% of the ICU patients most of them being septic patients (Vincent et al, 2006). Moreover, they found a positive correlation between the number of organ systems failing and ICU mortality stressing the importance of MOF in the clinical outcome of critically ill patients (Vincent et al, 2006).

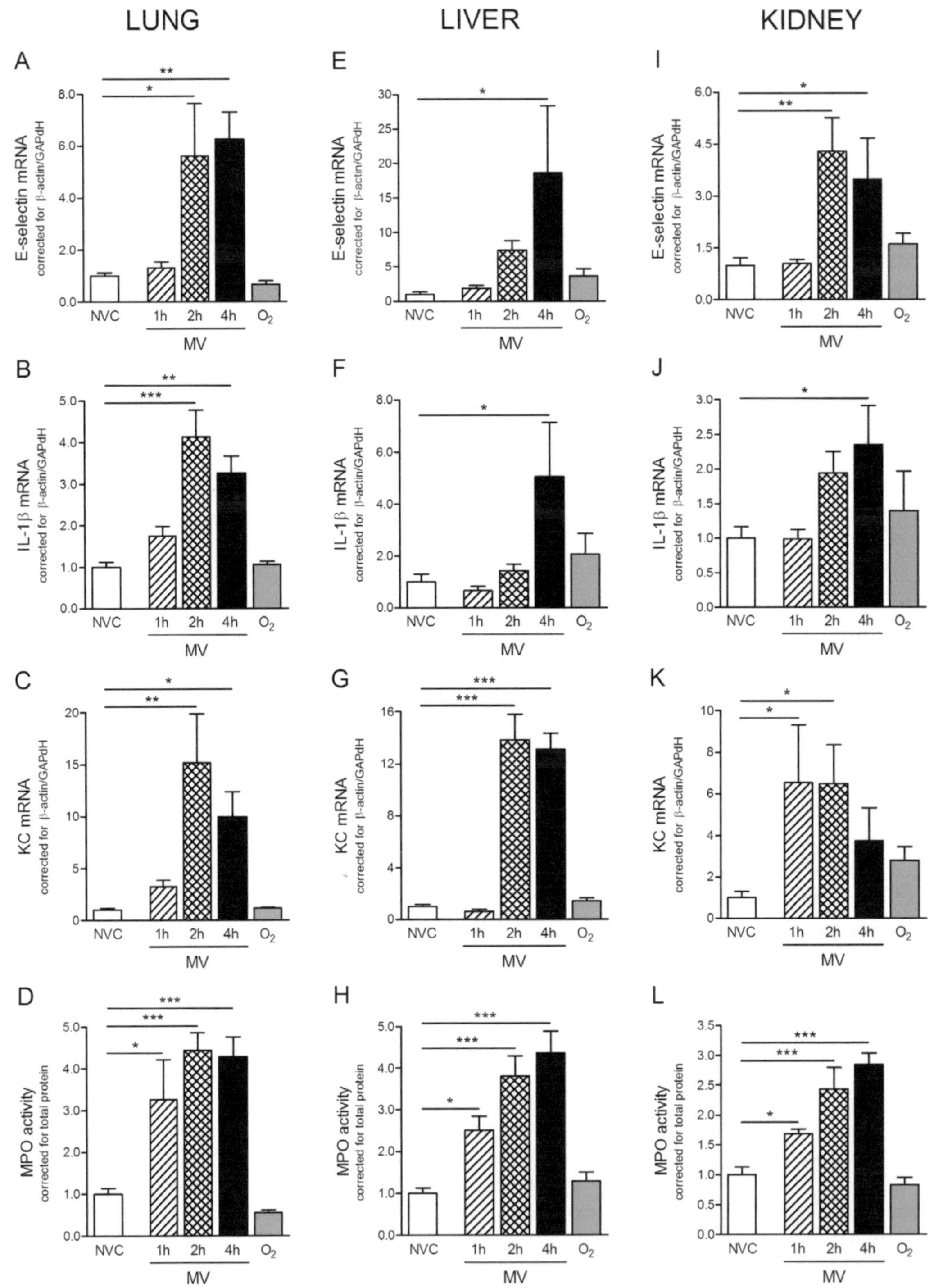

Fig. 1. Mechanical ventilation induces endothelial activation and inflammation in pulmonary, hepatic and renal tissue.

Reprinted with permission of Critical Care (Hegeman et al, 2009). To investigate whether alveolar stretch may cause endothelial activation and inflammation in the lung and distal organs, healthy mice were mechanically ventilated for 1, 2 or 4 hours with high pressures (i.e. high level of alveolar stretch). Non-ventilated mice served as a reference group. Spontaneous breathing animals were placed in an oxygen saturated box for 4 hours (FiO_2 of 1.0, hyperoxia) to evaluate whether the high FiO_2 associated with our ventilation strategy may contribute to changes in the immune response. **A, E, I:** In total lung, liver and kidney homogenates, respectively, mRNA expression of the adhesion molecule E-selectin was determined by real-time RT-PCR. **B-C, F-G, J-K:** In addition, mRNA expression of the pro-inflammatory cytokine interleukin (IL)-1β and the chemokine keratinocyte-derived chemokine (KC) was determined. Levels were normalized for expression of internal controls, i.e. the average value of β-actin and glyceraldehyde 3-phosphate dehydrogenase (GAPdH). **D, H, L:** In total lung, liver and kidney homogenates, respectively, myeloperoxidase (MPO) activity was determined as a measure of granulocyte infiltration. Levels were normalized for total protein concentration. Data are depicted relative to NVC and expressed as mean ± SEM for n = 4-8 animals. * $p<0.05$, ** $p<0.01$, *** $p<0.001$ (parameters were analyzed by one-way ANOVA with least significant difference (LSD) post-hoc test). NVC = non-ventilated controls; 1h, 2h, 4h = ventilated for either 1, 2 or 4 hours; O_2 = hyperoxia for 4 hours; MV = mechanical ventilation.

There is convincing evidence that leukocyte-endothelial interactions are not only important in the pathogenesis of pulmonary disorders (Abraham, 2003; Moraes et al, 2003) but also in systemic events like sepsis and MOF (Whalen et al, 2000). It has been proposed that an elevation of adhesion molecule expression might contribute to tissue injury and ultimately to MOF by facilitating leukocyte activation and migration (Bone, 1991; Parrillo, 1993). In this regard, we examined whether alveolar stretch due to mechanical ventilation results in endothelial activation and inflammation in healthy mice, not only in the lung but also in organs distal to the lung (Hegeman et al, 2009). We observed that 4 hours of mechanical ventilation with high pressures, i.e. high level of alveolar stretch, induced *de novo* synthesis of various adhesion molecules in pulmonary but also in hepatic and renal tissue (figures 1a, e, i). In addition, increased cytokine and chemokine mRNA levels were found in the lung and distal organs after mechanical ventilation (figures 1b-c, f-g, j-k) accompanied by enhanced granulocyte infiltration (figures 1d, h, l). Our data imply that ventilator-induced endothelial activation in the lung, liver and kidney facilitates migration and adhesiveness of activated immune cells to inflamed tissue, which in turn may lead to tissue injury in these organs (Hegeman et al, 2009).

Since we observed increased endothelial activation and inflammation after mechanical ventilation in the lung and distal organs, it seems plausible that mechanical ventilation plays a significant role in the development of both VILI and MOF (Hegeman et al, 2009). Supporting this hypothesis, earlier experimental research provided evidence that mechanical ventilation evokes detrimental effects in distal organs (Imai et al, 2003; Nin et al, 2006). Imai et al. demonstrated that mechanical ventilation with high tidal volumes induces epithelial cell apoptosis in the kidney and small intestine (Imai et al, 2003). Moreover, these authors showed that mechanical ventilation leads to elevated levels of serum markers such as creatinine indicative for renal failure (Imai et al, 2003). Ventilator-induced cardiovascular and hepatic injury has been described as well (Nin et al, 2006). It should be noted that these previous studies used animals with *pre-existing* lung injury whereas our study used *healthy* animals, suggesting that already existing inflammation is not a prerequisite for unveiling the negative effects of mechanical ventilation on distal organs. In line with this notion, a recent clinical trial showed that mechanical ventilation contributes to the development of acute kidney injury (AKI) in critically ill patients without ALI at onset of mechanical ventilation (Cortjens et al, 2011). Nonetheless, infectious events are known to aggravate ventilator-induced effects (Imai et al, 2003; O'Mahony et al, 2006) and possibly underlie the high incidence of MOF in critically ill patients ventilated with high tidal volumes and/or inspiratory pressures (Schultz, 2008).

It remains to be determined which underlying mechanisms initiate the onset of endothelial activation and inflammation in distal organs during mechanical ventilation. Haitsma et al. and Tutor et al. demonstrated that ventilator-induced permeability of alveolar-capillary barriers provokes inflammatory mediator release into the blood circulation (Haitsma et al, 2000; Tutor et al, 1994). Although there is quite some evidence that inflammatory mediators will be released from inflamed pulmonary tissue into the systemic environment, a causal relationship between ventilator-induced spill-over and the pathogenesis of MOF has not been confirmed yet.

Our experimental data indicate that ventilator-induced changes in *de novo* expression of adhesion molecules, cytokines and chemokines occur simultaneously in the lung, liver and kidney (Hegeman et al, 2009). Moreover, granulocyte recruitment to the liver and kidney was already observed after 1 hour of mechanical ventilation (Hegeman et al, 2009). In view of this spatiotemporal pattern of inflammatory mediator expression, we suggest that release or spill-over of cytokines and chemokines from the lung into the blood circulation is probably not the only cause of the enhanced pro-inflammatory environment in distal organs during mechanical ventilation. It cannot be excluded, however, that inflammatory mediators released into the circulation may contribute to *de novo* synthesis of adhesion molecules, cytokines and chemokines in distal organs, since cytokines like IL-1β and TNF-α are known to induce the production of a host of inflammatory mediators (Goodman et al, 2003). Since cytokines have in general only a very short half-life in plasma (± 20 minutes), it is more logical that *locally* produced mediators dictate the level of distal organ involvement. Local induction of cytokines by e.g. oxygen-based free radicals may be another important pro-inflammatory source in distal organs.

Previously, it has been suggested that the physical stress of mechanical ventilation may trigger the sympathetic nervous system leading to an increase in catecholamine secretion (Plotz et al, 2004). Locally released catecholamines have been described to activate transcription factors like nuclear factor (NF)-κB in macrophages and promote production of IL-1β, TNF-α and IL-8 (Elenkov et al, 2000; Flierl et al, 2009; Spengler et al, 1990). These findings imply that stimulation of sympathetic nerve terminals in e.g. the liver and kidney may evoke a pro-inflammatory response in these peripheral organs (Elenkov et al, 2000; Straub et al, 2000). Subsequently, the presence of IL-1β, TNF-α and IL-8 may result in an acute phase response in the liver possibly via α–adrenergic activation (Elenkov et al, 2000; Flierl et al, 2009; Spengler et al, 1990). Based on these notions, we would like to propose that ventilator-induced activation of sympathetic nerve terminals in distal organs may contribute to the pro-inflammatory state of these organs. In turn, this pro-inflammatory state in distal organs may prime for the development of MOF in the critically ill patient (Imai et al, 2003; O'Mahony et al, 2006; Schultz, 2008). If so, modulation of adrenergic receptor function might be advantageous for the outcome of patients with MOF. Supporting this hypothesis, Miksa et al. showed in experimental models of sepsis that an α_{2A}-adrenocepter antagonist reduced plasma levels of aspartate aminotransferase (AST), alanine aminotransferase (ALT) and creatinine, indicative for attenuated liver and kidney injury (Miksa et al, 2009). Moreover, these authors showed that inhibition of α_{2A}-adrenocepter activation significantly improved survival in septic animals from 45 to 75% (Miksa et al, 2009).

Another pathway of neuroimmune regulation is considered to be involved in the pathogenesis of VILI and MOF as well. In various inflammatory diseases, the efferent vagus nerve mediates anti-inflammatory action by downregulating pro-inflammatory immune responses (Kumar & Sharma, 2010). Recently, dos Santos et al. showed that disruption of the vagus nerve aggravates pulmonary wet-to-dry ratio, neutrophil infiltration, IL-6 production and apoptotic cell death, whereas stimulation of the vagus nerve was attenuating these parameters of VILI (dos Santos et al, 2011). These recent findings imply that the immunoregulatory function of the vagus nerve is of importance in VILI (dos Santos et al, 2011). Also in systemic diseases like sepsis, vagus-mediated neuroimmune signaling has been suggested to be important (Kumar & Sharma, 2010). In this respect, Pavlov et al. revealed that pharmacological activation of the vagus nerve improved survival of septic mice by inhibiting pro-inflammation (Pavlov et al, 2007). Taken together, stimulating the cholinergic anti-inflammatory pathway by pharmacological agents may represent potential therapeutic intervention strategies in patients diagnosed with VILI and/or MOF.

Besides an enhanced systemic pro-inflammatory milieu, it has been hypothesized that suppression of the peripheral immune system may also be crucially involved in the pathogenesis of MOF (Pinsky et al, 1993; Syrbe et al, 1994). Initially, suppression of the peripheral immune function may provide a compensatory mechanism to restore homeostasis under physiological circumstances (Bone, 1996). Yet, the compensatory reaction may become maladaptive when existing for prolonged periods of time consequently leading to excessive suppression of peripheral lymphocytes and augmented susceptibility to infections. In this respect, Angele and Faist reported that many ventilated, critically ill patients suffer from unexplained immune suppression and thus have an associated increased risk for infections and MOF (Angele & Faist, 2002). Therefore, locally enhanced production of cytokines by e.g. endothelial cells, hepatic or renal cells in the distal organs - in combination with a hampering immune function - may be detrimental for the patient to survive.

Previously, we demonstrated that mechanical ventilation suppresses lymphocyte function outside the lung (Plotz et al, 2002; Vreugdenhil et al, 2004). In children without lung pathology, the functional capacity of peripheral blood leukocytes to produce TNF-α, IL-6 and IFN-γ *in vitro* was significantly reduced after 2 hours of mechanical ventilation (Plotz et al, 2002). This was accompanied by a reduction in natural killer (NK) cell activity (Plotz et al, 2002). Also in healthy rats, we observed that 4 hours of mechanical ventilation with high pressures suppressed peripheral immune functioning, i.e. reduced NK cell activity, mitogen-induced splenocyte proliferation and cytokine production (Vreugdenhil et al, 2004). Supporting these earlier findings, 5 hours of HV_T-ventilation resulted in diminished mitogen-induced splenocyte proliferation compared to NVC in our murine model of VILI (figure 2).

Taken together, our data indicate that mechanical ventilation does not only induce a pro-inflammatory environment in organs distal to the lung, but also impairs the functioning of peripheral lymphocytes. Whether organ failure results from ongoing pro-inflammation of the environment (Pinsky et al, 1993) and/or persistent suppression of the immune function (Syrbe et al, 1994), these dysregulated immune responses may contribute to the development of MOF and subsequently cause increased morbidity and mortality in the critically ill patient (Rittirsch et al, 2008).

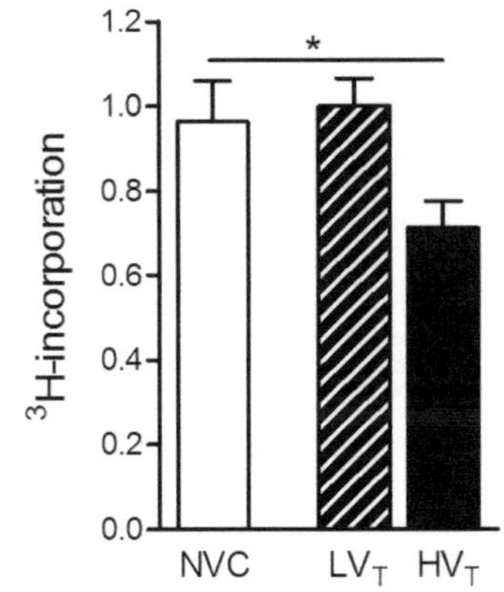

Fig. 2. Mechanical ventilation with high tidal volumes induces suppression of splenocyte proliferation.

To investigate whether mechanical ventilation suppressed functioning of peripheral lymphocytes, healthy mice were mechanically ventilated for 5 hours with either low or high tidal volumes. Non-ventilated mice served as a reference group. *In vitro* mitogen-induced splenocyte proliferation was assessed as a measure of peripheral lymphocyte functioning. Splenocytes were stimulated *in vitro* with αCD3 (1μg/ml), a T cell specific antibody. After 48 hours ^{3}H-thymidine was added and 16 hours later incorporation of ^{3}H-thymidine was determined. Data are depicted relative to LV_T and expressed as mean ± SEM for n = 10-16 animals. * $p<0.05$ (parameter was analyzed by one-way ANOVA with least significant difference (LSD) post-hoc test). NVC = non-ventilated controls; LV_T, HV_T = ventilated with either low or high tidal volumes.

2.2 Alveolar-capillary permeability

The primary site of pulmonary gas exchange is the < 0.2 μm thin part of the alveolar-capillary membrane, consisting of alveolar epithelial and capillary endothelial cells (Burns et al, 2003; Weibel, 1984). Back in the 1980s, investigators observed that mechanical ventilation and the subsequent stretch of pulmonary tissue induces damage to epithelial-endothelial barriers thereby impairing gas exchange (Dreyfuss et al, 1985; Egan, 1982; Parker et al, 1984). In addition, Dreyfuss et al. demonstrated that enhanced microvascular permeability was responsible for the formation of pulmonary edema during mechanical ventilation with high tidal volumes (Dreyfuss et al, 1985). Besides apoptotic and/or necrotic cell death, loss of alveolar epithelial and capillary endothelial cell integrity is thought to play a crucial role in the ventilator-induced disruption of alveolar-capillary barriers (Pugin, 2003).

2.2.1 Cell death

Apoptosis is distinguished by cell shrinkage and nuclear fragmentation, while cell organelles and plasma membrane maintain their integrity for a prolonged period (Chang & Yang, 2000; Rossi & Gaidano, 2003). Apoptotic cell death is primarily regulated by cysteine aspartyl-specific proteases (caspases) and consists of two distinct routes: the intrinsic (mitochondria-mediated) and extrinsic (death receptor-mediated) pathway (Lavrik et al, 2005a). In response to oxidative stress, DNA damage and other types of severe intracellular stress, mitochondria undergo marked changes in membrane integrity and activate the *intrinsic* apoptotic pathway (Denecker et al, 2001; Festjens et al, 2004). Enhanced mitochondrial membrane permeability leads to release of pro-apoptotic proteins, like cytochrome *c*, from the mitochondria into the cytosol. Cytochrome *c* associates with apoptototic protease-activating factor (APAF)-1 and procaspase-9 to generate an apoptosome complex (Acehan et al, 2002; Jiang & Wang, 2000). In the apoptosome, procaspase-9 is cleaved to its mature form and activates the executioner caspase-3. Consequently, caspase-dependent DNAses are activated thereby causing chromatin condensation and DNA degradation (Chang & Yang, 2000). The *extrinsic* apoptotic pathway is initiated by triggering cell surface death receptors like the TNF receptor (TNFR)-1 and Fas (Lavrik et al, 2005b). Triggering of death receptors evokes formation of a death-inducing signaling complex (DISC) (Danial & Korsmeyer, 2004). The DISC brings procaspase-8 molecules in close proximity to each other resulting in their autoproteolytic activation (Chang et al, 2003). After autocleavage of procaspase-8, active caspase-8 is released into the cytosol and cleaves important executioner caspases (Chang et al, 2003). Caspase-8 is also involved in an indirect pathway linking the extrinsic and intrinsic routes of apoptotic cell death (Korsmeyer et al, 2000; Zamzami & Kroemer, 2003). In this pathway, activation of caspase-8 leads to the cleavage of Bid to truncated Bid (tBid) which induces permeability of the mitochondrial membrane. An important mediator of both the intrinsic and extrinsic apoptotic pathway is p53, a tumor suppressor molecule (Haupt et al, 2003). P53 is a transcription factor for several Bcl-2 family genes, including Bid and Bax, thereby promoting cytochrome *c* release from mitochondria and initiating the intrinsic apoptotic pathway (Haupt et al, 2003). In addition, p53 induces APAF-1 expression which is required for formation of the apoptosome complex (Kannan et al, 2001). P53 may also initiate the extrinsic apoptotic pathway through induction of Fas and activation of caspase-8 (Ding et al, 2000).

Necrosis is characterized by irreversible plasma membrane damage, cytoplasmic swelling, organelle breakdown and, ultimately, cell rupture with leakage of cellular contents into the extracellular space (Fiers et al, 1999; Kroemer et al, 2005). Consequently, this type of cell death is associated with a marked inflammatory response. It has been proposed that necrosis might provide a backup suicide mechanism when caspase-dependent pathways of apoptosis cannot be properly activated (Fiers et al, 1999; Leist & Jäättelä, 2001) although this hypothesis may be too simplistic. Depletion of adenosine triphosphate (ATP) for instance may favor a switch from apoptosis to necrosis, in part because ATP is necessary for optimal activation of caspases (Leist et al, 1997). For many years, necrosis has been considered to be an uncontrolled process. However, recent evidence suggests that the course of necrotic cell death might be as tightly regulated as apoptotic cell death (Festjens et al, 2006; Golstein & Kroemer, 2007). It has to be kept in mind though, that necrotic and apoptotic traits might co-exist (Kroemer et al, 2009) and that the same cell death inducers may promote either necrosis or apoptosis depending on the specific environmental setting (Galluzzi et al, 2009). In this regard, previous research showed that triggering of TNFR-1 by TNF does not only lead to activation of the extrinsic pathway of apoptosis but also to programmed necrosis involving receptor-interacting protein (RIP) kinases (Galluzzi et al, 2009; Hitomi et al, 2008). Data from Cho et al., He et al. and Zhang et al. implicate RIP3 as a pivotal switch between TNF-induced apoptosis and necrosis (Cho et al, 2009; He et al, 2009; Zhang et al, 2009a). Based on this notion, the protein complex containing RIP1/RIP3 has been proposed to function as a "necrosome" (Declercq et al, 2009). In this setting, RIP3 promotes mitochondrial dysfunction, subsequent production of reactive oxygen species (ROS) and eventually necrotic cell death. Besides the production of ROS, necrotic cell death is associated with sustained elevation of cytosolic calcium levels (Harwood et al, 2005). Calcium overload leads to activation of calcium-dependent cysteine proteases, calpains. Active calpains promote release of lysosomal catabolic aspartyl proteases, cathepsins, which cleave essential cytoskeletal components like spectrin (also known as fodrin), microtubule subunits and microtubule-associated proteins thereby resulting in enhanced destabilization of the cell and ultimately in necrotic cell death (Artal-Sanz & Tavernarakis, 2005; Zhang et al, 2009b).

Apart from necrosis, autophagy has been recognized as a distinct form of non-apoptotic cell death. Authophagy is the main cellular pathway for degradation of damaged cytoplasmic organelles or denatured proteins (Levine & Klionsky, 2004). In response to stress (e.g. hyperoxia, oxidative stress, pro-inflammation), autophagic vacuoles sequester damaged organelles or proteins. Subsequently, autophagic vacuoles fuse with lysosomes where the internalized contents will be degraded by lysosomal enzymes like cathepsins (Ryter & Choi, 2010). While basal activation of autophagy ascertains the physiological turnover of cytoplasmic organelles and proteins, dysregulation or excessive activation of autophagy may induce non-apoptotic cell death (Galluzzi et al, 2008; Maiuri et al, 2007). A potential cross-talk has been proposed between the mechanisms that regulate autophagy and those regulating apoptosis or necrosis (Galluzzi et al, 2008).

Cell death has been considered to play a crucial role in the disruption of alveolar-capillary barriers (Pugin, 2003). Previously, *in vitro* studies demonstrated that mechanical stretch may activate apoptotic cell death (dos Santos et al, 2004; Edwards et al, 1999; Hammerschmidt et al, 2004). Moreover, several investigators reported enhanced apoptosis after 2 to 5 hours of mechanical ventilation with high tidal volumes (Chiang et al, 2011; Le et al, 2008; Li et al, 2007). Although the precise role of necrotic cell death has not been elucidated in VILI yet, it has been demonstrated *in vitro* that mechanical stretch as such induces necrosis (Hammerschmidt et al, 2004; Tschumperlin et al, 2000). Therefore, we investigated whether apoptotic and/or necrotic cell death pathways were activated in lungs of healthy mice exposed to either 5 hours of LV_T or HV_T-ventilation. Protein expression of cleaved caspase-8, -9 and -3 was determined in total lung homogenates as measures of caspase-dependent cell death. Protein expression of cleaved α-fodrin (145/150kDa fragments yielded by calcium-activated calpains) was determined as a measure of caspase-independent cell death. Our data demonstrate unequivocally that basal cleavage of caspase-8 was not enhanced by LV_T or HV_T-ventilation (figure 3a). Furthermore, cleaved caspase-9 and -3 were below detection level in all experimental groups implying that caspase-dependent pathways of apoptosis were not activated. Cleaved α-fodrin levels, however, were significantly increased in lungs of ventilated mice in comparison to NVC, which was independent of ventilation strategy (figure 3b). On the basis of these findings, it is tempting to speculate that 5 hours of mechanical ventilation induces cell death primarily via caspase-independent necrotic pathways. In contrast to our present data, Wolthuis et al. observed in a comparable model of VILI that the number of caspase 3-positive cells on lung sections was higher in HV_T-ventilated mice than in control animals although this increase did not reach statistical significance ($p=0.055$) (Wolthuis et al, 2009a). Taken together, we propose that apoptosis is not the major executive mechanism of cell death in our experimental model of VILI. Nonetheless, we cannot exclude that caspase-dependent pathways of cell death are modestly activated which - together with necrotic activities induced in the target cell - will determine the level of cell death.

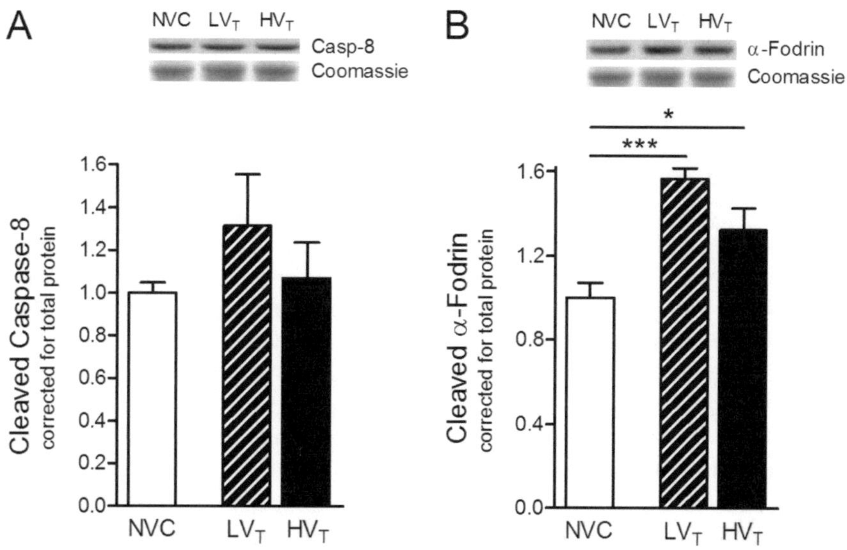

Fig. 3. Mechanical ventilation activates caspase-independent pathways of cell death.
To investigate whether mechanical ventilation activated caspase-dependent and/or caspase-independent pathways of cell death, healthy mice were mechanically ventilated for 5 hours with either low or high tidal volumes. Non-ventilated mice served as a reference group. **A:** In total lung homogenates, protein expression of cleaved caspase-8 was determined by Western blotting as a measure for activation of caspase-dependent cell death pathways. Cleaved caspase-9 and -3 were below detection level in all experimental groups. **B:** In addition, protein expression of cleaved α-fodrin (145/150kDa fragments yielded by calcium-activated calpains) was determined as a measure for activation of caspase-independent cell death pathways. Levels were normalized for total protein levels (Coomassie staining). Inset: representative Western blot depicting immunodetectable cleaved capase-8 and α-fodrin, respectively. Data are depicted relative to NVC and expressed as mean ± SEM for n = 5-8 animals. * $p<0.05$, *** $p<0.001$ (parameters were analyzed by one-way ANOVA with least significant difference (LSD) post-hoc test). NVC = non-ventilated controls; LV_T, HV_T = ventilated with either low or high tidal volumes.

2.2.2 Loss of vascular integrity

Under normal conditions, quiescent vascular endothelium establishes a tight barrier which controls the movement of plasma and/or leukocytes from the circulation into the underlying tissue (Cines et al, 1998). To achieve this barrier function, tight cell-cell contacts are formed by junctional transmembrane proteins such as vascular endothelial (VE)-cadherin (Dejana, 2004). Vascular leakage is an important feature of inflammatory disorders and is predominately caused by hyperpermeability of the endothelial barrier (Lentsch & Ward, 2000; Michel & Curry, 1999).

One of the crucial systems regulating vascular cell integrity is the angiopoietin (Ang)-Tie2 system (Fiedler & Augustin, 2006). Ang-1 and Ang-2 are, respectively, an agonist and antagonist of the tyrosine kinase receptor Tie2 (Fiedler et al, 2003). Constitutive Ang-1 expression and Tie2 phosphorylation in adult vasculature implies that Ang-1–mediated Tie2 signaling is required to maintain endothelial cell integrity and quiescence (Fiedler &

Augustin, 2006). Binding of Ang-1 leads to autophosphorylation of Tie2, subsequently activating several intracellular signaling pathways and maintaining endothelial cell integrity (Fiedler & Augustin, 2006). One of the signal transduction routes initiated upon Tie2 activation is the phosphatidylinositol 3 kinase (PI3K)–Akt pathway, which in general promotes cell survival (DeBusk et al, 2004; Kim et al, 2000; Papapetropoulos et al, 2000). In this regard, it has been shown that Ang-1–mediated Tie2 signaling may prevent endothelial cell apoptosis by activating Akt and upregulating survivin, an apoptosis inhibitor (Papapetropoulos et al, 2000). Daly et al. proposed a molecular mechanism through which Ang-1–mediated Akt activation may promote vascular stability (Daly et al, 2004). These authors demonstrated that Akt activation inactivates the forkhead transcription factor FKHR (FOXO1) which regulates genes associated with endothelial cell apoptosis (survivin) and vascular destabilization (Ang-2) (Daly et al, 2004). These findings imply that Ang-1–mediated Tie2 signaling prevents Ang-2 expression and subsequent loss of vascular integrity. Another signal transduction route that may be influenced upon Tie2 phosphorylation is the NF-κB pathway. Hughes et al. showed that Tie2 interacts with A20-binding inhibitor of NF-κB (ABIN)-2, a NF-κB regulatory protein (Hughes et al, 2003). As a consequence of ABIN-2 recruitment, Ang-1-mediated Tie2 signaling inhibits activation of the NF-κB pathway and results in an anti-inflammatory and quiescent status of the endothelial barrier (Hughes et al, 2003). Finally, Gavard et al. described that Ang-1–mediated Tie2 signaling protects against vascular endothelial growth factor (VEGF)-stimulated endothelial permeability by inhibiting VEGF-triggered endocytosis of VE-cadherin, a junctional transmembrane protein establishing tight cell-cell contacts (Gavard et al, 2008). Until now, an increase in Ang-2 levels has been recognized to be the modulating factor of the Ang-Tie2 system. In situations of endothelial activation, Ang-2 proteins are released from endothelial specific storage granules (Weibel-Palade bodies) and compete with Ang-1 for binding to the Tie2 receptor (Fiedler & Augustin, 2006). Accordingly, Ang-2 may exert antagonistic functions on Ang-1–mediated Tie2 signaling and alter vascular integrity, destabilize the endothelial barrier and prime the endothelium to attain responsiveness to pro-inflammatory mediators (Fiedler & Augustin, 2006). In line with this, van der Heijden et al. demonstrated that circulating Ang-2 and increased Ang-2/Ang-1 ratios are related to pulmonary permeability edema and severity of ALI/ARDS in ventilated patients with or without sepsis (van der Heijden et al, 2008). Furthermore, Gallagher et al. showed that high circulating Ang-2 levels in ALI/ARDS patients are associated with a poor outcome (Gallagher et al, 2008). Since 67% of these ALI/ARDS patients were mechanically ventilated, the authors proposed that ventilatory support alone does not cause enhanced Ang-2 levels (Gallagher et al, 2008). However, there is also conflicting evidence that Ang-2 may induce Tie2 activation in stressed endothelial cells (Daly et al, 2006).

Both clinical and experimental studies recognized the importance of the Ang-Tie2 system in the pathogenesis of lung diseases related to VILI, like ALI and ARDS (van der Heijden et al, 2009). Karmpaliotis et al. demonstrated that vascular permeability and pulmonary edema were accompanied by reduced Ang-1 and enhanced VEGF levels in lungs of lipopolysaccharide (LPS)-challenged mice (Karmpaliotis et al, 2002). The same authors proposed that changes in the balance between Ang-1 (anti-leakage) and VEGF (pro-leakage) might contribute to the pathophysiology of ALI (Karmpaliotis et al, 2002).

It may well be that a disturbed balance between Ang-1 and VEGF plays an indispensable role in VILI as well. Therefore, we examined whether 5 hours of either LV_T or HV_T-ventilation would influence the Ang-Tie2 system and VEGF expression in lungs of healthy mice (Hegeman et al, 2010). Particularly in lungs of HV_T-ventilated mice, marked changes in the Ang-Tie2 system were observed. We demonstrated that Ang-1, Ang-2 and Tie2 mRNA expression was significantly reduced in HV_T-ventilated mice in comparison with NVC (figures 4a-c). At this time point, Ang-1 and Ang-2 protein expression also tended to decrease (figures 4d-f). Moreover, we observed that HV_T-ventilation caused increased expression of VEGF (figure 4g) which is in agreement with a prior report (Nin et al, 2008). Our findings strongly suggest that changes in the Ang-Tie2 system, together with elevated VEGF expression, are involved in the development of VILI (Hegeman et al, 2010).

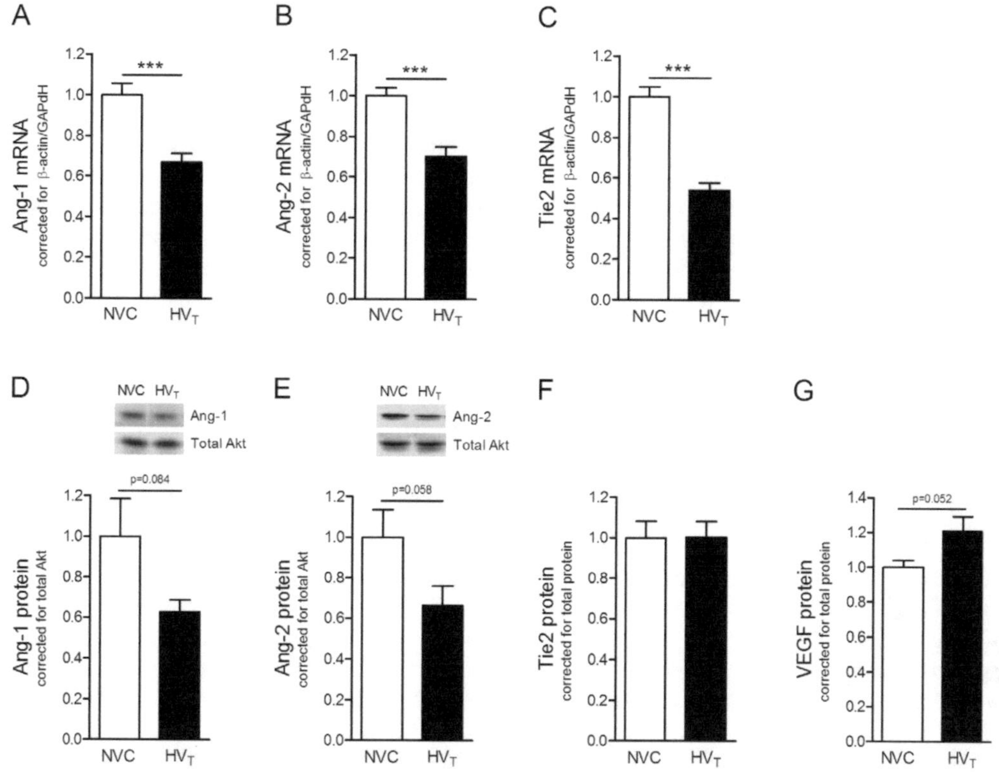

Fig. 4. Mechanical ventilation affects the angiopoietin (Ang)-Tie2 system and vascular endothelial growth factor (VEGF) expression.
Reprinted with permission of PLoS One (Hegeman et al, 2010). To investigate whether mechanical ventilation influences the Ang-Tie2 system, healthy mice were mechanically ventilated for 5 hours with high tidal volumes. Non-ventilated mice served as a reference group. **A-C**: In total lung homogenates, mRNA expression of Ang-1, Ang-2 and Tie2 was determined by real-time RT-PCR. Levels were normalized for expression of internal controls, i.e. the average value of β-actin and glyceraldehyde 3-phospate dehydrogenase (GAPdH). **D-E**: In total lung homogenates, protein expression of Ang-1 and Ang-2 was determined by Western blotting. Membranes were reprobed with antibody recognizing total Akt (Akt1/PKBα) to control for equal loading. No group differences in total Akt were found. Inset: representative Western blot depicting immunodetectable Ang-1 and Ang-2, respectively. **F-G**: In total lung homogenates, protein expression of Tie2 and VEGF was determined by ELISA. Levels were normalized for total protein concentrations. Data are

depicted relative to NVC and expressed as mean ± SEM for n = 6-12 animals. *** $p<0.001$ (parameters were analyzed by independent T-test). NVC = non-ventilated controls; HV_T = ventilated with high tidal volumes.

In addition to the Ang-Tie2 system, Rho guanosine triphosphatases (GTPases) are recognized to be crucially involved in the mechanosensitive regulation of vascular permeability (Birukov, 2009; Spindler et al, 2010). Rho GTPases act as molecular switches that regulate a wide variety of signal transduction pathways involved in cell behavior (Schmidt & Hall, 2002; Wojciak-Stothard & Ridley, 2002). Rho GTPases cycle between an active guanosine triphosphate (GTP)-bound and an inactive guanosine diphosphate (GDP)-bound conformational state. Switching between the active and inactive form is tightly regulated. Guanine nucleotide exchange factors (GEFs), for example, promote the exchange from GDP to GTP leading to activation of Rho GTPases (Wojciak-Stothard & Ridley, 2002).
Rac1 and Cdc42 are the main Rho GTPases needed for maintaining endothelial barrier function, whereas RhoA primarily has a destabilizing effect on endothelial barrier properties (Spindler et al, 2010). RhoA activation has been described to induce formation of stress fibers comprising actin and myosin (Ridley & Hall, 1992; Wojciak-Stothard et al, 1998). Consequently, actin-myosin contractility is suggested as the major mechanism of RhoA-mediated impairment of endothelial barrier properties (Spindler et al, 2010). RhoA signals through a downstream effector kinase, so-called Rho-kinase or Rho-associated coiled-col forming kinase (ROCK) (Liao et al, 2007). Activation of ROCK by RhoA inhibits myosin phosphatase acitivty subsequently leading to myosin light chain phosphorylation and stress fiber formation (Amano et al, 1997; Kimura et al, 1996).

3. Therapeutic interventions in critically ill patients with ventilator-induced lung injury

The recognition that conventional mechanical ventilation itself provokes detrimental effects in ventilated patients has led to the introduction of "lung-protective" ventilation strategies (Gillette & Hess, 2001). So far, mechanical ventilation with reduced tidal volumes is the only therapeutic approach effectively attenuating pulmonary injury and subsequent morbidity and mortality in critically ill ALI/ARDS patients (Amato et al, 1998; the ARDS network, 2000; Villar et al, 2006). In this regard, the ARDS Network revealed a 22% relative risk reduction in mortality rate when ventilating ALI/ARDS patients with "lung-protective" strategies, i.e. mechanical ventilation with tidal volumes of 6 ml/kg instead of with 12 ml/kg (the ARDS network, 2000). Notably, Determann et al. showed mechanical ventilation with lower tidal volumes also to attenuate development of lung injury in patients without ALI at the onset of mechanical ventilation (Determann et al, 2010). Recent research however, provided striking evidence that even "lung-protective" ventilator settings may result in the development of important aspects of VILI (Cobelens et al, 2009; Vaneker et al, 2007; Wolthuis et al, 2009b). We confirmed these prior reports in a murine model of VILI. We observed that not only conventional ventilation strategies with high tidal volumes but also clinically relevant ventilation strategies with low tidal volumes causes inflammation and vascular leakage in the lung (Hegeman et al, 2010; Hegeman et al, 2011b). Interestingly, a recent clinical trial revealed that mechanical ventilation with tidal volumes of 6ml/kg did not protect against the development or worsening of AKI in critically ill patients without ALI at onset of mechanical ventilation (Cortjens et al, 2011).
Apart from preserving alveolar integrity by reducing tidal volumes, additional therapeutic intervention strategies that prevent the detrimental effects of mechanical stretch are therefore

urgently needed. Based on the mechanisms that may underlie the pathogenesis of VILI (as mentioned above), therapies manipulating the course of inflammation and/or alveolar-capillary permeability might be advantageous for the clinical outcome of ventilated patients.

3.1 Inhibition of ventilator-induced lung inflammation: does it preclude lung injury?

It has been recognized that granulocytes and inflammatory mediators are important in the pathogenesis of VILI (Haitsma et al, 2003; Wilson et al, 2003; Wilson et al, 2005). Consequently, anti-inflammatory agents like glucocorticoids are suggested to attenuate or prevent the detrimental effects induced by mechanical ventilation (Brower et al, 2001; Luce, 2002). Glucocorticoids are a class of steroid hormones that exert their anti-inflammatory and immunosuppressive effects by binding to intracellular glucocorticoid receptors (GRs). After binding, the GR complex migrates from the cytosol to the nucleus where it regulates a wide range of gene activity, including inhibition of NF-κB and activator protein (AP)-1 driven expression of inflammatory genes (Barnes, 2006). Furthermore, glucocorticoids are known to suppress granulocyte recruitment and activation, preserve endothelial cell integrity and control vascular permeability (Ohta et al, 2001; Thompson, 2003). Although the efficacy of synthetic glucocorticoids to treat ALI/ARDS in critically ill patients is still under debate (Agarwal et al, 2007; Fernandes et al, 2005; Meduri et al, 2008), previous experimental research demonstrated that glucocorticoid treatment has the potential to attenuate ventilator-induced lung inflammation (Held et al, 2001; Ohta et al, 2001).

Unfortunately, the anti-inflammatory effects of synthetic glucocorticoids cannot be separated from their metabolic effects. In particular when given at higher doses and for longer periods, systemic administration of glucocorticoids is associated with severe side effects like elevated blood glucose levels, deposition of body fat, suppressed systemic immunity and increased susceptibility to infections (Schacke et al, 2002). One way to reduce the unwanted side effects of glucocorticoid treatment is to selectively deliver these therapeutic agents into the diseased tissue (Asgeirsdottir et al, 2007). In this respect, liposomal formulations are valuable drug delivery systems as they can act as a depot from which the encapsulated drug will be slowly released to enable prolonged, local drug exposure at low concentrations (Storm & Crommelin, 1998). Moreover, liposomes preferably extravasate into tissues with increased capillary permeability (Storm & Crommelin, 1998) facilitating delivery at sites of inflammation and/or mechanical stretch. Previously, Ásgeirsdóttir et al. clearly showed that delivery of liposome-encapsulated dexamethasone inhibits pro-inflammatory gene expression without affecting blood glucose levels (Asgeirsdottir et al, 2007), one of the first clinically relevant side effects of free dexamethasone treatment (Feldman-Billard et al, 2006; Weinstein et al, 1995). Because local delivery of glucocorticoids by liposomal formulations could be of therapeutic importance in the context of VILI as well, we studied whether liposomes containing dexamethasone (Dex-liposomes) inhibited ventilator-induced lung inflammation (Hegeman et al, 2011a). We observed that administration of Dex-liposomes at initiation of ventilation diminished crucial inflammatory parameters of VILI such as IL-1β, IL-6 and KC mRNA expression, especially in LV_T-ventilated mice (Hegeman et al, 2011a). Yet, this formulation was not as effective as free dexamethasone in preventing granulocyte infiltration into pulmonary tissue (Hegeman et al, 2011a). As granulocytes are considered to be important in the development of VILI (Kawano et al, 1987), we hypothesized that phagocytosis of liposomes by *activated* granulocytes may be advantageous and should therefore be enhanced (Hegeman et al, 2011a). We proposed that IgG-modified Dex-liposomes (IgG-Dex-liposomes) may be more efficient in attenuating ventilator-induced lung inflammation than Dex-liposomes due to interaction with Fcγreceptors (FcγRs) on activated granulocytes and macrophages (McKenzie & Schreiber, 1998). Indeed, IgG-Dex-liposomes were pharmacologically more effective than Dex-liposomes particularly in preventing granulocyte infiltration induced by either LV_T or HV_T-ventilation (Hegeman et al, 2011a). Additionally, IgG-Dex-liposomes inhibited most parameters of ventilator-induced lung inflammation as efficient as free dexamethasone. Our experimental data imply that conjugation of IgG to Dex-liposomes significantly improves their efficacy in attenuating ventilator-induced lung inflammation (Hegeman et al, 2011a). Importantly, the use of liposomes may favor local release of dexamethasone thereby preventing unwanted systemic side effects (Asgeirsdottir et al, 2007).

At present, it is thought that ventilator-induced lung inflammation may precede lung injury. Therefore, we hypothesized that reducing the inflammatory response by therapeutic intervention strategies would prevent vascular leakage and impaired gas exchange associated with mechanical ventilation. We observed, however, that the potent anti-inflammatory agent dexamethasone did not prevent occurrence of the more crude parameters of VILI like the elevation in BALf protein level, the increase in pulmonary wet-to-dry ratio and the reduction in PaO_2/FiO_2 ratio (Hegeman et al, 2011b). Our findings oppose previous studies describing protective effects of glucocorticoid therapy on lung injury (Nin et al, 2006; Ohta et al, 2001). In a rat model of VILI, dexamethasone was shown to restore pulmonary function after 75 minutes of mechanical ventilation as indicated by improved PaO_2/FiO_2 ratios (Nin et al, 2006). Moreover, Ohta et al. demonstrated that administration of methylprednisolone caused a marked leftward shifting of the pressure-volume (P-V) curve of rats ventilated for 40 minutes (Ohta et al, 2001). However, the deterioration of the P-V curve was still evident regardless of the significant reduction in granulocyte infiltration (Ohta et al, 2001). Ohta et al. explained these findings by the effects of mechanical stretch on lung tissue like stress failure of pulmonary capillaries, which may contribute to lung injury to a great extent (Ohta et al, 2001; West et al, 1991). Since mice were exposed to 5 hours of mechanical ventilation in our experimental model of VILI, it is tempting to speculate that the progressive lung injury induced by prolonged mechanical stretch may not be influenced by the anti-inflammatory action of dexamethasone (anymore).

Similar to dexamethasone, administration of the vessel protective factor Ang-1 only inhibits inflammatory aspects of VILI (Hegeman et al, 2010). In a murine model of VILI, we observed that intravenous Ang-1 treatment at initiation of ventilation inhibited granulocyte infiltration and inflammatory mediator release, and completely abolished the increase in VEGF protein in lungs of HV_T-ventilated mice (Hegeman et al, 2010). Although Ang-1 was preventing development of these important aspects of VILI, it did not influence the end points of VILI such as vascular leakage and impaired gas exchange (Hegeman et al, 2010). Our data are in apparent contrast with previously reported protective effects of Ang-1 on vascular leakage in endotoxin-challenged animals (Huang et al, 2008; McCarter et al, 2007; Mei et al, 2007; Witzenbichler et al, 2005). Using a similar dosing and administration procedure of Ang-1, David et al. showed that Ang-1 therapy also stabilized endothelial barrier function in an murine model of polymicrobiological abdominal sepsis as evidenced by attenuation of protein leakage from lung capillaries into the alveolar compartment (David et al, 2011). These findings underline that the pathways involved in sepsis- and ventilator-induced lung injury are different. An explanation for this discrepancy might be that the enhanced inflammation is not the primary inducer of vascular leakage and impaired gas exchange during HV_T-ventilation as is the case in the induction of lung injury by sepsis. Indeed, it has been shown that ventilator-induced mechanical stretch itself may destabilize alveolar-capillary barrier function thereby resulting in increased vascular permeability and pulmonary edema (Dreyfuss et al, 1985; Egan, 1982; Parker et al, 1984). Ang-1 treatment will probably affect the capillary-endothelial but not the alveolar-epithelial barrier since the Tie2 receptor is mainly expressed on endothelial cells (Lemieux et al, 2005). Thus, the possibility remains that Ang-1 treatment is not capable of restoring lung injury induced by HV_T-ventilation as it only modulates endothelial inflammation (Hegeman et al, 2010). The fact that Ang-1 prevents pulmonary vascular leakage in animals exposed to LPS, which induces a generalized inflammation primarily in the endothelial cells of the lung (Weppler & Issekutz, 2008), supports this hypothesis. In this respect, it is of interest that the TNF-α inhibitor Etanercept diminished inflammation and coagulation in the lungs of ventilated mice without affecting alveolar-capillary permeability and pulmonary edema (Wolthuis et al, 2009a), which is in line with our findings.

Taken together, we would like to suggest that prevention of lung inflammation does not preclude a loss of pulmonary function in our experimental model of VILI, in contrast to what has been shown in models of endotoxin- or sepsis-induced ALI. Probably the mechanism of injury caused by mechanical ventilation is different from the injury caused by endotoxin-challenge. In this regard, our *in vivo* studies revealed that endotoxin-challenge provokes lung injury via both caspase-dependent apoptosis and caspase-independent necrosis (unpublished data by Kooijman et al.). Lung injury induced by either LV_T or HV_T-ventilation, however, is for the greater part caspase-independent and probably executed by pathways involving destabilization of the cytoskeleton via proteolytic activity of calpains (figure 3). Thus, the primary functional deficit induced by mechanical ventilation may be more geared at early cellular death due to alveolar (over)stretch which will most likely not be counteracted by anti-inflammatory intervention strategies.

3.2 Focus of future therapeutic interventions

We have clearly shown that anti-inflammatory intervention strategies do not prevent aspects of VILI driven by mechanosensitive alterations in barrier properties but will only regulate the pulmonary inflammation (Hegeman et al, 2010; Hegeman et al, 2011b). It may well be that it is difficult to diminish the effect of mechanical stretch on lung injury solely by anti-inflammatory therapy. So, we now propose that anti-inflammatory agents should not be applied to combat the mechanosensitive aspects of VILI. However, anti-inflammatory intervention strategies may well be considered when inflammation is the primary inducer of lung injury like in non-ventilated patients diagnosed with ALI or ARDS.

3.2.1 Inhibitors of RhoA and/or ROCK

Our findings imply that future therapeutic interventions in the ventilated, critically ill patient should aim at attacking the ventilator-induced impairment of alveolar-capillary barrier function. As Rho GTPases have been described to be important in the mechanosensitive regulation of endothelial barrier function (Birukov, 2009), inactivation of RhoA and/or ROCK may have a protective effect on endothelial barrier function in the context of VILI. In this respect, we investigated the effects of the selective ROCK inhibitor Y-27632 in a rat model of LPS-induced ALI (unpublished data by Kooijman et al.). ROCK inhibition significantly diminished endothelial permeability in LPS-challenged lungs, which was associated with decreased pulmonary inflammation and suppressed activation of caspase-dependent and caspase-independent cell death pathways. Our results are supported by previous studies in experimental models of ALI. Tasaka et al. showed that treatment with the ROCK inhibitor Y-27632 attenuated pulmonary edema formation and neutrophil infiltration induced by LPS (Tasaka et al, 2005). Also in an experimental model of oleic acid-induced ALI, ROCK inhibition resulted in diminished lung injury as demonstrated by improved lung histology and reduced myeloperoxidase (MPO) activity (Koksel et al, 2005). Together these data imply that ROCK inhibition might be a beneficial therapeutic strategy in preventing lung injury, at least in the absence of mechanosensitive aspects of mechanical ventilation.

GEF inhibitors may be superior to direct pharmacological inhibitors of RhoA or ROCK (Birukova et al, 2010). Pharmacological targeting of GEF enables inhibition of excessive Rho signaling resulting from pathological conditions, while basal RhoA activity will remain unchanged. GEF factor H1 (GEF-H1) has been characterized as a RhoA-specific GEF (Ren et al, 1998). Consequently, (excessive) activation of GEF-H1 is associated with endothelial permeability. Evidence for the importance of GEF-H1 in endothelial barrier dysfunction has been provided by Birkova et al. (Birukova et al, 2006; Birukova et al, 2010). These authors showed that small interfering (si)RNA-based knockdown of GEF-H1 abolished Rho signaling, stress fiber formation and permeability in an *in vitro* model of cell stretch (Birukova et al, 2010). Depletion of GEF-H1 also showed to attenuate vascular leakage in a murine model of VILI (Birukova et al, 2010). In view of these findings, GEF-H1 might be an attractive target to prevent the detrimental effects induced by the pathological mechanosensitive aspects associated with mechanical ventilation.

3.2.2 Inhibitors of cell death

Pulmonary cell death is thought to be involved in the ventilator-induced disruption of alveolar-capillary barriers and thus in the impairment of alveolar-capillary barrier function (Pugin, 2003). In lungs of LV_T and HV_T-ventilated mice, we observed elevated protein levels of cleaved α-fodrin, but not of cleaved caspases, signifying that 5 hours of mechanical ventilation primarily activates the caspase-independent cell death pathway (figure 2). In view of this notion, it would be of interest to evaluate the effects of calpain inhibitors in our experimental model of VILI. Protective effects of calpain inhibitors have already been shown in experiment models of inflammation (Cuzzocrea et al, 2000; Cuzzocrea et al, 2002; Rose et al, 2006). Cuzzocrea et al. described that treatment with calpain inhibitors diminishes granulocyte infiltration, lipid peroxidation and the degree of lung injury caused by intrapleural injection of carrageenan, a polysaccharide extracted from seaweed (Cuzzocrea et al, 2000). In addition, the same research group demonstrated that calpain inhibitors may decrease the degree of lung inflammation and injury induced by zymosan, which leads to the formation of reactive oxygen species (Cuzzocrea et al, 2002). More importantly, these authors demonstrated that inhibition of calpain activity did not only attenuate inflammation and injury in the lung but also in organs like the liver and intestine (Cuzzocrea et al, 2002). As we observed that mechanical ventilation with high pressures induces marked inflammation in both the lung and distal organs (Hegeman et al, 2009), treatment with calpain inhibitors may be beneficial in ventilated patients suffering from respiratory failure and/or MOF.

For many years, necrosis has been considered to be an uncontrolled process. However, recent evidence suggests that the course of necrotic cell death might be as tightly regulated as apoptotic cell death (Festjens et al, 2006; Golstein & Kroemer, 2007). It has to be kept in mind though, that necrotic and apoptotic traits may co-exist (Kroemer et al, 2009) and the same cell death inducers may promote either necrosis or apoptosis depending on the specific environmental setting (Galluzzi et al, 2009). Triggering of TNFR-1 by TNF-α does not only lead to activation of the extrinsic pathway of apoptosis but also to programmed necrosis involving RIP-kinases (Galluzzi et al, 2009; Hitomi et al, 2008). Necrostatin has been described as a small molecule inhibitor of programmed cell necrosis which prevents RIP1 kinase activation (Degterev et al, 2005). Importantly, previous research already showed that inhibition of programmed cell necrosis by necrostatin protects against the development of brain injury (Degterev et al, 2005; Northington et al, 2011; You et al, 2008). Northington et al. described that necrostatin exerts its protective effects by inhibition of the RIP1-RIP3 interaction, decreased oxidative injury and suppression of the pro-inflammatory response (Northington et al, 2011). The effect of necrostatin has not yet been evaluated in models of lung injury which are clearly associated with increased cell death, oxidative injury and pro-inflammation. Since mechanical ventilation in our experimental model of VILI primarily activated the caspase-independent route of cell death, treatment with necrostatin might be a preventive strategy for the devastating mechanosensitive effects of mechanical ventilation.

3.2.3 Mesenchymal stem cells

Adult stem cells have retained the ability to differentiate into a variety of cell lineages (McCulloch & Till, 2005). One of the most well characterized adult stem cells are the mesenchymal stem cells (MSCs) (Pittenger et al, 1999). MSCs can be isolated from various tissues such as bone marrow, placenta and adipose tissue. MSCs have been described to home to injured tissue beds, interact with injured cells and secrete multiple paracrine factors that regulate endothelial and epithelial permeability, decrease inflammation, enhance tissue repair and inhibit bacterial growth (Lee et al, 2011). In addition, MSC therapy may support endogenous stem cells residing in pulmonary tissue (Lee et al, 2011). In view of these notions, cell-based therapy with MSCs has been proposed as a potential intervention strategy for severe lung diseases.

Previously, MSCs have been shown to restore function of damaged tissue in experimental models of lung disease. To our knowledge, the effecs of MSCs were primarily studied in rodent models of ALI. In this regard, intravenous MSC administration reduced lung inflammation and prolonged survival in a murine model of bleomycin-induced lung injury and fibrosis (Ortiz et al, 2003; Rojas et al, 2005). Similar effects of MSC treatment have been described in murine models of endotoxin-induced lung injury (Mei et al, 2007; Xu et al, 2007; Xu et al, 2008). Xu et al. observed that intravenous MSC administration prevents endotoxin-induced lung injury, edema formation and inflammation in mice (Xu et al, 2007). Moreover, genetic engineering of MSCs showed to improve the protective effects of MSCs even more (Mei et al, 2007; Xu et al, 2008). Mei et al. evaluated the integrity of the alveolar-capillary membrane barrier by measuring total protein, albumin and IgM concentration in BALf in a murine model of LPS-induced ALI (Mei et al, 2007). They showed that treatment with MSCs alone already partially reduced these indicators of lung injury in LPS-exposed mice. MSCs overexpressing the vessel protective factor Ang-1, however, restored total protein, albumin and IgM to levels not different from naive control animals (Mei et al, 2007). It should be noted though, that mechanical ventilation provokes a different spectrum of pulmonary injury compared to LPS-challenge as demonstrated by the difference in efficacy of Ang-1 treatment in our model of VILI (Hegeman et al, 2010). Nonetheless, it is tempting to speculate that autologous stem cell transplantation could become a beneficial approach to protect ventilated patients against detrimental effects induced by mechanical ventilation.

4. Conclusions

Although mechanical ventilation is a life-saving procedure in the ICU, it has the potential to aggravate or even induce detrimental effects (Dreyfuss & Saumon, 1998; Slutsky, 1999). Our previous studies aimed at evaluating the mechanisms that may underlie the pathogenesis of VILI and MOF (figure 5). To summarize, we demonstrated that both LV_T and HV_T-ventilation increased pulmonary cytokine, chemokine and adhesion molecule expression accompanied by significant granulocyte infiltration (Hegeman et al, 2011b). We observed that 5 hours of either LV_T or HV_T-ventilation primarily induced caspase-independent pathways of cell death (figure 3). In addition, our findings strongly suggest that changes in the Ang-Tie2 system, together with elevated VEGF expression, are involved in the development of VILI (figure 4) (Hegeman et al, 2010). An intriguing clinical observation is that most critically ill ALI/ARDS patients do not succumb to acute lung failure but rather to progressive non-pulmonary organ dysfunction, so-called MOF (Ferring & Vincent, 1997; Montgomery et al, 1985; Valta et al, 1999). In this respect, we showed that mechanical ventilation with high pressures increased the pro-inflammatory state of the lung but also of the liver and kidney (figure 1) (Hegeman et al, 2009). Moreover, we observed that HV_T-ventilation impairs functioning of peripheral lymphocytes (figure 2). Together, these data indicate that ventilator-induced alveolar (over)stretch may play a significant role in the pathogenesis of both VILI and MOF.

Based on the hypothesis that a ventilator-induced inflammatory response may precede lung injury, we evaluated the effects of different anti-inflammatory intervention strategies on various aspects considered to be important in the development of VILI. One of the most potent drugs to downregulate inflammatory responses are glucocorticoids (Brower et al, 2001; Luce, 2002). Despite the successful inhibitory effect on lung inflammation, we observed that glucocorticoid therapy did not prevent the elevation in BALf total protein levels, the increase in pulmonary wet-to-dry ratio and reduction of PaO_2/FiO_2 ratio during mechanical ventilation (Hegeman et al, 2011b). Similarly, the vessel protective factor Ang-1 did not protect ventilated mice against these more crude aspects of VILI even though granulocyte infiltration, inflammatory mediator and VEGF expression were markedly diminished (Hegeman et al, 2010). Thus, prevention of inflammation does not preclude loss of pulmonary function implying that lung inflammation and injury are two independent components of VILI.

In view of these most recent findings, we propose that anti-inflammatory therapy may not prevent the aspects of VILI driven by mechanosensitive alterations in barrier properties, like vascular leakage and impaired gas exchange, but will only regulate pulmonary inflammation. Therefore, future therapeutic intervention strategies in the ventilated, critically ill patient should aim at attacking the ventilator-induced impairment of alveolar-capillary barrier function. As Rho GTPases have been described to be important in the mechanosensitive regulation of endothelial barrier function (Birukov, 2009), ROCK or GEF-H1 inhibitors might be an attractive target to prevent the detrimental effects induced by the alveolar (over)stretch associated with mechanical ventilation. In addition, the attenuation of caspase-independent cell death - via calpain inhibitors or RIP-kinase inhibitors such as necrostatin - might also be a preventive strategy in maintaining alveolar-capillary barrier function. Moreover, restoring function of damaged tissue by autologous stem cell transplantation could become a beneficial approach to treat the critically ill patient as well. Nonetheless, preventing prolonged exposure to mechanical stretch by reducing tidal volumes remains of utmost importance.

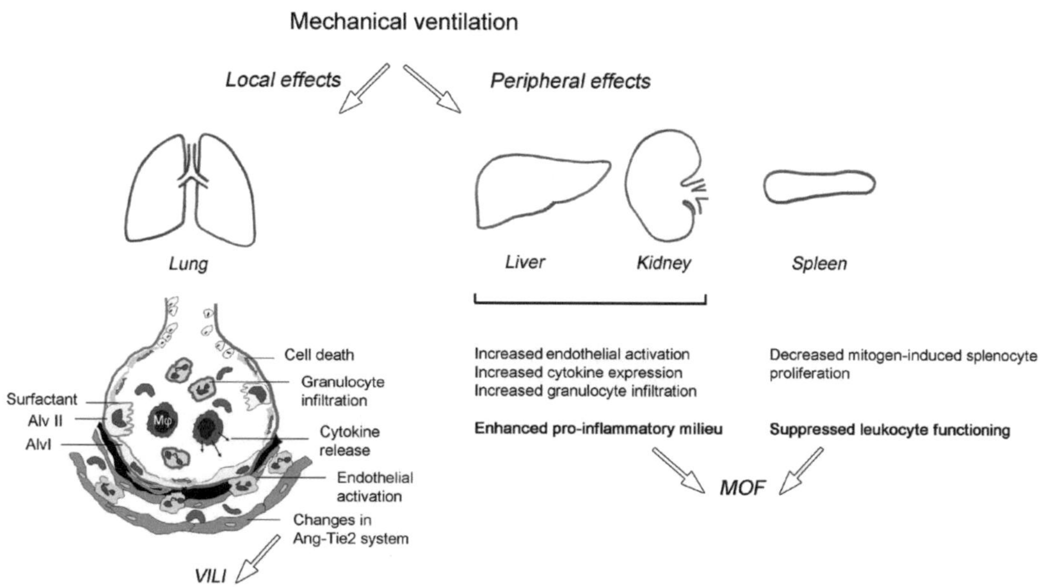

Fig. 5. Possible mechanisms that may underlie the pathogenesis of ventilator-induced lung injury (VILI) and multiple-organ failure (MOF).
Part of illustration adapted with permission of H.A.E. Vreugdenhil (Thesis "Mechanical ventilation and immune function" by H.A.E. Vreugdenhil, 2003). Although life-saving, mechanical ventilation may cause harm by itself. Our previous studies investigated the mechanisms that may underlie the pathogenesis of VILI and MOF in healthy mice. We showed that mechanical ventilation provokes endothelial activation (including changes in the angiopoietin (Ang)-Tie2 system), inflammation and cell death (primarily via activation of the caspase-independent route) in pulmonary tissue. Besides these local effects of mechanical ventilation, we also demonstrated enhanced endothelial activation and inflammation in hepatic and renal tissue (enhanced pro-inflammatory milieu of distal organs). In addition, we observed reduced mitogen-induced splenocyte proliferation after mechanical ventilation with high tidal volumes (suppressed peripheral lymphocyte functioning). Alv = alveolar epithelial cell; Mφ = macrophage.

5. Acknowledgements

The studies were financially supported by the Catharijne Foundation (University Medical Center Utrecht, Utrecht, the Netherlands). For their contribution to abovementioned studies, the authors thank: A. Kavelaars, E. Kooijman, I. den Hartog, J. Zijlstra, K. Amarouchi, M.P. Hennus, N.J.G. Jansen & P.M. Cobelens (University Medical Center Utrecht, Utrecht, the Netherlands); G. Molema, H. Moorlag, H. Morselt, J.A.A.M. Kamps, M. van Meurs & R. Jongman (University Medical Center Groningen, Groningen, the Netherlands); B. Lachmann & P.A.C. Specht (Erasmus Medical Center, Rotterdam, the Netherlands).

6. References

Abraham, E. (2003) Neutrophils and acute lung injury. *Crit Care Med* 31: S195-S199.

Acehan, D., Jiang, X., Morgan, D. G. *et al.* (2002) Three-dimensional structure of the apoptosome: implications for assembly, procaspase-9 binding, and activation. *Mol Cell* 9: 423-432.

Agarwal, R., Nath, A., Aggarwal, A. N. *et al.* (2007) Do glucocorticoids decrease mortality in acute respiratory distress syndrome? A meta-analysis. *Respirology* 12: 585-590.

Amano, M., Chihara, K., Kimura, K. *et al.* (1997) Formation of actin stress fibers and focal adhesions enhanced by Rho-kinase. *Science* 275: 1308-1311.

Amato, M.B., Barbas, C.S., Medeiros, D.M., *et al.* (1998) Effect of a protective-ventilation strategy on mortality in the acute respiratory distress syndrome. *N Engl J Med* 338: 347-354.

Angele, M. K. & Faist, E. (2002) Clinical review: immunodepression in the surgical patient and increased susceptibility to infection. *Crit Care* 6: 298-305.

Artal-Sanz, M. & Tavernarakis, N. (2005) Proteolytic mechanisms in necrotic cell death and neurodegeneration. *FEBS Lett* 579: 3287-3296.

Ásgeirsdóttir, S. A., Kamps, J. A., Bakker, H. I. *et al.* (2007) Site-specific inhibition of glomerulonephritis progression by targeted delivery of dexamethasone to glomerular endothelium. *Mol Pharmacol* 72: 121-131.

Ashbaugh, D. G., Bigelow, D. B., Petty, T. L. *et al.* (1967) Acute respiratory distress in adults. *Lancet* 2: 319-323.

Barnes, P. J. (2006) How corticosteroids control inflammation: Quintiles Prize Lecture 2005. *Br J Pharmacol* 148: 245-254.

Birukov, K. G. (2009) Small GTPases in mechanosensitive regulation of endothelial barrier. *Microvasc Res* 77: 46-52.

Birukova, A. A., Adyshev, D., Gorshkov, B. *et al.* (2006) GEF-H1 is involved in agonist-induced human pulmonary endothelial barrier dysfunction. *Am J Physiol Lung Cell Mol Physiol* 290: L540-L548.

Birukova, A. A., Fu, P., Xing, J. *et al.* (2010) Mechanotransduction by GEF-H1 as a novel mechanism of ventilator-induced vascular endothelial permeability. *Am J Physiol Lung Cell Mol Physiol* 298: L837-L848.

Bone, R. C. (1991) The pathogenesis of sepsis. *Ann Intern Med* 115: 457-469.

Bone, R. C. (1996) Immunologic dissonance: a continuing evolution in our understanding of the systemic inflammatory response syndrome (SIRS) and the multiple organ dysfunction syndrome (MODS). *Ann Intern Med* 125: 680-687.

Bregeon, F., Roch, A., Delpierre, S. *et al.* (2002) Conventional mechanical ventilation of healthy lungs induced pro-inflammatory cytokine gene transcription. *Respir Physiol Neurobiol* 132: 191-203.

Brower, R. G., Ware, L. B., Berthiaume, Y. *et al.* (2001) Treatment of ARDS. *Chest* 120: 1347-1367.

Burns, A. R., Smith, C. W. & Walker, D. C. (2003) Unique structural features that influence neutrophil emigration into the lung. *Physiol Rev* 83: 309-336.

Carlos, T. M. & Harlan, J. M. (1994) Leukocyte-endothelial adhesion molecules. *Blood* 84: 2068-2101.

Chang, D. W., Xing, Z., Capacio, V. L. *et al.* (2003) Interdimer processing mechanism of procaspase-8 activation. *EMBO J* 22: 4132-4142.

Chang, H. Y. & Yang, X. (2000) Proteases for cell suicide: functions and regulation of caspases. *Microbiol Mol Biol Rev* 64: 821-846.

Chiang, C. H., Chuang, C. H., Liu, S. L. *et al.* (2011) Apocynin attenuates ventilator-induced lung injury in an isolated and perfused rat lung model. *Intensive Care Med.* 37:1360-1367.

Cho, Y. S., Challa, S., Moquin, D. *et al.* (2009) Phosphorylation-driven assembly of the RIP1-RIP3 complex regulates programmed necrosis and virus-induced inflammation. *Cell* 137: 1112-1123.

Cines, D. B., Pollak, E. S., Buck, C. A. *et al.* (1998) Endothelial cells in physiology and in the pathophysiology of vascular disorders. *Blood* 91: 3527-3561.

Cobelens, P. M., van Putte, B. P., Kavelaars, A. *et al.* (2009) Inflammatory Consequences of Lung Ischemia-Reperfusion Injury and Low-Pressure Ventilation. *J Surg Res* 153: 295-301.

Copland, I. B., Martinez, F., Kavanagh, B. P. *et al.* (2004) High tidal volume ventilation causes different inflammatory responses in newborn versus adult lung. *Am J Respir Crit Care Med* 169: 739-748.

Cortjens, B., Royakkers, A. A., Determann, R. M. *et al.* (2011) Lung-protective mechanical ventilation does not protect against acute kidney injury in patients without lung injury at onset of mechanical ventilation. *J Crit Care.*

Cuzzocrea, S., Chatterjee, P. K., Mazzon, E. *et al.* (2002) Effects of calpain inhibitor I on multiple organ failure induced by zymosan in the rat. *Crit Care Med* 30: 2284-2294.

Cuzzocrea, S., McDonald, M. C., Mazzon, E. *et al.* (2000) Calpain inhibitor I reduces the development of acute and chronic inflammation. *Am J Pathol* 157: 2065-2079.

Daly, C., Pasnikowski, E., Burova, E. *et al.* (2006) Angiopoietin-2 functions as an autocrine protective factor in stressed endothelial cells. *Proc Natl Acad Sci U S A* 103: 15491-15496.

Daly, C., Wong, V., Burova, E. *et al.* (2004) Angiopoietin-1 modulates endothelial cell function and gene expression via the transcription factor FKHR (FOXO1). *Genes Dev* 18: 1060-1071.

Danial, N. N. & Korsmeyer, S. J. (2004) Cell death: critical control points. *Cell* 116: 205-219.

David, S., Park, J. K., van Meurs, M. *et al.* (2011) Acute administration of recombinant Angiopoietin-1 ameliorates multiple-organ dysfunction syndrome and improves survival in murine sepsis. *Cytokine* 55: 251-259.

DeBusk, L. M., Hallahan, D. E. & Lin, P. C. (2004) Akt is a major angiogenic mediator downstream of the Ang1/Tie2 signaling pathway. *Exp Cell Res* 298: 167-177.

Declercq, W., Vanden Berghe, T. & Vandenabeele, P. (2009) RIP kinases at the crossroads of cell death and survival. *Cell* 138: 229-232.

Degterev, A., Huang, Z., Boyce, M. *et al.* (2005) Chemical inhibitor of nonapoptotic cell death with therapeutic potential for ischemic brain injury. *Nat Chem Biol* 1: 112-119.

Dejana, E. (2004) Endothelial cell-cell junctions: happy together. *Nat Rev Mol Cell Biol* 5: 261-270.

Denecker, G., Vercammen, D., Declercq, W. *et al.* (2001) Apoptotic and necrotic cell death induced by death domain receptors. *Cell Mol Life Sci* 58: 356-370.

Determann, R.M., Royakkers, A., Wolthuis, E.K., *et al.* (2010) Ventilation with lower tidal volumes as compared with conventional tidal volumes for patients without acute lung injury: a preventive randomized controlled trial. *Crit Care* 14: R1.

Ding, H. F., Lin, Y. L., McGill, G. *et al.* (2000) Essential role for caspase-8 in transcription-independent apoptosis triggered by p53. *J Biol Chem* 275: 38905-38911.

Donnelly, S. C., Strieter, R. M., Kunkel, S. L. *et al.* (1993) Interleukin-8 and development of adult respiratory distress syndrome in at-risk patient groups. *Lancet* 341: 643-647.

dos Santos, C. C., Han, B., Andrade, C. F. *et al.* (2004) DNA microarray analysis of gene expression in alveolar epithelial cells in response to TNFalpha, LPS, and cyclic stretch. *Physiol Genomics* 19: 331-342.

dos Santos, C. C., Shan, Y., Akram, A. *et al.* (2011) Neuroimmune regulation of ventilator-induced lung injury. *Am J Respir Crit Care Med* 183: 471-482.

Dreyfuss, D., Basset, G., Soler, P. *et al.* (1985) Intermittent positive-pressure hyperventilation with high inflation pressures produces pulmonary microvascular injury in rats. *Am Rev Respir Dis* 132: 880-884.

Dreyfuss, D. & Saumon, G. (1998) From ventilator-induced lung injury to multiple organ dysfunction? *Intensive Care Med* 24: 102-104.

Dreyfuss, D., Soler, P., Basset, G. *et al.* (1988) High inflation pressure pulmonary edema. Respective effects of high airway pressure, high tidal volume, and positive end-expiratory pressure. *Am Rev Respir Dis* 137: 1159-1164.

Edwards, Y. S., Sutherland, L. M., Power, J. H. *et al.* (1999) Cyclic stretch induces both apoptosis and secretion in rat alveolar type II cells. *FEBS Lett* 448: 127-130.

Egan, E. A. (1982) Lung inflation, lung solute permeability, and alveolar edema. *J Appl Physiol* 53: 121-125.

Elenkov, I. J., Wilder, R. L., Chrousos, G. P. *et al.* (2000) The sympathetic nerve--an integrative interface between two supersystems: the brain and the immune system. *Pharmacol Rev* 52: 595-638.

Feldman-Billard, S., Du Pasquier-Fediaevsky, L. & Heron, E. (2006) Hyperglycemia after repeated periocular dexamethasone injections in patients with diabetes. *Ophthalmology* 113: 1720-1723.

Fernandes, A. B., Zin, W. A. & Rocco, P. R. (2005) Corticosteroids in acute respiratory distress syndrome. *Braz J Med Biol Res* 38: 147-159.

Ferring, M. & Vincent, J. L. (1997) Is outcome from ARDS related to the severity of respiratory failure? *Eur Respir J* 10: 1297-1300.

Festjens, N., van Gurp, M., van Loo, G. *et al.* (2004) Bcl-2 family members as sentinels of cellular integrity and role of mitochondrial intermembrane space proteins in apoptotic cell death. *Acta Haematol* 111: 7-27.

Festjens, N., Vanden Berghe, T. & Vandenabeele, P. (2006) Necrosis, a well-orchestrated form of cell demise: signalling cascades, important mediators and concomitant immune response. *Biochim Biophys Acta* 1757: 1371-1387.

Fiedler, U. & Augustin, H. G. (2006) Angiopoietins: a link between angiogenesis and inflammation. *Trends Immunol* 27: 552-558.

Fiedler, U., Krissl, T., Koidl, S. *et al.* (2003) Angiopoietin-1 and angiopoietin-2 share the same binding domains in the Tie-2 receptor involving the first Ig-like loop and the epidermal growth factor-like repeats. *J Biol Chem* 278: 1721-1727.

Fiers, W., Beyaert, R., Declercq, W. *et al.* (1999) More than one way to die: apoptosis, necrosis and reactive oxygen damage. *Oncogene* 18: 7719-7730.

Flierl, M. A., Rittirsch, D., Nadeau, B. A. *et al.* (2009) Upregulation of phagocyte-derived catecholamines augments the acute inflammatory response. *PLoS ONE* 4: e4414.

Gallagher, D. C., Parikh, S. M., Balonov, K. *et al.* (2008) Circulating angiopoietin 2 correlates with mortality in a surgical population with acute lung injury/adult respiratory distress syndrome. *Shock* 29: 656-661.

Galluzzi, L., Kepp, O. & Kroemer, G. (2009) RIP kinases initiate programmed necrosis. *J Mol Cell Biol* 1: 8-10.

Galluzzi, L., Vicencio, J. M., Kepp, O. *et al.* (2008) To die or not to die: that is the autophagic question. *Curr Mol Med* 8: 78-91.

Gando, S., Kameue, T., Matsuda, N. *et al.* (2004) Systemic inflammation and disseminated intravascular coagulation in early stage of ALI and ARDS: role of neutrophil and endothelial activation. *Inflammation* 28: 237-244.

Gavard, J., Patel, V. & Gutkind, J. S. (2008) Angiopoietin-1 prevents VEGF-induced endothelial permeability by sequestering Src through mDia. *Dev Cell* 14: 25-36.

Gillette, M. A. & Hess, D. R. (2001) Ventilator-induced lung injury and the evolution of lung-protective strategies in acute respiratory distress syndrome. *Respir Care* 46: 130-148.

Golstein, P. & Kroemer, G. (2007) Cell death by necrosis: towards a molecular definition. *Trends Biochem Sci* 32: 37-43.

Goodman, R. B., Pugin, J., Lee, J. S. *et al.* (2003) Cytokine-mediated inflammation in acute lung injury. *Cytokine Growth Factor Rev* 14: 523-535.

Haitsma, J. J., Uhlig, S., Goggel, R. *et al.* (2000) Ventilator-induced lung injury leads to loss of alveolar and systemic compartmentalization of tumor necrosis factor-alpha. *Intensive Care Med* 26: 1515-1522.

Haitsma, J. J., Uhlig, S., Verbrugge, S. J. *et al.* (2003) Injurious ventilation strategies cause systemic release of IL-6 and MIP-2 in rats in vivo. *Clin Physiol Funct Imaging* 23: 349-353.

Hammerschmidt, S., Kuhn, H., Grasenack, T. *et al.* (2004) Apoptosis and necrosis induced by cyclic mechanical stretching in alveolar type II cells. *Am J Respir Cell Mol Biol* 30: 396-402.

Harwood, S. M., Yaqoob, M. M. & Allen, D. A. (2005) Caspase and calpain function in cell death: bridging the gap between apoptosis and necrosis. *Ann Clin Biochem* 42: 415-431.

Haupt, S., Berger, M., Goldberg, Z. *et al.* (2003) Apoptosis - the p53 network. *J Cell Sci* 116: 4077-4085.

He, S., Wang, L., Miao, L. *et al.* (2009) Receptor interacting protein kinase-3 determines cellular necrotic response to TNF-alpha. *Cell* 137: 1100-1111.

Headley, A. S., Tolley, E. & Meduri, G. U. (1997) Infections and the inflammatory response in acute respiratory distress syndrome. *Chest* 111: 1306-1321.

Hegeman, M. A., Cobelens, P. M., Kamps, J. A. *et al.* (2011a) Liposome-encapsulated dexamethasone attenuates ventilator-induced lung inflammation. *Br J Pharmacol* 163: 1048-1058.

Hegeman, M. A., Hennus, M. P., Cobelens, P. M. *et al.* (2011b) Inhibition of pulmonary inflammation by dexamethasone does not prevent ventilator-induced lung injury. *Accepted as abstract for the 24th Annual Congress of the European Society of Intensive Care Medicine (ESICM), Berlin, Germany.*

Hegeman, M. A., Hennus, M. P., Heijnen, C. J. *et al.* (2009) Ventilator-induced endothelial activation and inflammation in the lung and distal organs. *Crit Care* 13: R182.

Hegeman, M. A., Hennus, M. P., van Meurs, M. *et al.* (2010) Angiopoietin-1 treatment reduces inflammation but does not prevent ventilator-induced lung injury. *PLoS ONE* 5: e15653.

Held, H. D., Boettcher, S., Hamann, L. *et al.* (2001) Ventilation-induced chemokine and cytokine release is associated with activation of nuclear factor-kappaB and is blocked by steroids. *Am J Respir Crit Care Med* 163: 711-716.

Hitomi, J., Christofferson, D. E., Ng, A. *et al.* (2008) Identification of a molecular signaling network that regulates a cellular necrotic cell death pathway. *Cell* 135: 1311-1323.

Huang, Y. Q., Sauthoff, H., Herscovici, P. *et al.* (2008) Angiopoietin-1 increases survival and reduces the development of lung edema induced by endotoxin administration in a murine model of acute lung injury. *Crit Care Med* 36: 262-267.

Hudson, L. D., Milberg, J. A., Anardi, D. *et al.* (1995) Clinical risks for development of the acute respiratory distress syndrome. *Am J Respir Crit Care Med* 151: 293-301.

Hughes, D. P., Marron, M. B. & Brindle, N. P. (2003) The antiinflammatory endothelial tyrosine kinase Tie2 interacts with a novel nuclear factor-kappaB inhibitor ABIN-2. *Circ Res* 92: 630-636.

Ikegami, M., Jobe, A., Jacobs, H. *et al.* (1984) A protein from airways of premature lambs that inhibits surfactant function. *J Appl Physiol* 57: 1134-1142.

Imai, Y., Parodo, J., Kajikawa, O. *et al.* (2003) Injurious mechanical ventilation and end-organ epithelial cell apoptosis and organ dysfunction in an experimental model of acute respiratory distress syndrome. *JAMA* 289: 2104-2112.

Iwaki, M., Ito, S., Morioka, M. *et al.* (2009) Mechanical stretch enhances IL-8 production in pulmonary microvascular endothelial cells. *Biochem Biophys Res Commun* 389: 531-536.

Jiang, X. & Wang, X. (2000) Cytochrome c promotes caspase-9 activation by inducing nucleotide binding to Apaf-1. *J Biol Chem* 275: 31199-31203.

Kannan, K., Kaminski, N., Rechavi, G. *et al.* (2001) DNA microarray analysis of genes involved in p53 mediated apoptosis: activation of Apaf-1. *Oncogene* 20: 3449-3455.

Karmpaliotis, D., Kosmidou, I., Ingenito, E. P. *et al.* (2002) Angiogenic growth factors in the pathophysiology of a murine model of acute lung injury. *Am J Physiol Lung Cell Mol Physiol* 283: L585-L595.

Kawano, T., Mori, S., Cybulsky, M. *et al.* (1987) Effect of granulocyte depletion in a ventilated surfactant-depleted lung. *J Appl Physiol* 62: 27-33.

Kelley, J. (1990) Cytokines of the lung. *Am Rev Respir Dis* 141: 765-788.

Kim, I., Kim, H. G., So, J. N. *et al.* (2000) Angiopoietin-1 regulates endothelial cell survival through the phosphatidylinositol 3'-Kinase/Akt signal transduction pathway. *Circ Res* 86: 24-29.

Kimura, K., Ito, M., Amano, M. *et al.* (1996) Regulation of myosin phosphatase by Rho and Rho-associated kinase (Rho-kinase). *Science* 273: 245-248.

Koksel, O., Yildirim, C., Tiftik, R. N. *et al.* (2005) Rho-kinase (ROCK-1 and ROCK-2) upregulation in oleic acid-induced lung injury and its restoration by Y-27632. *Eur J Pharmacol* 510: 135-142.

Korsmeyer, S. J., Wei, M. C., Saito, M. *et al.* (2000) Pro-apoptotic cascade activates BID, which oligomerizes BAK or BAX into pores that result in the release of cytochrome c. *Cell Death Differ* 7: 1166-1173.

Kroemer, G., El-Deiry, W. S., Golstein, P. *et al.* (2005) Classification of cell death: recommendations of the Nomenclature Committee on Cell Death. *Cell Death Differ* 12 Suppl 2: 1463-1467.

Kroemer, G., Galluzzi, L., Vandenabeele, P. *et al.* (2009) Classification of cell death: recommendations of the Nomenclature Committee on Cell Death 2009. *Cell Death Differ* 16: 3-11.

Kumar, V. & Sharma, A. (2010) Is neuroimmunomodulation a future therapeutic approach for sepsis? *Int Immunopharmacol* 10: 9-17.

Lachmann, B., Eijking, E. P., So, K. L. *et al.* (1994) In vivo evaluation of the inhibitory capacity of human plasma on exogenous surfactant function. *Intensive Care Med* 20: 6-11.

Lachmann, B., Hallman, M. & Bergmann, K. C. (1987) Respiratory failure following anti-lung serum: study on mechanisms associated with surfactant system damage. *Exp Lung Res* 12: 163-180.

Lavrik, I. N., Golks, A. & Krammer, P. H. (2005a) Caspases: pharmacological manipulation of cell death. *J Clin Invest* 115: 2665-2672.

Lavrik, I. N., Golks, A. & Krammer, P. H. (2005b) Death receptor signaling. *J Cell Sci* 118: 265-267.

Le, A., Damico, R., Damarla, M. *et al.* (2008) Alveolar cell apoptosis is dependent on p38 MAP kinase-mediated activation of xanthine oxidoreductase in ventilator-induced lung injury. *J Appl Physiol* 105: 1282-1290.

Lee, J. W., Fang, X., Krasnodembskaya, A. *et al.* (2011) Concise review: mesenchymal stem cells for acute lung injury: role of paracrine soluble factors. *Stem Cells* 29: 913-919.

Lee, W. L. & Downey, G. P. (2001) Neutrophil activation and acute lung injury. *Curr Opin Crit Care* 7: 1-7.

Leist, M. & Jäättelä, M. (2001) Four deaths and a funeral: from caspases to alternative mechanisms. *Nat Rev Mol Cell Biol* 2: 589-598.

Leist, M., Single, B., Castoldi, A. F. *et al.* (1997) Intracellular adenosine triphosphate (ATP) concentration: a switch in the decision between apoptosis and necrosis. *J Exp Med* 185: 1481-1486.

Lemieux, C., Maliba, R., Favier, J. *et al.* (2005) Angiopoietins can directly activate endothelial cells and neutrophils to promote proinflammatory responses. *Blood* 105: 1523-1530.

Lentsch, A. B. & Ward, P. A. (2000) Regulation of inflammatory vascular damage. *J Pathol* 190: 343-348.

Levine, B. & Klionsky, D. J. (2004) Development by self-digestion: molecular mechanisms and biological functions of autophagy. *Dev Cell* 6: 463-477.

Li, L. F., Liao, S. K., Ko, Y. S. *et al.* (2007) Hyperoxia increases ventilator-induced lung injury via mitogen-activated protein kinases: a prospective, controlled animal experiment. *Crit Care* 11: R25.

Liao, J. K., Seto, M. & Noma, K. (2007) Rho kinase (ROCK) inhibitors. *J Cardiovasc Pharmacol* 50: 17-24.

Luce, J. M. (2002) Corticosteroids in ARDS. An evidence-based review. *Crit Care Clin* 18: 79-89, vii.

Luscinskas, F. W. & Gimbrone, M. A., Jr. (1996) Endothelial-dependent mechanisms in chronic inflammatory leukocyte recruitment. *Annu Rev Med* 47: 413-421.

Maiuri, M. C., Zalckvar, E., Kimchi, A. *et al.* (2007) Self-eating and self-killing: crosstalk between autophagy and apoptosis. *Nat Rev Mol Cell Biol* 8: 741-752.

Marshall J.C. (2001). The multiple organ dysfunction syndrome. In: *Holzheimer RG, Mannick JA, eds. Surgical Treatment: Evidence-based and problem-oriented.* Munich: Zuckschwerdt Verlag, 780-785.

McCarter, S. D., Mei, S. H., Lai, P. F. *et al.* (2007) Cell-based angiopoietin-1 gene therapy for acute lung injury. *Am J Respir Crit Care Med* 175: 1014-1026.

McCulloch, E. A. & Till, J. E. (2005) Perspectives on the properties of stem cells. *Nat Med* 11: 1026-1028.

McKenzie, S. E. & Schreiber, A. D. (1998) Fc gamma receptors in phagocytes. *Curr Opin Hematol* 5: 16-21.

Mead, J., Takishima, T. & Leith, D. (1970) Stress distribution in lungs: a model of pulmonary elasticity. *J Appl Physiol* 28: 596-608.

Meduri, G. U., Headley, S., Kohler, G. *et al.* (1995) Persistent elevation of inflammatory cytokines predicts a poor outcome in ARDS. Plasma IL-1 beta and IL-6 levels are consistent and efficient predictors of outcome over time. *Chest* 107: 1062-1073.

Meduri, G. U., Marik, P. E., Chrousos, G. P. *et al.* (2008) Steroid treatment in ARDS: a critical appraisal of the ARDS network trial and the recent literature. *Intensive Care Med* 34: 61-69.

Mei, S. H., McCarter, S. D., Deng, Y. *et al.* (2007) Prevention of LPS-induced acute lung injury in mice by mesenchymal stem cells overexpressing angiopoietin 1. *PLoS Med* 4: e269.

Michel, C. C. & Curry, F. E. (1999) Microvascular permeability. *Physiol Rev* 79: 703-761.

Miksa, M., Das, P., Zhou, M. *et al.* (2009) Pivotal role of the alpha(2A)-adrenoceptor in producing inflammation and organ injury in a rat model of sepsis. *PLoS ONE* 4: e5504.

Montgomery, A. B., Stager, M. A., Carrico, C. J. *et al.* (1985) Causes of mortality in patients with the adult respiratory distress syndrome. *Am Rev Respir Dis* 132: 485-489.

Moraes, T. J., Chow, C. W. & Downey, G. P. (2003) Proteases and lung injury. *Crit Care Med* 31: S189-S194.

Nin, N., Lorente, J. A., de Paula, M. *et al.* (2008) Rats surviving injurious mechanical ventilation show reversible pulmonary, vascular and inflammatory changes. *Intensive Care Med* 34: 948-956.

Nin, N., Penuelas, O., de Paula, M. *et al.* (2006) Ventilation-induced lung injury in rats is associated with organ injury and systemic inflammation that is attenuated by dexamethasone. *Crit Care Med* 34: 1093-1098.

Northington, F. J., Chavez-Valdez, R., Graham, E. M. *et al.* (2011) Necrostatin decreases oxidative damage, inflammation, and injury after neonatal HI. *J Cereb Blood Flow Metab* 31: 178-189.

O'Mahony, D. S., Liles, W. C., Altemeier, W. A. *et al.* (2006) Mechanical ventilation interacts with endotoxemia to induce extrapulmonary organ dysfunction. *Crit Care* 10: R136.

Ohta, N., Shimaoka, M., Imanaka, H. *et al.* (2001) Glucocorticoid suppresses neutrophil activation in ventilator-induced lung injury. *Crit Care Med* 29: 1012-1016.

Orfanos, S. E., Mavrommati, I., Korovesi, I. *et al.* (2004) Pulmonary endothelium in acute lung injury: from basic science to the critically ill. *Intensive Care Med* 30: 1702-1714.

Ortiz, L. A., Gambelli, F., McBride, C. *et al.* (2003) Mesenchymal stem cell engraftment in lung is enhanced in response to bleomycin exposure and ameliorates its fibrotic effects. *Proc Natl Acad Sci U S A* 100: 8407-8411.

Papapetropoulos, A., Fulton, D., Mahboubi, K. *et al.* (2000) Angiopoietin-1 inhibits endothelial cell apoptosis via the Akt/survivin pathway. *J Biol Chem* 275: 9102-9105.

Parker, J. C., Townsley, M. I., Rippe, B. *et al.* (1984) Increased microvascular permeability in dog lungs due to high peak airway pressures. *J Appl Physiol* 57: 1809-1816.

Parrillo, J. E. (1993) Pathogenetic mechanisms of septic shock. *N Engl J Med* 328: 1471-1477.

Pavlov, V. A., Ochani, M., Yang, L. H. *et al.* (2007) Selective alpha7-nicotinic acetylcholine receptor agonist GTS-21 improves survival in murine endotoxemia and severe sepsis. *Crit Care Med* 35: 1139-1144.

Petty, T. L. & Ashbaugh, D. G. (1971) The adult respiratory distress syndrome. Clinical features, factors influencing prognosis and principles of management. *Chest* 60: 233-239.

Pinsky, M. R., Vincent, J. L., Deviere, J. *et al.* (1993) Serum cytokine levels in human septic shock. Relation to multiple-system organ failure and mortality. *Chest* 103: 565-575.

Pittenger, M. F., Mackay, A. M., Beck, S. C. *et al.* (1999) Multilineage potential of adult human mesenchymal stem cells. *Science* 284: 143-147.

Plotz, F. B., Slutsky, A. S., van Vught, A. J. *et al.* (2004) Ventilator-induced lung injury and multiple system organ failure: a critical review of facts and hypotheses. *Intensive Care Med* 30: 1865-1872.

Plotz, F. B., Vreugdenhil, H. A., Slutsky, A. S. *et al.* (2002) Mechanical ventilation alters the immune response in children without lung pathology. *Intensive Care Med* 28: 486-492.

Pugin, J. (2003) Molecular mechanisms of lung cell activation induced by cyclic stretch. *Crit Care Med* 31: S200-S206.

Pugin, J., Dunn, I., Jolliet, P. *et al.* (1998) Activation of human macrophages by mechanical ventilation in vitro. *Am J Physiol* 275: L1040-L1050.

Ranieri, V. M., Suter, P. M., Tortorella, C. *et al.* (1999) Effect of mechanical ventilation on inflammatory mediators in patients with acute respiratory distress syndrome: a randomized controlled trial. *JAMA* 282: 54-61.

Ren, Y., Li, R., Zheng, Y. *et al.* (1998) Cloning and characterization of GEF-H1, a microtubule-associated guanine nucleotide exchange factor for Rac and Rho GTPases. *J Biol Chem* 273: 34954-34960.

Ridley, A. J. & Hall, A. (1992) The small GTP-binding protein rho regulates the assembly of focal adhesions and actin stress fibers in response to growth factors. *Cell* 70: 389-399.

Rittirsch, D., Flierl, M. A. & Ward, P. A. (2008) Harmful molecular mechanisms in sepsis. *Nat Rev Immunol* 8: 776-787.

Rojas, M., Xu, J., Woods, C. R. *et al.* (2005) Bone marrow-derived mesenchymal stem cells in repair of the injured lung. *Am J Respir Cell Mol Biol* 33: 145-152.

Rose, R., Banerjee, A. & Ramaiah, S. K. (2006) Calpain inhibition attenuates iNOS production and midzonal hepatic necrosis in a repeat dose model of endotoxemia in rats. *Toxicol Pathol* 34: 785-794.

Rossi, D. & Gaidano, G. (2003) Messengers of cell death: apoptotic signaling in health and disease. *Haematologica* 88: 212-218.

Ryter, S. W. & Choi, A. M. (2010) Autophagy in the lung. *Proc Am Thorac Soc* 7: 13-21.

Schacke, H., Docke, W. D. & Asadullah, K. (2002) Mechanisms involved in the side effects of glucocorticoids. *Pharmacol Ther* 96: 23-43.

Schmidt, A. & Hall, A. (2002) Guanine nucleotide exchange factors for Rho GTPases: turning on the switch. *Genes Dev* 16: 1587-1609.

Schultz, M. J. (2008) Lung-protective mechanical ventilation with lower tidal volumes in patients not suffering from acute lung injury: a review of clinical studies. *Med Sci Monit* 14: RA22-RA26.

Schwarz, M. A. (2001) Acute lung injury: cellular mechanisms and derangements. *Paediatr Respir Rev* 2: 3-9.

Seeger, W., Gunther, A., Walmrath, H. D. *et al.* (1993) Alveolar surfactant and adult respiratory distress syndrome. Pathogenetic role and therapeutic prospects. *Clin Investig* 71: 177-190.

Slutsky, A. S. (1993) Mechanical ventilation. American College of Chest Physicians' Consensus Conference. *Chest* 104: 1833-1859.

Slutsky, A. S. (1999) Lung injury caused by mechanical ventilation. *Chest* 116: 9S-15S.

Slutsky, A. S. & Tremblay, L. N. (1998) Multiple system organ failure. Is mechanical ventilation a contributing factor? *Am J Respir Crit Care Med* 157: 1721-1725.

Spengler, R. N., Allen, R. M., Remick, D. G. *et al.* (1990) Stimulation of alpha-adrenergic receptor augments the production of macrophage-derived tumor necrosis factor. *J Immunol* 145: 1430-1434.

Spindler, V., Schlegel, N. & Waschke, J. (2010) Role of GTPases in control of microvascular permeability. *Cardiovasc Res* 87: 243-253.

Storm, G. & Crommelin, D. J. A. (1998) Liposomes: quo vadis? *Pharm Sci Technol To* 1: 19-31.

Straub, R. H., Mayer, M., Kreutz, M. *et al.* (2000) Neurotransmitters of the sympathetic nerve terminal are powerful chemoattractants for monocytes. *J Leukoc Biol* 67: 553-558.

Syrbe, U., Meinecke, A., Platzer, C. *et al.* (1994). Improvement of monocyte function - a new therapeutic approach? In: *Reinhart K, Eyrich K, Sprung CL, eds. Sepsis: Current Perspectives in Pathophysiology and Therapy.*, Berlin: Springer-Verlag, 473-500.

Tasaka, S., Koh, H., Yamada, W. *et al.* (2005) Attenuation of endotoxin-induced acute lung injury by the Rho-associated kinase inhibitor, Y-27632. *Am J Respir Cell Mol Biol* 32: 504-510.

the ARDS network (2000) Ventilation with lower tidal volumes as compared with traditional tidal volumes for acute lung injury and the acute respiratory distress syndrome. The Acute Respiratory Distress Syndrome Network. *N Engl J Med* 342: 1301-1308.

Thompson, B. T. (2003) Glucocorticoids and acute lung injury. *Crit Care Med* 31: S253-S257.

Tobin, M. J. (2001) Advances in mechanical ventilation. *N Engl J Med* 344: 1986-1996.

Tremblay, L., Valenza, F., Ribeiro, S. P. *et al.* (1997) Injurious ventilatory strategies increase cytokines and c-fos m-RNA expression in an isolated rat lung model. *J Clin Invest* 99: 944-952.

Tremblay, L. N. & Slutsky, A. S. (1998) Ventilator-induced injury: from barotrauma to biotrauma. *Proc Assoc Am Physicians* 110: 482-488.

Tschumperlin, D. J., Oswari, J. & Margulies, A. S. (2000) Deformation-induced injury of alveolar epithelial cells. Effect of frequency, duration, and amplitude. *Am J Respir Crit Care Med* 162: 357-362.

Tsuno, K., Miura, K., Takeya, M. *et al.* (1991) Histopathologic pulmonary changes from mechanical ventilation at high peak airway pressures. *Am Rev Respir Dis* 143: 1115-1120.

Tutor, J. D., Mason, C. M., Dobard, E. *et al.* (1994) Loss of compartmentalization of alveolar tumor necrosis factor after lung injury. *Am J Respir Crit Care Med* 149: 1107-1111.

Valta, P., Uusaro, A., Nunes, S. *et al.* (1999) Acute respiratory distress syndrome: frequency, clinical course, and costs of care. *Crit Care Med* 27: 2367-2374.

van der Heijden M., van Nieuw Amerongen, G. P., Koolwijk, P. *et al.* (2008) Angiopoietin-2, permeability oedema, occurrence and severity of ALI/ARDS in septic and non-septic critically ill patients. *Thorax* 63: 903-909.

van der Heijden M., van Nieuw Amerongen, G. P., Chedamni, S. *et al.* (2009) The angiopoietin-Tie2 system as a therapeutic target in sepsis and acute lung injury. *Expert Opin Ther Targets* 13: 39-53.

Vaneker, M., Halbertsma, F. J., van Egmond, J. *et al.* (2007) Mechanical ventilation in healthy mice induces reversible pulmonary and systemic cytokine elevation with preserved alveolar integrity: an in vivo model using clinical relevant ventilation settings. *Anesthesiology* 107: 419-426.

Verbrugge, S. J., Sorm, V. & Lachmann, B. (1997) Mechanisms of acute respiratory distress syndrome: role of surfactant changes and mechanical ventilation. *J Physiol Pharmacol* 48: 537-557.

Villar, J., Kacmarek, R.M., Perez-Mendez, L., *et al.* (2006) A high positive endexpiratory pressure, low tidal volume ventilatory strategy improves outcome in persistent acute respiratory distress syndrome: a randomized, controlled trial. *Crit Care Med* 34: 1311-1318.

Vincent, J. L., Sakr, Y., Sprung, C. L. *et al.* (2006) Sepsis in European intensive care units: results of the SOAP study. *Crit Care Med* 34: 344-353.

Vlahakis, N. E., Schroeder, M. A., Limper, A. H. *et al.* (1999) Stretch induces cytokine release by alveolar epithelial cells in vitro. *Am J Physiol* 277: L167-L173.

Vreugdenhil, H. A., Heijnen, C. J., Plotz, F. B. *et al.* (2004) Mechanical ventilation of healthy rats suppresses peripheral immune function. *Eur Respir J* 23: 122-128.

Ware, L. B. & Matthay, M. A. (2000) The acute respiratory distress syndrome. *N Engl J Med* 342: 1334-1349.

Webb, H. H. & Tierney, D. F. (1974) Experimental pulmonary edema due to intermittent positive pressure ventilation with high inflation pressures. Protection by positive end-expiratory pressure. *Am Rev Respir Dis* 110: 556-565.

Weibel, E.R. (1984). The Pathway for Oxygen: Structure and Function in the Mammalian Respiratory System. In: *Harvard Univ.Press*. Cambridge, MA, 425.

Weinstein, S. P., Paquin, T., Pritsker, A. *et al.* (1995) Glucocorticoid-induced insulin resistance: dexamethasone inhibits the activation of glucose transport in rat skeletal muscle by both insulin- and non-insulin-related stimuli. *Diabetes* 44: 441-445.

Weppler, A. & Issekutz, A. C. (2008) Alveolar epithelium down-modulates endotoxin-but not tumor necrosis factor alpha-induced activation of endothelium and selectively inhibits neutrophil transendothelial migration. *Exp Lung Res* 34: 425-453.

West, J. B., Tsukimoto, K., Mathieu-Costello, O. *et al.* (1991) Stress failure in pulmonary capillaries. *J Appl Physiol* 70: 1731-1742.

Whalen, M. J., Doughty, L. A., Carlos, T. M. *et al.* (2000) Intercellular adhesion molecule-1 and vascular cell adhesion molecule-1 are increased in the plasma of children with sepsis-induced multiple organ failure. *Crit Care Med* 28: 2600-2607.

Wilson, M. R., Choudhury, S., Goddard, M. E. *et al.* (2003) High tidal volume upregulates intrapulmonary cytokines in an in vivo mouse model of ventilator-induced lung injury. *J Appl Physiol* 95: 1385-1393.

Wilson, M. R., Choudhury, S. & Takata, M. (2005) Pulmonary inflammation induced by high-stretch ventilation is mediated by tumor necrosis factor signaling in mice. *Am J Physiol Lung Cell Mol Physiol* 288: L599-L607.

Witzenbichler, B., Westermann, D., Knueppel, S. *et al.* (2005) Protective role of angiopoietin-1 in endotoxic shock. *Circulation* 111: 97-105.

Wojciak-Stothard, B., Entwistle, A., Garg, R. *et al.* (1998) Regulation of TNF-alpha-induced reorganization of the actin cytoskeleton and cell-cell junctions by Rho, Rac, and Cdc42 in human endothelial cells. *J Cell Physiol* 176: 150-165.

Wojciak-Stothard, B. & Ridley, A. J. (2002) Rho GTPases and the regulation of endothelial permeability. *Vascul Pharmacol* 39: 187-199.

Wolthuis, E. K., Vlaar, A. P., Choi, G. *et al.* (2009a) Recombinant human soluble tumor necrosis factor-alpha receptor fusion protein partly attenuates ventilator-induced lung injury. *Shock* 31: 262-266.

Wolthuis, E. K., Vlaar, A. P., Choi, G. *et al.* (2009b) Mechanical ventilation using non-injurious ventilation settings causes lung injury in the absence of pre-existing lung injury in healthy mice. *Crit Care* 13: R1.

Xu, J., Qu, J., Cao, L. *et al.* (2008) Mesenchymal stem cell-based angiopoietin-1 gene therapy for acute lung injury induced by lipopolysaccharide in mice. *J Pathol* 214: 472-481.

Xu, J., Woods, C. R., Mora, A. L. *et al.* (2007) Prevention of endotoxin-induced systemic response by bone marrow-derived mesenchymal stem cells in mice. *Am J Physiol Lung Cell Mol Physiol* 293: L131-L141.

You, Z., Savitz, S. I., Yang, J. *et al.* (2008) Necrostatin-1 reduces histopathology and improves functional outcome after controlled cortical impact in mice. *J Cereb Blood Flow Metab* 28: 1564-1573.

Zamzami, N. & Kroemer, G. (2003) Apoptosis: mitochondrial membrane permeabilization--the (w)hole story? *Curr Biol* 13: R71-R73.

Zhang, D. W., Shao, J., Lin, J. *et al.* (2009a) RIP3, an energy metabolism regulator that switches TNF-induced cell death from apoptosis to necrosis. *Science* 325: 332-336.

Zhang, Z., Larner, S. F., Liu, M. C. *et al.* (2009b) Multiple alphaII-spectrin breakdown products distinguish calpain and caspase dominated necrotic and apoptotic cell death pathways. *Apoptosis* 14: 1289-1298.

19

Optimizing Perioperative Ventilation Support with Adequate Settings of Positive End-Expiratory Pressure

Zhanqi Zhao[1], Claudius Stahl[2], Ullrich Müller-Lisse[3],
Inéz Frerichs[4] and Knut Möller[1]
[1]*Department of Biomedical Engineering, Furtwangen University,*
[2]*Department of Anesthesiology, University Medical Center of Freiburg,*
[3]*Department of Radiology, University of Munich,*
[4]*Department of Anesthesiology and Intensive Care Medicine,*
University Medical Center of Schleswig-Holstein Campus Kiel,
Germany

1. Introduction

1.1 Mechanical ventilation

Mechanical ventilation is often employed to replace spontaneous breathing of patients under general anesthesia. Even after operation, the patient still needs ventilation support until the respiratory muscles regain full function. A ventilator delivers a certain amount of air flow through a facial mask or tracheal tube to the patient whose respiratory system fails to function properly due to the effects of anesthetics or diseases. Based on the difference in breath initiation, mechanical ventilation can be divided into two categories: controlled ventilation and assisted ventilation. In this chapter, we focus on controlled mechanical ventilation, under which the patient is not able to trigger a valid breath and the ventilator overtakes all the workload of respiratory muscles. Respiratory parameters such as respiratory rate (RR), inspiratory–to-expiratory time ratio (I:E), tidal volume (V_t) (or minute volume) are controlled by the ventilator.

Traditionally, controlled mechanical ventilation can either be volume controlled (VCV) or pressure controlled (PCV). Ideal respiratory signals obtained in a healthy human during VCV and PCV are shown in Fig. 1. In the VCV mode, a patient receives constant flow from the ventilator until a preset V_t is reached. A severe drawback of VCV is missing control of the peak airway pressure. Airway pressure (P_{aw}) depends on respiratory system compliance and resistance. In patients with certain lung diseases, such as acute lung injury (ALI), the same setting of V_t as in patients with healthy lungs may lead to a higher peak P_{aw} with the potential to further injure the lung. Therefore, VCV is often applied with a pressure limitation. Once the peak P_{aw} rises above this limit, the ventilator will stop delivering gas even if the preset V_t is not yet reached. In the PCV mode, a maximum airway pressure (P_{max}) is defined. Inspiration ends when P_{max} is reached i.e. the flow driven by the pressure difference decreases to zero. PCV may be superior to VCV in patients requiring one-lung anesthesia (Tuğrul *et al.*, 1997). However, the V_t is not controlled by the ventilator in the PCV mode, but determined by the preset maximum pressure and respiratory system mechanics. There is no guarantee that sufficient gas will be delivered into the lung. Hence, V_t and minute volume that the patient receives must be monitored. In reality, the respiratory signals measured by the ventilator do not look exactly like the ideal tracings shown in Fig. 1. Signals are subjected to various error sources, such as environmental noise, sense dysfunction, and calibration failure and they also depend on individual physiological or pathophysiological properties of the patient's respiratory system.

Respiratory signal analysis is helpful for the clinician and beneficial to the patient. Lung diseases influence tidal ventilation, which is reflected in the P_{aw}, air flow and respiratory volume signals. Based on a shape analysis of respiratory signals, clinical diagnosis can be supported. For example, the flow-volume curve of a patient with cystic fibrosis during forced respiration, measured by body plethysmography, is plotted in Fig. 2. Low expiratory flow rates compared to the normal values at 75%, 50% and 25% of volume capacity indicate airway obstruction in this patient.

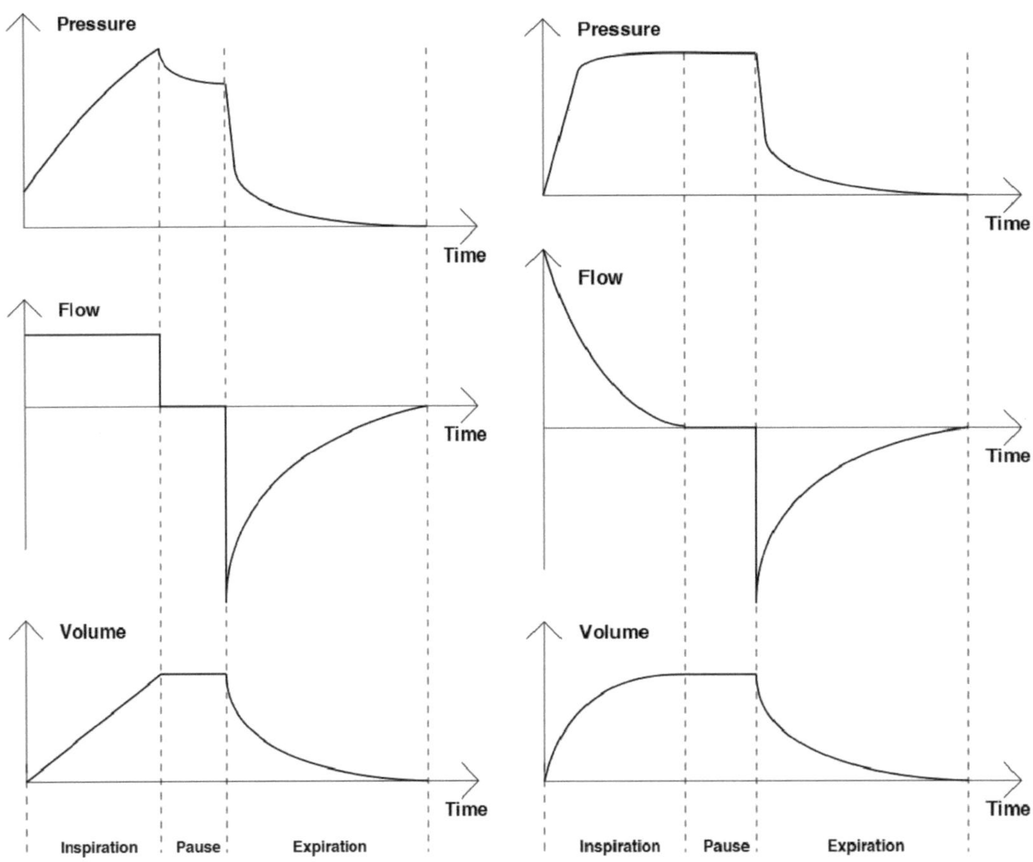

Fig. 1. Ideal respiratory signals (airway pressure, air flow and respiratory volume) of a healthy human under volume controlled (left) and pressure controlled (right) ventilation mode.

To better understand the respiratory system, many mathematical models were proposed (Gillis and Lutchen, 1999, Lutchen and Costa, 1990). The simplest one is based on the first order equation of motion:

$$P_{aw}(t) = V(t) / C_{rs} + V'(t) \times R_{rs} + P_0 \tag{1}$$

where P_{aw}, V and V' denote airway pressure, volume and airway flow, C_{rs} and R_{rs} represent respiratory system compliance and resistance, respectively; P_0 is the pre-existing pressure in the lung. With the measured respiratory signals, lung mechanics (C_{rs} and R_{rs}) can be calculated. These measures provide a better insight into the lung status and thereby help the physicians to establish diagnosis and make adequate therapeutical decisions.

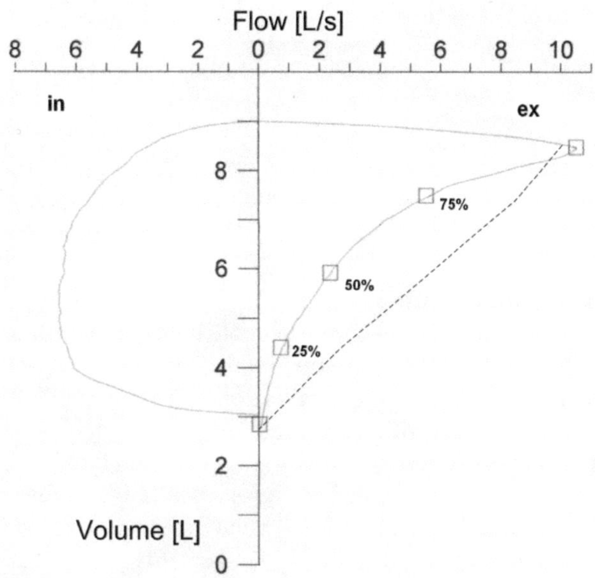

Fig. 2. Flow-volume curve of a patient with cystic fibrosis during forced respiration. The inspiration phase is depicted on the left side and expiration on the right side of the vertical axis. Rectangle points indicate maximal expiratory flow, expiratory flow at 75%, 50%, 25% of vital capacity and the end of expiration, from top to bottom respectively. The dashed-line shows the normal reference of expiratory flow rate with respect to this patient's age, height and weight.

At different locations i.e. the airway opening, the trachea or at the alveoli, pressure measurements are of interest. If the patient is intubated, tracheal pressure (P_{trach}) is sometimes more desired than P_{aw} since the endotracheal tube contributes significantly to total airflow resistance, and thus affects the R_{rs} calculation (Guttmann *et al.*, 1993). Alveolar pressure (P_{alv}) is a decisive factor of alveolar recruitment/derecruitment. P_{alv} is usually calculated by subtracting total resistive pressure from P_{aw} or P_{trach}. Typical examples of different pressure-volume curves based on P_{aw}, P_{trach} and P_{alv} are plotted in Fig. 3. Note that at the start of inspiration and expiration, the signals are disturbed due to the non-ideal mechanics of the ventilator.

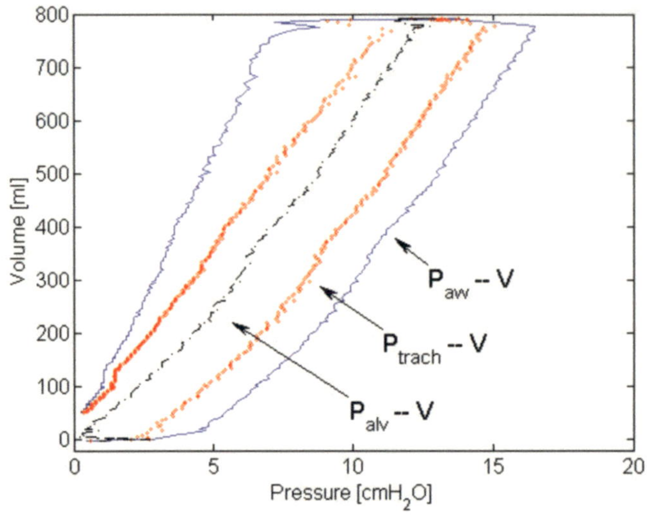

Fig. 3. Three pressure-volume curves obtained in a lung healthy patient undergoing orthopedic surgery. P_{aw} (blue line): airway pressure; P_{trach} (red circle): tracheal pressure; P_{alv} (black dashed line): alveolar pressure.

1.2 Lung protective ventilation strategy

When patients are generally anesthetized, the alveoli in the dependent lung regions may collapse while non-dependent regions remain open. With the help of sufficient external pressure delivered by a ventilator during inspiration, some of the collapsed lung regions may be opened up (i.e. they are recruited) but already open regions may be overinflated. Neither atelectasis nor hyperinflation of lung regions is beneficial in most clinical cases, however, one or the other or a mixture of both processes is inevitable to a certain degree. During expiration, while gas is exhaled, the alveolar pressure drops, which may lead to alveolar collapse (i.e. derecruitment) of the dependent lung regions. Different types of ventilator-induced lung injury (VILI) are therefore observed during mechanical ventilation (Dreyfuss and Saumon, 1998, Uhlig and Frerichs, 2008), such as shear stress trauma caused by cyclic recruitment/derecruitment, barotrauma and pulmonary edema caused by high ventilation pressure. As one of many perioperative complications, acute respiratory distress syndrome (ARDS) was found developed in 3.1% of patients after thoracic surgery and carrying a high mortality rate of over 30% (Grichnik and D'Amico, 2004, Phua *et at.*, 2009). Various lung protective ventilation strategies have therefore been proposed, including high positive end-expiratory pressure (PEEP) combined with low V_t (Brower *et al.*, 2004, Brochard *et al.*, 1998, The Acute Respiratory Distress Syndrome Network, 2000), permissive hypercapnia (Hickling *et al.*, 1990), and recruitment maneuvers (Lachmann, 1992), to reduce the adverse consequences of mechanical ventilation. In this chapter, we focus on optimization of PEEP.

PEEP was introduced to maintain the once recruited atelectatic areas open and thereby reduce the risk of hypoxemia, cyclic recruitment/derecruitment and biotrauma (Gattinoni *et al.*, 2001, Slutsky and Tremblay, 1998). Figure 4 illustrates the effect of PEEP on keeping the lung open. In healthy subjects, although the pulmonary alveoli increase their size at the end of inspiration and decrease at the end of expiration, the shape of alveoli doesn't change thanks to the pulmonary surfactant. However, in patients with lung injury or with other types of lung disease as well as during thoracic surgery, some alveoli collapse at the end of expiration when the pressure drops below a critical value, and reopen in the next inspiration when the pressure rises above a certain opening pressure. To avoid cyclic recruitment/derecruitment (open/collapse) and to "keep the lung open", an adequate PEEP is applied (Fig. 4B). At the end of expiration, P_{aw} doesn't drop to 0 cmH_2O (relative to atmospheric pressure). Instead, the pressure is held by the ventilator at a preselected positive level. The recruited lung regions remain aerated, which leads to a better oxygenation.

2. PEEP optimization

2.1 History

In 1960's, Ashbaugh *et al.* proposed the use of PEEP to improve oxygenation in a clinical syndrome characterized by atelectasis and hypoxemia (Ashbaugh *et al.*, 1967). The use of PEEP has become widespread ever since that study. Suter and his colleagues later published the concept of "optimal" PEEP (Suter *et al.*, 1975). Because at that time, cardiac output and blood gas measurements were not always available, they suggested that maximizing tidal compliance could be used to identify a PEEP level, at which oxygen delivery was optimized. In the past three decades, a multitude of physicians and scientists dedicated themselves to identify the best PEEP levels for patients under surgeries (Beiderlinden *et al.*, 2003, Berendes *et al.*, 1996, Bensenor *et al.*, 2007), as well as patients with variable diseases, such as ALI or ARDS (Badet *et al.*, 2009, Huh *et al.*, 2009), morbid obesity (Bohm *et al.*, 2009, Erlandsson *et al.*, 2006), chronic obstructive pulmonary disease (COPD) (Glerant *et al.*, 2005, Mancebo *et al.*, 2000), brain-injury (Shapiro and Marshall, 1978, Huynh *et al.*, 2002), including infants (Greenough *et al.*, 1992, Dimitriou *et al.*, 1999). Although different terminologies and end-points for optimizing PEEP were used (Villar, 2005), most of the approaches tried to obtain the best oxygenation while minimizing VILI as outcome. A lower mortality rate and a better quality of life would be the most desirable goals of therapies. While PEEP has experimentally been shown to reduce VILI, there is no consent in the literature if a suitable PEEP is able to reduce mortality (Miller *et al.*, 1992, DiRusso *et al.*, 1995, Brower *et al.*, 2004), due to the fact that the effect of PEEP is hard to be assessed independently.

It remains under debate how to titrate an adequate PEEP level in individual patients, despite the widely used application of PEEP in clinical practice (Rouby *et al.*, 2002). Increase of PEEP may prevent alveolar derecruitment in dependent areas but may lead to hyperinflation in the non-dependent areas, which may trigger pulmonary inflammation (Terragni *et al.*, 2007). Besides, high PEEP levels may reduce cardiac output (Baigorri *et al.*, 1994) and impair the hemodynamic stability (Herff *et al.*, 2008). Therefore, as also stated by Rouby and Brochard in an editorial (Rouby and Brochard, 2007), one goal of setting PEEP is to find a suitable level, high enough to keep the lung open while minimizing adverse side effects.

Generally speaking, the current available methods of PEEP titration can be mainly divided into three categories: They are based on 1) arterial blood gases such as partial pressure of oxygen in arterial blood (PaO_2) and oxygen saturation (SpO_2); 2) lung mechanics such as dynamic compliance and static pressure-volume (P/V) curve; 3) imaging techniques such as computed tomography (CT) and electrical impedance tomography (EIT). In the following, representative methods within these three categories are introduced and their assets and drawbacks discussed.

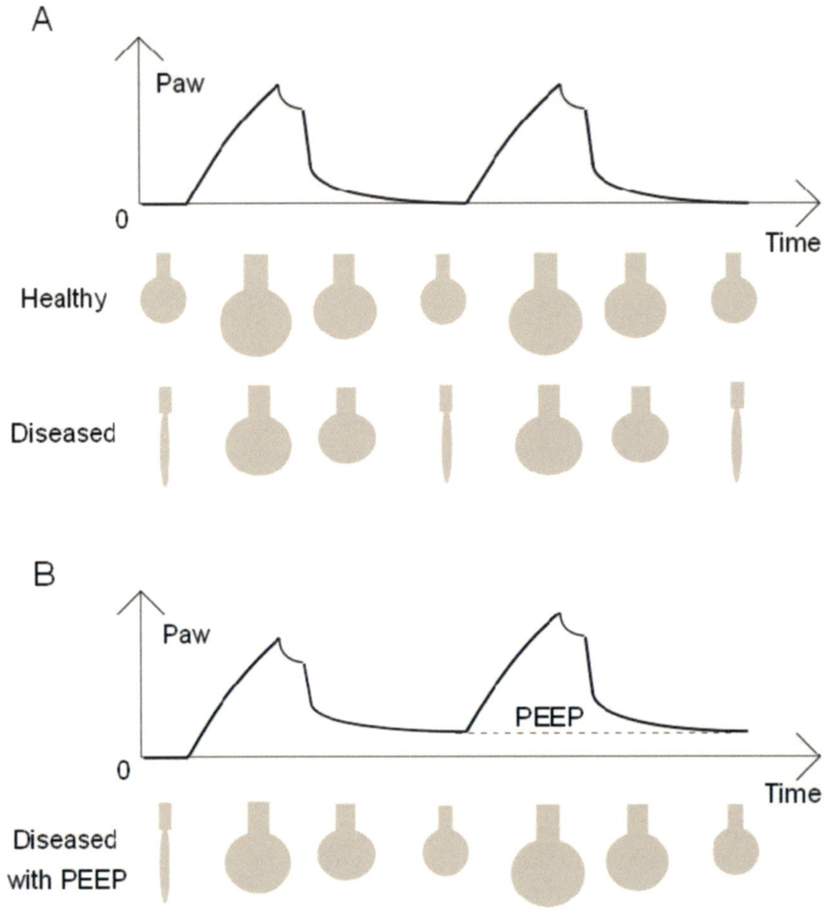

Fig. 4. The effect of positive end-expiratory pressure (PEEP) on keeping the alveoli open. A: Under controlled mechanical ventilation without PEEP, alveoli of a healthy subject stay open throughout the whole breathing cycle, while the alveoli of a patient with lung disease collapse at the end of expiration. B: When PEEP is applied, the recruited alveoli will no longer collapse at the end of expiration in a patient with lung disease.

2.2 Optimizing PEEP with blood gas analysis

One of the main goals of PEEP selection is to optimize oxygenation. Therefore, it is reasonable to guide the PEEP settings by analyzing blood gases (Girgis *et al.*, 2006, Borges *et al.*, 2006, Luecke *et al.*, 2005). It was suggested that "best" PaO_2 (maximum value) indicates the "optimal" PEEP in many studies (Borges *et al.*, 2006, Suarez-Sipmann *et al.*, 2007). Toth *et al.* suggested setting PEEP at the level where PaO_2 starts to drop rapidly during a decremental PEEP trial (Toth *et al.*, 2007). A typical course of PaO_2 values obtained during a decremental PEEP trial in an experimental model of ALI is shown in Fig. 5. PEEP decreased from 30 cmH_2O to 5 cmH_2O in steps of 5 cmH_2O. Decrease of PaO_2 implies worse aeration and oxygenation. Optimal PEEP is defined at the pressure level before PaO_2 decreases significantly.

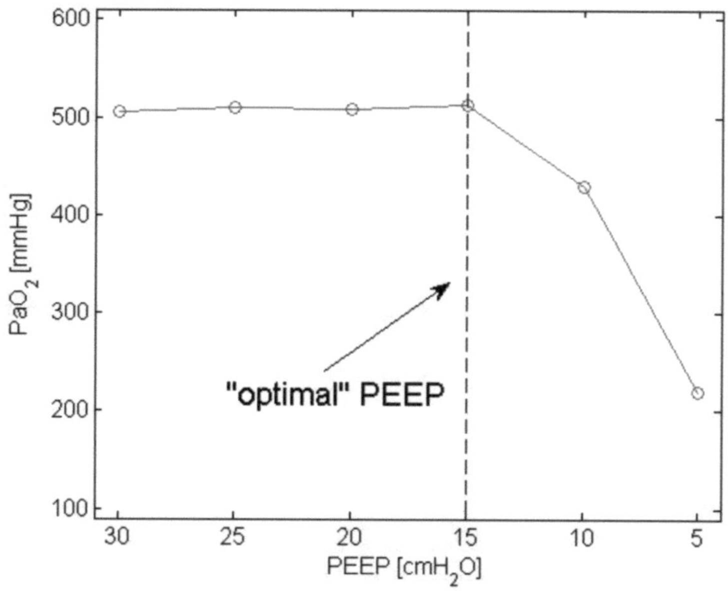

Fig. 5. Change of PaO_2 during a decremental PEEP trial in a porcine model of acute lung injury. Vertical dashed line indicates the optimal PEEP level with respect to PaO_2.

Luecke *et al.* argued that improving only PaO_2 was not good enough, the elevation of $PaCO_2$ should not be ignored (Luecke *et al.*, 2005). Girgis *et al.* have shown in twenty ALI/ARDS patients that the PaO_2/FiO_2 ratio was improved by tuning FiO_2 after a recruitment maneuver and monitoring the SpO_2 changes during decremental PEEP titration (Girgis *et al.*, 2006). SpO_2 values were measured by pulse oximetry, which is a noninvasive method, however, less precise than direct measurement of arterial oxygen saturation. Rouby concluded in a review that the highest PaO_2 and SaO_2 at the lowest FiO_2 indicated the right PEEP level (Rouby *et al.*, 2002). Caramez *et al.* have compared ten different parameters for setting PEEP following a recruitment maneuver, including blood gas analysis and lung mechanics (Caramez *et al.*, 2009). The results of PEEP selection using C_{rs}, PaO_2 with or without $PaCO_2$ were statistically indistinguishable (Caramez *et al.*, 2009). Statistically significant differences may have not been revealed due to the small number of studied subjects (n = 14) and high variation. Although these studies indicate that PaO_2 is a possible criterion for setting PEEP, precise blood gas analysis is invasive and discontinuous and, thus, not suitable for continuous bedside monitoring.

2.3 Optimizing PEEP with lung mechanics

The P/V curve has been introduced to individualize V_t and PEEP settings in patients with ARDS by Matamis *et al.* in 1984 (Matamis *et al.*, 1984). In this concept, a lower inflection point (LIP) and an upper inflection point (UIP) are identified on the inflation limb of the P/V curve (Fig. 6B). The LIP was considered to be the pressure level at which massive alveolar recruitment occurs (Jonson and Svantesson, 1999); UIP was considered to be the pressure level indicating alveolar overdistension (Roupie *et al.*, 1995). In consequence, a ventilation strategy was developed to keep the lung open (by setting PEEP above LIP) and to minimize overdistension (by restricting V_t such that peak pressure is smaller than UIP)

(Dambrosio *et al.*, 1997, Hermle *et al.*, 2002). Takeuchi *et al.* proposed that setting PEEP at LIP + 2 cmH_2O might be more appropriate (Takeuchi *et al.*, 2002). However, studies indicate that LIP is only the beginning of recruitment and the UIP is not a reliable marker of overdistension (Crotti *et al.*, 2001, Hickling, 2002, Downie *et al.*, 2004). New findings suggest that it may be better to set PEEP according to UIP on the deflation limb of the P/V curve (Albaiceta *et al.*, 2004). In order to obtain quasi-static P/V curves, the normal ventilation process has to be interrupted by performing a specific respiratory maneuver such as low-flow inflation (Servillo *et al.*, 1997), super-syringe inflation (Matamis *et al.*, 1984) or SCASS, i.e. static compliance by automated single steps (Sydow *et al.*, 1991), (Fig. 6A). As pointed out by LaFollette *et al.*, the key to bedside application is acquiring a dynamic curve, which is easier and more applicable, instead of a static one (LaFollette *et al.*, 2007).
Respiratory system compliance C_{rs} or elastance E_{rs} (C_{rs}=1/E_{rs}) can be measured quasi-statically by airway occlusion (D'Angelo *et al.*, 1991) or dynamically by applying linear least-squares regression on the first order equation of motion (Eq. 1) (Iotti *et al.*, 1995). Considering the limitation of static C_{rs} (Stenqvist *et al.*, 2008) and the significant difference between static and dynamic C_{rs} (Stahl *et al.*, 2006), it is the dynamic lung mechanics that should be monitored. Many studies have shown that "optimal" PEEP may be obtained by identifying maximal dynamic C_{rs}, or minimal E_{rs} (Fig. 7) (Suter *et al.*, 1975, Carvalho *et al.*, 2008, Stahl *et al.*, 2006). Hickling demonstrated with a mathematical model of an ARDS lung that maximizing C_{rs} during a decremental PEEP trial may be more suitable to indicate the "optimal" PEEP (Hickling, 2001). Several studies support this result (Suarez-Sipmann *et al.*, 2007, Hanson *et al.*, 2009).

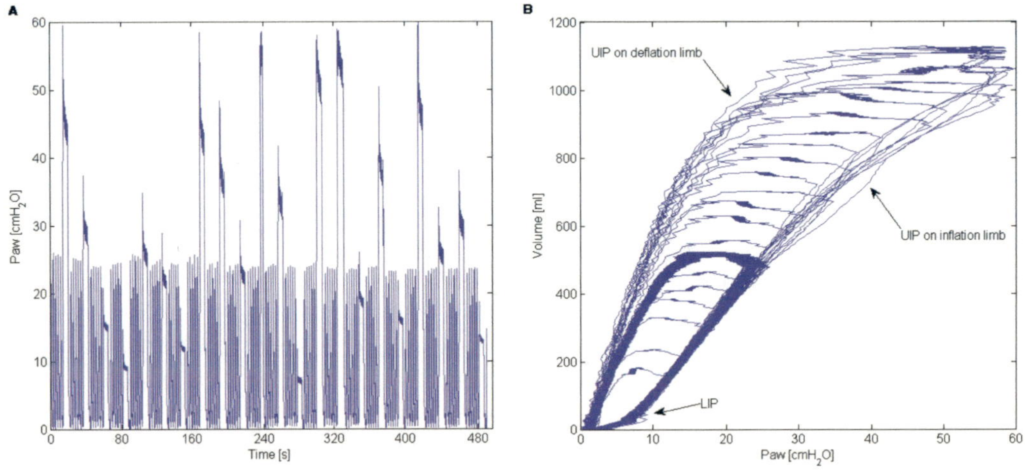

Fig. 6. A: Airway pressure (P_{aw}) of an ARDS patient during the SCASS maneuver to determine static compliance by automated single steps (Sydow *et al.*, 1991) and B: the corresponding P/V curves with lower inflection point (LIP) and upper inflection point (UIP) marked on both inflation and deflation limbs.

Methods other than P/V curve and maximum dynamic compliance are rarely used in clinical practice. Mols *et al.* suggested that the intra-tidal compliance-volume curve, calculated by the SLICE method (Guttmann *et al.*, 1994), was able to indicate the ongoing recruitment and overdistension of alveoli in the lung (Mols *et al.*, 1999). The shapes of the

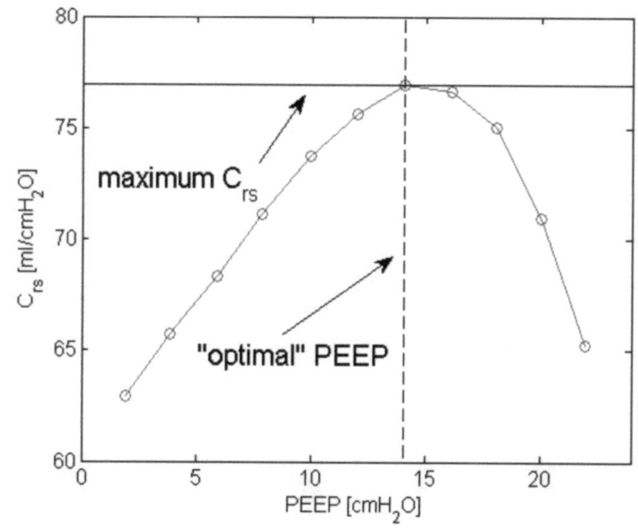

Fig. 7. Mean dynamic respiratory system compliances (C_{rs}) of a sedated patient under mechanical ventilation at different PEEP levels. Dashed line indicates the "optimal" PEEP level, at which C_{rs} is maximum.

compliance-volume curves are classified into three categories: 1) a decrease in slope indicates overdistension; 2) an increase in slope indicates recruitment; 3) a quasi-horizontal compliance-volume curve indicates a suitable PEEP setting (Mols *et al.*, 1999). However, the method has not yet been evaluated for clinical relevance. Ranieri *et al.* used the pressure-time curve as an index to predict pulmonary stress (Ranieri *et al.*, 2000). This method requires phases with constant air flow which limits its applicability. Nevertheless, these methods have brought the importance of pulmonary mechanical stress into focus. Talmor *et al.* estimated the transpulmonary pressure with help of esophageal balloon catheters and set PEEP to such a level that transpulmonary pressure stayed between 0 and 10 cmH_2O during end-expiratory occlusion, and less than 25 cmH_2O during end-inspiratory occlusion (Talmor *et al.*, 2008). They observed improvement of PaO_2/FiO_2 ratio and C_{rs} compared to the group guided according to the ARDS network standard-of-care recommendations. This finding is interesting, but the placement of esophageal balloon catheters needs additional effort in clinical care. Therefore, this method will only become accepted if advantages over other methods using C_{rs} and blood gas analysis are outweighing the extra burden of complex handling.

2.4 Optimizing PEEP with imaging techniques

CT has a very good spatial resolution and is able to show the distribution of the tissue density in the chest, thereby providing primarily morphological data. Hence, CT is the gold standard for assessment of tidal volume distribution in injured lungs and many validation studies were done by comparing various methods with the CT results (Gattinoni *et al.*, 2006, Carvalho *et al.*, 2008, Suarez-Sipmann *et al.*, 2007, Meier *et al.*, 2008). Figure 8 shows two chest CT images of a patient under mechanical ventilation at two different PEEP levels. Higher aeration and reversal of lung collapse in the dependent lung regions were detected at a PEEP level of 15 cmH_2O (Fig. 8, right) compared to that of 5 cmH_2O (Fig. 8, left).

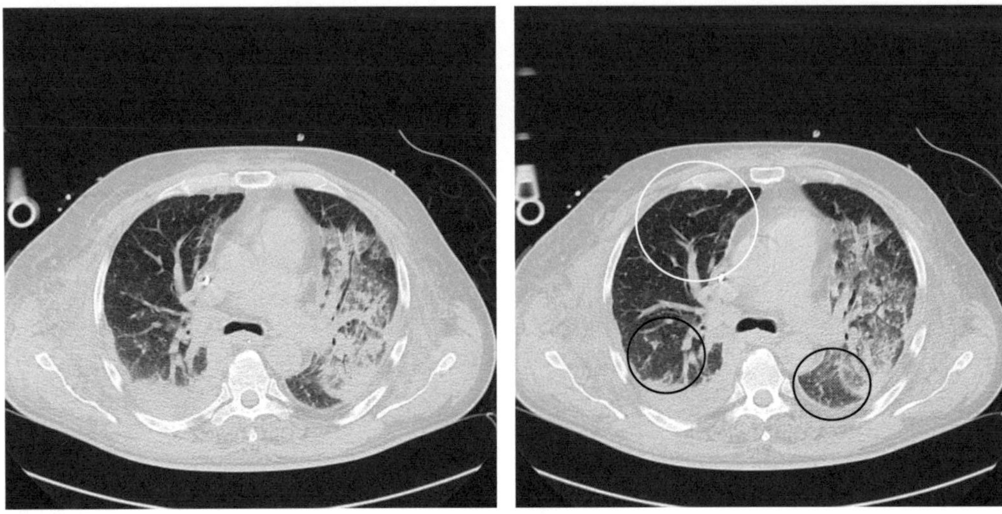

Fig. 8. CT images of a patient under mechanical ventilation at two different PEEP levels. Left: PEEP=5 cmH_2O; Right: PEEP=15 cmH_2O. Pneumonic infiltrates in the left lung and intrapleural fluid accumulation are discernible. Lung aeration is increased, e.g. in the anterior region of the right lung (white circle) and dependent lung regions are recruited (black circles) at the higher PEEP level.

Unfortunately, application of CT imaging for bedside monitoring is limited due to complex handling (e.g. large equipment) and radiation exposure of patients. Hertzog *et al.* have reported a case study using mobile CT scanners to optimize PEEP in a 6-month-old premature infant (Hertzog *et al.*, 2001). However, even with the development of low-dose CT, radiation exposure makes it practically impossible to use CT to guide PEEP titration at the bedside.

In contrast to CT, the relatively new imaging technique, electrical impedance tomography (EIT) is noninvasive and radiation-free. EIT utilizes the phenomenon that changes in regional air content modify electrical impedance of lung tissue (Nopp *et al.*, 1993). Small alternating electrical currents are applied at the chest wall surface during examination and the resultant potential differences are measured. The distribution of electrical impedance within the chest can be determined from these data. Although EIT has a relatively low resolution, it has the potential to monitor regional lung aeration and to visualize regional ventilation distribution dynamically at the bedside (Zhao *et al.*, 2010). Thus, EIT may provide additional information to individualize protective ventilation strategies by titrating PEEP.

Several applications of EIT for selecting PEEP were recently proposed. Erlandsson and colleagues used EIT to set PEEP in morbidly obese patients by maintaining a stable end-expiratory lung volume, and suggested that the corresponding PEEP level was optimal (Erlandsson *et al.*, 2006). Although the PaO_2/FiO_2 ratio and C_{rs} increased in these patients, this "optimal" PEEP need not be the best oxygenation point. Besides, the identification of stable, horizontal end-expiratory EIT values may be difficult. Luepschen and colleagues modified the centre of gravity index from Frerichs *et al.* (Frerichs *et al.*, 1998) to evaluate functional lung opening and overdistension of the lung tissue in an animal model of lavage-induced acute lung injury (Luepschen *et al.*, 2007). Dargaville *et al.* have applied EIT during an incremental and decremental PEEP trial to identify the PEEP level at which the most homogeneous distribution of regional C_{rs} and ventilation was observed in healthy, injured and surfactant-treated lungs (Dargaville *et al.*, 2010). Zhao and colleagues applied the global inhomogeneity (GI) index (Zhao *et al.*, 2009) to facilitate the PEEP titration in mechanically ventilated patients undergoing orthopedic surgery (Zhao *et al.*, 2010) (Fig. 9). Lowhagen et al proposed the assessment of intratidal ventilation distribution using EIT to identify optimal PEEP level in patients with ALI/ARDS (Lowhagen *et al.*, 2010). These results are promising but they still need to be confirmed in further larger studies on lung injured patients. Other EIT-based methods assessing regional lung filling characteristics (Grant *et al.*, 2009, Hinz *et al.*, 2007) have also shown potential to guide PEEP setting. As stated by Dueck in a review article, EIT is helpful in achieving the balance between alveolar recruitment and hyperinflation for patients with severe lung injury (Dueck, 2006). Although the use of EIT is limited to scientific research and clinical experiments, EIT has the potential to gain acceptance from more physicians and become a useful tool in clinical routine in the future.

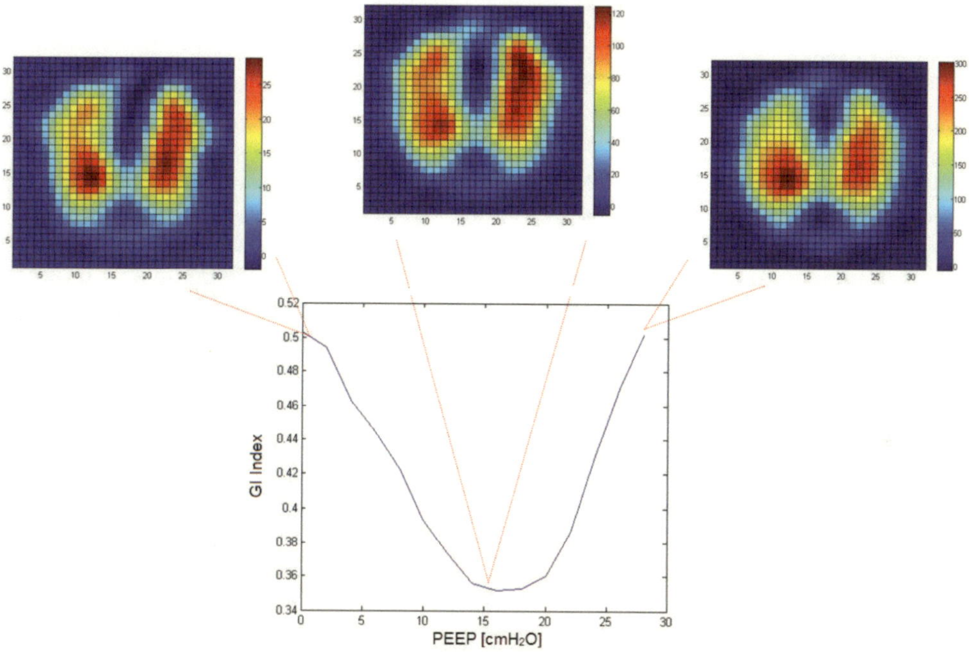

Fig. 9. PEEP titration guided by ventilation homogeneity based on electrical impedance tomography (EIT) (Zhao *et al.*, 2010). Top: EIT images at different PEEP levels (from left to right: PEEP = 0, 15, 28 cmH_2O). The color bars at the right side of each image indicate the magnitude of change in relative impedance during ventilation. Lung regions with the highest ventilation are coded in red. Bottom: global inhomogeneity (GI) index (Zhao *et al.*, 2009) versus PEEP. The minimum value of GI index implies the PEEP level at which ventilation distribution is most homogeneous.

2.5 Combination of PEEP setting indices

Individualized PEEP titration is important, especially in patients with severe lung injury (Kallet and Branson, 2007). Methods discussed in this chapter focused on different aspects: C_{rs} and P/V curves represent the global mechanical properties of the respiratory system;

blood gas analysis provides a direct view on the oxygenation status; CT and EIT evaluate the local ventilation distribution. Obviously, it is rational to combine these different variables to guide PEEP titration. We suggest selecting PEEP according to a weighted combination of C_{rs}, GI index (EIT analysis) and SpO_2 (or PaO_2) to include all available information on the patient's lung status. The disease state of the patient and strategic treatment goals may lead to different weighted combinations. A practical way to define these weighting factors is still warrant and should be achieved in the future with further studies.
Besides, ventilator settings, such as tidal volume (Suter *et al.*, 1978) and inspired oxygen concentration (FiO_2) (Rouby *et al.*, 2002) may strongly influence the "optimal" level of PEEP. The National Institutes of Health's ARDS Network has developed a recommendation in form of a PEEP/FiO_2 titration table to adjust these variables (Brower *et al.*, 2004). As mentioned before, lung protective ventilation strategies are more than just PEEP optimization. The patients will also benefit from adequate tidal volumes and body positioning which may additionally limit hyperinflation and reduce the amount of non-aerated lung tissue.

3. Summary

Perioperative ventilation support is indispensable for patients under thoracic surgery. Inadequate settings of ventilation support may cause a number of problems, including hypoxemia, shear stress trauma, barotraumas and pulmonary edema. A suitable PEEP level maintains dependent lung regions open and thereby improves oxygenation and reduces the risk of inflammation. The selection of optimal PEEP is still under debate. We propose to combine indices of lung mechanics, blood gas analysis and imaging techniques to titrate PEEP. Besides, application of PEEP should be complemented with other strategies (e.g. low tidal volume, appropriate body positioning, recruitment maneuver), to achieve the best outcome of the patient.

4. Acknowledgment

This review was developed within the project MOTiF-A supported by a grant (1781X08) of the German Research and Development Department (BMBF), and the project PAR supported by a grant (MO 579/1-2) of the German Research Foundation (DFG).

5. References

Albaiceta, G. M., Taboada, F., Parra, D., Luyando, L. H., Calvo, J., Menendez, R. & Otero, J. (2004). Tomographic study of the inflection points of the pressure-volume curve in acute lung injury. *Am J Respir Crit Care Med,* 170, pp. 1066-72.

Ashbaugh, D. G., Bigelow, D. B., Petty, T. L. & Levine, B. E. (1967). Acute respiratory distress in adults. *Lancet,* 2, 319-23.

Badet, M., Bayle, F., Richard, J. C. & Guerin, C. (2009). Comparison of optimal positive end-expiratory pressure and recruitment maneuvers during lung-protective mechanical ventilation in patients with acute lung injury/acute respiratory distress syndrome. *Respir Care,* 54, pp. 847-54.

Baigorri, F., De Monte, A., Blanch, L., Fernandez, R., Valles, J., Mestre, J., Saura, P. & Artigas, A. (1994). Hemodynamic responses to external counterbalancing of auto-positive end-expiratory pressure in mechanically ventilated patients with chronic obstructive pulmonary disease. *Crit Care Med,* 22, pp. 1782-91.

Beiderlinden, M., Groeben, H. & Peters, J. (2003). Safety of percutaneous dilational tracheostomy in patients ventilated with high positive end-expiratory pressure (PEEP). *Intensive Care Med,* 29, pp. 944-8.

Bensenor, F. E., Vieira, J. E. & Auler Junior, J. O. (2007). Thoracic sympathetic block reduces respiratory system compliance. *Sao Paulo Med J,* 125, pp. 9-14.

Berendes, E., Lippert, G., Loick, H. M. & Brussel, T. (1996). Effects of positive end-expiratory pressure ventilation on splanchnic oxygenation in humans. *J Cardiothorac Vasc Anesth,* 10, pp. 598-602.

Bohm, S. H., Maisch, S., Von Sandersleben, A., Thamm, O., Passoni, I., Martinez Arca, J. & Tusman, G. (2009). The effects of lung recruitment on the Phase III slope of volumetric capnography in morbidly obese patients. *Anesth Analg,* 109, pp. 151-9.

Borges, J. B., Okamoto, V. N., Matos, G. F., Caramez, M. P., Arantes, P. R., Barros, F., Souza, C. E., Victorino, J. A., Kacmarek, R. M., Barbas, C. S., Carvalho, C. R. & Amato, M. B. (2006). Reversibility of lung collapse and hypoxemia in early acute respiratory distress syndrome. *Am J Respir Crit Care Med,* 174, pp. 268-78.

Brochard, L., Roudot-Thoraval, F., Roupie, E., Delclaux, C., Chastre, J., Fernandez-Mondejar, E., Clementi, E., Mancebo, J., Factor, P., Matamis, D., Ranieri, M., Blanch, L., Rodi, G., Mentec, H., Dreyfuss, D., Ferrer, M., Brun-Buisson, C., Tobin, M. & Lemaire, F. (1998). Tidal volume reduction for prevention of ventilator-induced lung injury in acute respiratory distress syndrome. The Multicenter Trail Group on Tidal Volume reduction in ARDS. *Am J Respir Crit Care Med,* 158, pp. 1831-8.

Brower, R. G., Lanken, P. N., Macintyre, N., Matthay, M. A., Morris, A., Ancukiewicz, M., Schoenfeld, D. & Thompson, B. T. (2004). Higher versus lower positive end-expiratory pressures in patients with the acute respiratory distress syndrome. *N Engl J Med,* 351, pp. 327-36.

Caramez, M. P., Kacmarek, R. M., Helmy, M., Miyoshi, E., Malhotra, A., Amato, M. B. & Harris, R. S. (2009). A comparison of methods to identify open-lung PEEP. *Intensive Care Med,* 35, pp. 740-7.

Carvalho, A. R., Spieth, P. M., Pelosi, P., Vidal Melo, M. F., Koch, T., Jandre, F. C., Giannella-Neto, A. & De Abreu, M. G. (2008). Ability of dynamic airway pressure curve profile and elastance for positive end-expiratory pressure titration. *Intensive Care Med,* 34, pp. 2291-9.

Crotti, S., Mascheroni, D., Caironi, P., Pelosi, P., Ronzoni, G., Mondino, M., Marini, J. J. & Gattinoni, L. (2001). Recruitment and derecruitment during acute respiratory failure: a clinical study. *Am J Respir Crit Care Med,* 164, pp. 131-40.

D'angelo, E., Robatto, F. M., Calderini, E., Tavola, M., Bono, D., Torri, G. & Milic-Emili, J. (1991). Pulmonary and chest wall mechanics in anesthetized paralyzed humans. *J Appl Physiol,* 70, pp. 2602-10.

Dambrosio, M., Roupie, E., Mollet, J. J., Anglade, M. C., Vasile, N., Lemaire, F. & Brochard, L. (1997). Effects of positive end-expiratory pressure and different tidal volumes on alveolar recruitment and hyperinflation. *Anesthesiology,* 87, pp. 495-503.

Dargaville, P. A., Rimensberger, P. C. & Frerichs, I. (2010). Regional tidal ventilation and compliance during a stepwise vital capacity manoeuvre. *Intensive Care Med,* 36, pp. 1953-61.

Dimitriou, G., Greenough, A. & Laubscher, B. (1999). Appropriate positive end expiratory pressure level in surfactant-treated preterm infants. *Eur J Pediatr,* 158, pp. 888-91.

Dirusso, S. M., Nelson, L. D., Safcsak, K. & Miller, R. S. (1995). Survival in patients with severe adult respiratory distress syndrome treated with high-level positive end-expiratory pressure. *Crit Care Med,* 23, pp. 1485-96.

Downie, J. M., Nam, A. J. & Simon, B. A. (2004). Pressure-volume curve does not predict steady-state lung volume in canine lavage lung injury. *Am J Respir Crit Care Med,* 169, pp. 957-62.

Dreyfuss, D. & Saumon, G. (1998). Ventilator-induced lung injury: lessons from experimental studies. *Am J Respir Crit Care Med,* 157, pp. 294-323.

Dueck, R. (2006). Alveolar recruitment versus hyperinflation: A balancing act. *Curr Opin Anaesthesiol,* 19, pp. 650-4.

Erlandsson, K., Odenstedt, H., Lundin, S. & Stenqvist, O. (2006). Positive end-expiratory pressure optimization using electric impedance tomography in morbidly obese patients during laparoscopic gastric bypass surgery. *Acta Anaesthesiol Scand,* 50, pp. 833-9.

Frerichs, I., Hahn, G., Golisch, W., Kurpitz, M., Burchardi, H. & Hellige, G. (1998). Monitoring perioperative changes in distribution of pulmonary ventilation by functional electrical impedance tomography. *Acta Anaesthesiol Scand,* 42, pp. 721-6.

Gattinoni, L., Caironi, P., Pelosi, P. & Goodman, L. R. (2001). What has computed tomography taught us about the acute respiratory distress syndrome? *Am J Respir Crit Care Med,* 164, pp. 1701-11.

Gattinoni, L., Caironi, P., Valenza, F. & Carlesso, E. (2006). The role of CT-scan studies for the diagnosis and therapy of acute respiratory distress syndrome. *Clin Chest Med,* 27, pp. 559-70; abstract vii.

Gillis, H. L. & Lutchen, K. R. (1999). How heterogeneous bronchoconstriction affects ventilation distribution in human lungs: a morphometric model. *Ann Biomed Eng,* 27, pp. 14-22.

Girgis, K., Hamed, H., Khater, Y. & Kacmarek, R. M. (2006). A decremental PEEP trial identifies the PEEP level that maintains oxygenation after lung recruitment. *Respir Care,* 51, pp. 1132-9.

Glerant, J. C., Leleu, O., Rose, D., Mayeux, I. & Jounieaux, V. (2005). Oxygen consumption and PEEPe in ventilated COPD patients. *Respir Physiol Neurobiol,* 146, pp. 117-24.

Grant, C. A., Fraser, J. F., Dunster, K. R. & Schibler, A. (2009). The assessment of regional lung mechanics with electrical impedance tomography: a pilot study during recruitment manoeuvres. *Intensive Care Med,* 35, pp. 166-70.

Greenough, A., Chan, V. & Hird, M. F. (1992). Positive end expiratory pressure in acute and chronic respiratory distress. *Arch Dis Child,* 67, pp. 320-3.

Grichnik, K. P. & D'Amico, T. A. (2004). Acute lung injury and acute respiratory distress syndrome after pulmonary resection. *Semin Cardiothorac Vasc Anesth,* 8, pp. 317-34.

Guttmann, J., Eberhard, L., Fabry, B., Bertschmann, W. & Wolff, G. (1993). Continuous calculation of intratracheal pressure in tracheally intubated patients. *Anesthesiology,* 79, pp. 503-13.

Guttmann, J., Eberhard, L., Fabry, B., Zappe, D., Bernhard, H., Lichtwarck-Aschoff, M., Adolph, M. & Wolff, G. (1994). Determination of volume-dependent respiratory system mechanics in mechanically ventilated patients using the new SLICE method. *Technol Health Care,* 2, pp. 175-191.

Hanson, A., Gothberg, S., Nilsson, K., Larsson, L. E. & Hedenstierna, G. (2009). VTCO2 and dynamic compliance-guided lung recruitment in surfactant-depleted piglets: a computed tomography study. *Pediatr Crit Care Med,* 10, pp. 687-92.

Herff, H., Paal, P., Von Goedecke, A., Lindner, K. H., Severing, A. C. & Wenzel, V. (2008). Influence of ventilation strategies on survival in severe controlled hemorrhagic shock. *Crit Care Med,* 36, pp. 2613-20.

Hermle, G., Mols, G., Zugel, A., Benzing, A., Lichtwarck-Aschoff, M., Geiger, K. & Guttmann, J. (2002). Intratidal compliance-volume curve as an alternative basis to adjust positive end-expiratory pressure: a study in isolated perfused rabbit lungs. *Crit Care Med,* 30, pp. 1589-97.

Hertzog, J. H., Cartie, R. J., Hauser, G. J., Dalton, H. J. & Cleary, K. (2001). The use of a mobile computed tomography scanner in the pediatric intensive care unit to evaluate airway stenting and lung volumes with varying levels of positive end-expiratory pressure. *Pediatr Crit Care Med,* 2, pp. 346-8.

Hickling, K. G. (2001). Best compliance during a decremental, but not incremental, positive end-expiratory pressure trial is related to open-lung positive end-expiratory pressure: a mathematical model of acute respiratory distress syndrome lungs. *Am J Respir Crit Care Med,* 163, pp. 69-78.

Hickling, K. G. (2002). Reinterpreting the pressure-volume curve in patients with acute respiratory distress syndrome. *Curr Opin Crit Care,* 8, pp. 32-8.

Hickling, K. G., Henderson, S. J. & Jackson, R. (1990). Low mortality associated with low volume pressure limited ventilation with permissive hypercapnia in severe adult respiratory distress syndrome. *Intensive Care Med,* 16, pp. 372-7.

Hinz, J., Gehoff, A., Moerer, O., Frerichs, I., Hahn, G., Hellige, G. & Quintel, M. (2007). Regional filling characteristics of the lungs in mechanically ventilated patients with acute lung injury. *Eur J Anaesthesiol,* 24, pp. 414-24.

Huh, J. W., Jung, H., Choi, H. S., Hong, S. B., Lim, C. M. & Koh, Y. (2009). Efficacy of positive end-expiratory pressure titration after the alveolar recruitment manoeuvre in patients with acute respiratory distress syndrome. *Crit Care,* 13, R22.

Huynh, T., Messer, M., Sing, R. F., Miles, W., Jacobs, D. G. & Thomason, M. H. (2002). Positive end-expiratory pressure alters intracranial and cerebral perfusion pressure in severe traumatic brain injury. *J Trauma,* 53, pp. 488-92; discussion pp. 492-3.

Iotti, G. A., Braschi, A., Brunner, J. X., Smits, T., Olivei, M., Palo, A. & Veronesi, R. (1995). Respiratory mechanics by least squares fitting in mechanically ventilated patients: applications during paralysis and during pressure support ventilation. *Intensive Care Med,* 21, pp. 406-13.

Jonson, B. & Svantesson, C. (1999). Elastic pressure-volume curves: what information do they convey? *Thorax,* 54, pp. 82-7.

Kallet, R. H. & Branson, R. D. (2007). Respiratory controversies in the critical care setting. Do the NIH ARDS Clinical Trials Network PEEP/FIO2 tables provide the best evidence-based guide to balancing PEEP and FIO2 settings in adults? *Respir Care,* 52, pp. 461-75; discussion pp. 475-7.

Lachmann, B. (1992). Open up the lung and keep the lung open. *Intensive Care Med,* 18, pp. 319-21.

Lafollette, R., Hojnowski, K., Norton, J., Dirocco, J., Carney, D. & Nieman, G. (2007). Using pressure-volume curves to set proper PEEP in acute lung injury. *Nurs Crit Care,* 12, pp. 231-41.

Lowhagen, K., Lundin, S. & Stenqvist, O. (2010). Regional intratidal gas distribution in acute lung injury and acute respiratory distress syndrome--assessed by electric impedance tomography. *Minerva Anestesiol,* 76, pp. 1024-35.

Luecke, T., Herrmann, P., Kraincuk, P. & Pelosi, P. (2005). Computed tomography scan assessment of lung volume and recruitment during high-frequency oscillatory ventilation. *Crit Care Med,* 33, S155-62.

Luepschen, H., Meier, T., Grossherr, M., Leibecke, T., Karsten, J. & Leonhardt, S. (2007). Protective ventilation using electrical impedance tomography. *Physiol Meas,* 28, S247-60.

Lutchen, K. R. & Costa, K. D. (1990). Physiological interpretations based on lumped element models fit to respiratory impedance data: use of forward-inverse modeling. *IEEE Trans Biomed Eng,* 37, pp. 1076-86.

Mancebo, J., Albaladejo, P., Touchard, D., Bak, E., Subirana, M., Lemaire, F., Harf, A. & Brochard, L. (2000). Airway occlusion pressure to titrate positive end-expiratory pressure in patients with dynamic hyperinflation. *Anesthesiology,* 93, pp. 81-90.

Matamis, D., Lemaire, F., Harf, A., Brun-Buisson, C., Ansquer, J. C. & Atlan, G. (1984). Total respiratory pressure-volume curves in the adult respiratory distress syndrome. *Chest,* 86, pp. 58-66.

Meier, T., Luepschen, H., Karsten, J., Leibecke, T., Grossherr, M., Gehring, H. & Leonhardt, S. (2008). Assessment of regional lung recruitment and derecruitment during a PEEP trial based on electrical impedance tomography. *Intensive Care Med,* 34, pp. 543-50.

Miller, R. S., Nelson, L. D., Dirusso, S. M., Rutherford, E. J., Safcsak, K. & Morris, J. A., Jr. (1992). High-level positive end-expiratory pressure management in trauma-associated adult respiratory distress syndrome. *J Trauma,* 33, pp. 284-90; discussion pp. 290-1.

Mols, G., Brandes, I., Kessler, V., Lichtwarck-Aschoff, M., Loop, T., Geiger, K. & Guttmann, J. (1999). Volume-dependent compliance in ARDS: proposal of a new diagnostic concept. *Intensive Care Med,* 25, pp. 1084-91.

Nopp, P., Rapp, E., Pfutzner, H., Nakesch, H. & Ruhsam, C. (1993). Dielectric properties of lung tissue as a function of air content. *Phys Med Biol,* 38, pp. 699-716.

Phua, J., Badia, J. R., Adhikari, N. K., Friedrich, J. O., Fowler, R. A., Singh, J. M., Scales, D. C., Stather, D. R., Li, A., Jones, A., Gattas, D. J., Hallett, D., Tomlinson, G., Stewart, T. E. & Ferguson, N. D. (2009). Has mortality from acute respiratory distress syndrome decreased over time?: A systematic review. *Am J Respir Crit Care Med,* 179, 220-7.

Ranieri, V. M., Zhang, H., Mascia, L., Aubin, M., Lin, C. Y., Mullen, J. B., Grasso, S., Binnie, M., Volgyesi, G. A., Eng, P. & Slutsky, A. S. (2000). Pressure-time curve predicts minimally injurious ventilatory strategy in an isolated rat lung model. *Anesthesiology,* 93, pp. 1320-8.

Rouby, J. J. & Brochard, L. (2007). Tidal recruitment and overinflation in acute respiratory distress syndrome: yin and yang. *Am J Respir Crit Care Med,* 175, pp. 104-6.

Rouby, J. J., Lu, Q. & Goldstein, I. (2002). Selecting the right level of positive end-expiratory pressure in patients with acute respiratory distress syndrome. *Am J Respir Crit Care Med,* 165, pp. 1182-6.

Roupie, E., Dambrosio, M., Servillo, G., Mentec, H., El Atrous, S., Beydon, L., Brun-Buisson, C., Lemaire, F. & Brochard, L. (1995). Titration of tidal volume and induced hypercapnia in acute respiratory distress syndrome. *Am J Respir Crit Care Med,* 152, pp. 121-8.

Servillo, G., Svantesson, C., Beydon, L., Roupie, E., Brochard, L., Lemaire, F. & Jonson, B. (1997). Pressure-volume curves in acute respiratory failure: automated low flow inflation versus occlusion. *Am J Respir Crit Care Med,* 155, pp. 1629-36.

Shapiro, H. M. & Marshall, L. F. (1978). Intracranial pressure responses to PEEP in head-injured patients. *J Trauma,* 18, pp. 254-6.

Slutsky, A. S. & Tremblay, L. N. (1998). Multiple system organ failure. Is mechanical ventilation a contributing factor? *Am J Respir Crit Care Med,* 157, pp. 1721-5.

Stahl, C. A., Moller, K., Schumann, S., Kuhlen, R., Sydow, M., Putensen, C. & Guttmann, J. (2006). Dynamic versus static respiratory mechanics in acute lung injury and acute respiratory distress syndrome. *Crit Care Med,* 34, pp. 2090-8.

Stenqvist, O., Odenstedt, H. & Lundin, S. (2008). Dynamic respiratory mechanics in acute lung injury/acute respiratory distress syndrome: research or clinical tool? *Curr Opin Crit Care,* 14, pp. 87-93.

Suarez-Sipmann, F., Bohm, S. H., Tusman, G., Pesch, T., Thamm, O., Reissmann, H., Reske, A., Magnusson, A. & Hedenstierna, G. (2007). Use of dynamic compliance for open lung positive end-expiratory pressure titration in an experimental study. *Crit Care Med,* 35, pp. 214-21.

Suter, P. M., Fairley, B. & Isenberg, M. D. (1975). Optimum end-expiratory airway pressure in patients with acute pulmonary failure. *N Engl J Med,* 292, pp. 284-9.

Suter, P. M., Fairley, H. B. & Isenberg, M. D. (1978). Effect of tidal volume and positive end-expiratory pressure on compliance during mechanical ventilation. *Chest,* 73, pp. 158-62.

Sydow, M., Burchardi, H., Zinserling, J., Ische, H., Crozier, T. A. & Weyland, W. (1991). Improved determination of static compliance by automated single volume steps in ventilated patients. *Intensive Care Med,* 17, pp. 108-14.

Takeuchi, M., Goddon, S., Dolhnikoff, M., Shimaoka, M., Hess, D., Amato, M. B. & Kacmarek, R. M. (2002). Set positive end-expiratory pressure during protective ventilation affects lung injury. *Anesthesiology,* 97, pp. 682-92.

Talmor, D., Sarge, T., Malhotra, A., O'donnell, C. R., Ritz, R., Lisbon, A., Novack, V. & Loring, S. H. (2008). Mechanical ventilation guided by esophageal pressure in acute lung injury. *N Engl J Med,* 359, pp. 2095-104.

Terragni, P. P., Rosboch, G., Tealdi, A., Corno, E., Menaldo, E., Davini, O., Gandini, G., Herrmann, P., Mascia, L., Quintel, M., Slutsky, A. S., Gattinoni, L. & Ranieri, V. M. (2007). Tidal hyperinflation during low tidal volume ventilation in acute respiratory distress syndrome. *Am J Respir Crit Care Med,* 175, pp. 160-6.

The Acute Respiratory Distress Syndrome Network. (2000). Ventilation with lower tidal volumes as compared with traditional tidal volumes for acute lung injury and the acute respiratory distress syndrome. *N Engl J Med,* 342, pp. 1301-8.

Toth, I., Leiner, T., Mikor, A., Szakmany, T., Bogar, L. & Molnar, Z. (2007). Hemodynamic and respiratory changes during lung recruitment and descending optimal positive end-expiratory pressure titration in patients with acute respiratory distress syndrome. *Crit Care Med,* 35, pp. 787-93.

Tuğrul, M., Camci, E., Karadeniz, H., Sentürk, M., Pembeci, K. & Akpir, K. (1997). Comparison of volume controlled with pressure controlled ventilation during one-lung anaesthesia. *Br J Anaesth,* 79, pp. 306-10.

Uhlig, S. & Frerichs, I. (2008). [Lung protective ventilation - pathophysiology and diagnostics]. *Anasthesiol Intensivmed Notfallmed Schmerzther,* 43, pp. 438-45; quiz pp. 446.

Villar, J. (2005). The use of positive end-expiratory pressure in the management of the acute respiratory distress syndrome. *Minerva Anestesiol,* 71, pp. 265-72.

Zhao, Z., Moller, K., Steinmann, D., Frerichs, I. & Guttmann, J. (2009). Evaluation of an electrical impedance tomography-based global inhomogeneity index for pulmonary ventilation distribution. *Intensive Care Med,* 35, pp. 1900-6.

Zhao, Z., Steinmann, D., Frerichs, I., Guttmann, J. & Moller, K. (2010). PEEP titration guided by ventilation homogeneity: a feasibility study using electrical impedance tomography. *Crit Care,* 14, R8.

20

Perioperative Pulmonary Functional Assessment

Felipe Villar Álvarez[1],
Germán Peces-Barba Romero[1] and Miguel Ángel Palomero Rodríguez[2]
[1]Department of Pneumology, IIS Fundación Jiménez Díaz, CIBERES,
[2]Department of Anesthesiology, Hospital La Paz, Madrid,
Spain

1. Introduction

Pulmonary resection is the first therapeutic option of various lung pathologies, among which localized non-microcytic bronchogenic carcinoma is the most prevalent. Due to the fact that many patients who develop non-microcytic bronchogenic carcinoma present significant comorbidity, lung resection is associated with an increased risk (between 2 and 5%) of perioperative death (Little et al., 2005). Therefore, it is important to assess the patient's operability, which is defined as the ability to survive the lung resection without leaving any disabling sequelae.

As most of these patients are or have been smokers, many of them have varying degree of obstructive lung disease. It is known that the pulmonary obstruction increases the risk of lung resection (Miller et al., 1981), which is why the decision to perform resection depends largely on the functional integrity of the lung not affected by tumor. As the excision supposes a loss of lung function, many years of research have led to a reasonably solid scientific evidence that the postoperative risk depends on post-surgery lung function, which can be estimated preoperatively by knowing the amount of tissue to be resected basing on anatomical size or quantifying it by perfusion scintigraphy (Wernly et al., 1980).

On the other hand, it is also known that the functional capacity measured by exercise tests is associated with postoperative mortality (Puente & Ruiz., 2003). This has led to the development of integrated strategies in which basal functional tests are followed by postoperative function estimate and, in borderline patients, by stress testing (Marshall & Olsen 1993).

2. Perioperative pulmonary physiology

The major cardiopulmonary complications that alter normal lung function occur as a result of surgery (thoracotomy and resection of lung parenchyma) and anaesthesia (table 1). The thoracic surgery causes restrictive changes in the lung function characterized by moderate to severe reductions (50%) in vital capacity and up to 70% decrease of functional residual capacity (FRC). As a result of the FRC decrease, the volume of airway closure is shifted, so in the areas of pulmonary decline the end point of exhalation is below the closure volume, which causes an early closure of the airway and, therefore, of the areas of atelectasis. The factors that reduce FRC include supine position, pain, general anaesthesia and obesity. These functional changes occur without apparent obstruction of the airway, so that the ratio of forced expiratory volume in one second (FEV1) and forced vital capacity (FVC) does not decrease.

The action of the anaesthetic and the muscle relaxant used in the surgical procedure, involves a decrease in lung volumes. In addition, the effects of these drugs on the diaphragm and the bulbar center responsible for regenerating respiratory impulses are the main reasons that justify changes in lung volumes.

The cause of the diaphragm muscle dysfunction is not clear yet. Direct damage to the muscles during the surgical intervention has been proposed as one of possible mechanisms, but transdiaphragmatic pressure measurements during maximal phrenic nerve stimulation suggest that the depression of the central nervous system efferent traffic on the diaphragm occurs as a result of inhibitory reflexes associated with pain and other stimuli to sympathetic or vagal receptors.

Hypoxemia and arterial hypercapnia that appear, especially in the postoperative period, are mainly due to the effects of anaesthesia used during the surgery and cause a decrease in the interrelation ventilation/perfusion (V/Q), and besides lead to deterioration of hypoxic pulmonary vasoconstriction, alveolar hypoventilation or low cardiac output. The gas exchange disorder is intensified with combination of hypoventilation, increase in dead space ventilation, rapid shallow breathing and a decrease in mixed venous oxygen saturation due to low cardiac output, anemia and arterial desaturation and increased peripheral oxygen consumption with pain, fever or stress (Beckles et al., 2003).

Lung function changes with anesthesia and surgery
Impairment of gas exchange
Reduction in lung volumes
Dysfunction of the diaphragm
Depression of ventilatory control
Inhibition of cough and mucociliary system

Table 1. Mechanism of lung function changes with anesthesia and surgery (Swenson, 1999).

Ventilatory depression is also typical of the postoperative period and is marked by the residual effects of anaesthesia that inhibit normal response to hypoxia and hypercapnia. Analgesics and other sedatives may enhance these effects, and impede the implementation of pulmonary rehabilitation. They can rarely lead to episodes of sleep apnea.

The lung defends itself from attacks of infectious and environmental agents with cough and mucociliary clearance. The former is suppressed both with excessive and poor pain treatment. The latter can be altered by an ineffective cough, limited by restrictive changes and weakened respiratory muscles and also by atelectasis and dysfunction and ciliary damage caused by anaesthetic gases (Swenson, 1999).

Finally, it should be noted that many of these functional alterations may come as a result of postoperative complications such as atelectasis, infections, respiratory failure or exacerbations of chronic obstructive lung disease (table 2).

Postoperative pulmonary complications
General complications
Atelectasis
Infection (Pneumonia or bronchitis)
Bronchospam
Respiratory failure
Prolonged mechanical ventilation
Exacerbation of chronic lung disease
Pulmonary embolism
Obstructive sleep apnea
Specific thoracic surgical complications
Pleural effusion
Phrenic nerve injury
Bronchopleural fistula and empyema
Sternal wound infection
Gastroesophafeal anastomotic leak

Table 2. Postoperative pulmonary complications in patients with thoracic surgery (Swenson, 1999).

3. Lung function tests

In the preoperative thoracic surgery the functional assessment schemes have varied over the past 50 years. Most respirotary function tests which were utilized in order to minimize morbidity and postoperative mortality (table 3) are no longer used today, being replaced by simpler techniques that provide similar or better information. Today the process of lung function assessment is spread out over several phases comprising a series of breathing tests that the patients scheduled for thoracic surgery will be given according to their baseline pulmonary function and the amount of lung tissue for resection. These steps complement each other, so that the degree of severity of impairment of lung function is the fact that determines whether or not to go a step higher.

Pulmonary function test	**Parameter**
Spirometry	FVC, FEV1, ppo-FEV1
Lung volumes	TLC, RV, TLC/RV%
Diffusing capacity of the lung for CO	DLCO, ppo-DLCO
Arterial gasometry	PaO2, PaCO2
Pulmonary hemodynamic	PAP, PVR
Perfusion scintigraphy	% Perfusion en each lung
Ventilation scintigraphy	% Ventilation in each lung
Exercise test (6-min walking, shuttle walk and stair climbing)	Distance walked
Cardiopulmonary exercise test	VO2 peak

Table 3. Pulmonary function test used in the preoperative assessment. FVC: Forced vital capacity. FEV1: Forced expiratory volume in 1 second. ppo: postoperative. TLC: Total lung capacity. RV: Residual volumen. DLCO: Diffusion capacity of the lung for carbon monoxide. PaO2: Oxygen partial pressure of artery. PaCO2: Carbon dioxide partial pressure of artery. PAP: Pulmonary artery pressure. PVR: Pulmonary vascular resistance. VO2: Oxygen uptake.

3.1 Spirometry

Spirometry is a simple, inexpensive test of high reproducibility, easy to perform. From the standpoint of the preoperative evaluation the most important variables are the FEV1 and FVC. In the early 1950s spirometry was already considered as the most valid technique to assess morbidity and postoperative mortality in the thoracic surgery.

The first authors who used the predictive power of FEV1 in such surgery observed that the complications derived from the resection of bronchial carcinoma were associated with absolute values of FEV1 lower than 2 liters (Boushy et al., 1971). Subsequently, the measurements of spirometry were combined with those of lung volumes and there was observed an increase in complications with a FEV1 less than 1.20 liters, reserve volume (RV) greater than 3.30 liters and total lung capacity (TLC) greater than 7.90 liters (Lockwood, 1973). On the other hand, there was an attempt to link the value of FEV1 with the type of lung resection and it was noticed that the requirement for pneumonectomy was a FEV1 more than 2 liters, for lobectomy more than 1 liter and for segmentectomy or wedge resection more than 0.6 liter (Miller et al., 1981).

Considering FEV1 in absolute values can lead to errors in the estimation of lung function, especially in patients of advanced age or low height. In this sense, there have been some studies whose data contemplate a reduction in complications when the FEV1 is greater than 60% (Richter et al., 1997) or 89 ± 19% (Wang et al., 2000) of predicted values (table 4). Therefore, it is preferable to place greater emphasis on FEV1 percentage value in relation to its theoretical value than to the absolute one. In addition, the highest possible FEV1 will be chosen using the available therapeutic arsenal (smoking cessation, pulmonary rehabilitation or drug treatment with bronchodilators or corticosteroids). Finally, we could say that for thoracic surgery the advisable value of FEV1 is greater than or equal to 80%.

Variables	Complications (n = 19)	No Complications (n = 38)	p Value
FEV_1, L	2.15 ± 0.50	2.69 ± 0.66	< 0.01
FVC, L	3.39 ± 0.82	3.73 ± 0.79	ns
FEV_1% predicted	72 ± 14	89 ± 19	< 0.001
FVC% predicted	87 ± 16	97 ± 15	< 0.05
FEV_1/FVC, %	64 ± 11	72 ± 11	< 0.05
RV/TLC, %	40 ± 8 (n = 17)	36 ± 9 (n = 30)	ns
DL_{CO}, ml/min/mm Hg	15.31 ± 3.72 (n = 17)	21.98 ± 5.92 (n = 30)	< 0.001
DL_{CO}% predicted	62 ± 13 (n = 17)	87 ± 15 (n = 30)	< 0.001
DL_{CO}/VA, ml/min/mm Hg/L	3.05 ± 0.91 (n = 17)	4.03 ± 0.97 (n = 30)	< 0.01
DL_{CO}/VA% predicted	74 ± 23 (n = 17)	91 ± 17 (n = 30)	< 0.05

Table 4. Preoperative lung function variables in relation to complications. FEV1: Forced expiratory volume in 1 second. FVC: Forced vital capacity. RV: Residual volume. TLC: Total lung capacity. DLCO: Diffusion capacity of the lung for carbon monoxide. VA: Alveolar volume. ns: not significant (Wang et al., 2000).

In the algorithms used for the functional assessment of candidates for lung resection, the value of postoperative FEV1 (ppo-FEV1) plays an important role in the alternative to perform further tests or exclude patients from surgery without performing these tests (Wyser et al., 1999) (figure 1). In this sense, a value of ppo-FEV1 less than 40% of predicted increases the risk of perioperative complications and mortality by 16-50% (Pierce et al., 1994), being higher (60%) when ppo-FEV1 is less than 30% (Nakahara et al., 1985).

Even today there is a disagreement about whether ppo-FEV1 is a good predictor of perioperative complications or not. It has been seen that ppo-FEV1 is not a good predictor of complications in patients with preoperative FEV1 greater than 70%. In addition, among these patients, who also have ppo-FEV1 less than 40%, the mortality is 4.8%. These findings explain the so-called "lung volume reduction effect", which shows a reduction of functional loss in patients with airflow limitations, such as, for example, in patients with chronic obstructive lung disease (COPD) (Sekine et al., 2003).

A ppo-FEV1 value of 40% is currently being used to distinguish between normal and high risk of complications in thoracic surgery. However, due to improvements in surgical techniques and perioperative management, the value of ppo-FEV1 could fall to 30%.

Although the ppo-FEV1 is fairly accurate in predicting the final residual value of FEV1 within 3-6 months after thoracic surgery, the real value of FEV1 is overestimated in the first postoperative days, when most of the complications occur. In this regard, it has been shown that the first postoperative day and after a lobecctomia the real value of FEV1 was 30% lower than expected. Therefore, it would be a better predictor of complications than the ppo-FEV1 was (Varela et al., 2007).

The current recommendations of the ERS / ESTS Task Force are that the ppo-FEV1 should not only be used to select patients with pulmonary cancer for lung resection, especially in patients with moderate or severe COPD. It is known that in patients with COPD it is likely to overestimate the loss of lung function in the early postoperative stages and ppo-FEV1 does not seem to be a reliable predictor of complications. Finally, a value of ppo-FEV1 less than 30% predicted would be a high risk parameter when included in an algorithm for assessing pulmonary reserve before thoracic surgery (Brunelli et al., 2009).

3.2 Diffusing capacity of the lung for carbon monoxide

The DLCO represents the amount of carbon monoxide trapped by the lungs after inspiration of a small amount of this gas. This test provides us with information about the alveolo-capillary membrane, which is responsible for alveolar oxygen exchange. Thus, the DLCO is used to evaluate the surgical risk in patients scheduled for thoracic surgery.

Although DLCO is a technique which allows to estimate the risk of postoperative complications, it is not as well studied as FEV1. Several studies have shown that a preoperative DLCO less than 60% predicted was associated with increased mortality and postoperative complications were increased when the DLCO was less than 80% of predicted value (Ferguson et al., 1998). It has also been observed that patients with decreased DLCO (65.3 ± 5.0%) had more respiratory complications than those with normal DLCO (90.1 ± 5.9%) (Wang et al., 1999). In addition, decreased DLCO is related to an increase in the frequency of hospital readmissions and poor quality of life for the long term.

Therefore, the DLCO is an additional test to spirometry in which if a patient's preoperative functional evaluation has a FEV1 and DLCO greater than or equal to 80%, no additional testings are required. But if a patient has a DLCO lower than 80% despite a FEV1 greater than or equal to 80%, additional tests should be performed to make sure that it is a good candidate for thoracic surgery. This indicates that the DLCO is an important test to predict postoperative complications both in patients without COPD as well as in patients suffering from this pathology (Ferguson et al., 2008).

On the other hand, a value of postoperative DLCO (ppo-DLCO) of 40% is currently being used to distinguish between normal and high risk of complications in patients undergoing lung resection (Wyser et al., 1999) (figure 1). However, taking into account advances in perioperative care and surgical techniques, the allowed limit of ppo-DLCO should be lowered to 30%.

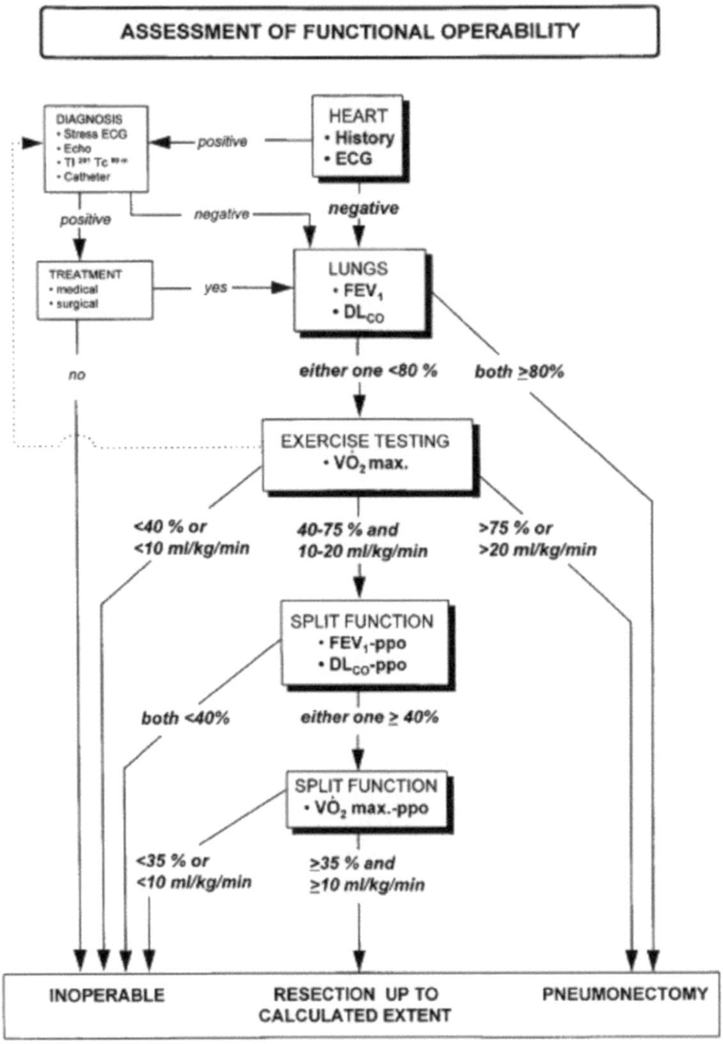

Fig. 1. Proposed algorithm for the assessment of the cardio-respiratory reserves of lung resection candidates. Tl 5 thallium; Tc 5 technetium. ECG: electrocardiogram. FEV1: Forced expiratory volume in 1 second. DLCO: Diffusion capacity of the lung for carbon monoxide. ppo: postoperative. VO2: Oxygen uptake. (Wyser et al., 1999).

The current recommendations of the ERS / ESTS Task Force indicate that the DLCO should be a routine measurement of functional evaluation of candidates for lung resection, especially if the spirometry is altered. The threshold value of ppo-DLCO of 30% is high risk when included in an algorithm for the assessment of pulmonary reserve before thoracic surgery (Brunelli et al., 2009).

3.3 Measurement of gas exchange

Arterial gasometry, is a test that is requested routinely in patients about to undergo thoracic surgery. Unlike spirometry, arterial blood gases values provide some more direct information about the problem with the gas exchange that is often present in this type of surgery. However, they do not provide as useful measurement as FEV1 or DLCO in the perioperative functional assessment.

In relation to arterial oxygen pressure (PaO2), few studies describe the exact role of this parameter in the assessment of perioperative risk. In some of them it has been shown that PaO2 below 50 mmHg is associated with postoperative complications (Mittman & Bruderman., 1977). Furthermore, sometimes hypoxemia in patients with bronchial carcinoma may be due to a shunt secondary to pulmonary atelectasis that is improved after the lung resection.

With regard to the blood pressure of CO2 (PaCO2), it has been postulated that hypercapnia (PaCO2 greater than 45 mmHg) involves an increase in postoperative complications (Meyer-Erkelenz et al., 1980). However, one study has demonstrated that patients with severe airflow obstruction (FEV1 40 ± 6%) and PaCO2 of 44 ± 4 mmHg, did not have any complications after lobectomy (Morice et al., 1992) (table 5). In this sense, other authors have also come to the conclusion that hypercapnia is not a risk factor for the presence of postoperative pulmonary complications (Miller et al., 1981). Therefore, although there is no consensus about the usefulness of the arterial gasometry in the perioperative functional assessment, it seems clear that hypercapnia should not exclude patients who are candidates for lung resection.

Subject No./ Age, yr/Sex	Height, cm	Weight, kg	FVC, %	FEV_1, L	FEV_1, %	FEV_1/FVC	Dco, %	TLC, %	Po_2, mm Hg	Pco_2, mm Hg	^{133}Xe FEV_1, %	$\dot{V}o_{2peak}$, ml/kg/min	Concomitant Heart Disease*
1/65/M	172.5	71	65	1.04	30	36	43	137	71	52	24	20.1	Cor pulmonale
2/76/M	170	65	49	1.05	39	60	50	185	74	36	26	15.1	None
3/75/M	175	61	61	1.37	45	58	66	85	89	43	32	19.2	RV enlargement
4/63/F	152.5	48	89	.95	44	40	62	140	86	42	32	16.2	None
5/70/M	170	60	78	1.27	47	52	49	107	69	49	37	16.1	Atrial fibrillation
6/72/M	167.5	66	68	1.14	41	55	56	169	76	48	31	15.2	RV enlargement
7/60/M	170	49	87	1.46	47	42	65	111	80	35	32	15.4	Cor pulmonale
8/64/M	180	96	72	1.14	33	35	40	133	65	43	31	16.5	RV enlargement
Mean 68	170	64	71	1.18	40	47	53	133	76	44	31	16.7	
SD 6	7.5	15	13	0.17	6	10	10	32	8	6	4	1.9	

Table 5. Relationship among spirometry, arterial blood gases and exercise testing in patients undergoing lung resection. FVC: Forced vital capacity. FEV1: Forced expiratory volume in 1 s. DCO: Diffusion capacity of the lung for carbon monoxide. TLC: Total lung capacity. PO2: Oxygen partial pressure of artery. PCO2: Carbon dioxide partial pressure of artery. VO2: Oxygen uptake. RV: Right ventricule. (Morice et al., 1992).

3.4 Quantitative ventilation/perfusion scintigraphy

The quantitative perfusion scintigraphy is based on the radiation emitted by an isotope that is taken up by the lungs after being injected intravenously. The percentage of radioactivity is associated with lung function, the right lung being the largest (55% of the total radiation). The left lung is responsible for the remaining 45% (figure 2).

The calculation of ppo-FEV1 in patients scheduled for pneumonectomy, from preoperative FEV1 and lung perfusion scintigraphy, is performed as follows (Kristersson et al., 1972):

$$\text{ppo} - \text{FEV1} = \text{preoperative FEV1 x \% of perfusion of the undisturbed lung}$$

Therefore, if such a patient is a candidate for left pneumonectomy and has a 3-liter preoperative FEV1 and the scintigraphy shows 30% perfusion in the left lung and 70% in the right, the value of FEV1 postpneumonectomy is:

$$\text{ppo} - \text{FEV1} = 3 \text{ litersx } 0{,}7 = 2{,}1 \text{ liters}$$

It has been shown that there is a good relationship between the ppo-FEV1 and real postoperative FEV1, while the ppo-FEV1 can be 10% lower than the measured FEV1 3 months after the surgery.
Wernley et al. applied the method of lung perfusion scintigraphy to calculate the FEV1 after lobectomy with the following formula (Wernly et al., 1980):

$$\text{Estimate of the FEV1 loss} = \text{preoperative FEV1 x \% affected lung perfusion x (number of segments in the lobe to be resected / number of segments in the lung)}$$

Perfusion scintigraphy has also been used to calculate ppo-DLCO, using the same formulas for estimating the ppo-FEV1. Therefore, the ppo-DLCO is calculated using the following formula:

$$\text{ppo} - \text{DLCO} = \text{preoperative DLCO x \% de perfusion of the unresected lung}$$

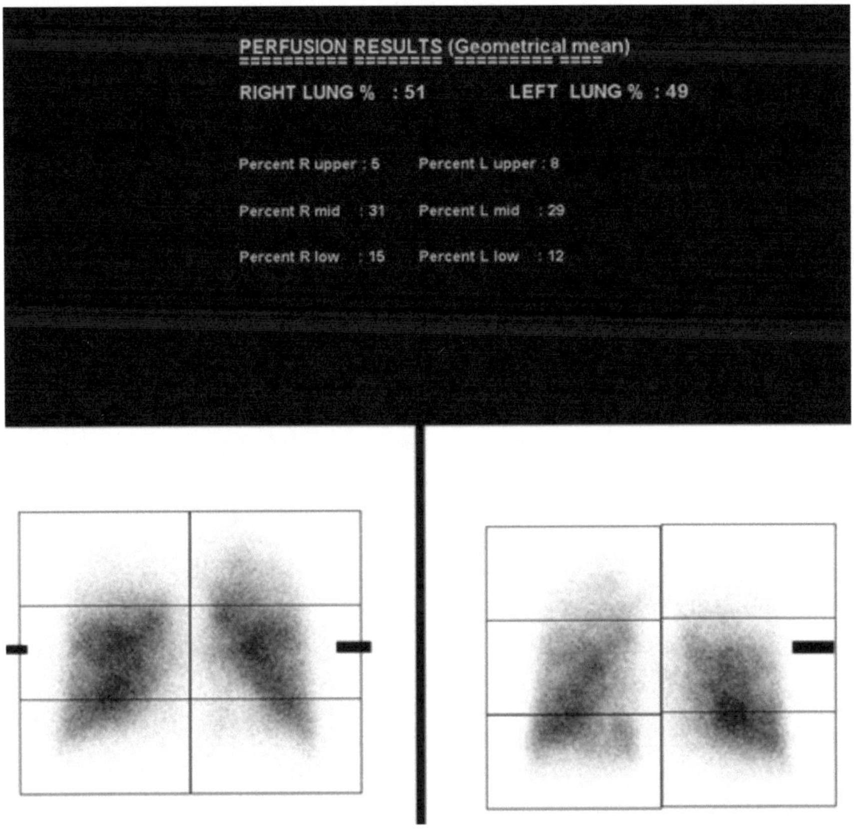

Fig. 2. Anterior and posterior images from perfusion scintigram. Three equally sized regions of interest over lungs are shown. Counts in each zone are measured. Geometric means of anterior and posterior images are then used to calculate relative perfusion and ventilation for each zone for each lung. By this method, percentages are obtained for upper, middle, and lower zones of right and left lungs for both perfusion and ventilation. (Win et al., 2006).

It is difficult to establish a definitive cut-off of ppo-FEV1 or ppo-DLCO above which resection of lung parenchyma will be safe. Some authors have estimated 0.8 liters as the limit below which it is unreasonable to perform the resection of the pulmonary parenchyma (Olsen et al., 1974). As an absolute value it can lead to errors, which is why it is better to use the percentage with respect to the theoretical value.

Several studies have shown that in candidates for lung resection, when ppo-FEV1 is greater than 40%, postoperative mortality is reduced (Markos et al., 1989), but other authors did not observe its increase when ppo-FEV1 is less than 40% (Morice et al., 1992). In relation to the ppo-DLCO it has also been noticed that the risk of postoperative complications is greater when the ppo-DLCO is less than 40% (Markos et al., 1989), and even one study estimates that this parameter is the best assessment of mortality and postoperative complications (Ferguson et al., 2008).

In practice, the scintigraphy has not been widely used in the functional assessment of patients about to undergo a lobectomy because of the difficulty in interpreting the individual contribution of each of the lobes to the whole of ventilation and perfusion. This could explain why several researchers consider that the simple calculation of the lung segments can predict the ppo-FEV1 as accurately as the ventilation perfusion scintigraphy does (Win et al., 2004). The ventilation scintigraphy has been widely used to predict postoperative lung function in patients with lung cancer who are scheduled for pneumonectomy (Colice et al., 2007).

The correlation between current and predicted ppo-FEV1 using the ventilation/perfusion scintigraphy has been variable with r between 0.67 and 0.9 (Win et al., 2006a). Both the ventilation and perfusion scintigraphies offer a good prediction of postoperative lung function individually, but it seems that there is no additional benefit in the performance of both (Win et al., 2006). However, the interpretation of the results should take into account that these techniques may underestimate the actual postoperative value (Zeiher et al., 1995).

3.5 Exercise test

During the exercise the patient is subjected to physical stress so that the whole system that regulates the uptake, transport and use of oxygen can be studied through the exercise test. When the latter is started, the lung increases the ventilation, oxygen uptake (VO2), CO2 production and blood flow similar to that which occurs during the postoperative period following the lung resection.

Among all the variables mentioned above, the most important is the peak oxygen uptake (VO2 peak), which gives us an idea of the global response to the effort and is defined as the maximum amount of oxygen a subject can capture, transport and use during the exercise. In addition, during the preoperative evaluation process the VO2 peak is the parameter that estimates the probability of complications best of all. Despite this, the exercise test should be performed only in selected cases (decrease in FEV1 and/or in DLCO below 80%) (Wayser et al., 1999).

3.5.1 Low-technology exercise; stair climbing, shuttle walk, and 6-min walk tests

Six-minute walk, stair climbing and shuttle walk tests have proved to be useful for preoperative risk stratification. In this sense, the 6-min walk test has a high reliability in the estimation of VO2 peak in healthy subjects and patients with COPD or those who are about to undergo lung transplantation and, therefore, in assessing the postoperative risk after thoracic surgery (Brunelli et al, 2009).

The shuttle walk test appears more reproducible and highly correlated with VO2 peak, estimating that 25 routes in this test are equivalent to a VO2 peak of 10 mL/kg/min (Singh et al, 1994). This cutoff point has been included in the algorithm proposed by the British Thoracic Society (BTS, 2001). However, no statistically significant differences have been found in the shuttle walk test among patients with and without complications after lung resection (Win et al., 2006b). This test tends to overestimate the exercise capacity in its range of lower values compared to VO2 peak, concluding that it should not be used alone to exclude patients from surgery (BTS, 2001). It has also been observed that patients who walk more than 400 meters in the shuttle walk test have a VO2 peak higher than 15 mL/kg/min (BTS, 2001).

The effectiveness of stair climbing test to predict serious cardiopulmonary complications following the lung resection surgery has already been demonstrated (Olsen et al., 1991). Against this background, the patients who climb less than 12 meters have a 2-fold higher rate of complications and mortality 23 times higher when compared with those who climb more than 22 meters, with a mortality rate of less than 1% (Brunelli et al., 2008). It has also been noticed that in patients with ppo-FEV1 or ppo-DLCO less than 40%, who climed more than 22 meters, the mortality rate is nonexistent (Brunelli et al., 2008).

Oximetry during the exercise has been proposed as a useful test in the preoperative assessment of candidates for lung resection (Colice et al., 2007). The role of oxygen desaturation during the exercise in postoperative risk stratification has not been defined in relation to early complications after the resection. In addition, it has been seen that oxygen desaturation during the exercise is a good predictor of postoperative respiratory failure, need for admission to an Intensive Care Unit (ICU), prolonged hospital stays and home treatment with oxygen (Ninan et al., 1997). On the other hand, oxygen saturation below 90% during the exercise test with incremental protocol is not a good predictor of postoperative cardiopulmonary morbidity (Varela et al., 2001).

3.5.2 High-technology exercise; cardiopulmonary exercise testing

There are 2 types of exercise protocol that have been used to evaluate the surgical risk: incremental or submaximal. They are usually carried out on a bicycle or a treadmill. The incremental protocol is the most used and consists in increasing the work to be performed by each patient to the limit of his tolerance. The exercise ends when the symptoms do not allow the patient to continue performing the exercise or when the registered variables do not permit to continue the test (ATS, 2003) (table 6).

Chest pain suggestive of ischemia
Ischemic ECG changes
Complex ectopy
Second or third degree heart block
Fall in systolic pressure > 20 mm Hg from the highest value during the test
Hypertension (> 250 mm Hg systolic; > 120 mm Hg diastolic)
Severe desaturation: $Sp_{O_2} \leq 80\%$ when accompanied by symptoms and signs of severe hypoxemia
Sudden pallor
Loss of coordination
Mental confusion
Dizziness or faintness
Signs of respiratory failure

Table 6. Indications for exercise terminations. ECG: electrocardiogram. SpO2: arterial oxygen saturation. (ATS, 2003).

The reliability of the exercise test with incremental protocol has been confirmed by numerous studies. In 1982 it was already proved that the complication rate decreased in patients with VO2 peak more than 1 liter (Eugene et al., 1982). In 1984 it was observed that the rate of postoperative complications was 100% when the VO2 peak was less than 15 mL/kg/min, but if this parameter was greater than 20 mL/kg/min, the risk of complications was 10% (Smith et al., 1984).

In 1992 it was found that among the patients with preoperative FEV1 less than or equal to 40%, ppo-FEV1 less than or equal to 33% or PaCO2 more than or equal to 45 mmHg, those who did not undergo a exercise test and had a VO2 peak above 15 ml/kg/min were considered suitable for lung resection with less postoperative complications (Morice et al., 1992).

In 1995 with a larger group of patients, it was already found that the VO2 peak, expressed as a percentage of predicted, estimated better postoperative complications, and that the patients with a VO2 peak more than 75% had 10% probability of complications. In contrast, in patients with VO2 peak less than 43% this probability increased to 90%, using as the cutoff point the VO2 peak of 60% (Bolliger et al. 1995a). At the same time, it was observed that patients with complications had a VO2 peak lower than 62.8% and if postoperative VO2 peak (ppo-VO2 peak) was less than 10 mL/kg/min, the risk of complications was very high (Bolliger et al., 1995b).

Recently it has been noticed that patients with complications have a VO2 peak of 15 mL/kg/min, while those without complications, have a VO2 peak of 19.2 mL/kg/min (Wang et al., 1999). Therefore, we can say that patients with a VO2 peak less than 10 mL/kg/min are not candidates for lung resection surgery. On the contrary, they are candidates if the VO2 peak is more than 15 mL/kg/min. Furthermore, in connection with the completion of pneumonectomy, VO2 peak values above 20 mL/kg/min or 75% of predicted value indicate a low risk of postoperative complications, while values below 10 mL/kg/ min or 40% of predicted indicate a high risk (Bolliger et al., 1995b).

Trying to get a better tolerance for exercise testing, especially in patients with dyspnoea who were not able to reach their VO2 peak, the submaximal protocol was proposed. In it the patient performs a pre-defined level of work (ATS, 2003).

After studying the exercise test with submaximal protocol in candidates for lung resection surgery, it has been observed that the VO2 reached allowed to predict the risk of postoperative complications (Miyoshi et al., 1989). However, this type of protocol usually requires invasive techniques which are not tolerated so well, therefore, this type of protocol is usually replaced by the incremental one.

The current recommendations of the ERS / ESTS Task Force is that the cardiopulmonary exercise test is sure, reproducible and should be performed in a controlled environment. In addition, the VO2 peak measured during the test with incremental protocol should be considered as the most important parameter to assess, as a measure of exercise capacity and as a good predictor of postoperative complications after thoracic surgery. Finally, to perform pneumonectomy the value of 75% of predicted or more than 20 mL/kg/min should be considered as cutoff point. The risk of postoperative complications is high if the VO2 peak is less than 35% of predicted or less than 10 mL/kg/min for any resection. Instead, there is insufficient evidence to recommend cutoff points for lobectomy (Brunelli et al., 2009).

3.6 Other tests

Thoracic computed tomography (CT) has efficacy comparable to that of perfusion scintigraphy in the calculation of ppo-FEV1 (Wu et al., 2002). In one study that compared the usefulness of thoracic CT (figure 3), single photon emission computed tomography (SPECT) and magnetic resonance imaging (MRI) in patients with bronchogenic carcinoma who are candidates for lung resection, MRI proved to be more accurate than the other two techniques in the measurement of ppo-FEV1 (Ohno et al., 2007).

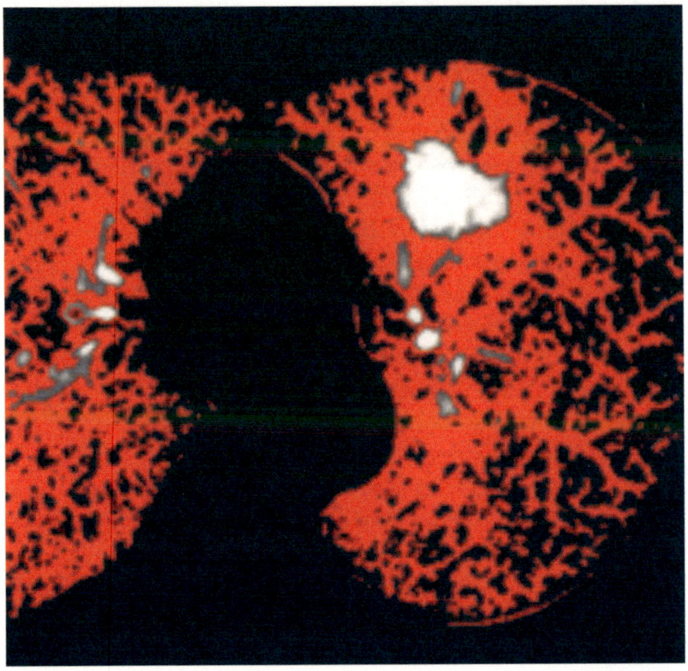

Fig. 3. Quantitative CT scan shows functional lung (*red*), pulmonary emphysema (*black*), and lung cancer (*white*). (Ohno et al., 2007).

The anatomical method is the calculation of postoperative lung function with the help of a formula that uses the preoperative FEV1 or FVC and the number of segments planned for resection (Zeiher et al., 1995). In case of lobectomy this formula estimates accurately the FEV1 postoperative and FCV which is not true in the case of pneumonectomy. That is why the latter is considered as inaccurate anatomical method.

The studies of pulmonary hemodynamics have also been used in the reseach of respiratory function in lung resection candidates. Perioperative risk is estimated by measuring the pulmonary arterial pressure and PaO2 during temporary occlusion of the pulmonary artery. This technique simulates the "physiological pneumonectomy" and is performed both at rest and during the exercise. It has been observed that growth in pressure in the pulmonary artery during the occlusion period increases the postoperative risk and complications (Gass & Olsen 1986). In addition, it has been observed that if the pulmonary arterial pressure is higher than 35 mmHg and PaO2 less than 45 mmHg, the patient is inoperable (Olsen et al., 1975). Another hemodynamic parameter used in the postoperative pulmonary assessment is the measurement of pulmonary vascular resistence (Schuurmans et al., 2002).

The main drawbacks of the use of pulmonary hemodynamics are the complexity of these techniques and the fact that they are invasive. Currently and in practice pulmonary hemodynamics is rarely used in respirotary assessing of candidates for thoracic surgery because the noninvasive tests have proved to have equal or superior efficacy.

4. Algorithms in the preoperative functional assessment

The use of algorithms in the evaluation of lung function in patients scheduled for thoracic surgery has as the main objective the step standardization of a series of diagnostic tests. These procedures avoid unnecessary costs, save time and allow you to gain experience in a more regulated way. This rationalization process contributes to improved patients care and decreased postoperative morbidity and mortality (Juliá Serdá et al., 2010).

Although several algorithms have been proposed to assess respiratory function in patients undergoing thoracic surgery, there are few validations of them. In addition, they depend on the patients population being served and the technical possibilities of each hospital or center where they are performed (Juliá Serdá et al., 2010).

One of the most widely accepted algorithms was proposed by Bolliger et al. and performed in 80 patients scheduled for resection of lung parenchyma (Bolliger et al. 1995a). This algorithm was validated later by Wyser et al. in 137 patients (figure 1), demonstrating a low postoperative complication rate (11%) and mortality (1.5%) (Wyser et al., 1999).

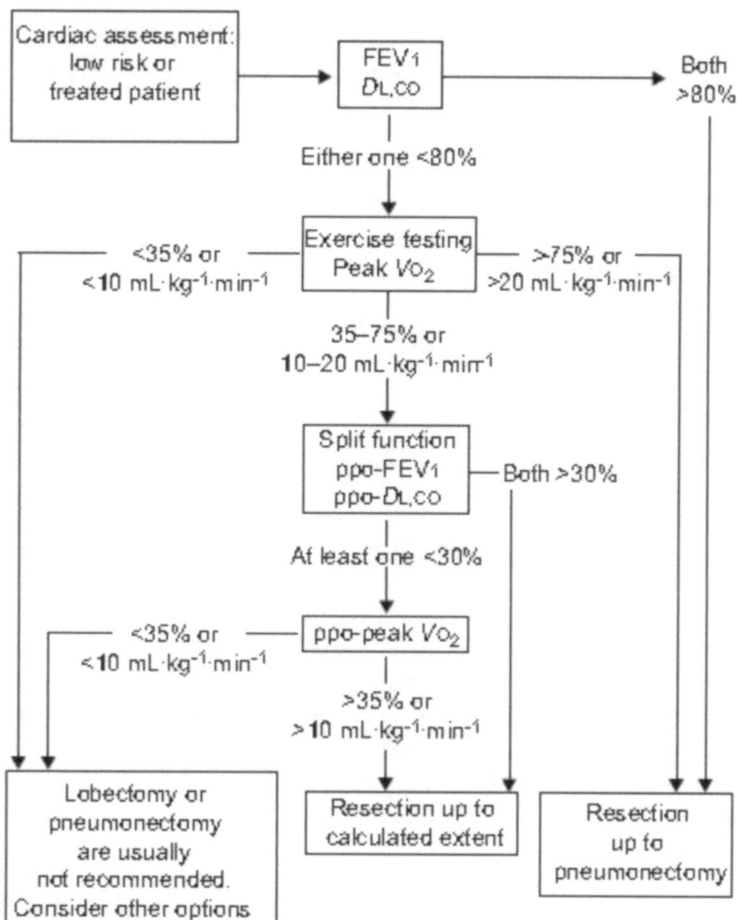

Fig. 4. Algorithm for assessment of cardiopulmonary reserve before lung resection in lung cancer patients. FEV1: Forced expiratory volume in 1 s. DLCO: Diffusion capacity of the lung for carbon monoxide. ppo: postoperative. VO2: Oxygen uptake. (Brunelli et al., 2009)

Taking into account these issues the ERS / ESTS Task Force has recently published its algorithm based fundamentally on the performance of exercise tests when preoperative FEV1 or DLCO is less than 80%. If in the exercise test VO2 peak is less than 35% or 10 mL/kg/min, it should not be recommendable to perform pneumonectomy or lobectomy, but if it is higher than 75% or 20 mL/kg/min, any resection (including pneumonectomy) would be indicated. If the VO2 peak is between these cutoff values, it would be advisable to calculate ppo-FEV1 and ppo-DLCO. If these are greater than 30%, lung resection would be indicated according to the calculated extension, and if, at least, one of these parameters is less than 30% it would be necessary to calculate the ppo-VO2 peak. After its calculation and if it is greater than 35% or 10 mL/kg/min, resection would be indicated depending on the calculated extension, and if its value is less than this cutoff, neither pneumonectomy nor lobectomy would be recommended. Finally, if it is impossible to perform cardiopulmonary exercise test and calculate the VO2 peak, it is recommendable to carry out the stair climbing test, but if the reached altitude is less than 22 meters, its calculation would be advisable (Brunelli et al., 2009) (figure 4).

One limitation in this type of algorithms, focusing on the completion of cardiopulmonary exercise testing, is that some candidates for lung resection are unable to execute any kind of exercise test due to the burden of concomitant comorbidities. These patients have demonstrated increased mortality after lung resection (Brunelli et al., 2005) and, after careful selection based on cardiopulmonary parameters they should be considered as high-risk patients and candidates to be perioperatively monitored.

5. Patient care managment

The use of bronchodilators, corticosteroids or a combination of both, as well as pulmonary rehabilitation and smoking cessation can help reduce postoperative complications occurring after thoracic surgery, especially in patients with comorbidities who present declining values of FEV1 or DLCO.

5.1 Smoking cessation

Smokers have significantly higher risk of postoperative complications, so an intervention for smoking cessation during the preoperative period may be effective to reduce the incidences of complications. Moreover, the time of surgery may be a unique opportunity for smoking cessation attempts to succeed (Moller & Villebro, 2005).

There is evidence that interventions for smoking cessation, which include nicotine replacement therapy (NRT), increase for a short term the rate of smoking cessation and decrease postoperative morbidity. In this process it remains unclear which treatment intensity is optimal. Derived from indirect comparisons, the interventions that begin from 4 to 8 weeks before surgery, based on weekly counselling and the NRT are the most effective to quit smoking and to prevent long-term postoperative complications (Moller & Villebro, 2005).

5.2 Pulmonary rehabilitation

Pulmonary rehabilitation, that includes exercise and education, is effective in candidates for lung volume reduction and in the pre-and postoperative period of lung transplantation (Nici et al., 2006). However, this effectiveness is not clearly demonstrated in surgical patients with lung cancer.

Before the surgery, the preoperative VO2 is inversely proportional to the probability of the presence of complications after lung resection (Wu et al., 2002), which, in turn, is associated with postoperative loss of lung function (Nagamatsu et al., 2007). In addition, pulmonary rehabilitation improves VO2 before the surgery in patients with COPD with low VO2 (less than 15 mL/kg/min), which reduces late complications without affecting the operability or the prognosis (Bobbio et al., 2008).

Preoperative training programs lead to a reduction of hospital stay and of complications in patients with COPD and lung cancer (Sekine et al., 2005). However, improved accessibility to intervention has been observed only in patients with "quasi normal" lung function (Lovin et al., 2006). Pulmonary rehabilitation in inpatients has shown benefits in exercise capacity and lung volumes (Cesario et al., 2007).

Therefore, in the light of the data presented, it seems logical that pulmonary rehabilitation may decrease the complication rate in candidates for lung resection, which is why future researches on the content and duration of rehabilitation programs are priorities.

5.3 Pharmacologic therapy

The diagnosis of COPD is often established during the preoperative functional assessment in patients scheduled for lung resection after the diagnosis of lung cancer. These patients, with a high percentage of respiratory complications, may be excluded from surgery if we fail to achieve, with proper treatment, a sufficient pulmonary function value.

The main guidelines for the management of COPD patients who are to undergo lung resection indicate that it is necessary that the patient quit smoking, do exercises in pulmonary rehabilitation and optimize proper treatment to improve lung function and reduce postoperative complications (Brunelli et al., 2009). However, the treatments indicated for patients with COPD and lung cancer do not differ from those which are recommended to patients who have only COPD, in which a short-term therapeutic effect is not expected.

In the scientific literature we have found only few studies that evaluate the short and long term effect of initiation of therapy in patients with COPD and lung cancer. Several of them value the effect of tiotropium on lung function, establishing its improvement up to 226ml in FEV1 (Kobayashi et al., 2009), but without any effect on post sugery complications (Ueda et al. 2010). In a recent study, the treatment with formoterol and budesonide added to tiotropium improved the FEV1 in 310ml and decreased the number of postoperative pulmonary complications (Bölükbas et al., 2011). One of the keys to these results is the improvement in lung function that occurs when adding corticosteroids to long-acting bronchodilators. Another key is the improvement in FEV1 due to these drugs, since its value, both pre-and postoperative, is associated with mortality and morbidity after the surgery. Therefore, an elevation of FEV1 can increase the number of candidates for surgical resection, thus optimizing the treatment of cancer and improve the prognosis of these patients.

6. Conclusion

A lot of scientific literature dedicated to pre-operative evaluation before surgical treatment of lung diseases has been published. The search for the ideal preoperative test to predict major perioperative risk of patients began with the use of spirometry in 1955. Since then, scientific evidence allowing the stratification of perioperative risk based in different preoperative pulmonary function tests, estimations of postoperative lung function, pulmonary circulation hemodynamics, arterial blood gases or exercise testing has been given. Therefore, the functional assessment has undergone major changes; apart from preoperative measurement of pulmonary function (FEV1, DLCO or VO2 peak) is getting more and more importance.

In the last few years, a number of decision-making algorithms interpreting the abundant literature on the issue have been described. These algorithms are mainly based on that postoperative FEV1 should not to be used alone to select patients for lung resection. DLCO should be routinely measured during pre-operative evaluation of lung resection candidates (regardless of whether the spirometric evaluation is abnormal or not). A postoperative FEV1 and DLCO values of 30% predicted is suggested to be a high risk threshold for this parameter when included in an algorithm for assessment of pulmonary reserve before surgery, exercise tests should be indicated for all the patients undergoing surgery with FEV1 or a DLCO < 80% of normal values and either ventilation scintigraphy or perfusion scintigraphy offer good prediction of post-operative lung function.

Finally, the main recommendation to the patients on which lung resection will be performed is to give up smoking for sufficient spell (at least 2–4 weeks) before the surgery, since it may decrease post-operative complications. Moreover, early pre- and post-operative rehabilitation should also be recommended, since it may produce functional benefits in patients with resected lung.

7. References

American Thoracic Society; American College of Chest Physicians. ATS / ACCP Statement on cardiopulmonary exercise testing. (2003). *Am J Respir Crit Care Med*, Vol.167, No.10, (May 2003), pp.211-77. ISSN 1073-449X.

Beckles, MA.; Spiro, SG.; Colice, GL. & Rudd, RM; American College of Chest Physician. (2003). The physiologic evaluation of patients with lung cancer being considered for resectional surgery Chest, Vol.123, No.1 Suppl, (January 2003), pp.105S-114S. ISSN 0012-3692.

Bobbio, A.; Chetta, A.; Ampollini, L.; Primomo, GL.; Internullo, E.; Carbognani, P.; Rusca, M. & Olivieri D. (2008). Preoperative pulmonary rehabilitation in patients undergoing lung resection for nonsmall cell lung cancer. *Eur J Cardiothorac Surg*, Vol.33, No.1, (November 2007), pp.95–98. ISSN 1010-7940.

Bolliger, C.; Jordan, P.; Soler, M.; Stulz, P.; Grädel, E.; Skarvan, K.; Elsasser, S.; Gonon, M.; Wyser, C. & Tamn, M. (1995). Exercise capacity as a predictor as postoperative complications in lung resection candidates. *Am J Respir Crit Care Med*, Vol.151 No.5, (May 1995), pp.1472-80. ISSN 1073-449X.

Bolliger, C.; Wyser, C.; Roser, H.; Soler, M. & Perruchoud, AP. (1995). Lung scanning and exercise testing for the prediction of postoperative perfonmance in lung resection candidates at increased risk for complications. *Chest*, Vol.108, No.2 (August 1995), pp.341-8. ISSN 0012-3692.

Bölükbas, S.; Eberlein, M.; Eckhoff, J. & Schirren, J. (2011). Short-term effects of inhalative tiotropium/formoterol/budesonide versus tiotropium/formoterol in patients with newly diagnosed chronic obstructive pulmonary disease requiring surgery for lung cancer: a prospective randomized trial. *European Journal of Cardio-thoracic Surgery*, Vol.39, No.6, (October 2010), pp.995-1000. ISSN 1010-7940.

Boushy, SF.; Biling, DM.; North, LB & Helgason, AH. (1971). Clinical course related to preoperative and postoperative pulmonary function in patients with bronchogenic carcinoma. *Chest*, Vol.59, No.4, (April 1971), pp.383-91. ISSN 0012-3692.

Brunelli, A.; Sabbatini, A.; Xiume, F.; Borri, A.; Salati, M.; Marasco, RD. & Finachini, A. (2005). Inability to perform maximal stair climbing test before lung resection: a propensity score analysis on early outcome. *Eur J Cardiothorac Surg*, Vol.27, No.3, (January 2005), pp.367–372. ISSN 1010-7940.

Brunelli, A.; Refai, M.; Xiume, F.; Salati, M.; Sciarra, V.; Socc, L. & Sabbatini,m A. (2008) Performance at symptom limited stair-climbing test is associated with increased ciardiopulmonary complications, mortality, and costs after major lung resection. *Ann Thorac Surg*, Vol.86, No.1 (July 2008), pp.240–247. ISSN 0003-4975.

Brunelli, A.; Charloux, A.; Bolliger, CT.; Rocco, G.; Sculier, JP.; Varela, G.; Licker, M.; Ferguson, MK.; FAivre-Finn, C.; Huber, RM.; Clini, EM.; Win, T.; De Ruysscher, D. & Goldman, L. on behalf of the European Respiratory Society and European Society of Thoracic Surgeons joint task force on fitness for radical therapy. (2009). ERS/ESTS clinical guidelines on fitness for radical therapy in lung cancer patients (surgery and chemo-radiotherapy). *Eur Respir J*, Vol.34, No.1 (September 2009), pp.17–41. ISSN 0903 - 1936.

BTS guidelines: guidelines on the selection of patients with lung cancer for surgery. (2001). *Thorax*, Vol.56, No.2, (February 2001), pp.89–108. ISSN 0040-6376.

Cesario, A.; Ferri, L.; Galetta, D.; Pasqua, F.; Bonassi, S.; Clini, E.; Biscione, G.; Cardaci, V.; di Toro, S.; Zarzana, A.; Margaritora, S.; Piraino, A.; Russo, P.; Sterzi, S. & Granone, P. (2007). Post-operative respiratory rehabilitation after lung resection for non-small cell lung cancer. *Lung Cancer*, Vol.57, No.2, (April 2007), pp.175–180. ISSN 0169-5002.

Colice, GL.; Shafazand, S.; Griffin, JP.; Keenan, R.; Bolliger, CT. & American College of Chest Physicians. (2007). Physiologic evaluation of the patient with lung cancer being considered for resectional surgery: ACCP evidenced-based clinical practice guidelines (2nd edition). *Chest*, Vol.132, Suppl.3, (September 2007), pp.161S–177S. ISSN 0012-3692.

Eugene J, Brown SE, Light RW. (1982). Maximun oxygen consumption: a physiologic guide to pulmonary serection. *Surg Forum*, Vol.33:,(1982), pp.260-2. ISSN 0071-8041.

Ferguson, MK.; Little, L.; Rizzo, L.; Popovich, KL.; Glonek, GF.; Leff, A.; Manjoney, D. & Little, AG. (1988). Diffusing capacity predicts morbidity and mortality after pulmonary resection. *J Thorac Cardiovasc Surg*, Vol.96, No.6, (December 1988), pp.894-900. ISSN: 0022-5223.

Ferguson, MK. & Vigneswaran, WT. (2008). Diffusing capacity predicts morbidity after lung resection in patients without obstructive lung disease. *Ann Thorac Surg*, Vol.85, No.4 (April 2008), pp.1158–1164. ISSN 0003-4975.

Gass, GD. & Olsen, GN. (1986). Preoperative pulmonary function testing to predict postoperative morbidity and mortality. *Chest*. Vol.89, No.1, (January 1986), pp.127-35. ISSN 0012-3692.

Juliá Serdá G, Ramírez Rodríguez R, Cabrera López C, Freixinet Gilart J. (2010) Aplicación de las pruebas de function cardiopulmonary en la práctica quirúrgica. In: *Tratado de Cirugía Torácica*, Fernández Fau L, Freisinet Gilart J, (Ed), pp.187-203, EDIMSA, ISBN 987-84-7714-341-3, Madrid, Spain.

Kobayashi, S.; Suzuki, S.; Niikawa, H.; Sugawara, T. & Yanai, M. (2009). Preoperative use of inhaled tiotropium in lung cancer patients with untreated COPD. *Respirology*, Vol.14, No.5, (May 2009), pp.675-9. ISSN 1323-7799.

Kristersson, S..; Lindell, SE, & Svanberg, L. (1972) Prediction of pulmonary function loss due to pneumonectomy using 133 Xe-radiospirometry. *Chest*, vol.62. No.6, (December 1972), pp.694-8. ISSN 0012-3692.

Little, AG.; Rusch, VW.; Bonner, JA.; Gaspar, LE.; Green, MR.; Webb, WR. & Stewart, AK. (2005). Patterns of surgical care of lung cancer patients. *Ann Thorac Surg*, Vol.80, No.6, (December 2005), pp.2051-6. ISSN 0003-4975.

Lockwood P. (1973). Lung function test results and the risk of post-thoracotomy complications. *Respiration*, Vol.30, No.6, (1973), pp.529-42. ISSN 0025-7931.

Lovin, S. ; Bouille, S. ; Orliaguet, O & Veale, D. (2006). [Preoperative rehabilitation in the surgical treatment of lung cancer]. *Pneumologia*, Vol.55, No.3, (July-September 2006), pp.109–112. ISSN 2067-2993.

Markos, J.; Mullan, BP.; Hillman, DR.; Musk, AW.; Antico, VF.; Lovegrove, FT.; Carter, MJ. & Finucane, KE. (1989). Preoperative assessment as a predictor of mortality and morbidity after lung resection. *Am Rev Respir Dis*, Vol.139, No.4, (April 1989), pp.902-10. ISSN 0003-0805.

Marshall, MC. & Olsen, GN. (1993). The physiologic evaluation of the lung resection candidate. *Clin Chest Med*, Vol.14, No.2, (June 1993), pp.305-20. ISSN 0272-5231.

Meyer-Erkelenz, JD.; Mösges, RW. & Sieverts, H. (1980). Speiroergometry (cardiopulmonary function under load). Reporto f the results of the 1979 colloquium in Aachen. *Prax Klin Pneumol*, Vo.34, No.10 (October 1980), pp.585-600. ISSN 0342-7498.

Miller, JI.; Grossman, GD. & Hatcher, CR. (1981). Pulmonary function test criteria for operability and pulmonary resection. *Surg Gynecol Obstet*, Vol.153. No.6, (December 1981), pp.893-5. ISSN 0039-6087.

Mittman, C. & Bruderman, I. (1977). Lung cancer: to operate or not? *Am Rev Respir Dis* Vol.116, No.3, (September 1977), pp.477-96. ISSN 0003-0805.

Miyoshi, S.; Nakahara, K.; Ohno, K.; Monden, Y. & Kawashima, Y. (1989). Exercise tolerance test in lung cancer patients: the relationship between exercise capacity and postthoracotomy hospital mortality. *Ann Thorac Surg*, Vol.44, (1989), pp.487-90. ISSN 0003-4975.

Moller, A. & Villebro, N. (2005). Interventions for preoperative smoking cessation. *Cochrane Database Syst Rev*, Vol.20, No.3, (July 2005), pp.CD002294. ISSN 1469-493X.

Morice, RC.; Peters, EJ.; Ryan, MB.; Putnam, JB.; Ali, MK. & Roth, JA. (1992). Exsercise testing in the evaluation of patiens at high risk for complications fron lung resection. *Chest*, Vol.101, No.2, (February 1992), pp.356-61. ISSN 0012-3692.

Nagamatsu, Y.; Maeshiro, K.; Kimura, NY.; Nishi, T.; Shima, I.; Yamana, H. & Shirouzo, K. (2007). Long-term recovery of exercise capacity and pulmonary function after lobectomy. *J Thorac Cardiovasc Surg*, Vol.134, No.5, (November 2005), pp.1273–1278. ISSN: 0022-5223.

Nakahara, K.; Monden, Y.; Ohno, K.; Miyoshi, S.; Maeda, H. & Kawashima, Y. (1985). A method for predicting postoperative lung function and its relation to postoperative complications in patients with lung cancer. *Ann Thorac Surg*, Vol.39, No.3, (March 1985), pp.260–265. ISSN 0003-4975.

Nici, L. & ATS/ERS Pulmonary Rehabilitation Writing Committee. (2006). American Thoracic Society/ European Respiratory Society statement on pulmonary rehabilitation. *Am J Respir Crit Care Med*, Vol.173, No.12, (June 2006), pp.1390–1413. ISSN 1073-449X.

Ninan, M. ; Sommers, KE.; Landreneau, RJ.; Weyant, RJ.; Tobias, J.; Luketich, JD.; Ferson, PF. & Kenan, RJ. (1997). Standardized exercise oximetry predicts postpneumonectomy outcome. *Ann Thorac Surg*, Vol.64, No.2, (August 1997), pp.328–332. ISSN 0003-4975.

Ohno, Y.; Koyama, H.; Nogami, M.; Takenaka, D.; Matsumoto, S.; Yoshinura, M.; Kotani, Y. & Sugimura, K. (2007). Postoperative lung function in lung cancer patients: comparative analysis of predictive capability of MRI, CT and SPECT. *AJR Am J Roentgenol*, 189, No.2, (August 2007), pp.400-8. ISSN 0361-803X.

Olsen, GN.; Block, AJ. & Tobias, JA. (1974). Prediction of postpneumonectomy pulmonary function using quantitative macroaggregate lung scaning. *Chest*, Vol.66, No.1, (July 1974), pp.13-6. ISSN 0012-3692.

Olsen, GN.; Block, AJ.; Swenson, EW.; Castle, JR. & Wynne, JW. (1975). Pulmonary function evaluation of the lung resection candidate: a prospective study. *Am Rev Respir Dis*, Vol.111, No.4, (April 1975), pp.379-87. ISSN 0003-0805.

Olsen, GN.; Bolton, JW.; Weiman, DS. & Hornung, GA. (1991). Stair climbing as an exercise test to predict the postoperative complications of lung resection. Two years' experience. *Chest*, Vol.99, No.3, (March 1991), pp.587–590. ISSN 0012-3692.

Pierce, RJ.; Copland, JM.; Sharpe, K. & Barter, CE. (1994). Preoperative risk evaluation for lung cancer resection: predicted postoperative product as a predictor of surgical mortality. *Am J Respir Crit Care Med*, Vol.150, No.4 (October 1994), pp.947–955. ISSN 1073-449X.

Puente Maestu, L. & Ruiz Martín, JJ. (2003). Stress testing and lung resection surgery. *Arch Bronconeumol*, Vol.39, No.3, (March 2003), pp.126-132. ISSN 0300-2896.

Richter Larsen, K.; Svendsen, UG.; Milman, N.; Brenoe, J. & Petersen, BN. (1997). Exercise testing in the preoperative evaluation of patients with bronchogenic carcinoma. *Eur Repir J*, Vol.10, No.7 (July 1997), pp.1559-65. ISSN 0903 - 1936.

Schuurmans, MM.; Diacon, AH. & Bolliger, CT. (2002). Functional evaluation before lung resection. *Clin Chest Med*, Vol.23, No.1 (March 2002), pp.159-72. ISSN 0272-5231.

Sekine, Y.; Iwata, T.; Chiyo, M.; Yasufuku, K.; Motohashi, S.; Yoshida, S.; Suzuki, M.; Iizasa, T.; Saitoh, Y. & Fujisawa, T. (2003). Minimal alteration of pulmonary function after lobectomy in lung cancer patients with chronic obstructive pulmonary disease. *Ann Thorac Surg*, Vol.76, No.2 (August 2003), pp.356–361. ISSN 0003-4975.

Sekine, Y.; Chiyo, M.; Iwata, T.; Yasufuku, K.; Furukawa, S.; Amada, Y.; Iyoda, A.; Shibuya, K.; Iizasa, T. & Fujisawa, T. (2005). Perioperative rehabilitation and physiotherapy for lung cancer patients with chronic obstructive pulmonary disease. *Jpn J Thorac Cardiovasc Surg*, Vol.53, No.5, (May 2005), pp.237–243. ISSN 0368-2811.

Singh, SJ.; Morgan, MD.; Hardman, AE.; Rowe, C. & Bardsley, PA. (1994). Comparison of oxygen uptake during a conventional treadmill test and the shuttle walking test in chronic airflow limitation. *Eur Respir J*, Vol.7, No.11, (November 1994). pp.2016–2020. ISSN 0903 - 1936.

Smith, TP.; Kinasewitz, GT.; Tucker, WY.; Spillers, WP. & George, RB. (1984). Exercise capacity as a predictor of post-thoracotomy morbidity. *Am Rev Respir Dis*, Vol.129. No.5, (May 1984), pp.730-4. ISSN 0003-0805.

Swenson ER, Swenson EW. (1999) Preoperative Pulmonary Evaluation. In: *Clinical Respiratory Medicine*, Albert RK, Spiro SG, Jett JR, (Ed), pp.229-234, Mosby, ISBN 0-323-02479-1, St. Louis, USA.

Ueda, K.; Tanaka, T.; Hayashi, M. & Hamano, K. (2010). Role of inhaled tiotropium on the perioperative outcomes of patients with lung cancer and chronic obstructive pulmonary disease. *Thorac Cardiovasc Surg*, Vol.58, No.1, (January 2010), pp.38-42. ISSN 0171-6425.

Varela, G..; Cordovilla, R.; Jimenez, MF. & Novoa, N. (2001). Utility of standardized exercise oximetry to predict cardiopulmonary morbidity after lung resection. *Eur J Cardiothorac Surg*, Vol.19, No.3, (March 2001), pp.351–354. ISSN 1010-7940.

Varela, G.; Brunelli, A.; Rocco, G.; Novoa, N.; Refai, M.; Jiménez, MF.; Salati, M. & Gatani, T. (2007) Evidence of lower alteration of expiratory volume in patients with airflow limitation in the immediate period after lobectomy. *Ann Thorac Surg*, Vol.84, No.3, (December 2006), pp.417–422. ISSN 0003-4975.

Wang, J.; Olak, J.; Ultmann, RE. & Ferguson, MK. (1999). Assessment of pulmonary complications after lung resection. *Ann Thorac Surg*, Vol.67, No.5, (May 1999), pp.1444-7. ISSN 0003-4975.

Wang, JS.; Abboud, RT.; Evans, KG.; Finley, RJ. & Graham, BL. (2000). Role of CO diffusing capacity during exercise in the preoperative evaluation for lung resection. *Am J Respir Crit Care Med.*, Vol.162, No.4, (October 2000), pp.1435-44. ISSN 1073-449X.

Wernly, JA.; DeMeester, TR.; Kirchner, PT.; Meyrowitz, PD.; Oxford, DE. & Golomb, HM. (1980). Clinical value of quantitative ventilation-perfusion lung scans in the surgical management of bronchogenic carcinoma. *J Thorac Cardiovase Surg*, Vol.80, No.4, (October 1980), pp.535-43. ISSN 0022-5223.

Win, T.; Laroche, CM.; Groves, AM.; White, C.; Wells, FC.; Ritchie, AJ. & Tasker, AD. (2004). Use of quantitative lung scintigraphy to predict postoperative pulmonary function in lung cancer patients undergoing lobectomy. *Ann Thorac Surg*, Vol. 78, No.4, (October 2004), pp.1215–1218. ISSN 0003-4975.

Win, T.; Tasker, AD.; Groves, AM.; White, C.; Ritchie, AJ.; Wells, FC. & Laroche, CM. (2006). Ventilation-perfusion scintigraphy to predict postoperative pulmonary function in lung cancer patients undergoing pneumonectomy. *AJR Am J Roentgenol*, Vol.187, No.5 (November 2006), pp.1260–1265. ISSN 0361-803X.

Win, T.; Jackson, A.; Groves, AM.; Sharples, LD.; Charman, SC. & Laroche, CM. (2006). Comparison of shuttle walk with measured peak oxygen consumption in patients with operable lung cancer. *Thorax*, Vol.61, No.1 (October 2005), pp.57–60. ISSN 0040-6376.

Wu, MT.; Pan, HB.; Chiang, AA.; Hsu. HK.; Chang, HC.; Peng, NJ.; Lai, PH.; Liang, HL. & Yang, CF. (2002). Prediction of postoperative lung function in patiens with lung cancer comparison of quantitative CT with perfusion scintigrafy. *Am J Roentgenol*, Vol.178, No.3, (March 2002), pp.667-72. ISSN 0361-803X.

Wyser, C.; Stulz, P.; Soler, M.; Tamm, M.; Muller-Brand, J.; Habicht, J.; Perrochoud, AP. & Bolliger, CT. (1999). Prospective Evaluation of an Algorithm for the Functional Assessment of Lung Resection Candidates. *Am J Respir Crit Care Med*, Vol.159, No.5, (May 1999), pp.1450-56. ISSN 1073-449X.

Zeiher, BG.; Gross, TJ.; Kern, JA..; Lanza, LA. & Peterson, MW. (1995). Predicting postoperative pulmonary function in patients undergoing lung resection. *Chest*, Vol.108, No.1, (July 1995), pp.68–72. ISSN 0012-3692.

21

Post Thoracotomy Pain Syndrome

F. Della Corte, C. Mendola, A. Messina and G. Cammarota
Azienda Ospedaliera Maggiore della Carità, Novara, Italia

1. Introduction

Post-thoracotomy pain is one of the most severe and long lasting complications after surgery (1-4) which acutely contributes to limit normal respiratory activity impairing the sputum clearance and reducing ventilatory function (5). Along with limb amputation, thoracotomy is the surgical procedure with the highest risk of severe and long lasting acute postoperative pain (6).

Moreover, a chronic post thoracotomy pain syndrome (PTPS) may delay the long term rehabilitation, worsening the quality of life because of the associated neuropathic pain even without recurrences of the primary disease (7). Lung cancer still remains the first cause of death for cancer (8) and prompt pulmonary surgery may be the only effective therapeutic strategy. Consequently, an increasing rate of thoracic surgery will be progressively associated with a higher PTPS incidence in the future.

The syndrome was firstly described in 1944 during the II world war when American surgeons reported persistent intercostal pain in soldiers submitted to thoracotomy (9). Until the end of the nineties, pain treatment was mainly based on intravenous opioids and the incidence of PTPS was about 61% one year after surgery (10).

2. Definition and incidence

The International Association for the Study of Pain (IASP) definition of Post Thoracotomy Pain Syndrome is the following: 'Pain that recurs or persists along a thoracotomy scar at least 2 months following surgical procedure' (7).

PTPS incidence between 11 and 80% has been reported in the literature (11-13). This variability is probably related to the setting of retrospective studies, the lack of an homogeneous definition of the severity and duration of the syndrome, the difference in anesthetic and analgesic protocols, the use of different pain evaluation scales and the time of postoperative follow-up. Moreover, the high variability in PTPS incidence may also be explained by the different attitude of patients towards discomfort (14).

3. Pain characteristics after thoracic surgery

PTPS is mostly described with the typical characteristics of neuropathic pain, often related to the surgical scar, since 82—90% of pain patients recognize the pain trigger directly to the surgical site (1, 10). Pain is primarily described as aching, tender, with numbness and to a lesser degree burning (1, 15); however, PTPS is sometimes described as tingling and pruritus sensation within the thoracic injured area. Finally, thoracic sensory deficits are referred by patients in terms of sensory loss and hypoesthesia to cold (16, 17). These neuropathic phenomena are principally located within mammary and sub mammary areas and ipsilateral scapular and interscapular regions.

Comparing to acute postoperative pain, PTPS does not specifically influence the respiratory function but may be able to limit daily activities. In other words, differences between acute and chronic pain are more related to the inability to restore the physiological functions of the organism to homeostatic pre-thoracotomy levels (18). Even if the pain intensity is moderate, normal daily activities might be hampered up to 50 % of cases and sleep disorders could be present in the 25% of patients (10); finally, severe pain could be present in 8% and can persist in more than 40% of cases (15). Unfortunately the social consequences and subsequent analgesic use have only been recorded in a minority of studies with different design (4, 13, 15, 19, 20) so that the actual impact of chronic pain on daily life remains undefined.

4. Pathogenetic features

The mechanisms that lead to PTPS are multiple and the pathogenesis is still unclear. The pathway of the painful experience related to thoracotomy is complex. Inputs from skin, muscles, ribs, and parietal pleura are conducted through intercostal nerves to the dorsal horn. Moreover, the vagus nerve and the autonomic system are involved in the conduction of noxious stimuli from visceral pleura and lung parenchyma; finally, the phrenic nerve is related to noxious stimuli from mediastinum, diaphragm and pericardial pleura (21, 22).

Although the pathogenesis of chronic neuropathic post thoracotomy pain syndrome is complex, the direct damage of intercostal nerves and the consequent effect on pain transmission seems to play a primary role (23). Many important peripheral and central nociceptive adaptions have been described after peripheral nerve injury (23).

Peripherally, ephaptic conduction or "cross-excitation" generated by neurons linked to injured nerves may trigger a distorted pathway of nociceptive stimuli which may be clinically relevant for the ongoing neuropathic pain (23, 24). Moreover, in these neurons the expression of sodium and calcium channels may be altered (23, 25, 26). A collateral sprouting of fibers from sensory axons into denervated areas has been also described in an animal model, but the degree of sprouting was not proportional to the degree of hyperalgesia after nerve section so that the role of this phenomenon seems to be limited (23, 27). Another important role may be played by direct coupling of the sympathic nerve system and the sensory nervous system in the dorsal root gangliation (28). The trigger signal of this sprouting is still unclear but the release of neurotrophic factors and cytokines following wallerian degeneration is likely to be decisive (29).

Central mechanisms are also implicated in the development of this syndrome (23). The nerve injury is coupled to a considerable degree of spinal cord reorganization. Large-diameter, low threshold A-beta fibres from mechanoceptors may wrongly sprout into lamina II, which is normally the termination of high-threshold A-delta and C fibres, leading to an erroneous interpretation of nociceptive stimuli (30). Peripheral nerve injury, similarly to chronic inflammation, is coupled to a persistent state of hyperexcitability of the dorsal horn neurons, a process called "central sensitization" (31, 32). The excitatory amino acid glutamate is known to be the major excitatory neurotransmitter related to noxious stimulation. Many postsynaptic receptors are linked to glutamate release but a strong evidence suggests that N-methyl-D-aspartate (NMDA) receptor subtype is the main involved in both inflammation and central sensitization (33). The gamma - amminobutirric acid (GABA) pathway represents the major inhibition system in the CNS. The suppression of this pathway with pharmacological inhibitors is associated with a dose-dependent allodynia (34). GABA receptors level is reduced after peripheral nerve axotomy, maybe because of primary degeneration of afferent neuron terminals on which the receptor is localized. The consequent reduction in GABA activity may play an important role in central sensitization (35). A separate pathway of nociceptive modulation in CNS is the purinergic system, including specifically adenosine. Neuropathic patients show a reduction in adenosine concentration in both circulating blood and CSF, suggesting a concurrent effect of adenosine in the modulation of chronic pain (36).

Finally, the reduced ability of opiates in relieving neuropathic pain is widely accepted but the exact extent of this phenomenon is controversial. The dose response function of opiates seems to be unfavorably shifted to the right (23). This clinical evidence may be explained by loss of peripheral opiate effect, loss of spinal opiate receptors and increased activity in physiological opioid antagonism system (23).

5. Factors influencing the prevalence of PTPS

5.1 Predisposing factors for the development of chronic pain are:

- Female gender (13, 37).
- Age under 60 years (37, 38)
- Genetic factors: genetic control of pain involves several genes such as catechol-Omethyltransferase (COMT), voltage-gated sodium channels, and GTP cyclohydrolase and tetrahydrobiopterin-related genes which are characterized by high level of variability in the population (39, 40).
- Psychological factors: anxiety, depression, malignant disease and social status, may play a determinant role in influencing perception and consequences of chronic pain (13, 41, 42). However the relationship between preoperative psychological factors and PTPS should be investigated with targeted study.
- Preoperative pain and analgesic consumption: the relationship between preoperative pain and analgesic consumption and the development of chronic pain is well established for some kinds of surgery (43, 44). Moreover, assessing the preoperative pain threshold of each patient may be useful to identify risking patients at risk of postoperative pain which may lead to chronification (electrical, heat, cold and pressure tests) (45-49). Unfortunately, the role of pre-surgical pain in PTPS recurrence is still controversial (13, 45, 50, 51).

5.2 Perioperative factors are the:

- Type and extent of surgery (intercostal nerve damage, resection of the chest wall, pleurectomy and pneumectomy)
- Intensity and duration of pain during the first postoperative day.

5.2.1 The type and extent of surgery

Many surgical approaches for thoracic cavity are described: median sternotomy, bilateral transverse thoracosternotomy, posterolateral thoractomy, muscle sparing thoracotomy and video-assisted thoracoscopy (VATS) (52).

Intercostal nerves are primarily involved in the rib cage pain transmission. The incision of the skin, soft tissue and muscles triggers an inflammatory response. The retraction of the intercostal space, and sometimes the resection of the ribs themselves, increases the damage to the costovertebral and costotrasversal ligaments with the subsequent involvement of the parietal pleura (53).

The intercostal nerve can be compressed by retractors or damaged during rib resection and closure of chest wall or can be trapped by sutures and healing processes. Nociception from mediastinic and diaphragmatic pleura is transmitted by different nervous pathways (phrenic and vagus nerves). This type of pain is deep and poorly localized. Moreover, this painful sensation triggered by diaphragmatic injury is also referred to the homolateral shoulder pain. Pleural drainage also produces deep pain due to both skin incision and pleural irritation.

In addition to surgical injury, the breathing cycle constantly involves the damaged structures, enhancing the trigger of thoracic pain.

The diagnosis of nerve injury is often associated with allodynia and/ or hyperalgesia plus numbness distributed in the area served by affected nerves.

The type of incision is strictly associated to post-thoracotomy pain and damage of intercostal nerves (54). The posterolateral thoracotomy, sparing serratus anterior and trapezius muscles, seems to minimize damaging in intercostal nerves compared to the standard posterolateral thoracotomy. Consequently, this technique is associated with a reduction of pain and improvement mobility of the ipsilateral shoulder in the first seven postoperative days.

However, several studies have questioned these results in terms of both acute and chronic pain after one year. An anterior axillary approach has been proposed to reduce the painful symptoms, but the benefit was not still confirmed by the literature. The technique used for closure of the chest wall may play a role in the intercostal nerve damage.

Nevertheless, all the different surgical approaches described above, may lead either to acute and chronic pain. This finding may be firstly explained by frequent anatomical variants in the intercostal nerves course so that their integrity is not ensured by any surgical choice. Moreover, the surgical retractor, used in all the techniques, may probably play an important role in the damage of the intercostal nerves.

The video-assisted thoracic surgery (VATS) seems to reduce the incidence of PTPS, probably because of multiple small incisions that produce a smaller nerve injury than open thoracotomy. However VATS does not preserve intercostal nerve from damage because the scope may crush nervous fibers against adjacent rib. Moreover the use of retractors to take away the lung section may also damage intercostals nerve (63-27). In conclusion VATS technique does not prevent the PTPS development but seems to reduce the PTPS incidence compared to muscle sparing incision (28)

5.2.2 The intensity and duration of pain during the first postoperative day

Several prospective studies show that the most important predictor for the development of PTPS is the persistent post surgical pain which is strictly related to the severity of acute postoperative pain. Acute postoperative pain, in fact, is related to the amount of intercostal nerves damaged (55, 56). However, some studies found no clear relationship between PTPS and intensity of acute postoperative pain (1, 4, 10). The literature is not exhaustive because no study evaluates overall preoperative, intraoperative and postoperative factors which can influence the incidence of PTPS. Undoubtely, the strict pain control is mandatory in this kind of surgery.

5.3 Postoperative factors

5.3.1 Social consequences

The social impact of PTPS as capability to influence daily activites and consequently quality of life were investigated by several studies (4, 10, 13, 15, 20). Commonly the effects of PTPS are registered in the following activities: standing, sitting, getting up, sleep. Even if the pain intensity is moderate, normal daily activities could be hampered up to 50 % of cases and sleep disorders could be present in the 25% of patients (10); finally severe pain could be present in 8% and it's not relieved in more than 40% of cases (50). However, because of lack of right evaluation of this kind of disabilities, the exact impact of PTPS on social field must be better investigated.

5.3.2 Disease relapse – chemo and radio therapy

Keller et all (57) suggest that relapse of disease can uncontrovertibly rise PTPS incidence. However, even if this data is obvious and well comprehensible, much more data are needed to support this evidence. Moreover, since no data are available about the effects of chemo and radio-therapy on PTPS incidence, several studies must be encouraged to understand their role on PTPS incidence.

6. Prevention and treatment strategies of PTPS

6.1 Intra and postoperative analgesia

Postoperative analgesia is commonly based on the use of regional anesthesia and systemic drug infusion. Different regional anesthesia techniques have been used: mostly thoracic epidural anesthesia (TEA) (58, 59), thoracic paravertebral block (PVB) (60), and, secondarily, pleural infusion or intercostal nerves block. The role of intrapleural infusion, intercostal nerve block and local infiltration in reducing PTPS is still unclear because studies evaluating this analgesic technique are confounding and lacking of exhaustive data (45).

TEA and PVB with opioids and local anesthetics mixture are the most used regional techniques. Nowadays, TEA is still considered the gold standard technique even if PVB has recently emerged as valid alternative to TEA (61).

However the role of TEA in reducing PTPS remains controversial and questionable. In any case, multimodal analgesia using different modalities as regional and systemic analgesic techniques is highly recommended (61).

On the contrary, there is no consensus on the drug to use for adjunct intravenous analgesia. Ketamine has been confirmed as a useful agent (62, 63) while COX-2 inhibitors, celecoxib i.e, were recently proposed as a valid alternative (64). Besides, only few studies reported about the efficacy of the S(+) - isomer of Ketamine (65) that has been demonstrated to have twice the anaesthetic and analgesic potency of the racemic ketamine preparation and is judged to induce less psychic emergence reactions, a reduced number of hallucinations (66) and to be followed by a more rapid recovery of vigilance (67, 68) preserving the hypoxic pulmonary vasoconstriction, enhancing oxygenation and decreasing shunt fractions in monopulmonary ventilation (52).

Only few trials have demonstrated the effect of iv ketamine as an adjunct to TEA. Suzuki et al (69) demonstrated the efficacy of 0,05 mg Kg^{-1} h^{-1} racemic ketamine combined with TEA with ropivacaine and morphine on acute pain control until 3 months postoperatively but not at 6 months follow-up. Dualé et al (63) confirmed that racemic ketamine (1mg $kg^{-1}h^{-1}$ during surgery and 1 mg $kg^{-1}h^{-1}$ in the first 24 hours) was effective in the immediate postoperative

pain but failed to prevent a reduction of chronic PTPS at 6 weeks and 4 months after surgery.
S-(+)-isomer of Ketamine has been demonstrated to be more effective than the racemic mixture with a lower incidence of side effects. Argiriadou et al (65) recently proposed the use of the S(+)-isomer of Ketamine in conjunction with thoracic paravertebral ropivacaine providing better early postoperative pain relief than ropivacaine alone or in adjunction with perecoxib.
In the last years a great interest has been elicited by the use of the preemptive analgesia and the administration of Ketamine during and after surgery to prevent and lessen the processes involved in the development of neuropathic pain (70) even if some contrasting results have been published on the use of Ketamine for postoperative pain control (71).
Patients treated with TEA in pre-empty modality with opioids and local anesthetics showed a lower incidence of chronic PTPS if compared to patients who received only intravenous opioids (72). Moreover, the exclusive intravenous administration of opioids may induce hyperalgesia and tolerance to opioids themselves, both processes NMDA receptors activation mediated (73).
NMDA receptors antagonists may prevent the acute tolerance to opioids and, among them, ketamine at a blood concentration of 30-120 ng ml^{-1} is able to strengthen the nociceptives effects of opioids without altering sedation indexes (74).
The preoperative administration of 0.1 mg/Kg epidural ketamine reduced the area affected by hyperalgesia and allodynia around the surgical wound in the first 30 days after incision; the same dosage given intramuscolarly did not produce the same effects (75). The limitations to these observations are that the neuropathic lesion and pain could appear after a period longer than expected (76).
The administration of NMDA receptors inhibition is hampered by the need of a prolonged administration which could be more efficient via an oral route administration (77).

7. Conclusions

Many progresses have been done in the identification and the pathophysiological understanding of PTPS even if we are far from a well defined understanding of this syndrome. From the clinical point of view the priority resides on the continuous collaboration among anesthetists, surgeons, pharmacists and nurses to guarantee to any patient the best approach and the most correct pharmacological therapy.
Multimodal analgesia using different modalities as regional and systemic analgesic techniques is highly recommended (61).
In our opinion, pain unit in the management of patients undergoing thoracotomy is likely to warrant intensive and aggressive pain control with multimodal strategy in order to assure high level of comfort in the perioperative period and consequently reduce the incidence of PTPS.

8. References

[1] *Kalso E, Perttunen K, Kaasinen S.* Pain after thoracic surgery. Acta Anaesthesiol Scand 1992; 36: 96-100.
[2] *Kavanagh BP, Katz J, Sandler AN.* Pain control after thoracic surgery. A review of current techniques. Anesthesiology 1994; 81: 737-59.

[3] *Richardson J, Smith T, Tsiamis A, Shah RD.* Postthoracotomy pain. Ann Thorac Surg 1998; 65: 300-2.

[4] *Tiippana E, Nilsson E, Kalso E.* Post-thoracotomy pain after thoracic epidural analgesia: a prospective follow-up study. Acta Anaesthesiol Scand 2003; 47: 433-8.

[5] *Fiore JF, Jr., Chiavegato LD, Denehy L, Paisani DM, Faresin SM.* Do directed cough maneuvers improve cough effectiveness in the early period after open heart surgery? Effect of thoracic support and maximal inspiration on cough peak expiratory flow, cough expiratory volume, and thoracic pain. Respir Care 2008; 53: 1027-34.

[6] *Nikolajsen L, Ilkjaer S, Kroner K, Christensen JH, Jensen TS.* The influence of preamputation pain on postamputation stump and phantom pain. Pain 1997; 72: 393-405.

[7] *Merskey H.* Classification of chronic pain syndromes and definition of pain terms. Pain 1986; suppl: S138-S9.

[8] *Shaw A, Keefe FJ.* Genetic and environmental determinants of postthoracotomy pain syndrome. Curr Opin Anaesthesiol 2008; 21: 8-11.

[9] *Blades B, Dugan DJ.* War wounds of the chest observed at the Thoracic Surgery Center, Walter Reed General Hospital. J Thorac Surg 1944; 13: 294-306.

[10] *Perttunen K, Tasmuth T, Kalso E.* Chronic pain after thoracic surgery: a follow-up study. Acta Anaesthesiol Scand 1999; 43: 563-7.

[11] *Rogers ML, Duffy JP.* Surgical aspects of chronic post-thoracotomy pain. Eur J Cardiothorac Surg 2000; 18: 711-6.

[12] *Gottschalk A, Cohen SP, Yang S, Ochroch EA.* Preventing and treating pain after thoracic surgery. Anesthesiology 2006; 104: 594-600.

[13] *Ochroch EA, Gottschalk A, Augostides J, et al.* Long-term pain and activity during recovery from major thoracotomy using thoracic epidural analgesia. Anesthesiology 2002; 97: 1234-44.

[14] *Landreneau RJ, Mack MJ, Hazelrigg SR, et al.* Prevalence of chronic pain after pulmonary resection by thoracotomy or video-assisted thoracic surgery. J Thorac Cardiovasc Surg 1994; 107: 1079-85; discussion 85-6.

[15] *Maguire MF, Ravenscroft A, Beggs D, Duffy JP.* A questionnaire study investigating the prevalence of the neuropathic component of chronic pain after thoracic surgery. Eur J Cardiothorac Surg 2006; 29: 800-5.

[16] *Gotoda Y, Kambara N, Sakai T, Kishi Y, Kodama K, Koyama T.* The morbidity, time course and predictive factors for persistent post-thoracotomy pain. Eur J Pain 2001; 5: 89-96.

[17] *Guastella V, Mick G, Soriano C, et al.* A prospective study of neuropathic pain induced by thoracotomy: incidence, clinical description, and diagnosis. Pain; 152: 74-81.

[18] *Erdek MA, Staats PS.* Chronic pain and thoracic surgery. Thorac Surg Clin 2005; 15: 123-30.

[19] *Hu JS, Lui PW, Wang H, et al.* Thoracic epidural analgesia with morphine does not prevent postthoracotomy pain syndrome: a survey of 159 patients. Acta Anaesthesiol Sin 2000; 38: 195-200.

[20] *Dajczman E, Gordon A., Kreisman H. Wolkove N.* Long-therm postthoracotomy pain. Chest 1991; 99: 270-4.

[21] *Klafta JM.* Impact of acute pain and its management for thoracic surgical patients. *In:* Ferguson MK (Ed.). Thoracic surgery clincs; 2005: 849-65.

[22] *Hazelrigg SR, Cetindag IB, Fullerton J.* Acute and chronic pain syndromes after thoracic surgery. Surg Clin North Am 2002; 82: 849-65.

[23] *Bridges D, Thompson SW, Rice AS.* Mechanisms of neuropathic pain. Br J Anaesth 2001; 87: 12-26.

[24] *Gracely RH, Lynch SA, Bennett GJ.* Painful neuropathy: altered central processing maintained dynamically by peripheral input. Pain 1992; 51: 175-94.

[25] *Dib-Hajj SD, Fjell J, Cummins TR, et al.* Plasticity of sodium channel expression in DRG neurons in the chronic constriction injury model of neuropathic pain. Pain 1999; 83: 591-600.

[26] *Waxman SG, Kocsis JD, Black JA.* Type III sodium channel mRNA is expressed in embryonic but not adult spinal sensory neurons, and is reexpressed following axotomy. J Neurophysiol 1994; 72: 466-70.

[27] *Devor M, Schonfeld D, Seltzer Z, Wall PD.* Two modes of cutaneous reinnervation following peripheral nerve injury. J Comp Neurol 1979; 185: 211-20.

[28] *Janig W, Levine JD, Michaelis M.* Interactions of sympathetic and primary afferent neurons following nerve injury and tissue trauma. Prog Brain Res 1996; 113: 161-84.

[29] *Ramer MS, Thompson SW, McMahon SB.* Causes and consequences of sympathetic basket formation in dorsal root ganglia. Pain 1999; Suppl 6: S111-20.

[30] *Woolf CJ, Shortland P, Coggeshall RE.* Peripheral nerve injury triggers central sprouting of myelinated afferents. Nature 1992; 355: 75-8.

[31] *Wall PD.* Neuropathic pain and injured nerve: central mechanisms. Br Med Bull 1991; 47: 631-43.

[32] *Coderre TJ, Katz J, Vaccarino AL, Melzack R.* Contribution of central neuroplasticity to pathological pain: review of clinical and experimental evidence. Pain 1993; 52: 259-85.

[33] *Doubell TP MR, Woolf CJ.* The dorsal horn: State-dependent sensory processing, plasticity and the generation of pain. *In:* Livingstone C (Ed.). Textbook of pain. London; 1999: 165-82.

[34] *Yaksh TL.* Behavioral and autonomic correlates of the tactile evoked allodynia produced by spinal glycine inhibition: effects of modulatory receptor systems and excitatory amino acid antagonists. Pain 1989; 37: 111-23.

[35] *Sivilotti L, Woolf CJ.* The contribution of GABAA and glycine receptors to central sensitization: disinhibition and touch-evoked allodynia in the spinal cord. J Neurophysiol 1994; 72: 169-79.

[36] *Guieu R, Peragut JC, Roussel P, et al.* Adenosine and neuropathic pain. Pain 1996; 68: 271-4.

[37] *Kehlet H, Jensen TS, Woolf CJ.* Persistent postsurgical pain: risk factors and prevention. Lancet 2006; 367: 1618-25.

[38] *Pluijms WA, Steegers MA, Verhagen AF, Scheffer GJ, Wilder-Smith OH.* Chronic post-thoracotomy pain: a retrospective study. Acta Anaesthesiol Scand 2006; 50: 804-8.

[39] *Diatchenko L, Nackley AG, Tchivileva IE, Shabalina SA, Maixner W.* Genetic architecture of human pain perception. Trends Genet 2007; 23: 605-13.

[40] *Tegeder I, Costigan M, Griffin RS, et al.* GTP cyclohydrolase and tetrahydrobiopterin regulate pain sensitivity and persistence. Nat Med 2006; 12: 1269-77.

[41] *Taenzer P, Melzack R, Jeans ME.* Influence of psychological factors on postoperative pain, mood and analgesic requirements. Pain 1986; 24: 331-42.

[42] *Axelrod DA, Proctor MC, Geisser ME, Roth RS, Greenfield LJ.* Outcomes after surgery for thoracic outlet syndrome. J Vasc Surg 2001; 33: 1220-5.
[43] *Brandsborg B, Nikolajsen L, Hansen CT, Kehlet H, Jensen TS.* Risk factors for chronic pain after hysterectomy: a nationwide questionnaire and database study. Anesthesiology 2007; 106: 1003-12.
[44] *Aasvang E, Kehlet H.* Chronic postoperative pain: the case of inguinal herniorrhaphy. Br J Anaesth 2005; 95: 69-76.
[45] *Wildgaard K, Ravn J, Kehlet H.* Chronic post-thoracotomy pain: a critical review of pathogenic mechanisms and strategies for prevention. Eur J Cardiothorac Surg 2009; 36: 170-80.
[46] *Nielsen PR, Norgaard L, Rasmussen LS, Kehlet H.* Prediction of post-operative pain by an electrical pain stimulus. Acta Anaesthesiol Scand 2007; 51: 582-6.
[47] *Werner MU, Duun P, Kehlet H.* Prediction of postoperative pain by preoperative nociceptive responses to heat stimulation. Anesthesiology 2004; 100: 115-9; discussion 5A.
[48] *Granot M, Lowenstein L, Yarnitsky D, Tamir A, Zimmer EZ.* Postcesarean section pain prediction by preoperative experimental pain assessment. Anesthesiology 2003; 98: 1422-6.
[49] *Lundblad H, Kreicbergs A, Jansson KA.* Prediction of persistent pain after total knee replacement for osteoarthritis. J Bone Joint Surg Br 2008; 90: 166-71.
[50] *Maguire MF, Latter JA, Mahajan R, Beggs FD, Duffy JP.* A study exploring the role of intercostal nerve damage in chronic pain after thoracic surgery. Eur J Cardiothorac Surg 2006; 29: 873-9.
[51] *Gwak MS, Yang M, Hahm TS, Cho HS, Cho CH, Song JG.* Effect of cryoanalgesia combined with intravenous continuous analgesia in thoracotomy patients. J Korean Med Sci 2004; 19: 74-8.
[52] *Koehler RP, Keenan RJ.* Management of postthoracotomy pain: acute and chronic. Thorac Surg Clin 2006; 16: 287-97.
[53] *Kaplan J SP.* Thoracic Anesthesia; 2003.
[54] *Benedetti F, Vighetti S, Ricco C, et al.* Neurophysiologic assessment of nerve impairment in posterolateral and muscle-sparing thoracotomy. J Thorac Cardiovasc Surg 1998; 115: 841-7.
[55] *d'Amours RH, Riegler FX, Little AG.* Pathogenesis and management of persistent postthoracotomy pain. Chest Surg Clin N Am 1998; 8: 703-22.
[56] *Perkins FM, Kehlet H.* Chronic pain as an outcome of surgery. A review of predictive factors. Anesthesiology 2000; 93: 1123-33.
[57] *Keller SM, Carp NZ, Levy MN, Rosen SM.* Chronic post thoracotomy pain. J Cardiovasc Surg (Torino) 1994; 35: 161-4.
[58] *Ali M, Winter DC, Hanly AM, O'Hagan C, Keaveny J, Broe P.* Prospective, randomized, controlled trial of thoracic epidural or patient-controlled opiate analgesia on perioperative quality of life. Br J Anaesth; 104: 292-7.
[59] *Joshi GP, Bonnet F, Shah R, et al.* A systematic review of randomized trials evaluating regional techniques for postthoracotomy analgesia. Anesth Analg 2008; 107: 1026-40.
[60] *Scarci M, Joshi A, Attia R.* In patients undergoing thoracic surgery is paravertebral block as effective as epidural analgesia for pain management? Interact Cardiovasc Thorac Surg; 10: 92-6.

[61] *Wenk M, Schug SA.* Perioperative pain management after thoracotomy. Curr Opin Anaesthesiol.

[62] *Nesher N, Ekstein MP, Paz Y, Marouani N, Chazan S, Weinbroum AA.* Morphine with adjuvant ketamine vs higher dose of morphine alone for immediate postthoracotomy analgesia. Chest 2009; 136: 245-52.

[63] *Duale C, Sibaud F, Guastella V, et al.* Perioperative ketamine does not prevent chronic pain after thoracotomy. Eur J Pain 2009; 13: 497-505.

[64] *Senard M, Deflandre EP, Ledoux D, et al.* Effect of celecoxib combined with thoracic epidural analgesia on pain after thoracotomy. Br J Anaesth; 105: 196-200.

[65] *Argiriadou H, Papagiannopoulou P, Foroulis CN, et al.* Intraoperative Infusion of S(+)-Ketamine Enhances Post-thoracotomy Pain Control Compared With Perioperative Parecoxib When Used in Conjunction With Thoracic Paravertebral Ropivacaine Infusion. J Cardiothorac Vasc Anesth.

[66] *Ihmsen H, Geisslinger G, Schuttler J.* Stereoselective pharmacokinetics of ketamine: R(-)-ketamine inhibits the elimination of S(+)-ketamine. Clin Pharmacol Ther 2001; 70: 431-8.

[67] *Himmelseher S, Durieux ME.* Ketamine for perioperative pain management. Anesthesiology 2005; 102: 211-20.

[68] *Doenicke A, Kugler J, Mayer M, Angster R, Hoffmann P.* [Ketamine racemate or S-(+)-ketamine and midazolam. The effect on vigilance, efficacy and subjective findings]. Anaesthesist 1992; 41: 610-8.

[69] *Suzuki M, Haraguti S, Sugimoto K, Kikutani T, Shimada Y, Sakamoto A.* Low-dose intravenous ketamine potentiates epidural analgesia after thoracotomy. Anesthesiology 2006; 105: 111-9.

[70] *De Kock M, Lavand'homme P, Waterloos H.* 'Balanced analgesia' in the perioperative 70period: is there a place for ketamine? Pain 2001; 92: 373-80.

[71] *Annetta MG, Iemma D, Garisto C, Tafani C, Proietti R.* Ketamine: new indications for an old drug. Curr Drug Targets 2005; 6: 789-94.

[72] *Senturk M, Ozcan PE, Talu GK, et al.* The effects of three different analgesia techniques on long-term postthoracotomy pain. Anesth Analg 2002; 94: 11-5, table of contents.

[73] *Mao J, Price DD, Mayer DJ.* Mechanisms of hyperalgesia and morphine tolerance: a current view of their possible interactions. Pain 1995; 62: 259-74.

[74] *Tucker AP, Kim YI, Nadeson R, Goodchild CS.* Investigation of the potentiation of the analgesic effects of fentanyl by ketamine in humans: a double-blinded, randomised, placebo controlled, crossover study of experimental pain[ISRCTN83088383]. BMC Anesthesiol 2005; 5: 2.

[75] *Ozyalcin NS, Yucel A, Camlica H, Dereli N, Andersen OK, Arendt-Nielsen L.* Effect of pre-emptive ketamine on sensory changes and postoperative pain after thoracotomy: comparison of epidural and intramuscular routes. Br J Anaesth 2004; 93: 356-61.

[76] *Obata K, Yamanaka H, Kobayashi K, et al.* The effect of site and type of nerve injury on the expression of brain-derived neurotrophic factor in the dorsal root ganglion and on neuropathic pain behavior. Neuroscience 2006; 137: 961-70.

[77] *Snijdelaar DG, Koren G, Katz J.* Effects of perioperative oral amantadine on postoperative pain and morphine consumption in patients after radical prostatectomy: results of a preliminary study. Anesthesiology 2004; 100: 134-41.